ADVANCES IN NEUROLOGY
Volume 84

Advances in Neurology

Advances in Neurology

Volume 84

Neocortical Epilepsies

Editors

Peter D. Williamson, M.D.
Section of Neurology
Dartmouth–Hitchcock Medical Center
Lebanon, New Hampshire

Adrian M. Siegel, M.D.
Department of Neurology
University Hospital of Zürich
Zürich, Switzerland

David W. Roberts, M.D.
Section of Neurosurgery
Dartmouth–Hitchcock Medical Center
Lebanon, New Hampshire

Vijay M. Thadani, M.D., Ph.D.
Section of Neurology
Dartmouth–Hitchcock Medical Center
Lebanon, New Hampshire

Michael S. Gazzaniga, Ph.D.
Center for Cognitive Neuroscience
Dartmouth College
Hanover, New Hampshire

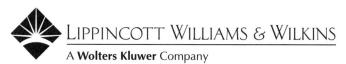
LIPPINCOTT WILLIAMS & WILKINS
A **Wolters Kluwer** Company
Philadelphia • Baltimore • New York • London
Buenos Aires • Hong Kong • Sydney • Tokyo

Acquisitions Editor: Anne M. Sydor
Developmental Editor: Julia Seto
Production Editor: Thomas Boyce
Manufacturing Manager: Benjamin Rivera
Cover Designer: Patricia Gast
Compositor: Lippincott Williams & Wilkins Desktop Division
Printer: Maple Press

© 2000 by LIPPINCOTT WILLIAMS & WILKINS
530 Walnut Street
Philadelphia, PA 19106-3780 USA
LWW.com

Library of Congress Cataloging-in-Publication Data

Neocortical epilepsies / editors, Peter D. Williamson ... [et al.].
    p. cm. — (Advances in neurology ; v. 84)
    Includes bibliographical references and index.
    ISBN 0-7817-1872-4
    1. Epilepsy. 2. Neocortex. I. Williamson, Peter D. II. Series.
RC372 .N36 2000
616.8'53—dc21
                                                                        00-030739

10 9 8 7 6 5 4 3 2 1

Advances in Neurology Series

Vol. 52: Brain Edema: Pathogenesis, Imaging, and Therapy: *D. Long, editor.* 640 pp., 1990.
Vol. 51: Alzheimer's Disease: *R. J. Wurtman, S. Corkin, J. H. Growdon, and E. Ritter-Walker, editors.* 308 pp., 1990.
Vol. 50: Dystonia 2: *S. Fahn, C. D. Marsden, and D. B. Calne, editors.* 688 pp., 1988.
Vol. 49: Facial Dyskinesias: *J. Jankovic and E. Tolosa, editors.* 560 pp., 1988.
Vol. 48: Molecular Genetics of Neurological and Neuromuscular Disease: *S. DiDonato, S. DiMauro, A. Mamoli, and L. P. Rowland, editors.* 288 pp., 1987.
Vol. 47: Functional Recovery in Neurological Disease: *S. G. Waxman, editor.* 640 pp., 1987.
Vol. 46: Intensive Neurodiagnostic Monitoring: *R. J. Gumnit, editor.* 336 pp., 1987.
Vol. 45: Parkinson's Disease: *M. D. Yahr and K. J. Bergmann, editors.* 640 pp., 1986.
Vol. 44: Basic Mechanisms of the Epilepsies: Molecular and Cellular Approaches: *A. V. Delgado-Escueta, A. A. Ward, Jr., D. M. Woodbury, and R. J. Porter, editors.* 1,120 pp., 1986.
Vol. 43: Myoclonus: *S. Fahn, C. D. Marsden, and M. H. VanWoert, editors.* 752 pp., 1986.
Vol. 42: Progress in Aphasiology: *F. C. Rose, editor.* 384 pp., 1984.
Vol. 41: The Olivopontocerebellar Atrophies: *R. C. Duvoisin and A. Plaitakis, editors.* 304 pp., 1984.
Vol. 40: Parkinson-Specific Motor and Mental Disorders, Role of Pallidum: Pathophysiological, Biochemical, and Therapeutic Aspects: *R. G. Hassler and J. F. Christ, editors.* 601 pp., 1984.
Vol. 39: Motor Control Mechanisms in Health and Disease: *J. E. Desmedt, editor.* 1,224 pp., 1983.
Vol. 38: The Dementias: *R. Mayeux and W. G. Rosen, editors.* 288 pp., 1983.
Vol. 37: Experimental Therapeutics of Movement Disorders: *S. Fahn, D. B. Calne, and I. Shoulson, editors.* 339 pp., 1983.
Vol. 36: Human Motor Neuron Diseases: *L. P. Rowland, editor.* 592 pp., 1982.
Vol. 35: Gilles de la Tourette Syndrome: *A. J. Friedhoff and T. N. Chase, editors.* 476 pp., 1982.
Vol. 34: Status Epilepticus: Mechanism of Brain Damage and Treatment: *A. V. Delgado-Escueta, C. G. Wasterlain, D. M. Treiman, and R. J. Porter, editors.* 579 pp., 1983.
Vol. 31: Demyelinating Diseases: Basic and Clinical Electrophysiology: *S. Waxman and J. Murdoch Ritchie, editors.* 544 pp., 1981.
Vol. 30: Diagnosis and Treatment of Brain Ischemia: *A. L. Carney and E. M. Anderson, editors.* 424 pp., 1981.
Vol. 29: Neurofibromatosis: *V. M. Riccardi and J. J. Mulvilhill, editors.* 288 pp., 1981.
Vol. 28: Brain Edema: *J. Cervós-Navarro and R. Ferszt, editors.* 539 pp., 1980.
Vol. 27: Antiepileptic Drugs: Mechanisms of Action: *G. H. Glaser, J. K. Penry, and D. M. Woodbury, editors.* 728 pp., 1980.
Vol. 26: Cerebral Hypoxia and Its Consequences: *S. Fahn, J. N. Davis, and L. P. Rowland, editors.* 454 pp., 1979.
Vol. 25: Cerebrovascular Disorders and Stroke: *M. Goldstein, L. Bolis, C. Fieschi, S. Gorini, and C. H. Millikan, editors.* 412 pp., 1979.
Vol. 24: The Extrapyramidal System and Its Disorders: *L. J. Poirier, T. L. Sourkes, and P. Bédard, editors.* 552 pp., 1979.
Vol. 23: Huntington's Chorea: *T. N. Chase, N. S. Wexler, and A. Barbeau, editors.* 864 pp., 1979.
Vol. 22: Complications of Nervous System Trauma: *R. A. Thompson and J. R. Green, editors.* 454 pp., 1979.
Vol. 21: The Inherited Ataxia: Biochemical, Viral, and Pathological Studies: *R. A. Kark, R. Rosenberg, and L. Schut, editors.* 450 pp., 1978.
Vol. 20: Pathology of Cerebrospinal Microcirculation: *J. Cervós-Navarro, E. Betz, G. Ebhardt, R. Ferszt, and R. Wüllenweber, editors.* 636 pp., 1978.
Vol. 19: Neurological Epidemiology: Principles and Clinical Applications: *B. S. Schoenberg, editor.* 672 pp., 1978.
Vol. 18: Hemi-Inattention and Hemisphere Specialization: *E. A. Weinstein and R. P. Friedland, editors.* 176 pp., 1977.
Vol. 17: Treatment of Neuromuscular Diseases: *R. C. Griggs and R. T. Moxley, editors.* 370 pp., 1977.
Vol. 16: Stroke: *R. A. Thompson and J. R. Green, editors.* 250 pp., 1977.
Vol. 15: Neoplasia in the Central Nervous System: *R. A. Thompson and J. R. Green, editors.* 394 pp., 1976.
Vol. 14: Dystonia: *R. Eldridge and S. Fahn, editors.* 510 pp., 1976.
Vol. 13: Current Reviews: *W. J. Friedlander, editor.* 400 pp., 1975.
Vol. 12: Physiology and Pathology of Dendrites: *G. W. Kreutzberg, editor.* 524 pp., 1975.
Vol. 11: Complex Partial Seizures and Their Treatment: *J. K. Penry and D. D. Daly, editors.* 486 pp., 1975.
Vol. 10: Private Models of Neurological Disorders: *B. S. Meldrum and C. D. Marsden, editors.* 270 pp., 1975.
Vol. 9: Dopaminergic Mechanisms: *D. B. Calne, T. N. Chase, and A. Barbeau, editors.* 452 pp., 1975.

Contents

III. The Epileptic Human Neocortex

IV. Clinical Characteristics of Neocortical Epilepsies

V. Evaluation in Neocortical Epilepsies

VI. Neuropsychological and Neuropsychiatric Aspects in Neocortical Epilepsies

VII. Neocortical Epilepsies in Pediatrics

Contributing Authors

C. Adam, M.D., Ph.D.
Department of Neurology
Clinique Paul Castaigne
Hôpital Pitié-Salpêtrière
Paris 75651
France

Frederick Andermann, M.D., F.R.C.P.(C)
Departments of Neurology and Neurosurgery
Montreal Neurological Institute
McGill University
3801 University Street
Montreal, Quebec H3A 2B4
Canada

Ralph G. Andrzejak
Department of Epileptology
Medical Center
University of Bonn
Sigmund-Freud-Strasse 25
D-53105 Bonn
Germany

Jochen Arnhold, Ph.D.
John von Neumann Institute for Computing
Research Center Jülich
D-52425 Jülich
Germany

Helen Barbas, Ph.D.
Professor
Department of Health Sciences
Boston University
635 Commonwealth Avenue
Boston, Massachusetts 02215

Helen I. Barkan, M.D.
Department of Neurology
Dartmouth–Hitchcock Medical Center
One Medical Center Drive
Lebanon, New Hampshire 03756

Alim Louis Benabid, M.D., Ph.D.
Service de Neurochirurgie
INSERM U318
CHU Régionale
B.P. 217
X-38043
Cedex 09 Grenoble
France

Emilia Berta, M.D.
Centro Regionale per la Chirurgia dell'Epilessia
Niguarda Hospital
3 Piazza Ospedale
20126 Milano
Italy

Ingmar Blümcke, M.D.
Department of Neuropathology
Medical Center
University of Bonn
Sigmund-Freud-Strasse 25
D-53105 Bonn
Germany

Warren T. Blume, M.D., F.R.C.P.(C)
Professor
Department of Clinical Neurological Sciences
University Hospital, Epilepsy Unit
339 Windermere Road
London, Ontario N6A 5A5
Canada

Warren W. Boling, Jr., M.D.
Department of Neurosurgery
Montreal Neurological Institute
McGill University
3801 University Street
Montreal, Quebec H3A 2B4
Canada

Susan Y. Bookheimer, Ph.D.
Department of Neurology
Brain Mapping Division
UCLA School of Medicine
710 Westwood Plaza
Los Angeles, California 90095-1769

Paul Boon, M.D., Ph.D.
Department of Neurology
EEG Laboratory–Epilepsy Monitoring Unit
University Hospital Gent
185 De Pintelaan
B-9000 Gent
Belgium

Richard Byrne, M.D.
Assistant Professor
Department of Neurosurgery
Rush-Presbyterian–St. Luke's Medical Center
1653 West Congress Parkway
Chicago, Illinois 60612-3833

Francesco Cardinale, M.D.
Centro Regionale per la Chirurgia dell'Epilessia
Niguarda Hospital
3 Piazza Ospedale
20126 Milano
Italy

Gregory D. Cascino, M.D.
Professor of Neurology
Mayo Medical School
Chair, Division of Epilepsy
Mayo Clinic
200 First Street, S.W.
Rochester, Minnesota 55905

Nicolas Chevassus au Louis, Ph.D.
Senior Research Scientist
INSERM U 29
Hôpital Port Royal
123 Boulevard de Port Royal
75674, Paris, France

Diane C. Chugani, Ph.D.
PET Center
Children's Hospital of Michigan
3901 Beaubien Boulevard
Detroit, Michigan 48201

Harry T. Chugani, M.D.
Pediatric Neurology Director
PET Center
Division of Pediatric Neurology
Children's Hospital of Michigan
3901 Beaubien Boulevard
Detroit, Michigan 48201

Mark S. Cohen, Ph.D.
Department of Neurology
Brain Mapping Division
UCLA School of Medicine
710 Westwood Plaza
Los Angeles, California 90095-1769

Barry W. Connors, Ph.D.
Professor
Department of Neuroscience
Brown University
Providence, Rhode Island 02912

Peter Crino, M.D., Ph.D.
Assistant Professor
Epilepsy Center
Hospital of the University of Pennsylvania
3400 Spruce Street
Philadelphia, Pennsylvania 19104

Nathan E. Crone, M.D.
Assistant Professor
Department of Neurology
The Johns Hopkins University School of Medicine
600 North Wolfe Street
Baltimore, Maryland 21287-7247

Terrance M. Darcey, Ph.D.
Section of Neurology
Dartmouth–Hitchcock Medical Center
One Medical Center Drive
Lebanon, New Hampshire 03756

M. D'Havé, M.Sc.
Department of Neurology
EEG Laboratory–Epilepsy Monitoring Unit
University Hospital Gent
185 De Pintelaan
B-9000 Gent
Belgium

Dennis J. Dlugos, M.D.
Division of Neurology
The Children's Hospital of Philadelphia
34th Street and Civic Center Boulevard
Philadelphia, Pennsylvania 19104

Heather A. Drury, M.S.
Senior Research Scientist
Department of Anatomy and Neurobiology
Washington University School of Medicine
660 South Euclid Avenue
St. Louis, Missouri 63110

Michael Duchowny, M.D.
Neuroscience Program
Miami Children's Hospital
3200 S.W. 60th Court
Miami, Florida 33155

Matthias Dümpelmann, Ph.D.
Department of Epileptology
Medical Center
University of Bonn
Sigmund-Freud-Strasse 25
D-53105 Bonn
Germany

John S. Ebersole, M.D.
Epilepsy Program
Department of Neurology
University of Chicago
5841 South Maryland Avenue
Chicago, Illinois 60637

Christian E. Elger, M.D., F.R.C.P.
Department of Epileptology
Medical Center
University of Bonn
Sigmund-Freud-Strasse 25
D-53105 Bonn
Germany

Jerome Engel, Jr., M.D., Ph.D.
Professor
Departments of Neurology and Neurobiology
UCLA School of Medicine
710 Westwood Plaza
Los Angeles, California 90095

Stefano Francione, M.D.
Centro Regionale per la Chirurgia dell'Epilessia
Niguarda Hospital
3 Piazza Ospedale
20126 Milano
Italy

Jacqueline A. French, M.D.
Associate Professor
Epilepsy Center
Hospital of the University of Pennsylvania
3400 Spruce Street
Philadelphia, Pennsylvania 19104

Hans-Joachim Freund, M.D.
Department of Neurology
Heinrich Heine University Düsseldorf
Moorenstrasse 5
D-40225 Düsseldorf
Germany

William D. Gaillard, M.D.
Associate Professor of Neurology and Pediatrics
The George Washington University School of
*   Medicine*
Director, Comprehensive Pediatric Epilepsy
*   Program*
Children's National Medical Center
111 Michigan Avenue, N.W.
Washington, D.C. 20010

Michael S. Gazzaniga, Ph.D.
Center for Cognitive Neuroscience
Dartmouth College
6162 Silsby Hall
Hanover, New Hampshire 03755-3547

Karen L. Gilbert, M.S.
Section of Neurology
Dartmouth–Hitchcock Medical Center
One Medical Center Drive
Lebanon, New Hampshire 03756

Melvyn A. Goodale, Ph.D.
MRC Group on Action and Perception
Department of Psychology
The University of Western Ontario
London, Ontario N6A 5C2
Canada

Jean Gotman, Ph.D.
Professor
Montreal Neurological Institute
McGill University
3801 University Street
Montreal, Quebec H3A 2B4
Canada

Peter Grassberger, Ph.D.
John von Neumann Institute for Computing
Research Center Jülich
D-52425 Jülich
Germany

Gregory L. Holmes, M.D.
Center for Research in Pediatric Epilepsy
Children's Hospital
300 Longwood Avenue
Boston, Massachusetts 02125

Joseph B. Hopfinger, Ph.D.
Department of Psychology
University of North Carolina, Chapel Hill
Chapel Hill, North Carolina 27516

Howard C. Hughes, Ph.D.
Department of Psychological and Brain Sciences
Dartmouth College
6207 Moore Hall
Hanover, New Hampshire 03755

Yushi Inoue, M.D.
Head, Clinical Research Division
National Epilepsy Center
Shizuoka Higashi Hospital
Shizuoka 420-8688
Japan

Amishi P. Jha, Ph.D.
Brain Imaging and Analysis Center
Duke University
Durham, North Carolina 27708

Barbara C. Jobst, M.D.
Section of Neurology
Dartmouth–Hitchcock Medical Center
One Medical Center Drive
Lebanon, New Hampshire 03756

Marilyn Jones-Gotman, Ph.D.
Departments of Neurology and Neurosurgery
Montreal Neurological Institute
McGill University
3801 University Street
Montreal, Quebec H3A 2B4
Canada

Sarang Joshi, Ph.D.
Center for Imaging Science
Johns Hopkins University
3400 North Charles Street
Baltimore, Maryland 21218

Philippe Kahane, M.D., Ph.D.
Clinique Neurologique
CHU Régionale
B.P. 217
X-38043
Cedex 09 Grenoble
France

Don W. King, M.D.
Professor
Department of Neurology
Medical College of Georgia
Augusta, Georgia 30912

Thomas Kral, M.D.
Department of Neurosurgery
Medical Center
University of Bonn
Sigmund-Freud-Strasse 25
D-53105 Bonn
Germany

Kenneth D. Laxer, M.D.
Professor
Department of Neurology
University of California, San Francisco
400 Parnassus Avenue
San Francisco, California 04143-0138

Sang-Ahm Lee, M.D.
Department of Neurology
Yale University School of Medicine
333 Cedar Street
New Haven, Connecticut 06520-8018

Sunghoon Lee, M.D.
Department of Neurosurgery
Yale University School of Medicine
333 Cedar Street
New Haven, Connecticut 06520-8082

Klaus Lehnertz, Ph.D.
Department of Epileptology
Medical Center
University of Bonn
Sigmund-Freud-Strasse 25
D-53105 Bonn
Germany

Ronald P. Lesser, M.D.
Professor
Departments of Neurology and
   Neurosurgery
The Johns Hopkins University
600 North Wolfe Street
Baltimore, Maryland 21287-7247

Petra Lewis, M.D.
Department of Radiology
Dartmouth–Hitchcock Medical Center
One Medical Center Drive
Lebanon, New Hampshire 03756

Giorgio Lo Russo, M.D.
Centro Regionale per la Chirurgia dell'Epilessia
Niguarda Hospital
3 Piazza Ospedale
20126 Milano
Italy

Giuseppe Luppino, M.D.
Istituto di Fisiologia Umana
Università di Parma
Via Volturno 39
43100 Parma
Italy

George R. Mangun, Ph.D.
Professor
Center for Cognitive Neuroscience
Duke University
Durham, North Carolina 27708

Miguel Marín-Padilla, M.D.
Molecular Neuroscience Program
Mayo Clinic
200 First Avenue, S.W.
Rochester, Minnesota 55906

Massimo Matelli, M.D.
Istituto di Fisiologia Umana
Università di Parma
Via Volturno 39
43100 Parma
Italy

Kazumi Matsuda, M.D.
Senior Neurosurgeon
Department of Neurosurgery
National Epilepsy Center
Shizuoka Higashi Hospital
Shizuoka 420-8688
Japan

Tadahiro Mihara, M.D.
Head, Department of Neurosurgery
National Epilepsy Center
Shizuoka Higashi Hospital
Shizuoka 420-8688
Japan

Michael B. Miller, Ph.D.
Center for Cognitive Neuroscience
Dartmouth College
6162 Silsby Hall
Hanover, New Hampshire 03755-3547

Michael I. Miller, Ph.D.
Center for Imaging Science
Johns Hopkins University
3400 North Charles Street
Baltimore, Maryland 21218

Claudio Munari, M.D. (deceased)
Centro Regionale per la Chirurgia dell'Epilessia
Niguarda Hospital
3 Piazza Ospedale
20126 Milano
and
Instituto di Clinica Neurochirurgica
University of Genoa
San Martino Hospital
10 Largo R. Benzi
16132 Genoa
Italy

George A. Ojemann, M.D.
Professor
Department of Neurological Surgery
University of Washington
1959 N.E. Pacific Street
Seattle, Washington 98195-6470

André Olivier, M.D., Ph.D.
Chairman, Department of Neurosurgery
Montreal Neurological Institute
McGill University
3801 University Street
Montreal, Quebec H3A 2B4
Canada

Yong D. Park, M.D.
Associate Professor
Department of Neurology
Medical College of Georgia
Augusta, Georgia 30912

Michael Petrides, Ph.D.
Professor
Departments of Neurology and Neurosurgery
Montreal Neurological Institute
McGill University
3801 University Street
Montreal, Quebec H3A 2B4
Canada

Roger J. Porter, M.D.
Wyeth-Ayerst Research
145 King of Prussia Road
Philadelphia, Pennsylvania 19101-8299

L. Felipe Quesney, M.D., Ph.D.
Division of EEG and Clinical Neurophysiology
Montreal Neurological Institute
McGill University
3801 University Street
Montreal, Quebec H3A 2B4
Canada

Pasko Rakic, M.D., Ph.D.
Professor and Chairman
Section of Neurobiology
Yale University School of Medicine
333 Cedar Street
New Haven, Connecticut 06510

David W. Roberts, M.D.
Section of Neurosurgery
Dartmouth–Hitchcock Medical Center
One Medical Center Drive
Lebanon, New Hampshire 03756

Andrew J. Saykin, Psy.D.
Director, Brain Imaging Lab
Department of Psychiatry
Dartmouth–Hitchcock Medical Center
One Medical Center Drive
Lebanon, New Hampshire 03756

J. Schramm, M.D.
Department of Neurosurgery
Medical Center
University of Bonn
Sigmund-Freud-Strasse 25
D-53105 Bonn
Germany

Masakazu Seino, M.D.
Honorary President
National Epilepsy Center
Shizuoka Higashi Hospital
Shizuoka 420-8688
Japan

Adrian M. Siegel, M.D.
Department of Neurology
University Hospital of Zürich
Frauenklinikstrasse 26
8091 Zürich
Switzerland

Alan H. Siegel, M.D.
Department of Radiology
Dartmouth–Hitchcock Medical Center
One Medical Center Drive
Lebanon, New Hampshire 03756

Joseph R. Smith, M.D.
Professor
Department of Surgery
Section of Neurosurgery
Medical College of Georgia
Augusta, Georgia 30912

Michael C. Smith, M.D.
Director, Rush Epilepsy Center
Associate Professor
Rush-Presbyterian–St. Luke's Medical Center
1653 West Congress Parkway
Chicago, Illinois 60612-3833

Dennis Spencer, M.D.
Professor and Chairman
Department of Neurosurgery
Yale University School of Medicine
333 Cedar Street
New Haven, Connecticut 06520-8082

Susan S. Spencer, M.D.
Professor
Department of Neurology
Yale University School of Medicine
333 Cedar Street
New Haven, Connecticut 06520-8018

Michael R. Sperling, M.D.
Jefferson Comprehensive Epilepsy Center
Department of Neurology
Jefferson Medical College of
  Thomas Jefferson University
111 South 11th Street
Philadelphia, Pennsylvania 19107

Laura Tassi, M.D.
Centro Regionale per la Chirurgia dell'Epilessia
Niguarda Hospital
3 Piazza Ospedale
20126 Milano
Italy

David C. Taylor, M.D., M.Sc., F.R.C.P.,
F.R.C.Psych.
Neurosciences Unit
Institute of Child Health
and
Great Ormond Street Hospital
The Wolfson Centre
Mecklenburgh Square
London WCIN 2AP
United Kingdom

Albert E. Telfeian, M.D., Ph.D.
Department of Neurosurgery
School of Medicine
University of Pennsylvania
3400 Spruce Street
Philadelphia, Pennsylvania 19104

Vijay M. Thadani, M.D., Ph.D.
Section of Neurology
Dartmouth–Hitchcock Medical Center
One Medical Center Drive
Lebanon, New Hampshire 03756

William H. Theodore, M.D.
Clinical Epilepsy Section
National Institute of Neurological Disorders
  and Stroke
National Institute of Health
Bethesda, Maryland 20892-1428

Takayasu Tottori, M.D.
Senior Neurosurgeon
Department of Neurosurgery
National Epilepsy Center
Shizuoka Higashi Hospital
Shizuoka 420-8688
Japan

David M. Treiman, M.D.
Department of Neurology
University of Medicine and Dentistry of New Jersey
Robert Wood Johnson Medical School
97 Paterson Street
New Brunswick, New Jersey 08901

T. Vandekerckhove, M.D.
Department of Neurosurgery
University Hospital Gent
185 De Pintelaan
B-9000 Gent
Belgium

David C. Van Essen, Ph.D.
Department of Anatomy and Neurobiology
Washington University School of Medicine
660 South Euclid Avenue
St. Louis, Missouri 63110

G. Van Hoey, M.Sc.
Department of Neurology
EEG Laboratory–Epilepsy Monitoring Unit
University Hospital Gent
185 De Pintelaan
B-9000 Gent
Belgium

B. Vanrumste, M.Sc.
Department of Neurology
EEG Laboratory–Epilepsy Monitoring Unit
University Hospital Gent
185 De Pintelaan
B-9000 Gent
Belgium

Kenneth Vives, M.D.
Department of Neurosurgery
Yale University School of Medicine
333 Cedar Street
New Haven, Connecticut 06520-8082

K. Vonck, M.D.
Department of Neurology
EEG Laboratory–Epilepsy Monitoring Unit
University Hospital Gent
185 De Pintelaan
B-9000 Gent
Belgium

W.R.S. Webber, Ph.D.
Director of Programming
Department of Neurology
The Johns Hopkins University
600 North Wolfe Street
Baltimore, Maryland 21287

Michael Westerveld, Ph.D.
Assistant Professor
Department of Neurosurgery
Yale University School of Medicine
333 Cedar Street
New Haven, Connecticut 06520-8082

James W. Wheless, M.D.
Associate Professor
Department of Neurology
University of Texas–Houston
6431 Fannin Street
Houston, Texas 77030

Guido Widman, M.D.
Department of Epileptology
Medical Center
University of Bonn
Sigmund-Freud-Strasse 25
D-53105 Bonn
Germany

Samuel Wiebe, M.D., F.R.C.P.(C)
Assistant Professor
Department of Clinical Neurological Sciences
London Health Sciences Centre–University Campus
The University of Western Ontario
339 Windermere Road
London, Ontario N6A 5A5
Canada

Heinz Gregor Wieser, M.D.
Neurology Clinic
University Hospital of Zürich
Frauenklinikstrasse 26
8091 Zürich
Switzerland

Peter D. Williamson, M.D.
Director, Dartmouth Epilepsy Program
Section of Neurology
Dartmouth–Hitchcock Medical Center
One Medical Center Drive
Lebanon, New Hampshire 03756

Allen R. Wyler, M.D.
Executive Medical Director
Neuroscience Institute
Swedish Medical Center
801 Broadway
Seattle, Washington 98122

Elaine Wyllie, M.D.
Department of Neurology
Pediatric Epilepsy Program
The Cleveland Clinic Foundation
9500 Euclid Avenue
Cleveland, Ohio 44195

Preface

The 1st International Dartmouth Symposium on Neocortical Epilepsies was held at the Dartmouth–Hitchcock Medical Center in September 1998. In the past decade, an enormous amount of new information has accumulated which elucidates not only the neuroanatomical development of the brain, but also its physiological and psychological functioning. Neocortical epilepsy, usually related to focal abnormalities of structure and function, illustrates better than most diseases how normal anatomy and normal neuronal activity are necessary for the brain to function as the organ of mind. Not only do patients with neocortical epilepsy have interictal disturbances of thought and behavior, but the seizures themselves produce transient disturbances of consciousness that demonstrate how fragile are the electrical patterns that underlie the normal mental state.

This volume brings together studies of anatomy, physiology, and psychology in the normal and the epileptic brain. Clinical contributions relating to precise anatomical and functional localization of seizure foci, as well as medical and surgical treatment are also included. Considerable emphasis is placed on state-of-the-art EEG and neuroimaging techniques including source localization, PET, and SPECT. Conventional MRI, functional MRI, and MRI spectroscopy play an increasingly important role in the understanding of normal brain function and the identification of seizure foci. Several authors describe progress in these areas. Advances in surgical technique and new medical therapies are also reviewed in depth. To avoid casting too wide a net, mesial temporal epilepsy and the primary generalized epilepsies were deliberately omitted.

So long as human beings think, basic science needs no apology. As Virgil said two thousand years ago, "Happy is he who knows the causes of things." However, the commitment of large resources merely to satisfy curiosity is difficult to justify. Physicians often believe, "Philosophers have only interpreted the world in various ways, but the real task is to alter it." We hope that this symposium, which juxtaposes the two types of work, will produce a cross-fertilization that leads to better understanding and better therapy.

The editors thank Abbott, Ortho-McNeil/Johnson & Johnson, GlaxoWellcome, Novartis, Ad-Tech, Elan, Elekta AB, Warner Lambert, Telefactor, Nicolet, and Cyberonics for corporate financial support that was generous and unrestricted. Special thanks are due to Deborah Holmes and Terri Farnham for administrative assistance and Carol Bruzewicz for secretarial support. We are also most grateful to Anne Sydor and Julia Seto at Lippincott Williams & Wilkins for their painstaking work, which turned a set of manuscripts into a volume that is part of a well-respected series.

As this volume was going to press, we learned the sad news of Dr. Claudio Munari's death. His contributions to the field of epilepsy surgery are a lasting memorial, and his inimitable personality will be greatly missed at future gatherings of neuroscientists.

Peter D. Williamson
Adrian M. Siegel
David W. Roberts
Vijay M. Thadani
Michael S. Gazzaniga
Lebanon, New Hampshire

ADVANCES IN NEUROLOGY
Volume 84

Neocortical Epilepsies.
Advances in Neurology, Vol. 84,
edited by P. D. Williamson, A. M. Siegel,
D. W. Roberts, V. M. Thadani, and M. S. Gazzaniga.
Lippincott Williams & Wilkins, Philadelphia © 2000.

1

Molecular and Cellular Mechanisms of Neuronal Migration: Relevance to Cortical Epilepsies

Pasko Rakic

Section of Neurobiology, Yale University School of Medicine, New Haven, Connecticut 06510

Neuronal cell migration as a major developmental phenomenon has been known since the end of the last century, but it did not receive much attention until the advent of ^{3}H-thymidine autoradiography and electron microscopy, which enabled determination of the rate and pathways of migrating neurons and examination of their ultrastructure and relationship to surrounding cells in situ. These studies led to concepts of inside-out gradient of neurogenesis, neuron–glial cell differential adhesion, the radial unit hypothesis of cortical development, and the protomap hypothesis of cortical parcellation.

In the past decade, methods of cellular biology and various in vitro approaches have provided an unprecedented opportunity to study the molecular mechanisms of neuronal migration. These studies revealed that directed, glial-guided neuronal migration requires the orchestration of multiple molecular events. These events include the selection of migratory pathways by cell-recognition receptors, the formation of adhesive interactions with cellular and extracellular substrates, and activation of specific ion channels that provide second messenger–mediated signals for the cytologic changes involved in motility. Understanding the role of individual molecular components that mediate neuronal migration, provides new insight into the pathogenesis of congenital cortical malformations.

Because all cortical neurons originate near the surface of the embryonic cerebral ventricle, they all must move to their final positions in the cortex, which develop within the outer territories of the cerebral wall, below the pia. The migratory pathways of individual neurons become particularly long in the large primate telencephalon. The size of a migratory neuron in the mouse and that in the human embryo are approximately the same, and negotiation of the tortuous, several-thousand-microns–long pathway in the gyrencephalic brain poses a daunting problem. Indeed, a massive migration of neurons in primates, including humans, occurs during midgestation and coincides with the rapid increase in the width of the cerebral wall and the buckling of its surface, beginning to form sulci and gyri (1). This is perhaps why the phenomenon of neuronal cell migration originally was inferred from the observation in histologic sections of human embryos by Wilhelm His (2). Relatively little progress was made in terms of the underlying cellular and molecular mechanisms of this phenomenon until the 1970s, however, when a combination of electron microscopic and ^{3}H-thymidine autoradiographic analyses revealed that postmitotic neurons migrate across the intermediate zone by following elongated shafts of nonneural elements called *radial glial cells* (3). These bipolar cells stretch their processes across the fetal cerebral wall from the onset of corticogenesis, but they become most prominent during midgestation, when many of them temporarily stop dividing (4). During the migratory period, cohorts of postmitotic cells originating in the proliferative mosaic follow a radial pathway consisting of single or, more often, multiple glial fibers, that span the developing cerebral wall (Fig. 1.1). While moving, migrating neurons may be in contact with many axonal and dendritic processes but, nevertheless, remain preferentially attached to glial fibers. This observation suggested a "gliophilic" mode of migration that is mediated by heterotypic adhesion molecules present on neuronal and glial cell surface (5,6; Rakic, 1990). The postmitotic cells that did not obey glial constraints and appeared to

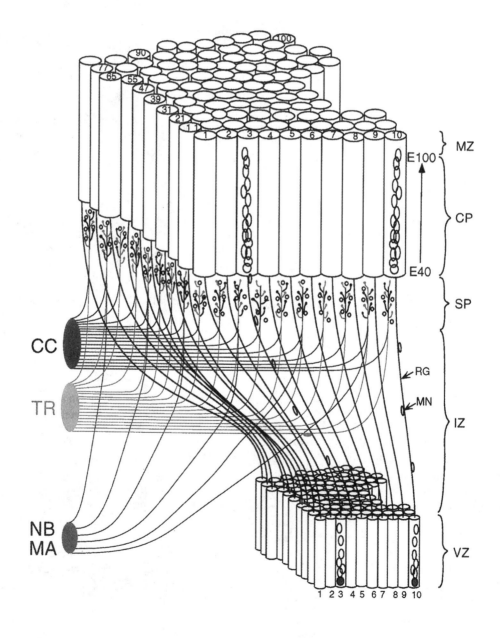

move along axonal tracts (e.g., red bipolar cell in Fig. 1.1) were considered *neurophilic* (5). Several initial observations suggested that a gliophilic class of migrating neurons may have the binding affinity for the surface of radial glial cells because they appear not to follow any other class of cellular processses that are present in the developing cerebral wall (3).

RADIAL UNIT HYPOTHESIS OF CORTICAL DEVELOPMENT

The adult neocortex consists of an array of iterative neuronal groups (called, interchangeably, *radial columns* or *modules*) that are interconnected in the vertical dimension, share a common extrinsic connectivity, and subserve the same function (7). The larger the cortex is in a given species, the larger the number of participating columnar units (1,8). Although the exact relationship between the functional columns in adult cortex and embryonic columns is not clear, the deployment of migrating neurons into radial columns during cortical development in a given individual and the large increase of cortical surface during evolution by the addition of such columns can be explained in the context of the *radial*

unit hypothesis (9). This hypothesis originally was based on the observation that postmitotic cells preserve their positions during movement by remaining attached to a given radial glial fascicle once they initiate their movement (3,10). Furthermore, the pattern of distribution of heavily and lightly ^{3}H-thymidine–labeled cells indicated that the columns likely consist of several clones (9). In the past decade, the *radial unit hypothesis* has served as a useful working model for research on the cellular and molecular mechanisms involved in normal and abnormal cortical development.

The proposal that cells in a given radial column may be clonally related became possible to test experimentally only after the introduction of the retrieval gene transfer method for in vivo analysis of cell lineages in the mammalian brain (11). Although the clonal relationship of labeled cells using this approach originally was based on the law of probability, cell distribution strongly suggested that most progenitors originating in the same site of the ventricular zone remain radially deployed in the cortex (12). A number of studies in chimeric and transgenic mice provided more direct evidence that

FIG. 1.1. A three-dimensional illustration of the basic developmental events and types of cell–cell interactions occurring during the early stages of corticogenesis, before formation of the final pattern of cortical connections. This cartoon emphasizes radial migration, a predominant mode of neuronal movement that, in primates, underlies the elaborate columnar organization of the neocortex. After their last division, cohorts of migrating neurons *(MD)* first traverse the intermediate zone *(IZ)* and then the subplate zone *(SP)*, where they have an opportunity to interact with "waiting" afferents arriving sequentially from the nucleus basalis and monoamine subcortical centers *(NB, MA)* from thalamic radiation *(TR)*, and from several ipsilateral and contralateral corticocortical bundles *(CC)*. After the newly generated neurons bypass the earlier generated ones situated in the deep cortical layers, they settle at the interface between the developing cortical plate *(CP)* and the marginal zone *(MZ)* and, eventually, form a radial stack of cells that share a common site of origin but are generated at different times. For example, neurons produced between embryonic day E40 and E100 in radial unit 3 follow the same radial gliala fasicle and form ontogenic column 3. Although some cells, presumably neurophilic in the nature of their surface affinities, may detach from the cohort and move laterally, guided by an axonal bundle (e.g., horizontally oriented, black cell leaving radial unit 3), most postmitotic cells are gliophilic (e.g., they have an affinity for the glial surface and strictly obey constraints imposed by transient radial glial *(RG)* scaffolding. This cellular arrangement preserves the relationships between the proliferative mosaic of the ventricular zone *(VZ)* and the corresponding protomap within the SP and CP, even though the cortical surface in primates shifts considerably during a massive cerebral growth encountered in mid-gestation (for details see Rakic 1988, 1995b).

most postmitotic, clonally related neurons move and remain radially distributed in the cortex [13–15; reviewed in Rakic (8)]. The use of the retroviral gene transfer method in the embryonic primate brain showed that, even in the large and highly convoluted cerebrum, radial deployment of many clones is remarkably preserved (16).

In addition to the clones that are distributed radially (12), certain populations of clonally related cortical cells do not obey strict radial constraints. Although lateral dispersion of postmitotic neurons was observed in the early Golgi studies [e.g., Fig. 1 of the report of the Boulder Committee (17)], this phenomenon has attracted renewed attention after advent of the retroviral method. Studies in rodents suggested widespread dispersion of some clonally related cortical cells (18). In the ferret telencephalon, about 15% of neurons appear to migrate nonradially (19), although it is not clear how many actually enter the cerebral cortex. The dispersion is more prominent at later developmental stages, suggesting that these cells may originate from the subventricular zone. It should be emphasized, however, that even those clonally related cells that disperse widely appear to migrate radially along glial fibers situated close to the site of their last mitotic division, a finding that is in full harmony with the radial unit hypothesis (20; Tan et al., 1998). In primates, it is likely that an even larger proportion of migrating neurons will obey the radial constraints imposed by a more elaborate radial glial scaffolding than in rodents (8,9).

The radial unit hypothesis provides an explanation for a large expansion of cortical surface without the significant increase in thickness that occurred during phylogenetic and ontogenetic development (9). It was proposed that the gene controlling the number of proliferative units at the ventricular surface sets a limit on the size of the cortical surface during individual development as well as during evolution of the mammalian species (21). A relatively small change in the timing of developmental cellular events could have large functional consequences. For example, a minor increase in the length of cell cycles or in the number of cell divisions in the ventricular zone can result in a large increase in the number of founder cells that form proliferative units (9). Proliferation in the ventricular zone initially proceeds exponentially by the prevalence of symmetric divisions; therefore, an additional round of mitotic cycles during this phase doubles the number of proliferative units and, consequently, the number of radial colums (21). According to this model, fewer than four extra rounds of cell divisions can account for the tenfold difference in size of cortical surface between monkey and human. In contrast, the 1,000-fold difference between the size of cerebral cortex in the mouse and human can be achieved by less than seven extra symmetric divisions in the ventricular zone before the onset of corticogenesis.

After the number of founder cells that will form individual radial units is set and corticogenesis has begun, many progenitor cells start to divide asymmetrically. Therefore, during this phase of development, an extra round of cell divisions would have a negligible effect on the thickness of the cortex [see Fig. 2 in Rakic (8)]. According to this model, one can predict that the about 2-week-longer duration of corticogenesis in human than in macaque should enlarge the cortical thickness by only 10% to 20%, which is actually observed (21). In contrast, even a small delay in the onset of the second phase of corticogenesis results in an order of magnitude larger cortical surface as a result of the increasing number of proliferative units at the ventricular zone.

MOLECULAR MECHANISM OF MIGRATORY PATHWAY RECOGNITION

The universality of neuronal guidance by radial glial scaffolding has been confirmed in a variety of mammalian species, including the human (22–26). Initially, based on inference from the neuron–glial relationship observed in situ, it was proposed that a single pair of binding, complementary molecules with gliophilic properties can account for the entire guidance phenomenon of radial migration (10). In the last decade, however, several putative recognition and adhesion molecules were identified (24,27–31). So far, accumulated evidence suggests that it is likely that more than one class of surface molecules must be involved to account for the phenomenon of recognition, adhesion, and cessation of neuronal cell migration (6).

An important feature of potential recognition molecules is that they should be expressed selectively and transiently in the leading process of postmitotic neurons at the surface adjacent to radial glial fibers (Fig. 1.2). Although the heterotypic recognition mechanism may be of low affinity, the molecules that are an integral part of the membrane can selectively recognize and bind to specific carbohydrate moieties on the adjacent cell. A major advance in this area was identification of the astrotactin, a molecule present on the surface of migrating neurons, blockage of the which curtails neuronal migration in vitro (32). We recently generated a polyclonal antiserum (D4) and monoclonal antibody (NJPA1) that recognizes polypeptide-forming plasmalemmal junctions situated between migrating neurons and adjacent radial glial fibers (27,33). The integrity of these junctional microdomains is maintained in the developing cerebral wall only during the phase of cell migration. In dissociated glial–neuronal cell cultures, these microdomains require intact microtubules and can be detected at the sites where the somal region of migrating neurons is in direct contact with elongated glial fibers. An addition of D4 and NJIA1 to the culture medium in imprint and slice preparation of the embryonic cerebral wall leads to withdrawal of the leading process, changes in microtubular organization, and finally, detachment of neurons from radial glial shafts (34).

After passing between previously generated neurons already settled in the deeper strata of cortical plate, migrating neurons abruptly stop their movement at the border of the marginal zone (Rakic, 1974, and MZ in Fig. 1.2). Actually, the leading process freely enters the marginal zone; it is the movement of the nucleus and surrounding cytoplasm that stops at this barrier (Fig. 1.2). Only in certain pathological conditions, such as exposure to alcohol, or in neurologic mutants, such as the reeler and New Zealand mice, do migrating cortical neurons invade the marginal zone (35,36); however, the mechanism that normally provides the CP/MZ barrier is not understood. We recently generated an additional antibody, PS2A1, that immunoreacts only with the segment of the radial glial fiber passing through the cortical plate and disappears abruptly at the interface to the marginal zone (31). This distribution stands in contrast to the distribution of reelin, the product of the *reeler* gene, that is abundant in immature Cajal–Retzius cells and is distributed predominantly within the marginal zone (37). Our preliminary results, using BrdU as a marker of neuronal birthdays, indicate that postmitotic migrating cells exposed to PS2A1 antibody fail to detach from the glial fibers at the interface between the cortical plate and the marginal zone; as a consequence, subsequently arriving neurons cannot come at the top and accumulate beneath the previously generated neurons, forming an outside-to-inside gradient of neurogenesis (31). A similar outside-to-inside sequence was observed in the cortex of the *reeler* mouse (35), although in this case a deficit of a different molecule is likely to be involved (37,38).

These studies revealed that the molecular mechanism for selection of a migratory pathway by postmitotic neurons is more complicated, and involves a larger number of molecular species than initially predicted. The fast growing body of data obtained from new experimental approaches is beginning to elucidate the mechanisms by which developmental genes regulate the temporal and spatial expression of adhesive proteins, controlling cell allocation to cerebral cortex.

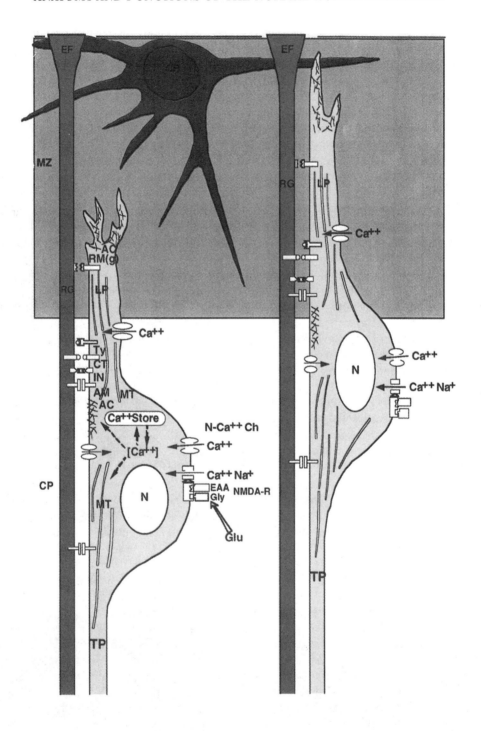

MOLECULAR CONTROL OF INITIATION, RATE, AND CESSATION OF SOMAL TRANSLOCATION

Active, directed migration of neurons across long distances involves the unidirectional translocation of the nucleus and somatic cytoplasm within the cytoplasmic cylinder of the growing leading processes. It also requires the signals controlling the cellular machinery involved in initiation and cessation of this movement. The mechanism of the actual physical displacement of cell perikarya has been sought only recently [reviewed in Rakic and Komuro (39)]. Voltage- and ligand-gated ion channels situated on the leading process and the cell soma of migrating neurons regulate the influx of calcium ions into migrating neurons (40). The influx and fluctuation of free Ca^{++}, in turn, may trigger polymerixation of cytoskeletal and contractile proteins essential for translocation of the nucleus and surrounding cytoplasm (Fig. 1.2). Using live slice and explant preparations of the developing neural tissue to measure the effect of various substances on the rate of cell migration, we found that the voltage-gated, N-type Ca^{++} channel (41) and ligand-gated, NMDA channel (42) are particulary active. The composition of the receptor/channel complexes on the surface of migrating neurons differs from the composition they have

after reaching their final destination (43). These receptor/channels can regulate Ca^{2+} levels in the migrating neurons (44). We have observed that the amplitude and frequency components of Ca^{2+} fluctuations are positively correlated with the rate of migrating granule cells in cerebellar microexplant cultures (40). Moreover, depression of the amplitude and frequency components of Ca^{2+} fluctuations by blockade of calcium influx across the plasma membrane results indicate that the combination of amplitude and frequency components of intracellular Ca^{2+} fluctuations may provide an intracellular signal controlling the rate of neuronal cell migration.

To explore the cellular machinery underlying translocation of the nucleus during neuronal migration, we determined the polarity of microtubule assemblies situated within the leading and trailing processes of migrating cerebellar granule cells in situ (45). Our analysis revealed that the newly assembled, positive ends of the microtubules situated in the leading process are uniformly facing the growing tip, whereas their disintegrating negative ends face the nucleus. In the trailing process, by contrast, microtubule arrays are of mixed polarity. Based on these results, we have proposed that the extension of the leading process, at least in part, may be created by the "push" force of the array of polymers built up in the direction of leading process exten-

FIG. 1.2. Model of a proposed cascade of molecular events that take place during migration of postmitotic across developing cerebral wall. Migrating cells extend a leading process *(LP)* that follows selectively the contours of the radial glial fiber *(RF)* as it spans the expanding cerebral wall. The cytoskeleton within the LP and trailing process *(TP)* contain prominent assemblies of microtubules *(MT)* and actin-like contractile proteins *(AC)* that are involved in elongation of the LP and translocation of the nucleus *(N)* and the surrounding cytoplasm. The LP enters the cortical plate *(CP)* and marginal zone *(MZ)*, but the nucleus stops at the CP/MZ interface *(gray area)*. Various intracellular, membrane-bound, and extracellular matrix molecules provide signals or are directly engaged in selection of migratory pathway, rate of cell movement, and finally in the cessation of migration at the CP/MZ borderline. Further explanation is in the text. *AC,* actin-like filaments; *AM,* homotypic adhesion molecule; *CR,* Cajal–Retzius cell; *CT,* catenin; *EAA,* excitatory amino acids; *EF,* endfoot of radial glial fiber; *Glu,* glutamate; *Gly,* glycine; *I,* integrine; *RM(g),* gliophilic recognition molecule; *RM(n),* neurophilic recognition molecule; *Ty,* site of increased tyrosine phosphorylation. (Reproduced from Rakic P. Intra- and extracellular control of neuronal migration: relevance to cortical malformations. In: Galaburda AM, Christen Y, eds. *Normal and abnormal development of cortex.* Berlin: Springer-Verlag, 1997, with permission.)

sion. In contrast, the nucleus and surrounding cytoplasm may be translocated within the membrane envelope because of the orchestrated dissociation of microtubules at their negative ends in front of the orchestrated dissociation of microtubules at their negative ends in front of the nucleus. Such a synchronized disintegration may create a cytoplasmic space devoid of stable cytoskeletal scaffolding as well as "pull" forces essential for this displacement (44). These "pull" forces are expected to be stronger in the leading process, where their orientation is mixed. A rapid, coordinated depolymerization of microtubule sheets alternating with a phase of relative stability at their negative ends, as observed during locomotion of nonneuronal cells (46), may underlie the alternation of movement and stationary periods observed during nuclear displacement in migrating neurons. Our hypothesis that the somatic translocation of the migrating cell, at least in part, may depend on the dynamics of polymerization, and depolymerization of the microtubule protein in the cytoplasm of the leading and trailing processes, is consistent with the finding that the slow extension of the leading process of migrating neurons precedes the phase of more rapid nuclear displacement (24,42,47). In addition, it is in harmony with the finding that the disruption of the microtubule structure results in the collapse of the migrating cell body and cessation of nuclear translocation (48). It should be underscored, however, that the proposed role of microtubules in nuclear displacement during neuronal migration does not exclude the synergistic action of actinlike contractile proteins, which also may participate in this event (5).

The signals that induce the onset and cessation of nuclear translocation are unknown, but repolarization of microtubules seems to be an essential prerequisite for this translocation. Caged by the cytoskeletal network, the nucleus could not move without rearrangement of microtubules. The rate of assembling the microtubule polymer depends on the concentration of cytosolic Ca^{2+}, which is delivered through specific voltage- and ligand-gated channels (Fig. 1.2). In addition, it has been suggested that the integrity and orientation of cytoskeletal proteins may be related to membrane-bound cell adhesion molecules (6) and to neuron–glial junctional complexes in migrating neurons (27). Identification of molecules that abruptly change their density at the interface of the cortical plate and marginal zone provides promising clues (34,37). Likewise, a sudden change in glutamate concentration at the interface to layer I can regulate channels/receptors that provide the signal for cytoskeletal stabilization (40). Interruption of the molecular messages in the chain of signals controlling assembly of the cytoskeleton in migrating neurons may explain abnormal neuronal placements in certain genetic and acquired brain malformations.

PROTOMAP HYPOTHESIS OF CYTOARCHITECTONIC DIVERSITY

A major challenge to developmental neurobiology is how individual and species-specific cytoarchitectonic areas have emerged from the initially seemingly uniform ventricular zone and cortical plate. Both intrinsic and extrinsic factors have been suggested. One attractive hypothesis is that all cortical neurons are equipotential and that laminar and areal differences are induced by extrinsic influences exerted through thalamic afferents (49). Indeed, the structural and functional homogeneity of the cortex emphasized by Lashley and colleagues in the middle of this century (e.g., 50) appears to be supported by the ostensible similarity in the laminar pattern of cell distribution in various cortical areas and by the acknowledged resemblance of their synaptic circuitry (7,51–53). This hypothesis is also in harmony with findings that a single-unit response with the typical visual receptive field properties can be elicited from the somatosensory cortex when input from the retina is experimentally rerouted to the somatosensory thalamus (54,55). Indeed, the evidence is overwhelming that the development of many features of cortical organization is highly dependent on interaction with thalamic afferents (10,56–59; Rakic, 1981).

Considerable evidence also has been found that the cells generated within the embryonic cerebral wall contain some basic programs of their prospective species-specific cortical organization. To reconcile existing experimental and descriptive data, we formulated a *protomap hypothesis* (9). This hypothesis suggests that the basic pattern of cytoarchitectonic areas emerges through synergistic, interdependent interactions between developmental programs intrinsic to cortical neurons and extrinsic signals supplied by specific input from the subcortical structures. According to this hypothesis, neurons of the embryonic cortical plate—indeed, even the proliferative ventricular zone where they originate—set up a primordial species-specific cortical map of areas that preferentially attract appropriate afferents and have a capacity to respond to this input in a specific manner. The prefix *proto* was introduced to emphasize the primordial, provisionary, and essentially malleable character of the protomap that is subject to considerable modification by the extrinsic influences exerted at later stages (9).

The initial indication that developmental events in the ventricular zone foreshadow prospective regional differences in the overlaying cerebral mantle comes from ^{3}H-thymidine labeling of dividing cells, which shows that the ventricular region subjacent to area 17 produces more neurons per radial unit (60) and that the region subjacent to area 17 has a substantially higher mitotic index than the adjacent area 18 (61). Therefore, certain region-specific differences in production of the ventricular zone can be detected even before neurons arrive at the cortex and become exposed to input from the periphery by means of the thalamic afferents (62,63). The development of correct topological connections in ophthalmic mice and in early enucleated animals indicates that a basic map can form in the absence of information from the periphery (9,64,65). Likewise, the primary visual cortex in the primate acquires a normal pattern of cytochrome oxidase (9,66,67) and major neuro-

transmitter receptors and synaptic density (68; Bourgeois et al., 1996) in the absence of any retinal input by means of the thalamus from the early embryonic stages. Finally, development of the orientation preference maps in the visual cortex is unaffected by either visual experience or the anatomic rearrangements of the geniculocortical connection into eye-specific domains (69).

The protomap hypothesis recently received support from several reports that show the emergence of area-specific antigens in the cortex before, or independent of, thalamic input (e.g., 70–75; Donoghue and Rakic, 1999; Rubenstein and Rakic, 1999). Recent in vivo and in vitro studies showed a high specificity of the growing thalamic axons for the selective regions of the embryonic cerebral cortex (76,77). It was also observed that specific functions can be restored only after transplantation of embryonic cells derived from the same, but not other, areas (78). It is likely, therefore, that regulatory genes that are differentially expressed in the cerebral wall could operate in the mammalian telencephalon, but only a few have been tested (79,80; Bishop et al., 2000; Miyashita-Lin et al., 1999). So far, perhaps the most compelling evidence in favor of the protomap hypothesis has been obtained using transgenic mice combined with transareal transplantation of the embryonic cerebral wall to other regions (81; Gitton et al., 1999) and rearrangement of thalamic input (Miyashita-Lin et al., 1999). This study indicates that certain genes are expressed selectively in the somatosensory cortex without, and irrespective of, the type of afferents that neurons destined for this region receive from the thalamus.

It should be underscored that, although the embryonic cerebral wall exhibits gradients of morphoregulatory molecules, as well as more specific area-specific molecular differences, the protomap within the embryonic crebrum provides only a set of species-specific genetic instructions and biologic constraints. The precise position of interareal borders, the overall size of each cytoarchitectonic area, and the details of their cellular and synaptic characteristics in the adult cerebral cortex are achieved through a cascade of reciprocal interactions between cortical neurons and cues they receive from afferents arriving from a variety of extracortical sources (9). Such afferents may serve to coordinate and adjust the ratio of various cell classes with the subcortical structures, as shown in the primary visual system (82). For example, the experimental manipulation of geniculocortical input to the visual cortex indicated that the size of a given cytoarchitectonic area can be regulated by afferents originating from subcortical structures (9,62,68,83). This extracortical control can be exerted on the rate of cell elimination as well as on cell production in the ventricular zone. In summary, the concept of the cortical protomap includes the role of both intrinsic and extrinsic determinants in shaping the final pattern and relative size of the cytoarchitectonic areas.

RELEVANCE OF NEURONAL MIGRATION TO CORTICAL MALFORMATION

Accumulated evidence suggests that specific communications between heterogeneous classes of cells play a major role in establishing their position, identity, and selection of migratory pathways before they arrive at their final destination in the cortex and form synaptic connections. Thus, multiple causes can produce similar migratory deficits and diverse forms of cortical malformations can be caused by the same molecular events. For example, the process of migration is highly sensitive to various physical (e.g., ionizing radiation, heat), chemical (e.g., various drugs, excessive use of alcohol), and biologic (some neurotropic viruses) agents, as well as to genetic mutations, and is thought to be the major cause of various gross brain malformations and also of more subtle abnormalities in neuronal positioning and in the pattern of synaptic circuits.

The most frequent migratory abnormalities are revealed in the mature brain by the presence of solitary ectopic neurons that have failed to reach their target and are scattered within the white matter. The cause for such

misplacements may be exposure to various exogenous agents, such as low doses of irradiation or drugs that interfere with signaling pathways (63,84). Despite their small number, such ectopic cells may be a major source of epileptic discharge by means of abnormal synaptic connections with the overlaying cortex. More massive malformations, known by descriptive terms such as *microencephaly, schizencephaly, lissencephaly, macrogyria, polymicrogyria,* or *double cortex,* may be fully or in part consequential to defective migration and abnormal settling of nerve cells during the formative stages of the human neocortex. The ectopic neurons in such malformations can serve as a focus of epileptic discharge. Advances made in developmental neurobiology allow some new interpretations of these malformations.

According to the radial unit hypothesis, the pathogenesis of major cortical malformations can be classified into two major categories. The first category comprises malformations in which the number of radial units in the cortex is reduced, whereas the number of neurons within each ontogenetic column remains relatively normal. It can be expected that defects in this category result from an early occurring event that alters the number of proliferative units at the time they are being formed in humans within the first 6 weeks of gestation. Once the number of proliferative units in the ventricular zone is established, albeit fewer, each unit can produce a normal or even greater number of neurons that become crowded in the diminished cerebral vesicle. It could be expected that the cortex would have a smaller surface area despite a normal or enlarged thickness and the presence of massive neuronal ectopias in the white matter. Identification of defective genes in humans that may cause a smaller cerebral surface with an absence of convolutions, presumably by disrupting neuronal migration, opens the prospect of unraveling the pathogenesis of such types of malformations at the molecular level (85).

The second category consists of malformations in which the initial formation of radial units is not affected, whereas the number of neurons within radial columns in the cortex is reduced. The defect in this category should begin after the sixth fetal week, when the normal complement of proliferative units in the human cerebrum already has been established. Such malformations can be caused by interference with cell proliferation through intrinsic (genetic) or extrinsic (irradiation or viral infection) factors. Diminished production of neurons in the proliferative units results in fewer neurons within ontogenetic columns, and the cortex is therefore thinner. It should be recognized that in most cases cortical malformations may have features of only one or the other category, but in practice most show a mixture of both.

The proposed classification of cortical malformations suggests possible developmental mechanisms by separating defects of unit formation from defects of ontogenetic column formation. In support of the radial unit hypothesis and the concept of a cortical protomap, experimental manipulations and neuropathological data reveal that each step (formation of proliferative units, formation of ontogenetic columns, and formation of cytoarchitectonic areas) can be separately affected by genetic defects or by extrinsic factors. This general model of the differential effect of early and late disturbance of corticogenesis on the surface and thickness of the cerebral cortex also has been tested by experimental manipulation of corticogenesis in primates. For example, targeted roentgenography before the onset of corticogenesis (E33-40), area 17, displayed only slight changes in cortical thickness, cell density, and area-specific cytoarchitectonic features, whereas the total surface devoted to area 17 was significantly diminished (63). In contrast, in animals irradiated with low doses during the period of corticogenesis, the surface of area 17 was not significantly altered, although the cortical layers generated at the time of irradiation had a significantly lower number of cells per radial unit. This interpretation has been supported by the mode of cortical development in the trisomy 16 mouse, which is considered to be an animal model of Down's syndrome (86). In this malformation, slow tangential expansion of neuroepithelium in Ts16 mice resulted in a reduction in the final telencephalic size that can be predicted by a reduction of radial units in early telencephalic development.

The number of neurons in radial columns also could be affected by excessive proliferation, diminished apoptosis, and a failure of neuronal migration. In such cases, supernumerary neurons may fail to reach the cortex and often survive in ectopic positions within the white matter. An instructive example in this category is the abnormal development of cerebral cortex in transgenic mouse, which was made using homologous recombination deficient in CPP32 protease that is essential for a normal process of programmed cell death [apoptosis (87)]. In homozygous mice, supernumerary cells were consistently located between the ventricular zone and the cerebral cortex in a remarkably similar fashion to the deployment in the "double cortex" (88).

The differential effect on the surface and thickness of the cortex can be observed in a variety of other malformations, although the pathogenesis in most cases remains obsure (89). Understanding the cellular and molecular mechanisms of neuronal proliferation and migration may help to explain the pathogenesis of the phenotype of previously inexplicable genetic and acquired conditions observed in mental retardation, schizophrenia, developmental dyslexia, as well as in childhood epilepsy (88–92).

ACKNOWLEDGMENTS

This work was suppported over the years by grants from the U.S. Public Health Service. This is an updated version of the review published in Research Perspectives in Neurosciences. Berlin: Springer-Verlag, 1997:81–89. I am indebted to the present and past members of my laboratory for their contributions and incisive discussion on this subject.

REFERENCES

1. Rakic P. Neuronal migration and contact interaction in primate telencephalon. *Postgrad Med J* 1978;54:25–40.

2. His W. *Unsere Körperform und das physiologische problem innerer entstehung.* Leipzig: Engelman, 1874.
3. Rakic P. Mode of cell migration to the superficial layers of fetal monkey neocortex. *J Comp Neurol* 1972;145: 61–84.
4. Schmechel DE, Rakic P. Arrested proliferation of radial glial cells during midgestation in rhesus monkey. *Nature* 1979;227:303–305.
5. Rakic P. Contact regulation of neuronal migration. In: Edelman GM, Thiery J-P, eds. *The cell in contact: adhesions and junctions as morphogenetic determinants.* New York: John Wiley & Sons, 1985:67–91.
6. Rakic P, Cameron RS, Komuro H. Recognition, adhesion, transmembrane signaling, and cell motility in guided neuronal migration. *Curr Opin Neurobiol* 1994;4:63–69.
7. Mountcastle VB. The columnar organization of the neocortex. *Brain* 1997;120:701–722.
8. Rakic P. Radial versus tangential migration of neuronal clones in the developing cerebral cortex. *Proc Natl Acad Sci USA* 1995;92:11323–11327.
9. Rakic P. Specification of cerebral cortical areas. *Science* 1988;241:170–176.
10. Rakic P. Neuron–glial interaction during brain development. *Trends Neurosci* 1981;4:184–187.
11. Sanes JR. Analyzing cell linages with a recombinant retrovirus. *Trends Neurosci* 1989;12:21–28.
12. Luskin MB, Pearlman AL, Sanes JR. Cell lineage in the cerebral cortex of the mouse studied in vivo and in vitro with a recombinant retrovirus. *Neuron* 1988;1:635–647.
13. Nakatsuji M, Kadokawa Y, Suemori H. Radial columnar patches in the chimeric cerebral cortex visualized by use of mouse embryonic stem cells expressing β-galactosidase. *Dev Growth Differ* 1991;33:571–578.
14. Tan S-S, Breen SJ. Radial mosaicism and tangential cell dispersion both contribute to mouse neocortical development. *Nature* 1993;362:638–640.
15. Soriano E, Dumesnil N, Auladell C, et al. Molecular heterogeneity of progenitors and radial migration in the developing cerebral cortex revealed by transgenic expression. *Proc Natl Acad Sci USA* 1995;92:11676–11680.
16. Kornack DR, Rakic P. Radial and horizontal deployment of clonally related cells in the primate neocortex: relationship to distinct mitotic lineages. *Neuron* 1995; 15:311–321.
17. Boulder Committee. Embryonic vertebrate central nervous system. Revised terminology. *Anat Rec* 1970; 166:257–261.
18. Walsh C, Cepko CL. Clonally related cortical cells show several migration patterns. *Science* 1988;241:1342–1345.
19. O'Rourke NA, Dailey ME, Smith SJ, et al. Diverse migratory pathways in the developing cerebral cortex. *Science* 1992;258:299–302.
20. Reid C, Liang I, Walsh C. Systematic widespread clonal organization in cerebral cortex. *Neuron* 1995;15:299–310.
21. Rakic P. A small step for the cell—a giant leap for mankind: a hypothesis of neocortical expansion during evolution. *Trends Neurosci* 1995b;18:383–388.
22. Sidman RL, Rakic P. Neuronal migration with special reference to developing human brain: a review. *Brain Res* 1973;62:1–35.
23. Kadhim HJ, Gadisseux J-F, Evrard P. Topographical and cytological evolution of the glial phase during prenatal development of the human brain: histochemical and electron microscopy study. *J Neuropathol Exp Neurol* 1988;47:166–188.

24. Hatten ME, Mason CA. Mechanism of glial-guided neuronal migration in vitro and in vivo. *Experimentia* 1990;46:907–916.
25. Misson JP, Austin CP, Takahashi T, et al. The alignment of migrating neural cells in relation to the murine neopallial radial glial fiber system. *Cereb Cortex* 1991; 1:221–229.
26. O'Rourke NA, Dulivan NA, Smith DP, et al. Tangential migration in developing cerebral cortex. *Development* 1995;1212:2165–2176.
27. Cameron RS, Rakic P. Polypeptides that comprise the plasmalemal microdomain between migrating neuronal and glial cells. *J Neurosci* 1994;14:3139–3155.
28. Edelman GM. Cell adhesion molecules. *Science* 1983; 219:450–457.
29. Hatten ME, Mason CA. Neuron–astroglia interactions in vitro and in vivo. *Trends Neurosci* 1986;9:168–174.
30. Schachner M, Faissner A, Fischer G. Functional and structural aspects of the cell surface in mammalian nervous system development. In: Edelman GM, Gall WE, Thiery JP, eds. *The cell in contact: adhesions and junctions as morphogenetic determinants.* New York: John Wiley & Sons, 1985:257–276.
31. Anton ES, Matthew WD, Rakic P. A regionally distributed radial glial antigen: a candidate for signaling an end to neuronal migration. *Soc Neurosci Abstr* 1996b; 22:1206.
32. Fishell G, Hatten ME. Astrotactin provides a receptor system for CNS neuronal migration. *Development* 1991;113:755–765.
33. Cameron RS, Ruffin JW, Cho NK, et al. Developmental expression, pattern of distribution, and effect on cell aggregation implicate a neuron–glial junctional domain polypeptide in neuronal migration. *J Comp Neurol* 1997;387:467–488.
34. Anton SA, Cameron RS, Rakic P. Role of neuro-glial junctional proteins in the maintenace and termination of neuronal migration across the embryonic cerebral wall. *J Neurosci* 1996;16:2283–2293.
35. Caviness VS Jr, Rakic P. Mechanisms of cortical development: a view from mutations in mice. *Ann Rev Neurosci* 1978;1:297–326.
36. Sherman GF, Galaburda AM, Geeschwind N. Cortical anomalies in brains of New Zealand mice: a neuropathologic model of dyslexia? *Proc Natl Acad Sci USA* 1985;82:8072–8074.
37. Ogawa M, Miyata T, Nakajima K, et al. The *reeler* gene-associated antigen on Cajal–Retzius neurons is a crucial molecule for laminar organization of cortical neurons. *Neuron* 1995;14:1–20.
38. Rakic P, Caviness VS. Cortical development: view from neurological muntants two decades later. *Neuron* 1995; 14:1101–1104.
39. Rakic P, Komuro H. The role of recepter-channel activity in neuronal cell migration. *J Neurobiol* 1995;26: 299–315.
40. Komuro H, Rakic P. Intracellular Ca^{2+} fluctuations modulate the rate of neuronal migration. *Neuron* 1996; 17:275–285.
41. Komuro H, Rakic P. Specific role of N-type calcium channels in neuronal migration. *Science* 1992;257: 806–809.
42. Komuro H, Rakic P. Modulation of neuronal migration by NMDA receptors. *Science* 1993;260:95–97.
43. Farrant M, Feldmeyer D, Takahashi T, et al. NMDA-re-

ceptor channel diversity in the developing cerebellum. *Nature* 1994;368:335–339.

44. Rossi D, Slater TN. The developmental onset of NMDA receptor channel activity during neuronal migration. *Neuropharmacology* 1993;32:1239–1248.

45. Rakic P, Knyihar-Csillik E, Csillik B. Polarity of microtubule assembly during neuronal migration. *Proc Natl Acad Sci USA* 1996;93:9218–9222.

46. Kirschner M, Mitchison T. Beyond self-assembly: from microtubules to morphogenesis. *Cell* 1986;45:329–342.

47. Komuro H, Rakic P. Dynamic of granule cell migration: a confocal microscopic study in acute cerebellar slice preparations. *J Neurosci* 1995;15:1110–1120.

48. Rivas RJ, Hatten MB. Motility and cytoskeletal organization of migrating cerebellar granule neurons. *J Neurosci* 1995;l15:981–989.

49. Creutzfeldt OD. Generality of the funtinal structure of the neocortex. *Naturwissenschaften* 1997;64:507–517.

50. Lashley KS, Clark G. The cytoarchitecture of the cerebral cortex of Ateles: a critical examination of cytoarchitectonic studies. *J Comp Neurol* 1946;85:223–305.

51. Eccles JC. The cerebral neocortex: a theory of its operation. In: Jones EG, Peters A, eds. *Cerebral cortex,* vol 2. New York: Plenum Press, 1984:1–36.

52. Rakic P, Singer W, eds. *Neurobiology of the neocortex.* New York: John Wiley & Sons, 1988.

53. Szentagothai J. The neuronal network of the cerebral cortex: a functional interpretation. *Prog Brain Res* 1987;201:219–248.

54. Frost DO, Metin C. Introduction of functional retinal projections to the somatosensory system. *Nature* 1985; 317:162–164.

55. Sur M, Geraghty PE, Roe AW. Experimentally induced visual projections in auditory thalamus and cortex. *Science* 1988;242:1434–1441.

56. Rakic P. Prenatal genesis of connections subserving ocular dominance in the rhesus monkey. *Nature* 1976;261: 467–471.

57. Hubel DH, Wiesel TN, LeVay S. Plasticity of ocular dominance columns in monkey striate cortex. *Philos Trans R Soc Lond B Biol Sci* 1977;278:377–409.

58. Schlagger BL, O'Leary DDM. Potential of visual cortex to develop an array of functional units unique to somatosensory cortex. *Science* 1992;266:1556–1560.

59. Shatz CJ. Emergence of order in visual system development. *Proc Natl Acad Sci USA* 1996;93:602–608.

60. Rakic P. Differences in the time of origin and in eventual distribution of neurons in areas 17 and 18 of the visual cortex in the rhesus monkey. *Exp Brain Res* 1976; 1(Suppl):244–248.

61. Dehay C, Giroud P, Berland M, et al. Modulation of the cell cycle contributes to the parcellation of the primate visual cortex. *Nature* 1993;366:464–466.

62. Kennedy H, Dehay C. Cortical specification of mice and men. *Cereb Cortex* 1993;3:171–186.

63. Algan O, Rakic P. Radiation-induced area- and lamina-specific deletion of neurons in the primate visual cortex. *J Comp Neurol* 1997;381:335–352.

64. Kaiserman-Abramov I, Graybiel A, Nauta WH. Thalamic projection to area 17 in a congenitally anophthalmic mouse strain. *Neuroscience* 1983;5:41–52.

65. Olivaria J, Van Sluyters RC. Callosal connections of the posterior neocortex in normal-eyed, congenitally anophthalmic and neonatally enucleated mice. *J Comp Neurol* 1984;230:249–268.

66. Kennedy H, Dehay C, Horsburgh G. Striate cortex periodicity. *Nature* 1990;384:494.

67. Kuljis RO, Rakic P. Hypercolumns in the monkey visual cortex can developin the absense of cues from photoreceptors. *Proc Natl Acad Sci USA* 1990;87:5303–5306.

68. Rakic P, Lidow MS. Distribution and density of neurotransmitter receptors in the absence of retinal input from early embryonic stages. *J Neurosci* 1995;15:2561–2574.

69. Chapman B, Stryker MP, Bonhoeffer T. Development of orientation preference maps in ferret primary visual cortex. *J Neurosci* 1996;16:6443–6453.

70. Arimatsu Y, Miyamoto M, Nihonmatsu I, et al. Early regional specification for a molecular neuronal phenotype in the rat neocortex. *Proc Natl Acad Sci USA* 1992;89: 8879–8883.

71. Ferri RT, Levitt P. Cerebral cortical progenitors are fated to produce region-specific neuronal populations. *Cereb Cortex* 1993;3:187–198.

72. Barbe MF, Levitt P. Attraction of specific thalamic input by cerebral grafts depends on the molecular identity of the implant. *Proc Natl Acad Sci USA* 1992;89:3706–3710.

73. Levitt P. Experimental approaches that reveal principles of cerebral cortical development. In: Gazzaniga M, ed. *Cognitive neurosciences.* Cambridge, MA: MIT Press, 1994:147–163.

74. Porteus MH, Brice EJ, Buffone A, et al. Isolation and characterization of a library of cDNA clones that are preferentially expressed in the embryonic telencephalon. *Mol Brain Res* 1992;12:7–22.

75. Buffone A, Kim HJ, Puelles L, et al. The mouse DLX-2 (Tes-1) Gbx-2 and Wnt-3 in the embryonic day 12.5 mouse forebrain defines potential transverse and longitudinal segmental boundaries. *Mech Dev* 1993;40:129–140.

76. Agmon AA, Yand LT, Jones GE, et al. Topological precision in the thalamic projection to the neonatal mouse. *J Neurosci* 1995;13:5365–5382.

77. Boltz J, Novak N, Staiger V. Formation of specific afferent connections in organotypic slice cultures fron rat visual cortex cocultured with lateral geniculate nucleus. *J Neurosci* 1992;12:3054–3070.

78. Barth TM, Stanfield BB. Homotopic, but not heterotopic, fetal cortical transplants can result in functional sparing following neonatal damage to the frontal cortex in rat. *Cereb Cortex* 1994;4:271–278.

79. Lu S, Bogorad LD, Murtha MT, et al. Expression pattern of a marine homeobox gene, Dbx, displays extreme spatial restriction in embryonic forebrain and spinal cord. *Proc Natl Acad Sci USA* 1992;89:8053.

80. Rubinstein JLR, Martinez S, Shimamura K, et al. The embryonic vertebrate forebrain: the prosomeric model. *Science* 1994;266:578–580.

81. Cohen-Tannoudji M, Babinet C, Wassef M. Early intrinsic regional specification of the mouse somatosensory cortex. *Nature* 1994;368:460–463.

82. Meissirel C, Wikler KC, Chalupa LM, et al. Early divergence of M and P visual subsystems in the embryonic primate brain. *Proc Natl Acad Sci USA* 1997;94: 5900–5905.

83. Rakic P, Suner I, Williams RW. Novel cytoarchitectonic areas induced experimentally within primate striate cortex. *Proc Natl Acad Sci USA* 1991;88:2083–2987.

84. Lidow MS. Prenatal cocaine exposure adversely affects the development of the primate cerebral cortex. *Synapse* 1995;21:332–341.

85. Reiner O, Carrozzo R, Shen Y, et al. Isolation of a

Miller–Dieker lissencephaly gene containing G protein b-subunit–like repeats. *Nature* 1993;364:717–721.

86. Haydar TF, Blue EB, Milliver ME, et al. Consequences of Trisomy 16 for mouse brain development: corticogenesis in a model of Down syndrome. *J Neurosci* 1996; 16:6175–6182.

87. Kuida K, Zheng TS, Na S, et al. Decreased apoptosis in the brain and premature lethatlity in CPP32-deficient mice. *Nature* 1996;384:368–372.

88. Palmini A, Andermann F, Aicardi J, et al. Diffuse cortical dysplasia or the "double cortex" syndrome. *Neurology* 1991;41:1656–1662.

89. Volpe JJ. *Neurology of the newborn,* 2nd ed. Philadelphia: WB Saunders, 1987.

90. Aicardi J. The agyria-pachygyria complex: a spectrum of cortical malformations. *Brain Dev* 1991;13:1–8.

91. Galaburda AM, Sherman GF, Rosen GD, et al. Developmental dyslexia: four consecutive patients with cortical abnormalities. *Ann Neurol* 1985;18:222–223.

92. Bloom RE. Advancing a neurodevelopmental origin of schizophrenia. *Arch Gen Psychiatry* 1993;50:224–227.

ADDITIONAL REFERENCES

Bishop KM, Gourdeau G, O'Leary DDM. Regulation of area identity in the mammalian neocortex by *Emx2* and *Pax6*. *Science* 2000;288:344–349.

Bourgeois J-P, Rakic P. Synaptoarchitecture of the occipital cortex in macaque monkeys devoid of retinal input from early embryonic stages. *Euro J Neurosci* 1996;8: 942–950.

Donoghue MJ, Rakic P. Molecular gradients and compartments in the embryonic primate cerebral cortex. *Cerebral Cortex* 1999;9:586–600.

Gitton Y, Cohen-Tannoudji M, Wassef M. Role of thalamic axons in the expression of H-2Z1, a mouse somatosensory cortex specific marker. *Cerebral Cortex* 1999;9: 611–620.

Miyashita-Lin EM, Hevner R, Montzka-Wassarman K, et al. Early neocortical regionalization in the absence of thalamic innervation. *Science* 1999;285:906–909.

Rakic P. Neurons in the monkey visual cortex: systematic relation between time of origin and eventual disposition. *Science* 1974;183:425–427.

Rakic P. Principles of neuronal cell migration. *Experientia* 1990;46:882–891.

Rakic P. Development of visual centers in the primate brain depends on binocular competition before birth. *Science* 1981;214:928–931.

Rubenstein JLR, Rakic P. Genetic control of cortical development. *Cerebral Cortex* 1999;9:521–523.

Tan S-S, Kalloniatis M, Sturm K, et al. Separate progenitors for radial and tangential cell dispersion during development of the cerebral neocortex. *Neuron* 1998;21: 295–304.

Neocortical Epilepsies.
Advances in Neurology, Vol. 84,
edited by P. D. Williamson, A. M. Siegel,
D. W. Roberts, V. M. Thadani, and M. S. Gazzaniga.
Lippincott Williams & Wilkins, Philadelphia © 2000.

2

Recovered Memory Function Following Lateralized Cortical Damage

Michael B. Miller and Michael S. Gazzaniga

Center for Cognitive Neuroscience, Dartmouth College, Hanover, New Hampshire 03755-3547

STRIVING FOR NORMALCY

We go to great lengths to cover the blemishes of our lives. Whether it is a pimple on our forehead or a word we avoid using because we have trouble pronouncing it, our goal is to appear normal, at the very least. Sometimes these actions are conscious, but at other times we are unaware that such a coverup is taking place. The mind seems particularly adept at covering shortcomings. Indeed, it seems also able to cover deficits caused by neurologic damage to particular regions of the brain.

The two cerebral hemispheres have predetermined functions, including language production, usually located in the left hemisphere, and face processing, usually located in the right hemisphere. It is also the case that the two hemispheres play different roles in managing the normal memory mechanisms of the human mind. This chapter addresses the uncovering of these processes and how the brain adapts to unilateral damage and hemispheric disconnection.

Split-brain patients, whose corpus callosum is severed to relieve severe convulsions caused by epileptic seizures, provide a unique opportunity to study the specialization of each hemisphere. Such studies have shown that the left hemisphere has the unique ability to interpret events and actions carried out by both sides of the brain. Whereas the right hemisphere may initiate an appropriate action based on what it perceives, the left hemisphere, not having perceived the same stimulus, will attempt to explain rationally its seemingly inappropriate behavior. The left hemisphere "interpreter" strives to make sense of the world, to build a continuous stream of coherent images, and to find causes for events. This interpretative ability can affect cognitive functioning, from basic perceptions to memory. Furthermore, the interpreter can cover certain brain deficits and create an illusion of plasticity.

A powerful demonstration of the left hemisphere's interpretative nature is the simultaneous concept test. In this task, a split-brain patient is shown a picture exclusively to the left hemisphere (e.g., a chicken) and another picture exclusively to the right hemisphere (e.g., a snow scene). The patient then is given an array of pictures and asked to point to one associated with the presented pictures; he or she is requested to use the left hand to point to a picture shown to the right hemisphere and right hand to point to a picture shown to the left. The left hemisphere chose a chicken claw; the right hemisphere chose a shovel. When asked to explain the choices, the patient responded, "Oh, that's simple. The chicken claw goes with the chicken, and you need a shovel to clean out the chicken shed." Because the right hemisphere cannot produce speech, it cannot explain its selection. The left hemisphere is unaware of the picture to which the right hemisphere is responding (i.e., the snow scene), and so it has to generate its own interpretation of why the left hand pointed to a shovel. It interprets the right brain's actions within the context of what it knows (i.e., a chicken claw) and generates an explanation for the shovel that is consistent with its knowledge (1).

The left hemisphere interpreter strives to make sense of the world even when it is detrimental to do so, such as inferring a cause for a random event. When presented with a random sequence of events, humans tend to look for a pattern and to infer a cause for the pattern (2). Wolford and colleagues, at Dartmouth College, recently conducted a probability-guessing experiment in which subjects tried to guess which of two events will occur next. Humans tend to match the frequency of previous occurrences in their guesses, despite the fact that this is a less than optimal strategy in that the probability of one event occurring by design is significantly higher than the other event occurring. Animals other than humans maximize or choose every time the option that has occurred the most frequently in the past, essentially outperforming humans. Wolford and colleagues extended this study to split-brain patients. They found that the right hemisphere maximizes much like other animals, whereas the left hemisphere matches. Similar results were obtained with lesion patients (3).

The interpretative nature of the left hemisphere also has its effects on memory. Metcalfe and associates (4) conducted a study on two split-brain patients. They used a lateralized recognition test of stimuli that included words, abstract figures, and faces. They found that the left hemisphere tended to recognize falsely newly presented stimuli that were related to the stimuli presented in the study session, whereas the right hemisphere was much more veridical in its recollection. In what follows, we outline how an intact left hemisphere with its powerful interpretive system can mask the cognitive deficits of a damaged right hemisphere.

FRONTAL LOBE MECHANISMS IN MEMORY

Many recent neuroimaging studies have correlated activations in the prefrontal cortex with episodic memory retrieval tasks (5–7). Although some of these activations are bilateral, from metanalysis studies we know that episodic retrieval tasks predominantly accompany blood flow activations in the right anterior prefrontal cortex, particularly Brodmann areas 10, 44, and 46 (7,8). These tasks include the retrieval of a wide range of stimuli, including words (5,9–11), pictures (10,11), and faces (12,13).

Even though these neuroimaging studies consistently show activations in the right prefrontal cortex, patients with damage specifically to that region—due either to stroke or surgery—do not have a lasting, significant memory impairment (14,15). They certainly would not be diagnosed as amnesic as would patients with damage to the medial temporal lobe (16). Swick and Knight from the University of California at Davis tested frontal lobe patients who have unilateral focal lesions to the left or right prefrontal cortex. They used the same memory test that produced blood flow activations to the same regions in normal subjects as those in which these patients have damage; they hypothesized that the patients should show deficits. Yet their performance on the tests fell well within the normal range. One interpretation is that because they tested the patients more than a year after their injury, their intact performance could be attributed to brain reorganization (14).

Should this lack of memory impairment be attributed to plasticity or brain reorganization? Alternatively, could deficits still exist but are masked by other cognitive processes? Patients do have cognitive deficits that are often considered peripheral to long-term memory, including deficits in strategic search and initiation necessary for free recall (17–19), temporal organization (15,20), source monitoring (21,

22), and on-line mnemonic processing or working memory (23,24). They also show deficits in attention and in the gating of irrelevant stimuli (25), an important factor to consider in this chapter. Nonetheless, despite all these deficits, these patients often appear normal on most standardized tests of memory, including the Wechsler Memory Scale, and most tests of recognition memory (18,26).

Our studies have demonstrated that these patients can have significant impairments in memory. At the same time, construction of a test that does not take into account the interpretative nature of the left hemisphere, actually can make the patients appear normal (27).

RECOVERY OF FUNCTION: MORE APPARENT THAN REAL

We recently showed normal subjects as well as patients with unilateral focal lesions to the right prefrontal cortex and to the left prefrontal cortex pictures of stereotypical scenes, such as a beach scene. We asked the subjects to study the pictures and to remember as much as they could about them. Later, we gave them a recognition test in which we asked whether they remembered seeing a beach ball or a teacher's chair or a spaceship, and so on in one of the study pictures. We found no difference in performance between normal subjects and the left and right frontal patients. That is, right frontal patients correctly recognized pictured items at the same rate as did the normal subjects. They also falsely recognized items not pictured but consistent with the theme of the picture—such as a beach umbrella—as often as normal subjects did. In addition, they produced a low rate of false alarms to items not pictured and completely unrelated to any of the pictures shown, such as a spaceship, as did the normal subjects. Therefore, according to the results of this simple recognition test, it might be concluded that their memory for specific items is completely intact.

Memory is a particularly malleable cognitive function that is filled with distortions and illusions and is quite open to interpreta-

tion. The conscious experience of remembering a single event is known to be a hodgepodge, that is, a conglomeration, of previously experienced sights, sounds, smells, emotions, all mixed in with a person's biases, imagination, and expectations that form a single coherent image or memory. Schemas can have a strong influence on this recollection. In 1981, Brewer and Treyens conducted a study in which they brought a subject into a graduate student's office and asked him or her to wait there while they set up the experiment (28). Ten minutes later, they brought the subject to another room and asked him or her to recall everything he or she could remember from the graduate student's office. The student often reported remembering seeing books, even though there were none. Books are often a part of an individual's schema of a graduate student's office, and this schema can have a powerful influence on recollection.

Schematic influences on memory have been studied since at least Bartlett's (29) investigation of subjects' recall of a story titled "The War of the Ghosts." After repeated recollections over a period of weeks, subjects often recalled vivid details about the story that never occurred but fit their stereotypes or schemas about Indian life. Since then, many studies have been conducted on how schemata can affect recollection by filling in the missing gaps of our memory (29–31).

We recently introduced a paradigm that uses the schematic influence of stereotypical scenes to produce a lot of false recognition accompanied by high ratings of vividness (32). The benefit of this paradigm, compared with previous false-memory paradigms, is that it can be used in a variety of laboratory settings. Many cognitive neuroscientists have investigated brain processes associated with true and false memories by using these kinds of paradigms in neuroimaging studies [see Schacter et al. (33) for review].

One conceptualization of recognition memory is that recognition taps into two dual processes (34–36). One is called *remembering,* the conscious recollection of elements of an experience. The other, *familiarity,* is a more vague recollection that something occurred based on a feeling of knowing. Familiarity has been linked to gist-based representations, or the storage of the general characteristics or associations of an event; remembering has been linked to verbatim, item-specific representations or remembering the element or feature of an event (37). These processes can be manipulated independently (35,38). Further, recognition memory and some cued recall can rely on one or the other process for normal performance.

THE LEFT HEMISPHERE AND GIST-BASED MEMORY

The left hemisphere's susceptibility to false alarms can be a result of its interpretive nature and consequent overreliance on gist-based or schematic-based memory. In 1992, Phelps and Gazzaniga showed two split-brain patients a sequence of slides that told a common story-such as a person getting out of bed and preparing to go to work (39). Later, the patients were given a recognition test in which they were shown three different kinds of pictures: pictures from the sequence shown during the study session, pictures not shown in the original sequence but consistent with the story line, and pictures not shown and irrelevant to the original sequence. Their responses were lateralized so the left and right hemispheres could be tested independently. They found that the left hemisphere falsely recognized the new, yet consistent pictures much more than they did with the right hemisphere. The left hemisphere sees these pictures, comprehends their connection to the original sequence, and concludes that they must have been seen before.

To illustrate left hemisphere involvement in memory distortion further, we conducted a functional magnetic resonance imaging (MRI) study of normal subjects and, by using a common word list paradigm, we compared the retrieval of true memories with the retrieval of false memories. In several subjects, we found that while the right hemisphere is active during the retrieval of true and false

items, the left hemisphere is active only during the retrieval of false items (40).

MEASURING THE TRUE STRENGTH OF MEMORY

We have developed several paradigms that effectively demonstrate the reconstructive nature of memory and that provide many instances of true and false recognition. For example, we again showed frontal patients and normal subjects pictures with strong, stereotypical scenes, such as a beach or a classroom scene. In one set of pictures, we removed the beach ball and beach blankets and left in the beach umbrella and the lifeguard's life preserver. In another set, we did just the opposite: removed the beach umbrellas and life preserver but left in the beach ball and blankets. Each picture that a subject saw, therefore, included two exemplars but not the other two exemplars. In another example, using a classroom, we removed the teacher's chair and the chalkboard erasers in one set and the chalkboard and the apples on a teacher's desk in another. In addition, an incongruent or novel item was added to each scene. The novel items were intended to be more memorable to the subject by being inconsistent with the picture's schema, for example, a gas pump on a beach or a barbecue grill in a classroom (41).

The purest measure of how strong a memory is for a particular item type is to measure the difference between *hit rates* (recognizing an item when it is presented) and *false-alarm rates* (falsely recognizing an item that was not presented) (42,43). To measure simply how often someonne claims to remember an item can be misleading because responses often are elevated by factors other than memory, such as a bias to say yes because of the context of the event. Recognition tests, such as the one discussed earlier in this chapter, often lead to wrong conclusions about how strong a subject's or patient's memory is for a particular item type (44). For example, we may have concluded that right frontal patients have just as strong a memory for items from a scene as normal subjects. The revised paradigm included presented and nonpre-sented conditions for each item type and al-lowed us to conduct a signal detection analy-sis on the results to determine the strength of memory for each item type, independent of response bias. So how did the memory of the right frontal patients measure up to normal subjects or left frontal patients? Was their memory really normal?

When we considered the performance on the schema-consistent items only (such as the beach ball in a beach scene or a teacher's chair in a classroom), we found that the right frontal lobe patients' performance was virtu-ally identical to normal subjects' performance and to left frontal patients (27). In both cases, they did well at recognizing the old items and also had many false alarms for new items. One might conclude that the right frontal pa-tients' memory for those items is completely normal, and that conclusion would be correct.

An important point to consider regarding these data was that even the normal subjects had virtually no memory for the items. In other words, with no difference between the hit rates and false-alarm rates, even normal subjects could not distinguish whether the items were presented, even though they re-ported vivid recollections of the missing items' presence (32). Currently, we are con-ducting other studies that suggest subjects do not bother encoding the details of scenes that are consistent with what they expect to be in the scene. Many investigators have reported that, when people face a complex visual scene, they rarely notice changes to objects that occur during an eye movement (45) or from one cut scene to the next in a video clip (46). Despite our conscious experience that we are viewing a detailed scene, when detect-ing changes to an object in a scene, our atten-tion must be focused on that object. There-fore, many details of a scene may never be encoded; or, if they are encoded, they are quickly forgotten. The mind, however, has an amazing capacity to fill the gaps. Later, when we try to recollect details about that scene, we reconstruct it based on what we expect to be there (28,32). Patients with damaged right prefrontal cortexes can do that as easily as can normal subjects and left frontal patients.

What we also found, however, was that right frontal patients could not remember novel items in a scene as well as could normal subjects or patients with damage restricted to the left prefrontal cortex. So, when we con-sidered the performance on schema-inconsis-tent items only (e.g., the barbecue grill in the classroom), normal subjects could remember these incongruent items easily and with large differences between the hit rates and false-alarm rates. Right frontal patients were signif-icantly impaired in their memory for these items, with small differences. So, even when the items were conspicuous in a scene, the pa-tients had difficulty remembering them (27). We concluded that the right frontal patients [the same patients tested by Swick and Knight (14)] did have a significant impairment in recognition memory but that the deficit was covered up in earlier recognition tests by their use of the event's general context.

In essence, these patients can remember the gist of an event. Particularly, right frontal pa-tients with an intact left hemisphere, the hemisphere of the interpreter, can use this in-formation to drive their recollection of the de-tails of the event. They can appear normal in many test situations, even though their item-specific memory is significantly impaired. The question remains: What causes this item-specific memory impairment? Is it a deficit in episodic memory retrieval, or is it an atten-tional deficit, like the inability to detect novel stimuli? Further research should pinpoint the source of these deficits.

CONCLUSION

In conclusion, it appears that patients with damage to the right prefrontal cortex do have significant memory impairments. Although the specific nature of these impairments is un-known, it is likely that the same mechanism could be producing the blood flow activations during episodic retrieval tasks. The point we would like to make is that these deficits can be masked by other cognitive processes. Memory is a malleable function that is susceptible to the interpretative nature of the left hemisphere. Therefore, appropriately sensitive psychological measures must be used before assuming plasticity or recovery of function.

Damage to the neocortex can have devastating effects on people's lives. The recovery of cognitive functions through brain plasticity is an exciting and promising area of research; however, it is important to keep in mind that the mind has an amazing ability to cover many deficits of the brain, thus enabling the patient to appear normal.

ACKNOWLEDGMENTS

Aided by NIH 2 P50 NS17778-18.

REFERENCES

1. Gazzaniga MS. Organization of the human brain. *Science* 1988;245:947–952.
2. Gilovich T, Vallone R, Tversky A. The hot hand in basketball: on the misperception of random sequences. *Cognitive Psychology* 1985;17:295–314.
3. Wolford GL, Miller MB, Gazzaniga MS. The left hemisphere's role in hypothesis formation. *Journal of Neuroscience* 2000;20(RC64):1–4.
4. Metcalfe J, Funnell M, Gazzaniga MS. Right-hemisphere memory superiority: studies of a split-brain patient. *Psychological Science* 1995;6:157–164.
5. Tulving E, Kapur S, Craik FIM, et al. Hemispheric encoding/retrieval asymmetry in episodic memory: positron emission tomography findings. *Proc Natl Acad Sci USA* 1994;91:2016–2020.
6. Nyberg L, Tulving E, Habib R, et al. Functional brain maps of retrieval mode and recovery of episodic information. *Neuroreport* 1995;6:249–252.
7. Buckner RL. Beyond HERA: contributions of specific prefrontal brain areas to long-term memory retrieval. *Psychonomic Bulletin Review* 1996;3:149–158.
8. Cabeza R, Nyberg L. Imaging cognition: an empirical review of PET studies with normal subjects. *J Cognitive Neuroscience* 1997;9:1–26.
9. Andreasen NC, O'Leary DS, Arndt S, et al. Short-term and long-term verbal memory: a positron emission tomography study. *Proc Natl Acad Sci USA* 1995;92:5111–5115.
10. Buckner RL, Raichle ME, Miezin FM, et al. PET studies of the recall of pictures and words from memory. *Society for Neuroscience Abstracts* 1995;21:1441.
11. Tulving E, Markowitsch HJ, Craik FIM, et al. Novelty and familiarity activations in PET studies of memory encoding and retrieval. *Cereb Cortex* 1996;6:71–79.
12. Grady CL, Maisog JM, Horowitz B, et al. Age-related changes in cortical blood flow activations during visual processing of faces and locations. *J Neurosci* 1994;14:1450–1462.
13. Haxby JV, Ungerleider LG, Horowitz B, et al. Face encoding and recognition in the human brain. *Proc Natl Acad Sci USA* 1996;93:922–927.
14. Swick D, Knight RT. Is prefrontal cortex involved in cued recall? A neuropsychological test of PET findings. *Neuropsychologia* 1996;34:1019–1028.
15. Shimamura AP, Janowsky JS, Squire LR. Memory for the temporal order of events in patients with frontal lobe lesions and amnesic patients. *Neuropsychologia* 1990;28:803–813.
16. Milner B, Squire LR, Kandel ER. Cognitive neuroscience and the study of memory. *Neuron* 1998;20:445–468.
17. Incisa della Rocchetta A, Milner B. Strategic search and retrieval inhibition: the role of the frontal lobes. *Neuropsychologia* 1993;31:503–524.
18. Janowsky JS, Shimamura AP, Kritchevsky M, et al. Cognitive impairment following frontal lobe damage and its relevance to human amnesia. *Behav Neurosci* 1989;103:548–560.
19. Jetter W, Poser U, Freeman RB, et al. A verbal long term memory deficit in frontal lobe damaged patients. *Cortex* 1986;22:229–242.
20. McAndrews MP, Milner B. The frontal cortex and memory for temporal order. *Neuropsychologia* 1991;29:849–859.
21. Janowsky JS, Shimamura AP, Squire LR. Source memory impairment in patients with frontal lobe lesions. *Neuropsychologia* 1989;27:1043–1056.
22. Johnson M, Raye C. False memories and confabulation. *Trends in Cognitive Science* 1998;2:137–145.
23. Goldman-Rakic PS. Cortical localization of working memory. In: McGaugh JL, Weinberger NM, Lynch G, eds. *Brain organization and memory: cells, systems, and circuits.* New York: Oxford University Press, 1990:285–298.
24. Petrides M. Lateral frontal cortical contribution to memory. *Seminars in the Neurosciences* 1996;8:57–63.
25. Knight RT. Evoked potential studies of attention capacity in human frontal lobe lesions. In: Levin HS, Eisenberg HM, Benton AL, eds. *Frontal lobe function and dysfunction.* New York: Oxford University Press, 1991:139–153.
26. Shimamura AP. Memory and frontal lobe function. In: Gazzaniga MS, et al., eds. *The cognitive neurosciences.* Cambridge, MA: MIT Press, 1995:803–813.
27. Miller MB, Wolford GL, Shimamura A, et al. Memory distortions and the frontal lobes. (Submitted.)
28. Brewer WF, Treyens JC. Role of schemata in memory for places. *Cognitive Psychology* 1981;13:207–230.
29. Bartlett F. *Remembering: a study in experimental and social psychology.* Cambridge: Cambridge University Press, 1932:63–94.
30. Bower GH, Black JB, Turner TJ. Scripts in memory for text. *Cognitive Psychology* 1979;11:177–220.
31. Alba JW, Hasher L. Is memory schematic? *Psychol Bull* 1983;93:203–231.
32. Miller MB, Gazzaniga MS. Creating false memories for visual scenes. *Neuropsychologia* 1998;36:513–520.
33. Schacter DL, Norman KA, Koutstaal W. The cognitive neuroscience of constructive memory. *Annu Rev Psychol* 1998;49:289–318.
34. Mandler G. Recognizing: the judgment of previous occurrence. *Psychol Rev* 1980;87:252–271.
35. Tulving E. Memory and consciousness. *Canadian Psychologist* 1985;26:1–12.
36. Gardiner JM, Java RI. Recognizing and remembering.

In: Collins A, Gathercole S, Morris P, eds. *Theories of memory.* Hillsdale, NJ: Erlbaum, 1993:189–206.

37. Brainerd CJ, Reyna VF. When things that were never experienced are easier to "remember" than things that were. *Psychological Science* 1998;9:484–489.

38. Gardiner J, Ramponi C, Richardson-Klavehn A. Experiences of remembering, knowing, and guessing. *Conscious Cogn* 1998;7:1–26.

39. Phelps EA, Gazzaniga MS. Hemispheric differences in mnemonic processing: the effects of left hemisphere interpretation. *Neuropsychologia* 1992;30:293–297.

40. Miller MB, Buonocore M, Wessinger CM, et al. Remembering false events rather than true events produces dynamic changes in underlying neural circuitry: a fMRI study. Abstract for the Society for Neuroscience 26th Annual Meeting, Washington, D.C., 1996.

41. Miller MB, Wolford GL, Gazzaniga MS. Schematic reconstructions: the thin line between true and false memories. (Submitted.)

42. Green DM, Swets JA. *Signal detection theory and psychophysics.* New York: John Wiley & Sons, 1966. Reprinted 1974 by Krieger, Huntington, NY.

43. Macmillan NA, Creelman CD. *Detection theory: a user's guide.* Cambridge: Cambridge University Press, 1991.

44. Miller MB, Wolford GL. The role of criterion shift in false memory. *Psychol Rev* 1999;106(2):398–405.

45. Rensink RA, O'Regan JK, Clark JJ. To see or not to see: the need for attention to perceive changes in scenes. *Psychological Science* 1997;8:368–373.

46. Simons DJ, Levin DT. Change blindness. *Trends in Cognitive Sciences* 1997;1:261–267.

Neocortical Epilepsies.
Advances in Neurology, Vol. 84,
edited by P. D. Williamson, A. M. Siegel,
D. W. Roberts, V. M. Thadani, and M. S. Gazzaniga.
Lippincott Williams & Wilkins, Philadelphia © 2000.

3

Functional and Structural Mapping of Human Cerebral Cortex: Solutions Are in the Surfaces

David C. Van Essen, Heather A. Drury, *Sarang Joshi, and *Michael I. Miller

*Department of Anatomy and Neurobiology, Washington University School of Medicine,
St. Louis, Missouri 63110; *Center for Imaging Science, Johns Hopkins University,
Baltimore, Maryland 21218*

The mammalian cerebral cortex contains numerous anatomically and functionally distinct areas arrayed in a complex mosaic across the cortical sheet. Efforts by cortical cartographers to determine the number, arrangement, and internal organization of these areas represent a major thrust in systems neuroscience over the entire twentieth century. Nonetheless, a precise and definitive charting of the entire neocortex has yet to be attained for any species. In the human neocortex, classic neuroanatomists identified ≈50 architectonic subdivisions (1). The actual number may be 100 or more areas, however, given the plethora of cortical areas recently discovered in nonhuman primates (2–6) coupled with the disproportionate expansion in cortical surface area in humans compared with nonhuman primates.

The prospects for accurately mapping the arrangement of functionally specialized areas in the human cerebral cortex have been enhanced greatly by recent advances in noninvasive neuroimaging techniques. Positron emission tomography allows localization of activation foci with an accuracy on the order of 1 cm, and functional magnetic resonance imaging (MRI) has even better spatial resolution, comparable to the 3-mm thickness of the cortical sheet. By combining functional MRI with structural MRI, it is possible to map activation patterns precisely in relation to the specific pattern of cortical folds in the same person.

The ability to chart function at near-millimeter resolution on a cortical sheet whose surface area is ≈80,000 mm^2/hemisphere poses major technical problems in the arenas of data analysis and visualization. The basic challenge is how best to visualize large amounts of complex experimental data with minimal loss of important information about spatial and topologic relationships. The problem is compounded by individual variability in cortical structure and function. This variability includes pronounced differences in the pattern of folding, in the size and shape of cortical areas, and in their location relative to these folds. Together, these factors introduce a degree of spatial uncertainty well in excess of the resolution available with current neuroimaging techniques.

To help meet this challenge, new visualization and analysis methods have been developed that emphasize surface representations and surface-based coordinates. Here we discuss three sets of recently developed tools that collectively offer major advantages over conventional methods that emphasize volume representations and stereotaxic coordinates. The first is surface-based visualization, which includes methods for reconstructing surfaces and changing the shape of the surface to facilitate the analysis of important geometric and topologic relationships. The second involves surface-based atlases in which reconstructions of particular hemispheres are used as standard substrates for analyzing data obtained from many subjects. The third involves surface-based warping, which uses surface representations to constrain the deformation from a source to a target hemisphere, thereby preserving critical topologic relationships when mapping data from individual subjects onto an atlas.

SURFACE-BASED VISUALIZATION OF CEREBRAL CORTEX

In the most common type of surface reconstruction, the cortex is represented by a wireframe meshwork running within the cortical sheet (or along its inner or outer margins). Figure 3.1A shows a reconstruction of a surface running midway through the cortical thickness of the right hemisphere of the Visible Man (7). The surface was generated from a digitized se-

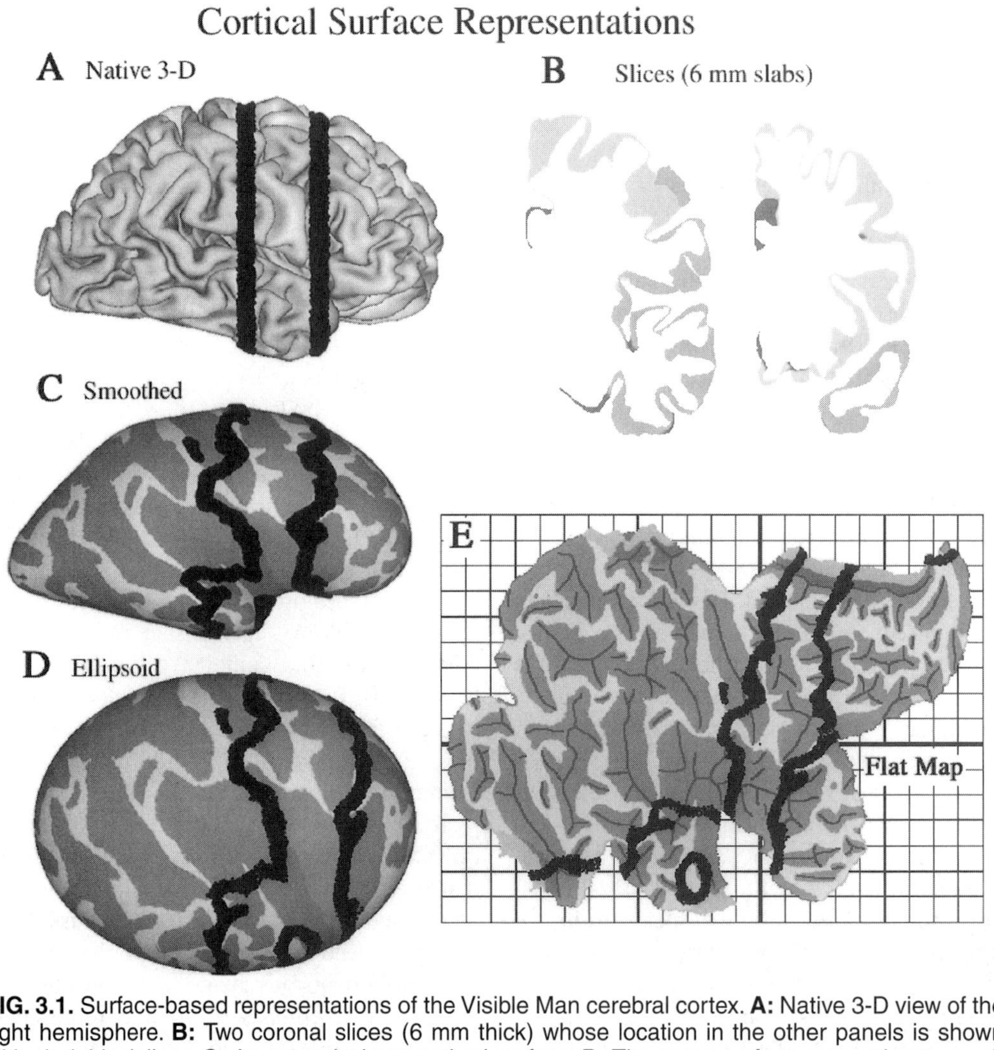

Cortical Surface Representations

FIG. 3.1. Surface-based representations of the Visible Man cerebral cortex. **A:** Native 3-D view of the right hemisphere. **B:** Two coronal slices (6 mm thick) whose location in the other panels is shown with *dark black lines.* **C:** An extensively smoothed surface. **D:** The same surface mapped onto an ellipsoid. **E:** A cortical flat map, with selected cuts to reduce distortions. The gridwork surrounding the map defines a surface-based coordinate system, with a grid spacing of 1 map-cm, equivalent to 1 cm along the cortical surface in regions that are not distorted.

ries of images through an entire brain (8) and has been rendered to show the frontal lobe in beige, the parietal lobe in green, the temporal lobe in blue, and the occipital lobe in pink. This native three-dimensional (3-D) display format, although providing a familiar view, has several inherent drawbacks. First, sulcal regions are largely occluded from view. Second, dimensions along the image are distorted by foreshortening wherever the surface is oblique to the viewing angle. Third, the stereotaxic coordinate system in which the cortex is embedded does not respect the topology of the cortical surface; points that are close together in 3-D space may be widely separated along the cortical surface.

Surfaces can be modified in several ways to address these problems. The major options include smoothing the surface, cutting it at suitable locations, and mapping it to a geometrically well-defined shape. Various combinations of these steps lead to four alternative display formats, shown in Fig. 3.1: (a) slices cut through the hemisphere (shown at two coronal levels in Fig. 3.1B); (b) an extensively smoothed surface, which makes buried regions visible (Fig. 3.1C); (c) a geometrically well-defined ellipsoidal representation (Fig. 3.1D); and (d) a cortical flat map (Fig. 3.1E). Darker shading represents cortex that is buried within sulci in the native 3-D configuration, thereby preserving an explicit representation of cortical geography. For each display format, Table 3.1

summarizes the tradeoffs between the improvements related to one set of characteristics (visibility, compactness, foreshortening, and parameterization) versus drawbacks that are introduced, including distortions of surface geometry, topological changes (cuts) in the surface, and shape changes that obscure relationships to the native 3-D configuration.

Slicing a surface into sections, such as the coronal slabs shown in Fig. 3.1B, reveals buried regions without changing the shape of the surface contours. This format has the advantage of familiarity, insofar as the contours have shapes similar to those shown in standard stereotaxic atlases. Moreover, with computerized reconstructions, it is feasible to slice a given surface in different sectioning planes (e.g., coronal or horizontal). On the other hand, slicing the surface makes it difficult to discern important topologic relationships within and between sections. This problem is exacerbated when sections are displayed only at sparse intervals, as is generally necessary because slices are not a compact display format.

Buried cortex is brought into full view in three formats that preserve surface continuity: extensively smoothed surfaces, ellipsoidal maps, and flat maps. Extensively smoothed surfaces (9) and ellipsoidal maps preserve all topologic relationships across the cortical surface, but they necessarily involve foreshortening around the perimeter, and they require

TABLE 3.1. Surface-based display formats for cerebral cortex[a]

	Native 3-D	Slices	Smoothed	Ellipsoid	Flat map
Visibility	Poor	Interval dependent	Good	Good	Excellent
Surface topology	Good	Many cuts	Good	Good	Some cuts
Compactness	Moderate	Poor	Moderate	Moderate	Excellent
Distortions	Low	Low	Moderate	Moderate	Moderate
Foreshortening	Poor	Axis dependent	Poor	Poor	Good
Parameterization	Stereotaxic (3-D)	Stereotaxic (3-D)	None	Surface-based (2-D ellipsoidal)	Surface-based (2-D Cartesian)
Ease of localization	—	Mixed	Good	Moderate	Mixed

3-D, three dimensional; 2-D, two-dimensional.

[a]Each surface display format is evaluated with respect to visibility (occlusion of buried cortex), topology (cuts in surface), compactness (number of views needed), distortion (fidelity of representing area on the modified surface), foreshortening (additional perspective distortions), parameterization (coordinate systems available), and localization (relative to the native 3-D configuration).

multiple views to see the entire hemisphere. Flat maps are the most compact representation because the entire hemisphere can be seen in a single view, and they have no foreshortening because the surface is planar; however, flat maps do entail the introduction of selected cuts to prevent severe distortions in surface area. Indeed, all the formats involving shape changes have modest distortions in surface area and in linear dimensions, which are inevitable because the cortex is not simply folded like a sheet of newspaper. Instead, it contains numerous "hot spots" of high intrinsic curvature (bumps and dents) analogous to the indentations on a golf ball (7). In general, such distortions are not a major drawback because accurate measurements of surface area can be made on the native 3-D surface even when the region of interest has been selected on a different format. Likewise, measurements of distance are best made by calculating geodesics along the native 3-D surface (10).

Mapping the cortex to a geometrically well-defined surface (ellipsoidal or planar) allows locations on the surface to be represented by a two-dimensional (2-D) coordinate system that respects the topology of the cortical surface. Just as latitude and longitude are more useful than volumetric (x, y, z) coordinates for describing locations on the earth's surface, surface-based coordinates have inherent advantages when describing locations in the cerebral cortex. Either polar or Cartesian coordinates can be used, but polar coordinates are a more natural parameterization for an ellipsoidal surface, and Cartesian coordinates are more natural for flat maps.

Shape changes and cuts tend to obscure the relationship between locations on a deformed surface and the corresponding locations in the native 3-D configuration. The extensively smoothed surface, which has no cuts and is shaped like a lissencephalic primate brain, is the least problematic in this regard. Other formats require more effort to recognize relationships with the native 3-D configuration, but the process is aided by software options for rapidly switching from one format to another while highlighting a particular point or domain of in-

terest. This is illustrated in Fig. 3.1 by showing the trajectories of the same two coronal slices (blue contours) on each of the display formats.

SURFACE-BASED ATLAS

When comparing experimental data obtained from different subjects, a standard approach is to display the results on a common anatomic substrate: an atlas. Some cerebral atlases in current use are based on histologic sections or MRI scans through a particular brain that is placed in a standard stereotaxic space, such as the Talairach stereotaxic space (11–13). Other atlases are based on MRIs averaged across many individual brains after initial transformation into stereotaxic space (14,15). This allows probabilistic descriptions regarding the location of different structures, but it is associated with considerable blurring of gyral and sulcal features because of residual variability in the position of any given sulcus.

Given the advantages of surface representations, it is important to have a cerebral atlas that includes an explicit surface reconstruction. To address this need, we used reconstructions of the left and right hemispheres of the Visible Man to establish a surface-based human cortical atlas (7,16). The Visible Man is a reasonable choice for such an atlas because its overall dimensions are similar to those of the Talairach atlas and because the pattern of convolutions for both hemispheres lies within the normal range of a population of normal brains (7,17). The atlas includes a complete map of major gyri and sulci in each hemisphere and is linked to multiple coordinate systems, including the Talairach stereotaxic space and Cartesian surface-based coordinate systems (Fig. 3.1).

Many types of experimental data can be visualized conveniently on the Visible Man atlas. Figure. 3.2 illustrates this by using published results on the functional organization of human visual cortex. The layout of topographically organized visual areas, including primary visual cortex (area V1) and surrounding extrastriate areas (V2, V3, VP, V3A, and V4v), is shown on a flat map of the occipi-

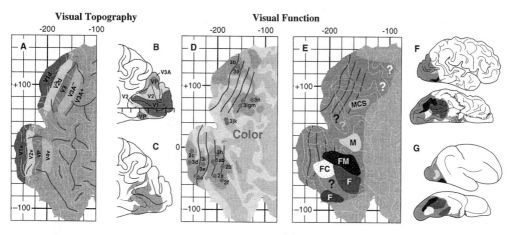

FIG. 3.2. Functional specialization in human visual cortex. **A:** Topographically organized visual areas shown on a flat map of occipitotemporal cortex in the Visible Man. **B:** The same areas on a medial view of the occipital lobe. **C:** The same regions on a lateral view of the hemisphere. **D:** Cortical regions implicated in processing of color. *Darker dots* denote centers of activation foci, and *lighter shading* denotes cortex with the 10-mm uncertainty limit. **E:** Cortical regions implicated in the processing of motion *(M);* form *(F);* form and color *(FC);* form and motion *(FM);* and motion, color, and spatial relations *(MCS).* Question marks denote additional regions potentially involved in processing of color *(dark),* motion *(medium),* and spatial relations *(light).* **F:** The same functional specializations shown on lateral and ventral 3-D views. **G:** The same pattern on extensively smoothed surfaces. (Adapted from Van Essen DC, Drury HA. Structural and functional analyses of human cerebral cortex using a surface-based atlas. *J Neurosci* 1997;17:7079–7102, with permission.)

totemporal cortex (Fig. 3.2A) and on a medial view of the occipital lobe (Fig. 3.2B). The most likely extent of area V1 in the Visible Man was estimated from a postmortem analysis of the architectonic borders of V1 (7,18). The boundaries of the extrastriate areas were estimated from their average widths determined in functional MRI studies and displayed on cortical flat maps (19,20). Although not indicated in Fig. 3.2, there are significant uncertainties (about ±1 cm) associated with the boundaries of each of these topographically organized areas, mainly because of individual variability in their size and location relative to geographic landmarks.

Complementing these maps of topographically organized areas are studies of regions activated by different aspects of visual processing. Figure 3.2C and D show regions implicated in color processing, and Fig. 3.2E through G summarize the specializations relating to color, motion, form, and spatial relationships. These results are based on positron emission tomography and functional MRI studies that did not include explicit surface reconstructions of the individual subjects from whom the data were acquired. Instead, the data were transformed into Talairach space by using conventional low-dimensional warping algorithms (involving only affine transformations), followed by averaging across multiple subjects and reporting the Talairach stereotaxic coordinates for the center of each activation focus. By using these coordinates, each activation focus can be mapped to the nearest point on the Visible Man surface (which itself has been transformed to Talairach space). For example, the distribution of activation foci implicated in color processing are plotted on a cortical flat map (Fig. 3.2C) and on a medial view of the hemisphere (Fig. 3.2D). Each green dot on the flat map shows the nearest point on the Visible Man surface to an activation focus reported by Lueck et al. (21) (foci 1a–c), Zeki et al. (22) (foci 2a–c), or Corbetta et al. (23) (foci 3a–n). It is deceptive, however, to view only the nearest point on the Visible Man surface because of individual variability that is not compensated by transforming each hemisphere into stereotaxic space.

When a given paradigm is repeated in many subjects, the centers of activation foci are scattered over a considerable range of stereotaxic space, but they lie primarily within 10 mm of the group mean (7,24,25). This scatter is attributable to biologic variability in the stereotaxic location of activation foci, although resolution limits of the neuroimaging techniques presumably contribute to some degree. The light green shading in Fig. 3.2C and D represents this spatial uncertainty by showing portions of the Visible Man surface that lie within 10 mm of one or another of the reported color activation foci. This represents geographic regions within which these foci probably would have been centered had the experiments been done on the Visible Man.

We extended this type of analysis to 118 activation foci from 12 studies reporting activation foci associated with processing of color, form, motion, and spatial relationships (7). In an intermediate stage of analysis (not illustrated here), all individual foci were superimposed on a single flat map. Figure 3.2E and F show summary representations generated from this superposition map, indicating which cortical regions are dominated by a single aspect of visual function and which involve overlap or close interdigitation of multiple functions. For example, the region of the lateral occipitotemporal cortex shaded red is associated largely or exclusively with motion processing (M), whereas the regions of the ventral occipitotemporal cortex shaded blue are associated largely or exclusively with form processing (F). Other regions involve overlap or close interdigitation of foci implicated in more than one function, including form and color analysis (FC, shaded blue–green) in or near areas VP and V4v; form and motion analysis (FM, shaded purple) in a ventrolateral portion of the occipitotemporal cortex; and motion, color, and spatial analysis (MCS, shaded orange) in or near area V3A in the dorsal extrastriate cortex. Although omitted in Fig. 3.2, this analysis also revealed numerous activation foci in areas V1 and V2, reflecting the involvement of both areas in multiple aspects of visual processing.

This example demonstrates the utility of a surface-based atlas as a substrate for objective analysis and compact visualization of large amounts of neuroimaging data; however, it also illustrates the limitations associated with the stereotaxic projection method and highlights the need for new methods to reduce spatial uncertainties when mapping data onto the atlas.

SURFACE-BASED WARPING

Here we introduce an approach that uses explicit surface representations to bring one hemisphere into better register with another. It is designed to achieve three general objectives, each motivated by key facts or plausible assumptions regarding cortical structure and function.

Surface Topology

A necessary (but by no means sufficient) condition for attaining optimal registration is to preserve surface topology in the mapping from one hemisphere (the *source*) to another (the *target*). This requires that neighboring points in the cortex of the source hemisphere always map to neighboring points in the cortex of the target hemisphere (and not, for example, to opposite banks of a sulcus or to locations lying outside the cortical gray matter). This constraint arises because the surface of the cortex (or of any layer within the cortex) is topologically equivalent to a simple disk and because the topologic arrangement of cortical areas (areal topology) across the cortical surface is thought to be identical, or at least similar, from one individual to the next.

Point-to-Neighborhood Correspondences

The deformation process aims to improve registration between locations that correspond in function, that is, that represent the same cortical area and an equivalent location within that area in the source and target hemispheres. There are inherent biological limits, however, as well as practical limits in identifying functionally corresponding locations in different hemispheres. The biologic limits arise because of individual variability in the size, shape, position, and internal organization of each cortical area. Individual cortical areas can vary in size by at least a factor of 2 (26,27), and many areas are characterized by internal compartments, or modules, whose total number and dimensions vary across individuals (28,29). Accordingly, it is unrealistic to expect functional correspondences to be identified more precisely than within a few millimeters for human cortex. Often the uncertainty is in the centimeter range because of resolution limits and sparseness in the available functional and structural data. It therefore makes sense to express functional correspondences in terms of "point-to-neighborhood" relationships, in which a given point in one hemisphere is associated not only with the most likely corresponding point in another hemisphere but also with a neighborhood whose extent reflects the degree of spatial uncertainty in this mapping. The deformation algorithm should force registration of corresponding landmarks only to a degree commensurate with this neighborhood size along the cortical surface.

Geographic landmarks provide valuable, albeit indirect, indicators of functional correspondences because the location of many cortical areas is correlated with the pattern of cortical folds. The tightness of this correlation differs from one region to another and tends to be stronger, for example, in the vicinity of primary sensory and motor areas than in most other regions (12,18,24). Also, the correlation is generally weaker in the highly convoluted human cortex than in less convoluted species such as the macaque monkey. Both the consistency and the variability of this relationship have a natural explanation in terms of a tension-based mechanism that may drive cortical folding during development (30).

Minimize Local Distortions

The functional and geographic landmarks available to guide the registration of any particular pair of hemispheres typically are distributed nonuniformly and often sparsely across the cortical surface. To achieve satisfactory registration of these landmarks, significant compression, expansion, or shearing of cortex in the intervening regions may be necessary. It is desirable, however, that such deformations be as smooth and regular as possible because it makes sense to assume similarity in the relative sizes and positions of cortical areas except where there is direct evidence to the contrary.

Surface-based warping offers an attractive general strategy for meeting all three of these objectives. Our approach involves a landmark-based deformation algorithm in which the surface is modeled as a viscoelastic fluid sheet (31,32). This approach is analogous to a 3-D viscoelastic model that has been used for high-dimensional volume deformations (32–35), but it is computationally much less demanding because of its lower dimensionality. The warping is driven by selected landmarks that are identifiable on both source and target maps and in this respect is analogous to the landmark-based approach of Bookstein (36). As landmarks, we use contours that are drawn explicitly along corresponding locations on the source and target maps, based on geographic or functional criteria. The warping algorithm deforms the source map so as to bring the landmarks more closely into register, but its viscoelastic characteristics tend to smooth out local distortions on the map, thereby allowing tradeoffs between these competing objectives.

Some issues that arise in judiciously selecting landmarks and in interpreting the results are illustrated in Fig. 3.3. The top panels (Fig. 3.3A,B) show cortical flat maps of the left and right hemispheres of the Visible Man, with the left hemisphere map mirror-flipped to facilitate comparison of their shapes. Our objective in this example was to warp the left hemisphere map to match the right hemisphere map by using only geographic landmarks to constrain the deformation.

To ensure a complete point-to-point mapping between hemispheres, the warping algorithm requires landmarks along the perimeter of each map, including not only the natural terminations of cortex but also the artificial

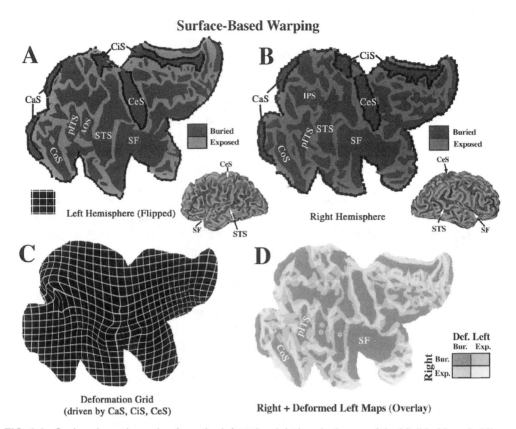

FIG. 3.3. Surface-based warping from the left to the right hemispheres of the Visible Man. **A:** Mirror-flipped flat map of the left hemisphere, with selected sulci labeled, and geographic landmarks used to constrain the deformation shown in black. **B:** Equivalently labeled flat map of the right hemisphere. **C:** Deformation field associated with a warping of the left hemisphere map to match the right hemisphere map. **D:** Overlay of right and deformed left hemisphere maps, color-coded as shown in inset to indicate buried *(Bur)* cortex or exposed *(Exp)* cortex in each hemisphere.

cuts that were made in geographically corresponding locations in the two hemispheres. As internal geographic landmarks, we used the central sulcus and calcarine sulcus, which are similar in shape and location on the two maps, and also the cingulate sulcus, whose local irregularities differ in the two hemispheres and was therefore assigned a weighting factor that tolerates less precise registration achieved by the deformation. The deformation grid in Fig. 3.3C shows the shape changes needed to make the left hemisphere map conform to the shape of the right hemisphere map. Because the warping algorithm ensures a diffeomorphic mapping, no topologic irregularities *(tangles)* are found in this

deformation field. This satisfies the objective of preserving surface topology, except for the discontinuities tolerated along the cuts. Relative to the original grid size (Fig. 3.3, inset), the deformations involve only modest compression or expansion and relatively little shear except in a few locations.

In Fig. 3.3D, the right hemisphere and deformed left hemisphere maps are directly superimposed and are color-coded to reveal the degree of geographic registration achieved by deformation. Brown denotes cortex that is buried (Bur) in both the right and deformed left hemisphere maps; yellow denotes exposed (externally visible) cortex (Exp) in both maps; and orange and light green denote regions in which exposed cortex on one map overlies buried cortex in the other and thus are not in geographic register. If buried cortex were completely in register between the source and target, the overlay would include only brown and yellow shading. This is impossible to achieve, however, because the two hemispheres differ considerably in the topologic pattern of buried versus exposed cortex, that is, their geographic topology.

As expected, the warping did achieve nearly complete overlap of buried cortex for the central sulcus and calcarine sulcus, whose perimeters were forced to be in tight register, and less overlap along the margins of the cingulate sulcus, where greater misalignment was tolerated. In regions distant from these landmarks, several patterns are evident. The easiest to interpret are regions such as the collateral sulcus, where there is good registration between sulci that are in obvious geographic correspondence. In contrast, in the vicinity of the posterior inferior temporal sulcus, a region known for the variability of its folds (17,24), the geographic correspondence is much weaker (mainly green and orange instead of brown and yellow in the overlay). Nonetheless, the deformation grid is notably regular in this region, which is desirable if the arrangement of cortical areas is similar on the left and right hemisphere maps despite the marked differences in folding.

Surface-based warping also can reveal unexpected geographic relationships that may be functionally significant, as exemplified by the region in and around the superior temporal sulcus (STS). The single asterisk in Fig. 3.3D indicates where the deformed left STS is aligned with the posterior sylvian fissure in the right hemisphere; the double asterisk indicates where the right STS is aligned with the deformed left anterior occipital sulcus, a sulcus that is altogether absent in the Visible Man right hemisphere. If the left and right STS are occupied by functionally corresponding areas not only in general but in the particular brain of the Visible Man, the geographic misregistration in Fig. 3.3D would signify an inadequacy of the landmarks used to constrain this particular deformation. An alternative inter-

pretation is that there are major left–right differences in the arrangement of cortical areas relative to geographic landmarks in the temporal lobe of the Visible Man related either to a consistent hemispheric asymmetry or to chance differences in how the cortex was folded in these two hemispheres. To distinguish between such possibilities would require neuroimaging or other functional data that obviously no longer can be obtained for the Visible Man, but this limitation will not apply to future studies that involve cortical reconstructions made from in vivo structural MRI scans.

More generally, surface-based warping should become an important tool in analyzing consistency as well as variability of cortical function and its relation to cortical geography. As progressively more areas and regions of functional specialization become routinely identifiable, they can be added to the repertoire of landmarks that help to constrain surface-based deformations while exploring the functional organization of less well-charted regions. Because reconstructing and flattening an entire hemisphere is a major endeavor with current technology, it is worth noting that surface-based warping can be profitably applied at a regional level by warping a map, say, of just the parietal lobe to match the corresponding region of an atlas.

INTERSPECIES COMPARISONS

Surface-based representations have obvious utility when comparing functional organization across species (19). Figure 3.4 illustrates one such example by using maps of functional organization in the macaque monkey (Fig. 3.4A) and the Visible Man (Fig. 3.4B). The macaque map shows the layout of 79 cortical areas identified in the summary partitioning scheme of Felleman and Van Essen (2). Selected visual areas (V1, V2, and V4) are assigned individual colors, as are the inferotemporal complex (IT) and a complex of motion-related areas (M), which includes areas MT, MSTd, and MSTl. These, plus the other areas implicated in vision (light blue), together occupy slightly more than half of the macaque neocortex, whereas only

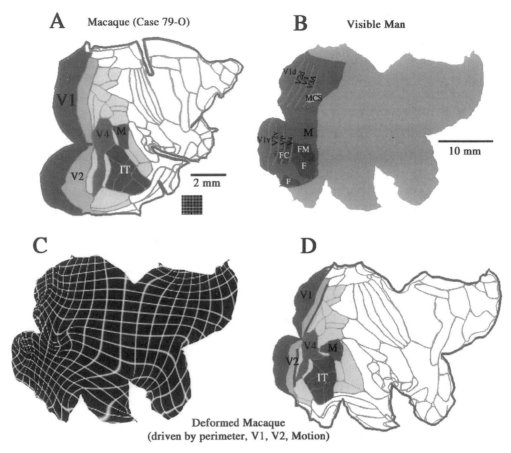

FIG. 3.4. Surface-based warping from macaque to human cortex. **A:** Flat map of cortical areas in the macaque, with visual areas indicated in various colors. **B:** Flat map of the Visible Man, with areas and functional specializations for vision indicated. **C:** Deformation grid that warps the macaque map to the shape of the human, constrained by the perimeter and selected functional regions. **D:** Deformed macaque cortical areas for comparison with the functional specializations of human visual cortex in (B).

20% to 25% of the human neocortex is known to be visual in function (dark gray in Fig. 3.4B). This twofold difference in relative extent of visual cortex impedes the evaluation of possible homologies, and the problem is exacerbated by the limited utility of geographic landmarks for interspecies comparisons. Although some areas have roughly the same location (e.g., much of V1 lies in the calcarine sulcus), other candidate homologies differ considerably in location (e.g., the motion-related complex, which lies within the STS in the macaque but well posterior to it in humans).

Surface-based warping is well suited for interspecies comparisons because it can preserve surface topology while tolerating highly nonuniform expansion or compression and also allowing functionally irrelevant differences in folding patterns to be ignored. For example, Fig. 3.4C,D shows a warping from macaque to human cortex, in which the deformation was driven by a combination of geographic landmarks along the perimeter plus several functionally based landmarks (areas V1, V2, and the motion-related complex). Because the normal cuts along the perimeter of the macaque map are fewer and shallower than those in the Visible Man, we added "virtual cuts" extending into the interior of the macaque map to attain better geographical correspondence.

The deformed macaque map is shown with the associated deformation grid in Fig. 3.4C and with cortical areas in Fig. 3.4D. As expected from the tenfold overall disparity in surface area, all regions of the deformed macaque become expanded (note the initial grid spacing in Fig. 3.4A, inset), but the expansion is relatively modest (≈twofold) for areas V1 and V2, intermediate (≈fivefold) for visual cortex as a whole, and much larger in the temporal and frontal lobes (more than 30-fold in some regions). Consequently, the deformation squeezes macaque V1 and V2 each into only a few percent of total cortex, compared with the ≈10% a piece they occupy in the native configuration. The motion complex is relatively more posterior in human cortex (to the left on the map) compared with its position in the macaque. The deformation brings the macaque inferotemporal complex into register with the larger of the human regions specialized for form analysis (including faces and inanimate forms), thus strengthening the argument for homology between these regions. Likewise, the ventral half of deformed macaque V4 is in register with human ventral V4, consistent with the homology presumed by this terminology. In contrast, dorsal V4 in the deformed macaque map lies over a region of human cortex whose function and topographic organization remains to be elucidated. In this and other regions, it is possible that human cortex contains areas that are altogether absent in the macaque (and in their common ancestor), perhaps reflecting a process analogous to gene duplication at the molecular level (37). Specific hypotheses along such lines can be explored by using surface-based warping after introducing appropriate internal cuts *(slits)* that allow nonexistent cortex in one species to expand into one or more areas in another species.

IMPLEMENTATION ISSUES

The various software packages needed for carrying out the different approaches illustrated here are in different stages of maturity and availability. Surface reconstruction and visualization software (CARET) is now available for Silicon Graphics workstations (http://v1.wustl.edu/caret.html). Digital copies of the Visible Man atlas are available for viewing and analyzing any data of interest, and the atlas is also accessible via an interactive Web site (http://v1.wustl.edu/CARETdaemon).

A major impediment to surface-based analyses has been the difficulty in automatically generating accurate surface reconstructions, particularly from high-resolution volume representations available using structural MRI. Software for key aspects of this process has become available recently (http://white.stanford.edu/html/teo/mri/mri.html), and additional software is under development in several laboratories. Progress also has been made in making robust flattening algorithms available (http://white.stanford.edu/~brian/mri/mrUnfold.html; http://v1.wustl.edu/software.html).

These methods all can be expected to undergo continued refinement that will include qualitative enhancements as well as improvements in speed and robustness. For example, our current surface-based warping algorithm operates only on cortical flat maps. A future objective is to warp ellipsoidal maps rather than flat maps, which will circumvent the limitations imposed by the artificial cuts present on flat maps. Once the warping is done on ellipsoids, it will still be easy to view the results on flat maps that include standard cuts.

The approaches discussed here represent important components of the emerging field of computational neuroanatomy (38,39). These and related developments will help usher in a new era of high-resolution brain mapping, which in turn will greatly improve our understanding of the organization and function of the cerebral cortex in a variety of species, most notably in humans.

ACKNOWLEDGMENTS

We thank Dr. C.H. Anderson for valuable suggestions. This project was supported by National Institutes of Health Grant EY02091 (D.C.V.E), National Science Foundation Grant BIR9424264 (M.I.M.), and joint funding from the National Institute of Mental Health, National Aeronautics and Space Administration, and National Institute on Drug Abuse under the Human Brain Project MHIDA52158. This article is reprinted, with permission from the authors, from the Proc Natl Acad Sci 1998;95: 788–795.

REFERENCES

1. Brodmann K. *Vergleichende Lokalisationslehre der Grosshirnrinde*. Leipzig: Barth, 1909:1–324.
2. Felleman DJ, Van Essen D. Distributed hierarchical processing in the primate cerebral cortex. *Cereb Cortex* 1991;1:1–47.
3. Preuss TM, Goldman-Rakic PS. Myelo- and cytoarchitecture of the granular frontal cortex and surrounding regions in the strepsirhine primate *Galago* and the anthropoid primate *Macaca*. *J Comp Neurol* 1991;310: 429–474.
4. Preuss TM, Goldman-Rakic PS. Ipsilateral cortical connections of granular frontal cortex in the strepsirhine primate Galago, with comparative comments on anthropoid primates. *J Comp Neurol* 1991;310:475–506.
5. Carmichael ST, Price JL. Architectonic subdivision of the orbital and medial prefrontal cortex in the macaque monkey. *J Comp Neurol* 1994;346:366–402.
6. Lewis JL. The intraparietal sulcus of the macaque and connected cortical regions: anatomical parcellation and connections throughout the hemisphere. Ph.D. thesis (California Institute of Technology, Pasadena, CA), 1997.
7. Van Essen DC, Drury HA. Structural and functional analyses of human cerebral cortex using a surface-based atlas. *J Neurosci* 1997;17:7079–7102.
8. Spitzer V, Ackerman MJ, Scherzinger AL, et al. The visible human male: a technical report. *J Am Med Inform Assoc* 1996;3:118–130.
9. Dale A, Sereno M. Improved localization of cortical activity by combining EEG and MEG with MRI cortical surface reconstruction: a linear approach. *J Cognitive Neuroscience* 1993;5:162–176.
10. Schwartz EL, Shaw A, Wolfson E. *IEEE Trans Patterns Anal Mach Intell* 1989;11:1005–1008.
11. Talairach J, Tournoux P. *Coplanar stereotaxic atlas of the human brain*. New York: Thieme Medical, 1988.
12. Roland PE, Zilles K. Brain atlases—a new research tool. *Trends Neurosci* 1994;17:458–467.
13. Toga AW, Ambach KL, Quinn B, et al. Postmortem anatomy from cryosectioned whole human brain. *J Neurosci Methods* 1994;54:239–252.
14. Andreasen NC, Arndt S, Swayze V II, et al. Thalamic abnormalities in schizophrenia visualized through magnetic resonance image averaging. *Science* 1994;226:294–298.
15. Evans AC, Kamber M, Collins DL, et al. In: Shorvon SD, Fish DR, Andermann F, Bydder GM, eds. *Magnetic resonance scanning and epilepsy*. New York: Plenum Press, 1994:263–274.
16. Drury HA, Van Essen DC. Functional specializations in human cerebral cortex analyzed during the visible man surface-based atlas. *Human Brain Mapping* 1997;5: 233–237.
17. Ono M, Kubick S, Abernathey CD. *Atlas of the cerebral sulci*. New York: Thieme Medical, 1990.
18. Rademacher J, Caviness VS Jr, Steinmetz H, et al. Topographical variation of the human primary cortices: implications for neuroimaging, brain mapping, and neurobiology. *Cereb Cortex* 1993;3:313–329.
19. Sereno MI, Dale AM, Reppas JB, et al. Borders of multiple visual areas in humans revealed by functional magnetic resonance imaging. *Science* 1995;268:889–893.
20. DeYoe EA, Carman G, Bandetinni P, et al. Mapping striate and extrastriate visual areas in human cerebral cortex. *Proc Natl Acad Sci USA* 1996;93:2382–2386.
21. Lueck CJ, Zeki S, Friston KJ, et al. The colour centre in the cerebral cortex of man. *Nature* 1989;340:386–389.
22. Zeki S, Watson JDG, Lueck CJ, et al. A direct demonstration of functional specialization in human visual cortex. *J Neurosci* 1991;11:641–649.
23. Corbetta M, Miezin F, Dobmeyer S, et al. Selective attention modulates extrastriate visual regions in humans during visual feature discrimination and recognition. *J Neurosci* 1991;11:2383–2402.
24. Watson JDG, Myers R, Frackowiak RSJ, et al. Area V5 of the human brain: evidence from a combined study using positron emission tomography and magnetic resonance imaging. *Cereb Cortex* 1993;3:37–94.
25. McCarthy G, Spencer M, Adrignolo A, et al. *Human Brain Mapping* 1995;2:234–243.
26. Filiminof IN. Über die variabilitat der grosshirnrindenstruktur. Mitteilung II. Regio occipitalis beim erwachsenen Menshchen. *J Psychol Neurol* 1932;44:1–96.
27. Van Essen DC, Newsome WT, Maunsell JHR. The visual field representation in striate cortex of the macaque monkey: asymmetries, anisotropies, and individual variability. *Vision Res* 1984;24:429–448.
28. Horton JC, Hocking DR. Intrinsic variability of ocular dominance column periodicity in normal macaque monkeys. *J Neurosci* 1996;16:7228–7339.
29. Olavarria JF, Van Essen DC. The global pattern of cytochrome oxidase stripes in visual area V2 of the macaque monkey. *Cereb Cortex* 1997;7:395–404.
30. Van Essen DC. A tension-based theory of morphogenesis and compact wiring in the central nervous system. *Nature* 1997;385:313–318.
31. Joshi SC. Large deformation landmark based differeomorphic for image matching. Ph.D. thesis (Sever Institute, Washington University, St. Louis, MO), 1997.
32. Joshi SC, Miller MI, Grenander U. On the geometry and shape of brain sub-manifolds. *Int J Pattern Recog Artif Intell* 1997;11:1317–1343.
33. Christensen GE, Rabbit RD, Miller MI. 3D brain mapping using a deformable neuroanatomy. *Phys Med Biol* 1994;39:609–618.
34. Joshi SC, Miller MI, Christensen GE, et al. In: Melter RA, Wu AY, Bookstein FL, Green WD, eds. *Vision geometry IV*. Bellingham, WA: International Society for Optical Engineering, vol 2573, 1995:278–289.
35. Christensen GE, Rabbit RD, Miller MI. *IEEE Trans Image Processing* 1996;5:1435–1447.
36. Bookstein FL. Biometrics, biomathematics, and the morphometric synthesis. *Bull Math Biol* 1995;58:313–365.
37. Allman J. In: Jones EG, Peters A. *Cerebral cortex,* vol 8A. New York: Plenum Press, 1990:269–283.
38. Grenander U, Miller MI. Statistical methods in computational anatomy. *Stat Comput Graph* 1996;7:1.
39. Miller MI, Banerjee A, Christensen G, et al. *Stat Methods Med Res* 1997;6:267–299.

Neocortical Epilepsies.
Advances in Neurology, Vol. 84,
edited by P. D. Williamson, A. M. Siegel,
D. W. Roberts, V. M. Thadani, and M. S. Gazzaniga.
Lippincott Williams & Wilkins, Philadelphia © 2000.

4

Integrating Electrophysiology and Neuroimaging in the Study of Brain Function

George R. Mangun, *Joseph B. Hopfinger, and †Amishi P. Jha

Center for Cognitive Neuroscience, Duke University, Durham, North Carolina 27708;
**Department of Psychology, University of North Carolina at Chapel Hill, Chapel Hill,*
North Carolina 27516; †Brain Imaging and Analysis Center, Duke University,
Durham, North Carolina 27708

Human brain research involves a wide variety of approaches, ranging from studies of the molecular bases of cellular function to the psychophysical capabilities of the individual person. It is well accepted that no single approach or level of analysis will provide a complete picture of the brain and mind, and it is commonplace to integrate information across domains of knowledge and experimental approaches. Increasingly, the integration of information is being attempted directly within studies, as no single tool or approach alone can provide the necessary detail to understand fully the brain function of interest. This chapter reviews convergent approaches to the investigation of cognitive functions, with emphasis on our efforts to integrate electrophysiology and functional brain imaging in humans. The approaches described herein have applications beyond studies of normal brain function and are being extended for use in clinical investigations and diagnoses. The present chapter, however, focuses on how the integration of methods for measuring brain function can be used to dissect the neural architecture of a basic mental capacity: selective attention.

Attentional processes are hypothesized to serve many neurocomputational goals and are involved in a wide variety of perceptual and cognitive operations. One aspect of attentional processing that has received much interest is the role of top-down attentional processes on visual information processing. Voluntarily directing our attention to events in the world around us benefits our perceptions, as demonstrated psychophysically in target detection and discrimination tasks (1,2). In particular, humans respond faster and more accurately to attended versus unattended events. Over the past four decades, significant effort has been expended in the attempt to understand attentional benefits by elucidating the neural underpinnings of the human visual attention system (3,4).

A number of studies in humans have used event-related potentials (ERPs) to track information processing during selective attention. The earliest effects of attention to be reliably observed in the ERP recording are those revealed when observers selectively attend to some locations in the visual field while ignoring others; this is known as *selective spatial attention*. Sensory-evoked ERPs recorded from electrodes placed on the human scalp are modified by whether or not the eliciting visual stimulus occurred at an attended location. The amplitude of the P1 component (80–120 msec latency), a positive polarity ERP recorded over the lateral occipital scalp (Fig. 4.1), is the shortest latency visual ERP to be reliably affected by

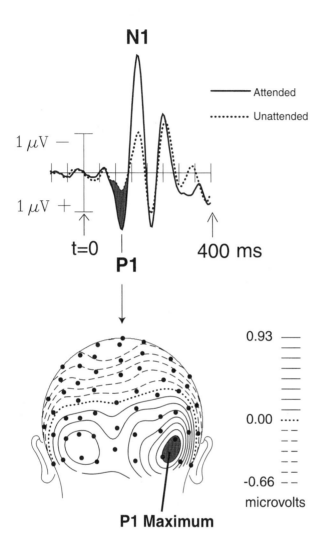

FIG. 4.1. Grand-average ERPs over eight subjects showing the occipital P1 attention effect. Subjects attended either the left or right visual field in separate blocks. **Top:** ERPs to a left field stimulus is shown when it is attended versus when ignored (during attend right conditions). ERPs are shown from the contralateral electrode location, where the P1 was maximal (electrode OR, located midway between O2 and T5 of the International 10–20 system). **Bottom:** Corresponding voltage topographic maps show the scalp location maxima of the attention effect in the time range of the P1 peak, 80–110 msec (from Mangun and Buck, unpublished).

spatial attention (5,6). Numerous studies demonstrated the reliability of this early attention effect and have clarified its properties (6–17). For example, it is now clear that any stimulus falling within an attended zone of visual space will elicit an enhanced P1 component, but attention to nonspatial properties of stimuli does not lead to modulations of the P1 component. That is, attending or ignoring stimuli based on their color (or other nonspatial feature) does not invoke changes in stimulus processing as early as the P1 component. Rather, nonspatial attention produces effects in the ERP waveform only at longer latencies (11,18,19). The shortest latency effect found for nonspatial

features has been for attention to color (18), where attention effects have poststimulus onset latencies of 120–150 msec (compared with 70–80 msec for spatial attention). Short-latency visual attention effects to other features, such as spatial frequency of stimuli, have been reported (20) but have not yet been replicated (21).

GAIN CONTROL OVER SENSORY PROCESSING

The modulation of early ERP components with spatial attention suggests a mechanism wherein top-down neural influences alter the gain on the processing of sensory signals at discrete stages of analysis. The idea of a gain-control model comes from the observations over many studies that spatial attention modulates ERP amplitudes but not latencies. That is, the P1 attention effect manifests only in the amplitude of the response. Moreover, the amplitude modulations in the P1 occur with little or no changes being observed in the wave shape or scalp distribution of the P1 component (for reviews, see 3,13). Indeed, the P1 component and other ERP components (such as the posterior scalp N1) are clearly elicited even when the stimulus is ignored or completely task irrelevant, albeit with reduced amplitudes. Thus, these ERP components behave as sensory responses to the physical features of the stimulus. Changes in luminance, spatial frequency, and location in the visual field all influence the P1, as would be expected if it reflected activity in visual–sensory processing areas. The pattern of attention effects on the P1 component are consistent with the idea that voluntary spatial attention acts to change the gain on sensory processing in a spatially specific manner (e.g., 5,23). This proposal is supported by recordings of single visual cortical neurons in monkeys indicating that spatial attention acts in a multiplicative fashion to enhance the firing of neurons coding attended stimuli (24). This is not to say that the only effect that voluntary attention can exert on visual processing is to change the gain of the neuronal response. This model is, however, consistent with the attention effects observed on the human P1 component and in single unit recordings in monkeys and furthermore is useful for describing how attention might aid visual processing.

It remains unclear, however, precisely how early during visual processing top-down attentional influences may be manifest. Whether this can occur at the level of primary sensory cortex, to act on the incoming sensory signal, is still under debate. Some studies reported that attention can influence processing in primary visual cortex (i.e., striate cortex or V1) during spatial (24,25 in monkeys), and nonspatial attention (20 in humans). Electrophysiologic findings remain inconsistent with other research arguing against visual attention effects in striate cortex (10,13,26,45). In part, some of

the difficulty in understanding how early in sensory processing attention may influence perceptual analyses comes from the fact that it is difficult to localize where in the brain a particular scalp-recorded ERP is generated.

FUNCTIONAL ANATOMY OF SELECTIVE ATTENTION

Modeling ERP Generators

Attempts to localize the intracranial generators of scalp-recorded ERPs all suffer from the same general limitation: The recordings are being made relatively far from their site of generation. Active neurons in the brain cause currents to flow passively through the tissues of the brain and the skull and finally to the scalp, where they are ultimately recorded. This is known as *volume conduction,* and it both helps and hinders ERP research. Volume conduction of ERPs is their main advantage because it permits signals generated within the brain, where one may not record in healthy subjects, to be measured noninvasively. Thus, tiny signals deep in the brain can become visible to us as they are passively conducted to the surface of the scalp; however, this fact also creates some difficulties for estimating where in the brain an ERP may be generated. Specifically, one cannot assume that the brain tissue directly underneath a particular recording electrode generated the recorded signal because it may have been volume conducted to that site from a distant locus. In addition, another aspect of the problem stems from what is known as the *inverse problem,* which refers to the dilemma that exists in inferring intracranial generators of scalp activity based on the pattern of voltages recorded over the scalp (i.e., the *scalp distribution*). Although a given distribution of charges inside the head will specify a unique pattern on the scalp (called the *forward solution*), the inverse is not true. A given pattern on the scalp might have been caused by any of a large number of possible configurations of charges inside the head. This is the basis of the inverse problem: that no unique solution can be obtained when going in the inverse direction from scalp recordings to neural generators. Nonetheless, inverse modeling using computer algorithms can be used to test possible models and can be especially useful when combined with additional sources of information.

Examples of the application of inverse modeling to studies of attention can be found in two studies in which the intracranial generators of visual ERPs in selective spatial attention tasks were modeled (26,28). These investigators identified several possible neural generators for visually evoked ERPs, including the P1 component and a shorter latency component known as the CI or NP80. The CI component was optimally localized to generators in primary visual (striate) cortex and was not affected by the direction of attention, which is consistent with prior studies (13). The later P1 component was affected by spatial attention, and it was localized to extrastriate generators. This group, therefore, concluded that extrastriate cortical activity reflected the earliest stage at which spatial attentional selection could be engaged.

Although the models derived from exercises of inverse modeling are plausible, the concern remains that it is difficult to falsify such models. This concern is based on the difficulty in verifying the accuracy of inverse dipole solutions in normal subjects. Occasionally, it is possible to work in neurologic patients who, for medical reasons, have electrodes placed inside their brains (29). These methods, interesting and useful as they have proven, nonetheless have limitations, the main ones being that electrodes are placed in only a few locations, determined by medical need, and that the subjects may currently be on medication, as in the case of patients with epilepsy. Thus, at present, the inverse problem remains a problem that is difficult to circumvent, limiting the conclusions that can be drawn on the basis of scalp-recorded electrophysiologic measures.

Functional Brain Imaging in Studies of Cognition

Functional neuroimaging methods such as positron emission tomography (PET) and func-

tional magnetic resonance imaging (fMRI) are able to provide relatively high spatial resolution pictures of human brain activity compared with scalp-recorded ERPs, which cannot. These methods now provide a means of viewing the living, thinking, acting, human brain. Thus, for studies of cognition that seek to identify the neural correlates of specific mental operations, functional imaging is the method of choice.

Functional imaging used in studies of cognition typically tracks changes in blood flow coupled to neural activity. These hemodynamic responses can be imaged by tracking radioactive water or other materials injected into the blood stream, as in PET, or by looking at changes in the magnetic properties of blood, as in the case of fMRI. With PET, because of the necessity of integrating data over many tens of seconds, there remains, however, essentially no temporal information in the resultant PET images. This level of temporal resolution is now being significantly improved using fMRI, especially event-related fMRI (30,46). At best, however, the timing information from any hemodynamic measure is still orders of magnitude poorer than the underlying neuronal events that trigger the blood flow response.

The debate discussed earlier concerning the earliest stage at which spatial attention affects visual processing appropriately illustrates the consequences of this limitation in hemodynamic (PET and fMRI) measures. Recent neuroimaging evidence in humans suggests that changes in neuronal processing with selective attention may occur in striate cortex (32). These findings, however, do not specify the time course of the activations. Therefore, it is not clear whether these attention-related blood flow changes in striate cortex reflect gating of stimulus inputs at short latencies or instead reflect changes in longer-latency activity mediated by reafferent modulations of striate neurons (33). Studies of subcortical brain structures provide evidence that attention-related modulations do not always reflect modulations of ascending sensory inputs. For example, the pulvinar nucleus of the thalamus, although not a sensory relay nucleus *per se,* is known to have visually responsive neurons that are affected by attention (see 4 and 31 for reviews). Furthermore, damage or blockade of these neurons leads to deficits in attentional orienting (35). Subcortical systems clearly are influenced by attention but may participate in attentional control circuitry rather than modulating sensory inputs within those same nuclei. Because the results of the studies finding hemodynamic modulation of striate neurons contain essentially no corresponding temporal information, interpretation of this activity remains limited in the conclusions that can be drawn about its role in attention processes.

To yield comprehensive and accurate information about sensory, motor, and cognitive processes, human brain research needs noninvasive measures of brain activity that have high spatial (i.e., on the order of millimeters or less) and high temporal (i.e., on the order of milliseconds) resolution. Although such measures are yet to be developed, perhaps based on unforeseen methods, at present we must make do with what is available, and currently no one measure alone suffices. Hence, integration of methods having complemen-

tary strengths is now being used (36). Next we describe several of our recent studies that combined PET or fMRI with ERP recordings in normal human subjects to investigate the neural mechanisms of human attention.

Integrating Event-related Potentials and Neuroimaging in Studies of Attention

In our first study using multimethodological integration, we combined ERP and PET methods to elucidate the time course and functional anatomy of spatial selective attention (10). The experimental design was similar to that used in several of our previous electrophysiological experiments (37). Subjects were presented with bilateral stimulus arrays, flashed at a rate of about 3 per second, that contained two nonsense symbols in each lateral hemifield. The subjects' task was to fixate a central point and to attend covertly to the symbol pairs in one hemifield, as specified beforehand by the experimenter. The subject was required to discriminate the symbols on the attended side and to respond with a rapid button press when the symbols were identical (Fig. 4.2, left panel).

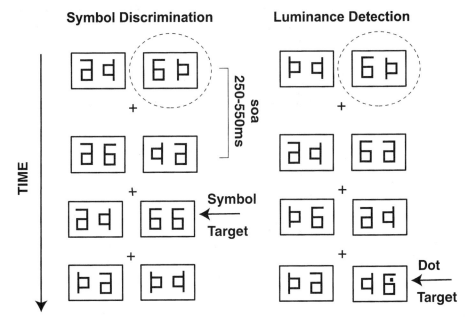

FIG. 4.2. Stimuli used in Heinze et al. (10) (left half of figure only) and Mangun et al. (38). See text for description of task.

The symbols in the opposite field were ignored during the entire block. In separate blocks, subjects were instructed to attend to the left or right hemifield stimuli.

The PET results revealed that spatial selective attention activated regions of the extrastriate visual cortex (posterior fusiform gyrus) in the hemisphere contralateral to the attended stimuli. In conjunction with the PET findings, ERP data obtained from the same subjects performing the same task indicated that changes in the ERPs with attention occurred as early as 80–130 msec after stimulus onset. The integration of the ERP and PET data involved asking whether the PET-defined brain activity might have produced the ERP attention effects we recorded at the scalp.

To address the foregoing question, the PET activations were used to infer the possible locations and numbers of active brain regions in our attention task. Forward modeling was used to ask whether electric activity within the PET-defined brain region possibly could have yielded our ERP effects. Forward modeling consists of using computer simulations to calculate the patterns of electric activity that would be obtained on the scalp surface from a particular type of electric activity located in a specific brain region. The regions we chose were those defined by the PET activations. We referred to the results of this modeling as *seeded forward solutions* because we placed (or seeded) the model neural sources within the PET-defined brain loci in the computer simulation. We found that dipoles located within the PET-defined loci yielded good accounts of the scalp-recorded ERP data, in the time range corresponding to the P1 component only (Fig. 4.3). Based on this pattern of findings, we argued that changes in input processing in extrastriate visual cortex (in the region of the posterior fusiform gyrus) were generating the P1 attention effect in the ERPs. As a result, we were able to localize in both time (80–130 msec poststimulus) and space (posterior fusiform gyrus) a cognitive operation related to early visual spatial attention.

Covariations in ERP and Functional Imaging Measures

In the foregoing, we described how ERP and PET measures of attention were related using experimental design and electric modeling. We suggested a relationship between activity at a particular time point in the ERP waveform and increased blood flow in the posterior fusiform gyrus, both related to attention. To the extent that these different measures of attentional modulation of stimulus processing are indeed related, one would anticipate that these measures also would covary with one another. In another study (38), we tested this directly by manipulating the perceptual load of the task and investigating whether the P1 attention effect and the posterior fusiform activations would be similarly affected. As before, subjects viewed bilateral stimulus arrays and in separate blocks they attended to either the right or left half of the arrays. In addition, however, two different tasks were included in this experiment. One task was identical to that of Heinze et al. (10) and involved a difficult symbol discrimination task in which subjects had to respond to matching symbols at the attended location. In the other, lower perceptual load task, only a simple luminance detection was required at the attended location. Specifically, subjects were required to respond to a small dot appearing within the confines of the bilaterally flashed symbol arrays (Fig. 4.2, left versus right panels). ERP and PET measures were obtained in separate sessions for each subject.

The results revealed a significant increase in the P1 component over contralateral scalp sites and a corresponding increase in blood flow in the contralateral posterior fusiform gyrus when subjects attended to one visual hemifield (Fig. 4.4, top). In addition to replicating our previous study (10), we found additional activations in the contralateral middle occipital gyrus. The key finding here, however, was that there was a significant interaction between the direction of attention (attend left versus right) and the task being performed (symbol matching versus luminance detection) for both the

Dipole-Fitting

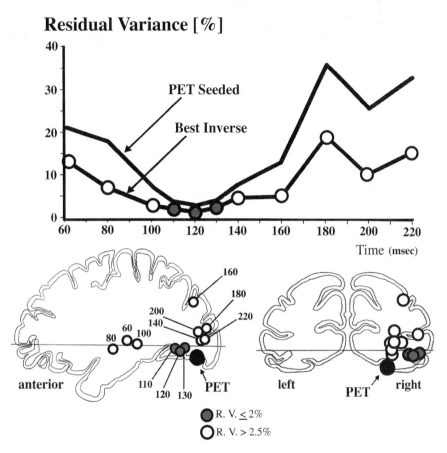

FIG. 4.3. Top: Residual variance of dipole solutions for seeded forward model and best-fitting inverse model (no constraints placed on the dipole locations or orientation). The minimum is in the time period near the peak of the P1 attention effect. **Bottom:** A sagittal section and coronal section from a stereotactic atlas showing the location of the right hemisphere activations at varying time points for the inverse modeling as well as the corresponding PET activation in the right posterior fusiform gyrus.

P1 component of the ERP and the PET activations in the posterior fusiform gyrus (Fig. 4.4, bottom). That is, both the P1 and the fusiform attention effects were affected further by the perceptual load of the task, and they covaried such that both were larger for the higher perceptual load task. This covariation between the P1 effect and the fusiform gyrus PET effect strengthens the hypothesis that the stage of visual processing indexed by the P1 component occurs in extrastriate cortex in the posterior fusiform gyrus. The method of using manipu-

lations of task parameters to examine covariations between effects observed in different recording modalities, is another means by which electrophysiological and blood flow measures can be linked together to provide high temporal and spatial resolution measures of cognitive functions.

Integrating ERPs and fMRI

One limitation of the PET studies described is that the method does not always permit in-

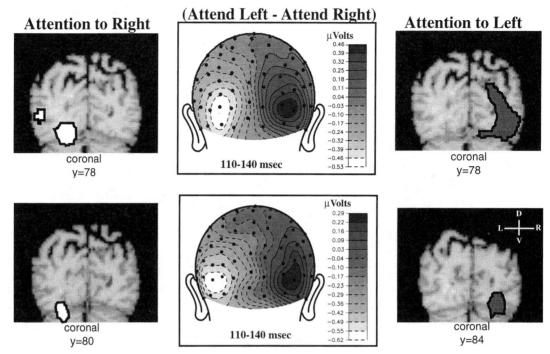

FIG. 4.4. Top left and right: Main effects of attending left versus attending right from PET data (38) mapped onto coronal MRI sections. PET activations, which showed a greater response for attending right than attending left, are shown in the upper left section (outlined in *black* and *filled-in white*). Activations that showed a greater response for attending left are shown in the upper right section (outlined in *black* and shaded *dark gray*). All PET activations shown are thresholded at Z > 2.33 (and are significant at the *p* <0.01 level, uncorrected). Activations of the posterior fusiform can be seen contralateral to the direction of attention. **Top middle:** The corresponding ERP attention effects for the P1 component shown as a voltage topographic map. **Bottom:** Activations and ERP attention effects that varied as a function of perceptual load. These included the posterior fusiform activation and the P1 component of the ERP.

vestigation of single subject data. Thus, any variations in the functional anatomy of cognitive mechanisms across individuals could not be assessed. The development of fMRI methods now permits functional imaging data to be acquired and evaluated in individual subjects, which may improve the resolution of neuroimaging, and hence the integration of ERPs and functional imaging, by taking into account the variation in gross anatomy and functional organization across subjects.

We recently undertook such an investigation using combined fMRI and ERP methods (22). We were able to observe significant spatial attention-related activity within individual subjects in ERPs and fMRI measures and to relate these activations to individual cortical anatomy. To provide a bridge to our former PET studies, we adapted the same spatial attention task used before: selective, covert attention to one half of bilaterally flashed symbol arrays (see Fig. 4.2); unlike prior PET studies, the direction of attention was cued by a central arrow to the left or right half of the arrays every 16 seconds. Thus, subjects were alternately attending to the left and right visual hemifield. ERPs also were obtained in identical attention conditions to provide high-resolution indices of the time course of attentional selection processes. These are shown as topographic voltage maps for the P1 component (Fig. 4.5, left column). FMRI results

Hemodynamic Effects (fMRI)

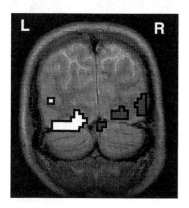

☐ **Attention Right**
■ **Attention Left**

Electrophysiological Effects (ERPs)

(Attend Left - Attend Right)

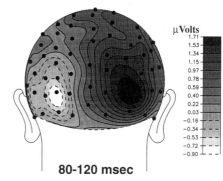

80-120 msec

FIG. 4.5. Left column: Main effects of attending left versus attending right from fMRI data for one subject [Mangun et al., 1998; (22)] showing activations in multiple areas of the occipital cortex. Activations are shown overlaid on high-density proton-density anatomic image for that subject; regions showing greater activation for attend left are shaded in *dark gray,* those showing greater activations for attend right are shown in *white,* outlined in *black.* The activations that are shown were thresholded at a statistical significance level of p <0.05, after background correction to remove effects of physiological noise, and were filtered using a 3×3 pixel median filter, which emphasizes clusters of activity. **Right column:** ERP attention effects for the same subject shown as a voltage topographic map, showing contralateral attention effects in the latency range of the P1 component (80–130 msec).

showed attention-related activity in a variety of cortical gyri, including the lingual, fusiform, inferior occipital, and middle occipital gyri (Fig. 4.5, right column). In general, the findings in individual subjects replicated our prior PET data, in which activations were observed following spatial normalization of individual subject data into a common coordinate space and averaging across subjects. Some variability was found between subjects in the fMRI results, which led us to investigate the relationship of our activations to the multiple visual areas of the brain. That is, when there is an activation in the area of the fusiform gyrus, does this reflect activation of a single visual cortical area, or, rather, is this a sign of activity across multiple, adjacent visual areas in the visual cortical hierarchy?

Mapping Attention Effects onto Functionally Defined Visual Areas

To relate scalp-recorded ERPs to underlying brain structures, it is important to be able to identify at what stage within the hierarchy of visual areas the attention-sensitive ERPs and neuroimaging activations are being generated. The presence of multiple visual areas is now well established in nonhuman primates based on single cell studies (40). Many early visual cortical areas in the primate show retinotopically organized representations of the visual field (41). In monkeys, these include the maps for lower visual field regions projecting dorsally in the brain, beginning with V1 (i.e., striate cortex) and continuing with successive re-representations, including

V2 and V3 (second and third visual areas, respectively). For upper-field stimuli, the maps from V1 project ventrally from V1 to V2, VP and ventral V4 (V4v). These visual cortical areas have now been studied using neuroimaging in humans (41–43), and the results show similar patterns to that in the macaque monkey (41).

To determine the relationship between the spatial attention effects within visual cortex and the multiple visual areas, we first functionally determined the borders of the early visual areas in each of our subjects using methods similar to those of Engel et al. (43) and Sereno et al. (41). Under passive viewing conditions, the upper and lower vertical meridia and left and right horizontal meridia were stimulated. We then reconstructed these activations onto anatomic templates derived for each of six subjects. Because visual borders between V1 and V2, V2 and VP/V3, and VP/V3 and V4 occur at the meridia of the visual field, this permitted the extent of the first few visual areas to be determined. This interpretation of the fMRI data for one subject is

shown in Fig. 4.6 (left column). Then it was possible to determine which visual areas were modulated during the spatial attention task by comparing the attention-related activations (attend left versus attend right) to the functionally defined visual areas for each subject. Evidence was found for activations in multiple visual areas, including V2, VP, and V4v (shown for one subject in Fig. 4.6).

Prior studies in humans using ERPs or functional imaging have been unable to identify the precise areas of visual cortex displaying attentional modulations. In this study, we used fMRI to define the borders of cortical visual areas V1 through V4 and were thus able to demonstrate that spatial attention modulates neuronal processing in multiple visual areas. The corresponding ERP recordings showed attentional modulations beginning at a latency of 80 to 90 msec after stimulus onset. This spatiotemporal pattern of attentional activations strongly supports a model of spatial selective attention that involves a tonic, gain control over human visual processing. Ongoing modeling studies are helping us to

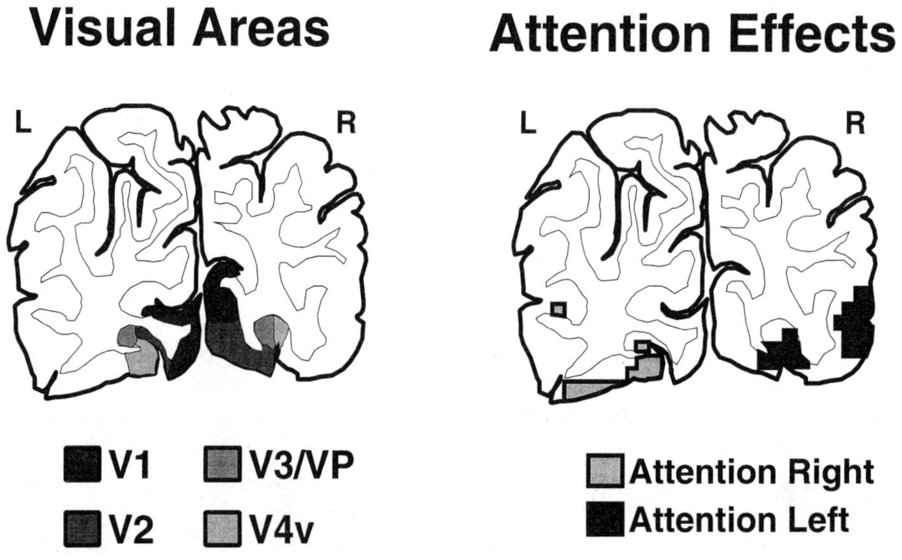

FIG. 4.6. Extent of visual areas and fMRI activations plotted onto templates derived from proton-density MRI scans. **Left column** shows interpretations of extent of visual areas V1, V2, V3/VP, and V4 for the subject shown in Fig. 4.5. **Right column** shows the locations of the attention effects in the same subject.

relate the P1 attention effect to specific, functionally defined visual areas.

Parametric Analyses of Functional Imaging Data

The analyses described previously were effective in isolating the lateralized selective attention effects in contralateral extrastriate regions. Other brain mechanisms, however, contribute to attentional processes that cannot be revealed with these types of analyses. The extrastriate attention effects identified before were obtained in analyses that controlled for global attention state by comparing one focused attention condition directly to another (i.e., attend left versus attend right conditions). If, however, some brain regions are similarly active in both conditions of attention (attend right and attend left), this will not be revealed in these types of analyses because it will be canceled out. This is an important control for nonspecific effects such as those attributable to behavioral/neural arousal, but creates barriers to investigations of some types of brain activity. Other types of analyses can help mitigate problems of cancellation of common activations across tasks, although they reintroduce the other problems noted (i.e., arousal confounds). One method is to look at comparisons of attended conditions to passive viewing conditions, as done by Corbetta et al. (44). Another approach is to test for parametric changes in brain activity over varying levels of task engagement. Such analyses are helping us to clarify neural circuits that contribute to the recruitment of attentional resources. These effects may be nonspecific with respect to selective attention but may provide clues about the brain regions involved in processes such as attentional control.

We performed a parametric analysis of the PET data described in the preceding section (38). As described, the degree of task difficulty was varied, whereas the stimuli were held constant. In addition to the symbol discrimination and dot detection conditions, a passive viewing condition also was included in that study and could be interpreted as hav-ing the lowest possible perceptual load for the given set of stimuli. Thus, analyses were performed to examine which PET activations and ERP components increased in a parametric fashion from passive viewing through simple luminance (dot) detection to complex symbol matching (form analysis). This analysis would capture changes in brain activity that were correlated with increasing attentional allocation, task involvement, or arousal.

Various brain regions were found to be activated or deactivated in the parametric analyses; we will not provide an exhaustive review here but instead will focus on two interesting effects. First, bilateral areas of inferior parietal cortex exhibited increasing levels of activation with increasing task demand. These parietal activations were extremely focal and thus not likely attributable to simple global behavioral and neural arousal. Rather, they may represent the global activation of these regions during spatial attention. These bilateral activations were not specific to attending left or right and therefore were canceled out during the selective attend left versus attend right comparisons described earlier (Fig. 4.4, top). The parietal activations were slightly more posterior to those reported by Corbetta et al. (44) in their attentional switching task. Nonetheless, the present pattern of results indicates that parietal as well as extrastriate cortex is activated during sustained visual spatial attention but in slightly different ways. As a result, the present findings are in line with the intuitions from neurologic observations that the parietal lobes should be involved in attentive behavior, perhaps as part of a widespread network of control circuitry. The result of this control is manifested in the visual cortex as the modulations of incoming sensory signals, as already described.

The second finding of interest here was a region in medial frontal cortex, including the supplementary motor area (SMA) and extending into the midcingulate gyrus, that showed systematically increasing blood flow with increasing task difficulty (Fig. 4.7). In conjunction with the parametric increase in SMA/cingulate activity measured by PET, a

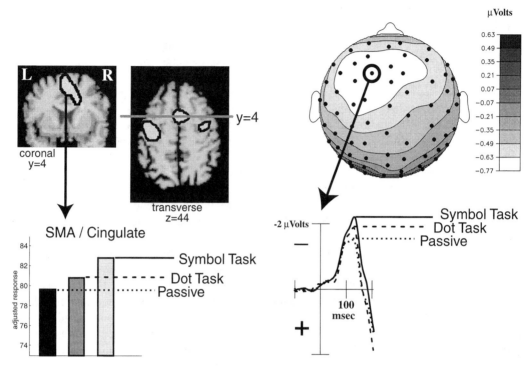

FIG. 4.7. Parametric analyses of PET attention effects and corresponding ERP effects with increasing levels of task difficulty. Changes in regional cerebral blood flow that increased systematically from passive viewing, to detecting simple luminance increments (dot task), to discriminating complex forms (symbol task) are shown for a region of frontal cortex (activations are outlined in *black,* and filled-in *light gray*—all activations thresholded at Z >2.33). The coronal section at left is taken at the anterior–posterior level indicated in the horizontal section displayed to the **right**. At the **bottom left**, the parametric pattern of increasing blood flow for the SMA/mid-cingulate activation is shown graphically. At **bottom right**, the waveform from a single frontocentral electrode site is displayed for the three levels of the task. An increase in the anterior N1 component (peaking at about 140 msec) can be seen with increasing task difficulty. The scalp distribution of this effect is shown at the **top right** and was determined by plotting the difference map for the symbol task minus passive viewing.

negative-polarity ERP component (anterior N1) with a widespread frontocentral scalp distribution peaking at 140 msec also showed a parametric increase in peak amplitude as a function of task difficulty (Fig. 4.7). The parametric pattern of activation as described for the SMA/cingulate permitted us to relate it to a brain potential with a frontocentral scalp distribution that covaried with the PET activations. This result was unexpected and provides a testable hypothesis about the role of the anterior N1 component in attentional control as well as its site of generation in the brain. The use of parametric analyses is therefore a powerful method for examining

the role of various brain regions in cognitive processing, especially as it may facilitate mapping between ERP and PET/fMRI measures of mental functions.

LOGIC AND CAVEATS OF MULTIMETHODOLOGIC INTEGRATION

The general logic inherent in our multimethodological integration studies revolves around several experimental design considerations. We refer to these as the frames of reference for relating the different forms of data. First, a common *experimental* frame of reference was used in our studies. That is, identical experimental conditions were used in both the functional imaging (PET/fMRI) and ERP sessions, and identical comparisons between conditions were used for analysis of the data (i.e., attend left minus attend right, parametric analyses, and manipulations of visual field location of the stimulus). A common *sensory* frame of reference was ensured by having identical stimuli in all recording sessions, thus preventing any differences from arising as a result of different stimulus parameters, and was accomplished by using the same computer monitors in the ERP/PET studies and the same magnetically safe goggle system in the ERP/fMRI studies. A common *physiologic* frame of reference was established by using the same participants in both the ERP and neuroimaging sessions. Thus, we can argue that both the ERP and PET (or fMRI) results are directly related to the same mental process of spatial selective attention.

In some studies, additional information was included from a *spatial* frame of reference by translating the results of the PET data into the spatial coordinate system defined for the ERP data. Specifically, this refers to the seeded-dipole modeling described previously. Thus, even though inverse modeling of ERP data alone cannot give one unique solution in many cases, the addition of constraints from neuroimaging can help to achieve physiologically and anatomically plausible models (see reference 34 for a related modeling approach). When used together, these multiple frames of reference enable stronger conclusions to be drawn from the experimental findings. Even so, fundamental questions remain about relating blood flow to electric activity, and these must be taken into account when attempting to integrate ERPs and functional imaging data.

Relationship of Electric to Blood Flow Measures

Relatively little is actually known about the nature of the mapping between electromag-

netic recordings and activations derived using functional neuroimaging. It is true, of course, that neuronal activity triggers a coupled hemodynamic response, but for any given observed hemodynamic response, the question remains as to what form of neuronal activity triggered it. Neurons display spontaneous background firing, and this may be modulated by various factors (e.g., arousal). Of course, neurons also show transient activity elicited by synaptic inputs (e.g., due to sensory stimulation). Both these forms of neural activity can be assumed to trigger hemodynamic responses. The difficulty arises when we attempt to associate a particular form of neuronal activity (as measured at the scalp) to a particular hemodynamic activation.

How might ERP and blood flow measures map onto one another for any sensory, motor, or cognitive process in a particular experiment? One possibility is a direct one-to-one mapping wherein the ERP and blood flow measures both may be reflections of identical neuronal activity; that is, both measured effects are produced as the result of the stimulus evoked activity, or both measured effects are produced as the result of the changes in background firing rate. Another possibility is that the ERP and blood flow measures may be reflecting different aspects of neuronal activity, but in the same neuronal populations. For example, a population of neurons may have increased background firing rates that drive increased blood flow, but this may not be easily recorded as ERPs. These same neurons, however, also may generate an enhanced transient-evoked responses that is recorded in the ERPs but that may be difficult to detect using blood flow measures. In this case, the same population of neurons may be responsible for both the ERP and PET/fMRI effects, and yet different processes underlie what each is recording. Another possibility is that the ERP and blood flow measures arise from distinct populations of neurons, even though both are reflections of attentional processing. If these populations were nearby (e.g., within the same cortical area), this might not present a problem for most types of analyses, but if they were in different brain regions (e.g., two adjacent visual cortical areas), then the type of modeling we have described could lead to errors. A final possibility is that ERPs and blood flow measures are not related in any manner. This possibility can be rejected for the studies reviewed here because the ERP and blood flow measures are related by the experimental circumstances under which they were isolated (i.e., the frames of reference described previously) and thus, at the very least, are both informative about the mental process of interest. It seems likely that any of these possibilities might be true for any given experimental effects, and thus, the precise relationship between an ERP data set and a functional imaging data set will have to be established on a case-by-case basis.

GENERAL CONCLUSIONS

We have reviewed a methodology for combining electrophysiologic and hemodynamic measures of brain activity that results in an improved temporal and spatial resolution relative to that which either method alone can produce. Through such integrative methods, human brain function can be studied with the resolution necessary to elucidate both the component neural structures and the stages of processing at which they are active. With such knowledge in hand, significant strides can be made toward understanding complex human functions. Here we have described evidence for the time course of activity and functional anatomy of neural systems involved in visual spatial attention. Selective attention was found to modulate activity in multiple visual areas in the human brain. It is now clear that the top-down influence of voluntary spatial selective attention involves changes in the way incoming information is processed in these areas of extrastriate visual cortex because the ERP signatures related to these effects have relatively short latencies. Thus, these data support early selection models of attention in which attention appears to act as a gain control over early stages of vision to modulate stimulus processing prior to complete perceptual analysis. From the perspec-

tive of human brain research, the integration of temporally specific and anatomically precise methods promises to provide what amounts to a real-time view of human brain activity. This approach can be used to understand normal brain function during sensory, motor, and cognitive activity, but it also should prove useful in probing the disordered or damaged nervous system.

ACKNOWLEDGMENTS

This research was supported by grants to G.R.M. from the NIMH, NINDS, and HFSP. J.B.H. was supported by an NSF Fellowship and A.P.J. was supported by an NIMH Fellowship. We gratefully acknowledge L.A. Buck, M. Soltani, H. Hinrichs, M. Scholz, C.L. Kussmaul, M. Girelli, M.S. Gazzaniga, S.A. Hillyard, and H.J. Heinze for their important contributions to portions of the research discussed here.

REFERENCES

1. Downing CJ. Expectancy and visual-spatial attention: effects on perceptual quality. *J Exp Psychol Hum Percept Perform* 1988;14:188–202.
2. Hawkins HL, Hillyard SA, Luck SJ, et al. Visual attention modulates signal detectability. *J Exp Psychol Hum Percept Perform* 1990;16:802–811.
3. Mangun GR. Neural mechanisms of visual selective attention in humans. *Psychophysiology* 1995;32:4–18.
4. Posner MI, Petersen SE. The attention system of the human brain. *Annu Rev Neurosci* 1990;13:25–42.
5. Eason RG. Visual evoked potential correlates of early neural filtering during selective attention. *Bulletin of the Psychonomic Society* 1981;18:203–206.
6. Van Voorhis ST, Hillyard SA. Visual evoked potentials and selective attention to points in space. *Perception and Psychophysics* 1977;22:54–62.
7. Eimer M. Sensory gating as a mechanism for visuospatial orienting: electrophysiological evidence from trial-by-trial cuing experiments. *Perception and Psychophysics* 1994;55:667–675.
8. Harter MR, Aine C, Schroeder C. Hemispheric differences in the neural processing of stimulus location and type: effects of selective attention on visual evoked potentials. *Neuropsychologia* 1982;20:421–438.
9. Heinze HJ, Luck SJ, Mangun GR, et al. Visual event-related potentials index focussed attention within bilateral stimulus arrays. I. Evidence for early selection. *Electroencephalogr Clin Neurophysiol* 1990;75:511–527.
10. Heinze HJ, Mangun GR, Burchert W, et al. Combined spatial and temporal imaging of spatial selective attention in humans. *Nature* 1994;392:543–546.
11. Hillyard SA, Munte TF. Selective attention to color and

location: an analysis with event-related brain potentials. *Perception and Psychophysics* 1984;36:185–198.

12. Mangun GR, Hillyard SA. Allocation of visual attention to spatial locations: tradeoff functions for event-related brain potentials and detection performance. *Perception and Psychophysics* 1990;47:532–550.

13. Mangun GR, Hillyard SA, Luck SJ. Electrocortical substrates of visual selective attention. In: Meyer D, Kornblum S, eds. *Attention and performance XIV.* Cambridge, MA: MIT Press, 1993:219–243.

14. Mangun GR, Hillyard SA. Modulations of sensory-evoked brain potentials indicate changes in perceptual processing during visual-spatial priming. *J Exp Psychol Hum Percept Perform* 1991;17:1057–1074.

15. Mangun GR, Hopfinger J, Kussmaul C, et al. Covariations in ERP and PET measures of spatial selective attention in human extrastriate cortex. *Human Brain Mapping* 1997;5:273–279.

16. Neville HJ, Lawson D. Attention to central and peripheral visual space in a movement detection task: an event-related potential and behavioral study. I. normal hearing adults. *Brain Res* 1987;405:253–267.

17. Rugg MD, Milner AD, Lines CR, et al. Modulation of visual event-related potentials by spatial and non-spatial visual selective attention. *Neuropsychologia* 1987;25:85–89.

18. Anllo-Vento L, Luck SJ, Hillyard SA. Spatio-temporal dynamics of attention to color: evidence from human electrophysiology. *Human Brain Mapping* 1998;6:216–238.

19. Harter MR, Aine CJ. Brain mechanisms of visual selective attention. In: Parasuraman R, Davies Dr, eds. *Varieties of attention.* London: Academic Press, 1984:293–321.

20. Zani A, Proverbio AM. ERP signs of early selective attention effects to check size. *Electroencephalogr Clin Neurophysiol* 1995;95:277–292.

21. Heslenfeld DJ, Kenemans JL, Kok A, et al. Feature processing and attention in the human visual system: an overview. *Biol Psychol* 1997;45:183–215.

22. Mangun GR, Buonocore M, Girelli M, et al. ERP and fMRI measures of visual spatial selective attention. *Human Brain Mapping* 1998;6:383–389.

23. Hillyard SA, Mangun GR. Sensory gating as a physiological mechanism for visual selective attention. In: Johnson R Jr, Parasuraman R, Rohrbaugh JW, eds. *Current trends in event-related brain potentials.* New York: Elsevier, 1987:61–67.

24. McAdams CJ, Maunsell JHR. Effects of attention on orientation-tuning functions of single neurons in macaque cortical area V4. *J Neurosci* 1999;19:431–441.

25. Motter BC. Focal attention produces spatially selective processing in visual cortical areas V1, V2, and V4 in the presence of competing stimuli. *J Neurophysiol* 1993;70:909–919.

26. Clark VP, Hillyard SA. Spatial selective attention affects extrastriate but not striate components of the visual evoked potential. *Journal of Cognitive Neuroscience* 1996;8:387–402.

27. Luck SJ, Hillyard SA, Mouloua M, et al. Effects of spatial cuing on luminance detectability: psychophysical and electrophysiological evidence for early selection. *J Exp Psychol Hum Percept Perform* 1994;20:887–904.

28. Gomez Gonzalez CM, Clark VP, Fan S, et al. Sources of attention-sensitive visual event-related potentials. *Brain Topogr* 1994;7:41–51.

29. Nobre AC, Allison T, McCarthy G. Modulation of human extrastriate visual processing by selective attention to colours and words. *Brain* 1998;121:1357–1368.

30. Buckner RL, Goodman J, Burock M, et al. Functional–anatomic correlates of object priming in humans revealed by rapid presentation event-related fMRI. *Neuron* 1998;20:285–296.

31. LaBerge D. Computational and anatomical models of selective attention in object identification. In: Gazzaniga M, ed. *The cognitive neurosicences.* Cambridge, MA: MIT Press, 1995:649–665.

32. Worden M, Schneider W, Wellington R. Determining the locus of attentional selectivity with functional magnetic resonance imaging. *Cognitive Neuroscience Society Abstracts* 1996;3:101.

33. Roelfsema PR, Lamme VAF, Spekreijse H. Object-based attention in the primary visual cortex of the macaque monkey. *Nature* 1998;395:376–381.

34. Liu AK, Belliveau JW, Dale AM. Spatiotemporal imaging of human brain activity using functional MRI constrained magnetoencephalography data: Monte Carlo simulations. *Proc Natl Acad Sci USA* 1998;95:8945–8950.

35. Petersen SE, Robinson DL, Morris JD. Contributions of the pulvinar to visual spatial attention. *Neuropsychologia* 1987;25:97–105.

36. Fox P, Woldorff M. Integrating human brain maps. *Current Opinions in Neurobiology* 1994;4:151–156.

37. Heinze HJ, Mangun GR. Electrophysiological signs of sustained and transient attention to spatial locations. *Neuropsychologia* 1995;33:889–908.

38. Mangun GR, Hopfinger J, Kussmaul C, et al. Covariations in ERP and PET measures of spatial selective attention in human extrastriate cortex. *Human Brain Mapping* 1997;5:273–279.

39. Mangun GR, Hillyard SA. Spatial gradients of visual attention: behavioral and electrophysiological evidence. *Electroencephalogr Clin Neurophysiol* 1988;70:417–428.

40. Van Essen D, DeYoe E. Concurrent processing in the primate visual cortex. In: Gazzaniga MS, ed. *Cognitive neuroscience.* Cambridge, MA: MIT Press, 1995:383–400.

41. Sereno M, Dale A, Reppas J, et al. Borders of multiple visual areas in humans revealed by functional magnetic resonance imaging. *Science* 1995;268:889–893.

42. Zeki S, Watson J, Lueck C, et al. A direct demonstration of functional specialization in human visual cortex. *J Neurosci* 1991;11:641–649.

43. Engel SA, Rumerlhart D, Wandell B, et al. fMRI of human visual cortex. *Nature* 1994;370:106.

44. Corbetta M, Miezin F, Shulman G, et al. A PET study of visuospatial attention. *J Neurosci* 1993;13:1202–1226.

45. Luck SJ, Chelazzi L, Hillyard SA, et al. Neural mechanisms of spatial selective attention in areas V1, V2, and V4 of macaque visual cortex. *J Neurophysiology* 1997;77:24–42.

46. Josephs O, Turner R, Friston K. Event-related fMRI. *Human Brain Mapping* 1997;5:243–248.

Neocortical Epilepsies.
Advances in Neurology, Vol. 84,
edited by P. D. Williamson, A. M. Siegel,
D. W. Roberts, V. M. Thadani, and M. S. Gazzaniga.
Lippincott Williams & Wilkins, Philadelphia © 2000.

5

Parietofrontal Circuits: Parallel Channels for Sensory–Motor Integrations

Massimo Matelli and Giuseppe Luppino

Istituto di Fisiologia Umana, Università di Parma, 43100 Parma, Italy

The early anatomists subdivided the parietal cortex of primates into two major cytoarchitectonic types: the *heterotypical granular cortex (koniocortex),* which is located in the postcentral gyrus, and the *homotypical cortex,* which occupies the remaining portion of the parietal lobe. Functionally, the koniocortex corresponds to the primary somatosensory cortex, whereas the posterior parietal cortex, situated between sensory cortices and motor cortices, was thought to be a classic "association" area that combines information from different sensory modalities to construct a unified representation of the space and of the body schema (1).

In this functional view, more emphasis was placed on input characteristics, and little account was taken of output requirements. In particular, spatial perception was considered a unitary, monolithic process: the brain forms a single spatial representation of each object regardless of what action is going to be executed in relation to that object. In recent years, neurophysiologic and neuroanatomic research has challenged this view. In the scheme emerging from these studies, the posterior parietal cortex is composed of a mosaic of different areas endowed with specific input–output connectivity, the function of which is to transform the sensory information coded in the coordinates of sensory epithelia (e.g., retina, skin) into information for movement

(sensory–motor transformations). Instead of a single, multipurpose "space area," the posterior parietal cortex is now thought to encode multiple representations of an object in space, each related to the control of specific actions such as foveating, orienting, grasping, or reaching. Space perception derives from the joint activity of these parietal areas and the frontal areas to which they are connected and that control movements requiring space computation (for a review of the literature, see 2,3).

This chapter presents this new picture of the organization of the parietofrontal connections and discusses the possible functional role of these connections in motor control.

HOMOTYPICAL AREAS OF THE PARIETAL LOBE

Anatomically, the posterior parietal cortex is formed by two lobules: the superior parietal lobule (SPL) and the inferior parietal lobule (IPL). The areas forming the posterior parietal cortex are shown in Fig. 5.1.

An important finding that emerged from recent anatomic and functional experiments is that, in the posterior parietal areas, there are multiple representations of the arms, legs, and face (Fig. 5.1). A further notion that radically changed in recent years is that the SPL is the exclusive target of the somatosensory cor-

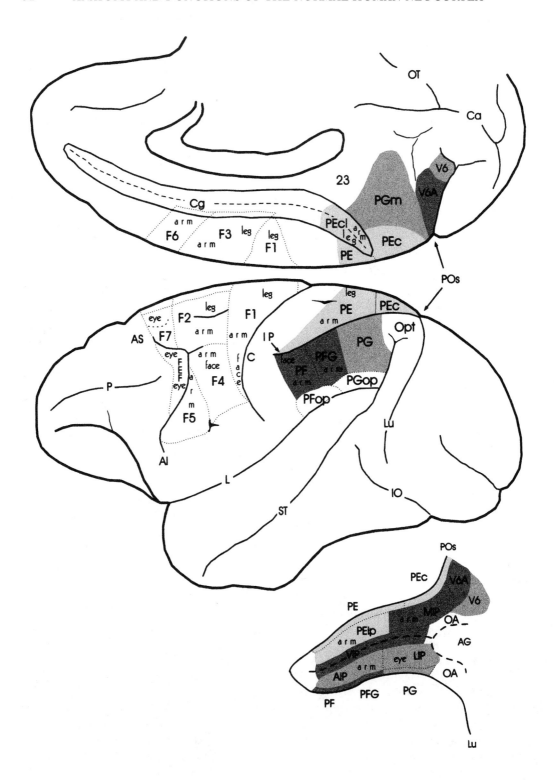

tices, whereas on IPL there is a convergence of both somatosensory and visual information (3,4). There is now evidence that both lobules receive somatosensory and visual inputs. The modern view is that only the anterior areas of the SPL (PE, PEc, PEci, and PEip) are related to somatosensory modality; posterior areas of both SPL (V6, PGm) and IPL (PG, LIP) process predominantly visual information. An integration of somatosensory and visual information occurs not only in the IPL (PF, PFG, and VIP) but also in SPL (MIP, V6A; for a review of the literature, see 3,4).

AGRANULAR AREAS OF THE FRONTAL LOBE

The classic view is that in the frontal lobe there are only two motor areas [primary motor area or M1 and supplementary motor area, SMA or M2, (5)]. A modern parcellation of the agranular frontal cortex (motor cortex) of the macaque monkey is shown in Fig. 5.1. The subdivision is based on cytoarchitectural and histochemical data (6). F1 basically corresponds to area 4 of Brodmann, and the other areas are subdivisions of Brodmann's area 6. F2 and F7, which lie in the superior part of area 6, are often referred to collectively as the *dorsal premotor cortex* (PMd); F4 and F5, which lie in the inferior area 6, are often referred to as the *ventral premotor cortex* (PMv). F3 (SMA) and F6 (pre-SMA) form the mesial area 6. (For a review of the various parcellations of the motor cortex, see 6.)

The anatomic subdivision shown in the figure is confirmed by functional data, showing that motor cortex contains many functional motor representations (motor fields), each located in different anatomic areas (Fig. 5.1). The dorsal part of F7 is devoted to the control of eye movements (supplementary eye field, SEF) (7), whereas the motor representation of lateral part of F7 is not fully established.

Recent studies of corticospinal projections (8,9) fully support the multiplicity of motor fields and confirm the presence of an arm representation in F1, F2, F3, F4, and F5 and of a leg representation in F1, F2, and F3. Areas F6 and F7 are virtually not connected with the spinal cord but project mainly to the brainstem (10).

The intrinsic connectivity of the various motor areas is consistent with the organization of corticospinal projections. Areas projecting to the spinal cord all send projections to F1, whereas F6 and F7 are connected only with the motor areas located rostral to F1 [F2, F3, F4, and F5 (11, 12)]. In contrast, F6 and F7 represent the main entrance of the prefrontal input to the motor cortex (11,12). Finally, the SEF has no connections with other motor (skeletomotor) fields. The frontal eye field (FEF) represents its main frontal target (13).

PARIETOFRONTAL CIRCUITS

The general pattern of parietofrontal circuits emerging from recent anatomic data is as follows. Each parietal area sends strong

---

FIG. 5.1. Mesial and lateral views of the macaque brain showing the cytoarchitectonic parcellation of the agranular frontal cortex and of the posterior parietal cortex. Motor areas are defined according to Matelli and Luppino (6). Parietal areas are defined according to Pandya and Seltzer (38) with the exclusion of those located within the intraparietal sulcus *(IP)*, which are defined according to physiologic data (for references, see text) and are shown in an unfolded view of the sulcus in the lowest part of the figure. On the basis of the available data, the various body parts representations are reported and the sensory modalities elaborated by the parietal areas displayed in different gray levels. *Light gray:* Somatosensory; *medium gray:* visual; *dark gray:* bimodal visual and somatosensory. In the prefrontal cortex, the frontal eye field (FEF) is also defined according to physiological criteria. *AG,* annectant gyrus; *AIP,* anterior intraparietal area; *C,* central sulcus; *Ca,* calcarine fissure; *Cg,* cingulate sulcus; *IO,* inferior occipital sulcus; *L,* lateral fissure; *LIP,* lateral intraparietal area; *Lu,* lunate sulcus; *NIP,* neutral intraparietal area; *OT,* occipitotemporal sulcus; *P,* principal sulcus; *POs,* parieto-occipital sulcus; *ST,* superior temporal sulcus.

TABLE 5.1. *Parietofrontal circuits in the macaque monkey*

Posterior parietal areas	Motor areas	Proposed function
AIP	F5 bank	Visual transformation for grasping
PF	F5 convexity	Internal representation of actions
VIP	F4	Peripersonal space coding for arm neck and face movements
LIP	FEF	Visual transformation for eye movements
PE	F1	Somatosensory transformation for movements
PEci	F3	Somatosensory transformation for posture
Pec–PEip	F2 dimple region	Somatosensory transformation for reaching
MIP	F2 ventrorostral	Visual and somatosensory transformation for reaching
PGm	F7	Unknown

projections (*predominant connections*) to a single motor area and weak projections (*additional connections*) to other motor areas. In turn, each motor area is the target of a specific set of parietal areas, among which only one has privileged connections.

Taking into account the predominant connections between parietal and motor areas, a series of segregated parietofrontal circuits can be identified. It has been proposed that, given the functional properties of parietal and motor areas, each circuit is involved in a specific sensory–motor transformation for action, and thus, it represents the basic element of the cortical motor system (14). Table 5.1 lists the parietofrontal circuits originating from the IPL and SPL and their putative role in motor control.

PARIETOFRONTAL CIRCUITS OF THE IPL

The major target of the IPL is the PMv. Recent anatomic and functional data showed that these projections are organized into at least four main visuomotor circuits. Figure 5.2A,B shows these connections.

AIP–F5 bank Circuit

Area AIP is located in the rostral part of the lateral bank of the intraparietal sulcus (IP) in front of area LIP (Fig. 5.1). Neurons of this area discharge during the grasping of specific objects and were classified into three groups: *motor-dominant, visual and motor,* and *visual-dominant neurons*. Motor-dominant neurons do not show any significant difference in activity when a monkey executes grasping in dark or light; visual and motor neurons are less active during grasping in dark than in light; visual-dominant neurons fire vigorously only when the object is visible. Many visually responsive neurons also discharge during fixation of the objects, even when fixation was not followed by a subsequent grasping movement. Finally, in most visual and motor neurons, the intrinsic characteristics of the object, effective in triggering a neuron and the type of grip coded by that neuron, coincided (15).

FIG. 5.2. Summary view of the main posterior parietal projections to the motor cortex in the macaque monkey (see also Table 5.1). **A:** Predominant parietal projections from areas located in the lateral bank and in the fundus of the intraparietal sulcus. To show these areas, the intraparietal sulcus has been opened and the occipital lobe removed. *Dashed line* marks the fundus of the sulcus. **B:** Predominant parietal projections from areas located on the convexity of the inferior parietal lobule. **C:** Predominant parietal projections from areas located in the superior parietal lobule. In this view of the brain, the inferior parietal lobule and the occipital lobe have been removed to show the areas located in the medial bank of the intraparietal sulcus and in the anterior bank of the parieto-occipital sulcus, respectively. Abbreviations as in Fig. 5.1.

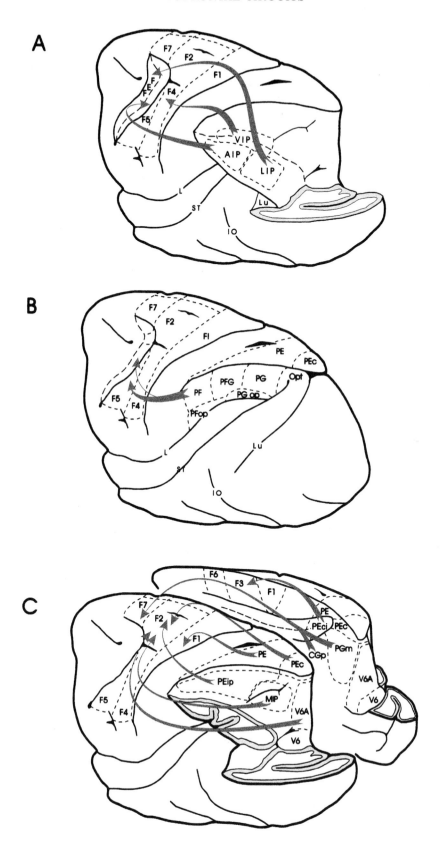

Area AIP is richly connected with F5, mostly with that part of F5 buried within the posterior bank of the inferior arcuate sulcus, where distal arm movements are represented (Fig. 5.2A) (16). F5 neurons discharge during specific goal-directed actions performed with the hand, mouth, or both. The most common action effective in triggering them is grasping. Most grasping neurons code specific types of hand prehension, such as precision grip, whole-hand prehension, and finger prehension (17). Similarly to AIP neurons, many F5 neurons are driven by the presentation of three-dimensional (3-D) objects, even when no immediate or subsequent action on the object is allowed (18). Taken together, these data suggest that AIP-F5 circuit plays a crucial role in transforming the intrinsic properties of the object into the appropriate hand movements (19).

Strong support for this hypothesis was recently provided by studies in which the two areas were inactivated separately (20). The main effect observed following independent inactivation of AIP and the bank of F5 was a disruption of the preshaping of the hand during grasping. The monkey, by relying on tactile information, still was able to grasp objects; therefore, the lesion of this circuit does not disrupt the ability to perform grasping movements, but rather it affects only the capacity to transform the 3-D properties of the object into appropriate hand movements.

PF–F5 convexity Circuit

Area PF lies in the rostral part of the convexity of the IPL. Previous physiologic studies showed that this area contains an arm and a face representation (Fig. 5.1). PF neurons are responsive to somatosensory or visual stimuli or both [bimodal neurons (21)]. The major motor target of area PF is the convexity of area F5 (Fig 5.2B).

Recently, it has been reported that neurons in this part of F5, although indistinguishable from those located within the bank of inferior arcuate sulcus in their motor properties, are markedly different in their visual properties.

The main characteristic of these neurons is that they discharge when the monkey observes another individual performing an action similar to that coded by the neuron. Object presentation is not sufficient to activate them. Because of this correspondence between visual and motor properties, these neurons were called "mirror neurons" (22).

The observed actions that most commonly activate the mirror neurons are: grasping, placing, manipulating objects. Most of them respond selectively when the monkey watches only one type of action (e.g., grasping). Typically, mirror neurons show congruence between the type of observed action and the action coded by the neuron.

Preliminary data showed that neurons with characteristics similar to those of mirror neurons are present in PF but their properties have not been yet studied in details (23).

These findings suggest an important cognitive role for the motor cortex that could be achieved in collaboration with area PF: that of representing actions internally. This internal representation, when evoked by an action made by others, should be involved in two related functions: action imitation and action recognition (for theoretic considerations, see 22).

VIP–F4 Circuit

Area VIP occupies the fundus of the IPL (Fig. 5.1) (26) and receives visual projections from various areas belonging to the dorsal visual stream [among them, areas medial superior temporal (MST) and middle temporal (MT)] MST involved in motion analysis (24). In addition, VIP receives somatosensory information from areas PEc and PFG (25).

Two main categories of VIP neurons are of interest with regard to spatial representation: (a) purely visual neurons and (b) bimodal, visual, and somatosensory neurons (26). Purely visual neurons are sensitive to moving stimuli. Bimodal neurons can be driven independently by visual and tactile stimuli. Their cutaneous receptive fields are located predominantly on the face, and their visual receptive fields are tied to the tactile ones. For many neurons, visual stimuli are effective only when located in the space around the body (*peripersonal space*). The visual receptive field of about 30% of visually responsive neurons is coded in egocentric, not in retinal coordinates (27).

The main motor target of area VIP is area F4 (Fig. 5.2A) (16). In F4, the arm, neck, face, and mouth movements are represented in a mediolateral topographic arrangement (28). As in area VIP, also in F4 bimodal and unimodal neurons can be identified (29). In contrast to VIP, however, unimodal neurons are typically driven by cutaneous stimulation, whereas pure visual sensitive neurons are extremely rare. Their tactile receptive fields, usually rather large, are predominantly located on the face, arm and the upper part of the body. The visual RFs of bimodal neurons are located in the peripersonal space, in register with the tactile fields. In about 70% of these neurons, the position of the visual receptive field does not change when the gaze moves. Similarly, the visual receptive field remains tied to the cutaneous receptive field when the body part, on which the tactile receptive field is located, is moved. Taken together, these properties indicate that in F4 the space is coded in coordinates centered on body parts (29,30). In conclusion, the functional properties of VIP–F4 circuit suggest that this circuit plays a crucial role in coding the peripersonal space and in transforming object locations into appropriate movements toward them.

LIP–FEF Circuit

Area LIP lies in the caudal sector of the lateral bank of the intraparietal sulcus (Fig. 5.1) is target of strong projections from several visual extrastriate areas [parieto–occipital area (PO), V3, V3a, V4, MT, and MST; (31)] and projects almost exclusively to area 8 (i.e., FEF) of the frontal lobe (Fig. 5.2A). Both LIP and FEF send descending projections to the superior colliculus (32).

Three main classes of neurons characterize the LIP–FEF circuit: neurons sensitive to the visual stimuli (*visual neurons*), neurons active

in relation with eye movements (*movement neurons*), and neurons showing both visual and movement-related activity [*visuomovement neurons* (33,34)]. Pure visual neurons usually have large receptive fields and respond strongly to stationary stimuli. Movement neurons discharge in association with saccades, more frequently before the saccade onset. Visuomovement neurons show both visual and saccade-related activity with the visual receptive fields in register with the "motor" field. In both LIP and FEF, the visual receptive fields are coded in a retinotopic frame of reference; when the eyes move, the receptive field also moves. A peculiar property of most LIP neurons is that their firing to visual stimuli is modulated by the position of the eyes (*gaze effect*). This property suggests that although the discharge intensity does not specify, *per se,* the spatial position, the absolute location of the triggering stimulus in space can be derived by the firing intensity of different neurons. These findings suggest that the LIP–FEF circuit plays an important role in transforming spatial information from retinocentric to craniocentric frame of reference for the oculomotor control.

PARIETOFRONTAL CIRCUITS OF THE SPL

The SPL is the major source of projections to PMd. These connections are organized into three skeletomotor and two visuomotor circuits. Figure 5.2C shows these connections.

PE–F1 Circuit

Since the classic studies by Sakata et al. (35) and Mountcastle et al. (36), area PE (area 5) is considered a higher-order somatosensory area whose neurons are mostly sensitive to specific combinations of multiple joint positions or combination of joint and skin stimuli. Lacquaniti et al. (37) provided evidence that area PE codes the location of the arm in space in a body-centered coordinate system. Therefore, the role proposed for PE–F1 circuit (Fig. 5.2C) is to transform information on body parts location into information necessary for the control of body parts movements. No visual inputs reach area PE (4).

PEci–F3 Circuit

The caudal part of the cingulate sulcus (Fig. 5.1) is occupied by area PEci, which, according to Pandya and Seltzer (38), is generally included in the SPL. Area PEci is connected with areas PE, PEc, and PGm. Although little functional evidence exists in this regard, this area is also known as a *supplementary sensory area* because it was reported to contain a complete somatosensory map of the body (39).

The main source of input to area F3 is PEci (Fig. 5.2C). Microstimulation studies showed that F3 contains a somatotopically organized representation of body movements (40).

Many neurons in F3 are sensitive to somatosensory stimuli (41). As in F1, the large majority of F3 neurons discharge in association with active movements; however, F3 differs from F1 because in F1 proximal and distal movements are anatomically segregated, whereas they are mixed in F3 (40). Furthermore, although there is some controversy (9), most authors agree that in F3 proximal movements are much more represented than distal movements (5,40). This is not the case for F1. On the basis of clinical data, Massion and co-workers (42) suggested that F3 is involved in the postural adjustments that precede voluntary movements. Taken together, these data suggest that the PEci–F3 circuit elaborates somatosensory information that is used mostly for postural purpose.

PEc/PEip–F2 dimple and MIP–F2 ventrorostral Circuits

The rostral part of the medial bank of IP is occupied by area PEip, defined as that part of the bank projecting to the spinal cord (43). In several studies, neurons were recorded from this area and showed that most of them respond to somatosensory stimuli and may become active in association with arm movements with directional selectivity (36,44). The directional tuning is usually broad.

Area PEc is located in the caudal sector of the dorsal aspect of SPL and is richly connected with area PE (38). It is likely that area PEc, like PE, is involved in the analysis of somatosensory stimuli for movement organization, whereas PEip and PEc appear to be involved mostly in somatosensory control of movements, both area MIP (45) and area V6A (46) use visual information for the same purpose.

Neurons responding both to visual and somatosensory stimulation were frequently recorded in MIP (45). Detailed information, however, about the functional properties of this area is lacking. More data are available on area V6A. About half of V6A neurons discharge in response to visual stimuli, whereas the remainder discharge mostly in association with eye or arm movements (46,47).

All four parietal areas described in this section project to area F2. Areas PEip and PEc project mostly to the dimple region of F2, whereas areas MIP and V6A project to the ventrorostral F2 (Fig. 5.2C).

The dimple region of F2 is somatotopically organized. Leg movements are represented dorsal to the dimple, whereas arm movements are located ventral to it (8,48). Functional studies of F2 have focused mostly on the motor properties of its neurons, showing that F2 neurons either discharge in association with movement onset or become active in advance of it. It is likely that neurons showing this anticipatory discharge play a role in motor preparation (4,49,50). There is little information about the responses of F2 neurons to sensory stimuli. Preliminary observations from our laboratory indicate that there is a differential distribution of sensory properties within F2. In the dimple region, most neurons respond to proprioceptive stimuli; in ventrorostral F2, neurons respond also to tactile and visual stimulation (51). This functional segregation of sensory modalities within F2 is consistent with the parietal input to the two F2 subregions.

In conclusion, the PEip/PEc–F2 dimple circuit appears to be involved in planning and controlling arm (and leg) movements on the basis of somatosensory information. In contrast, the MIP/V6A–F2 ventrorostral circuit uses somatosensory and visual information, probably for the same purpose. The optic ataxia symptoms, which typically result as a consequence of damage to superior parietal lobule (2), fit this hypothesis well.

PGm–F7 Circuit

Area PGm, which is located in the mesial wall of the SPL (Fig. 5.1) is cytoarchitecturally similar to area PG (38), from which it receives strong projections. Other connections are with areas PEc, MIP, V6, and LIP (for references, see 14); thus, on area PGm, visual and somatosensory information can converge. The physiologic properties of this area are, however, still largely unknown. Area PGm is the major source of parietal input to lateral F7 (Fig. 5.2C); but, given our limited knowledge about the functional properties of this frontal area, no speculations can be made about the role played by the PGm-F7 circuit in the sensory–motor transformation for action.

CONCLUSION

The existence in the posterior parietal cortex of multiple areas, with specific sensory inputs and privileged motor targets, indicates that the anatomic basis of the transformation of sensory information into actions is represented by several parallel parietofrontal circuits. Psychophysical studies showed the decomposition of reaching to a visual target into a projection of the arm (*transport phase*) and a phase in which the hand adapts to the spatial contours of the target (*grasping phase*). Analysis of the two components indicated that they rely on markedly different visuomotor transformations that are processed separately in the brain (52). These two phases have been selectively damaged by lesions located in different parts of the parietal lobe, suggesting that different circuits are involved in the vi-

suomotor transformations for reaching and grasping. Furthermore, the clinical observation that patients suffering from optic ataxia are impaired in reaching accurately toward a visual target, but still are able to perform correctly movements toward the body, indicates that reaching is not a unitary entity. Movements away and toward the body are possibly mediated by different circuits.

How do the parietofrontal circuits operate? The problem of sensory–motor integration has been addressed within the frame of a serial, hierarchical model of information processing. The result of the elaboration of converging sensory information performed by the posterior parietal cortex is conveyed to the executive areas of the frontal lobe. A copy (*corollary discharge*) of this command then may be sent back to the parietal cortex. This model assigns a fundamental role to parietal areas, leaving to frontal areas the role of motor execution. Perception and action then would be localized in separate cortical domains.

In a recent review of the neural characteristics of the F5–AIP cortical circuit for grasping, Gallese et al. (20) proposed a different model that assigns to the motor areas an important role in the visuomotor transformation for grasping. According to this model, AIP would translate the 3-D characteristics of the object into different grasping movements and send these options to F5, which, in turn, would choose the most suitable one on the basis of contextual information. Then, by means of recurrent connections, F5 would keep active in AIP only the set of neurons involved in the selected type of grasping. In other words, F5 instructs AIP about which, among the several possible grasping options, one is most appropriate. Therefore, the visuomotor transformation required for grasping objects is the result of the interplay between parietal and motor areas.

In conclusion, it is now clear that the neural activities of the posterior parietal cortex related to sensorimotor transformation for action and to higher cognitive functions are strongly influenced by the activity of the motor cortices. Therefore, for a better knowledge of the posterior parietal cortex functions, it will be necessary, in the future, to address specifically the issue of the role played by the frontoparietal projections in the information processing occurring in the posterior parietal cortex.

ACKNOWLEDGMENTS

Supported by European Community Contract n-BMH4-CT95-0789 and Ministers dell' Universita' e delle Ricerca Scientifica e Tecnologica (MURST).

REFERENCES

1. Critchley M. *The parietal lobes*. New York: Hafner Press, 1953:480.
2. Milner AD, Goodale MA. *The visual brain in action*. Oxford: Oxford University Press, 1995:248.
3. Rizzolatti G, Fogassi L, Gallese V. Parietal cortex: from sight to action. *Curr Opin Neurobiol* 1997;7:562–567.
4. Caminiti R, Ferraina S, Johnson PB. The sources of visual information to the primate frontal lobe: a novel role for the superior parietal lobule. *Cereb Cortex* 1996; 6:319–328.
5. Woolsey CN, Settlage PH, Meyer DR, et al. Patterns of localization in precentral and "supplementary" motor areas and their relation to the concept of a premotor area. *Res Publ Assoc Nerv Ment Dis* 1952;30:238–264.
6. Matelli M, Luppino G. Functional anatomy of human motor cortical areas. In: Boller F, Grafman J, eds. *Handbook of neuropsychology*, vol 11. Amsterdam: Elsevier, 1997:9–26.
7. Schlag J, Schlag-Rey M. Evidence for a supplementary eye field. *J Neurophysiol* 1987;57:179–200.
8. He SQ, Dum RP, Strick PL. Topographic organization of corticospinal projections from the frontal lobe: motor areas on the lateral surface of the hemisphere. *J Neurosci* 1993;13:952–980.
9. He SQ, Dum RP, Strick PL. Topographic organization of corticospinal projections from the frontal lobe: motor areas on the medial surface of the hemisphere. *J Neurosci* 1995;15:3284–3306.
10. Keizer K, Kuypers HGJM. Distribution of corticospinal neurons with collaterals to the lower brain stem reticular formation in monkey *(Macaca fascicularis)*. *Exp Brain Res* 1989;74:311–318.
11. Barbas H, Pandya DN. Architecture and frontal cortical connections of the premotor cortex (area 6) in the rhesus monkey. *J Comp Neurol* 1987;256:211–228.
12. Luppino G, Matelli M, Camarda R, et al. Corticocortical connections of area F3 (SMA-Proper) and area F6 (Pre-SMA) in the macaque monkey. *J Comp Neurol* 1993;338:114–140.
13. Huerta MF, Kaas JH. Supplementary eye field as defined by intracortical microstimulation: connections in Macaques. *J Comp Neurol* 1990;293:299–330.
14. Rizzolatti G, Luppino G, Matelli M. The organization of the cortical motor system: new concepts. *Electroencephalogr Clin Neurophsiol* 1998;106:283–296.
15. Sakata H, Taira M, Murata A, et al. Neural mechanisms of visual guidance of hand action in the parietal cortex of the monkey. *Cereb Cortex* 1995;5:429–438.
16. Luppino G, Murata A, Govoni P, et al. Independent parietofrontal circuits linking rostral intraparietal cortex (areas AIP and VIP) and the ventral premotor cortex (areas F5 and F4). *Exp Brain Res* 1999;128:181–187.
17. Rizzolatti G, Camarda R, Fogassi M, et al. Functional organization of inferior area 6 in the macaque monkey: II. Area F5 and the control of distal movements. *Exp Brain Res* 1988;71:491–507.
18. Murata A, Fadiga L, Fogassi L, et al. Object representation in the ventral premotor cortex (area F5) of the monkey. *J Neurophysiol* 1997;78:2226–2230.
19. Jeannerod M, Arbib MA, Rizzolatti G, et al. Grasping objects: the cortical mechanisms of visuomotor transformation. *Trends Neurosci* 1995;18:314–320.
20. Gallese V, Fadiga L, Fogassi L, et al. A parietal-frontal circuit for hand grasping movements in the monkey: evidence from reversible inactivation experiments. In: Thier P, Karnath H-O, eds. *Parietal lobe contributions to orientation in 3D space*. Heidelberg: Springer, 1997:255–270.
21. Hyvärinen J. Posterior parietal lobe of the primate brain. *Physiol Rev* 1982;62:1060–1129.
22. Rizzolatti G, Fadiga L, Gallese V, et al. Premotor cortex and the recognition of motor actions. *Cognitive Brain Research* 1996;3:131–141.
23. Fogassi L, Gallese V, Fadiga L, et al. Neurons responding to the sight of goal-directed hand/arm actions in the parietal area PF (7b) of the macaque monkey. *Soc Neurosci Abstr* 1998;24.
24. Boussaoud D, Ungerleider L, Desimone R. Pathways for motion analysis: cortical connections of the medial superior temporal and fundus of the superior temporal visual areas in the macaque. *J Comp Neurol* 1990;296: 462–495.
25. Seltzer B, Pandya DN. Posterior parietal projections to the intraparietal sulcus of the rhesus monkey. *Exp Brain Res* 1986;62:459–469.
26. Colby CL, Duhamel J-R, Goldberg ME. Ventral intraparietal area of the macaque: anatomic location and visual response properties. *J Neurophysiol* 1993;69: 902–914.
27. Bremmer F, Duhamel J-R, Ben Hamed S. Non-retinocentric coding of visual space in the macaque ventral intraparietal area (VIP). *Soc Neurosci Abstr* 1996;22: 666–668.
28. Gentilucci M, Fogassi L, Luppino G, et al. Functional organization of inferior area 6 in the macaque monkey: I. Somatotopy and the control of proximal movements. *Exp Brain Res* 1988;71:475–490.
29. Fogassi L, Gallese V, Fadiga L, et al. Coding of peripersonal space in inferior premotor cortex (area F4). *J Neurophysiol* 1996;76:141–157.
30. Graziano MSA, Yap GS, Gross CG. Coding of visual space by premotor neurons. *Science* 1994;266:1054–1057.
31. Andersen RA, Asanuma C, Essick G, et al. Corticocortical connections of anatomically and physiologically defined subdivisions within the inferior parietal lobule. *J Comp Neurol* 1990;296:65–113.
32. Lynch JC, Graybiel AM, Lobeck LJ. The differential projection of two cytoarchitectonic subregions of the inferior parietal lobule of macaque upon the deep layers of the superior colliculus. *J Comp Neurol* 1985;235: 241–254.

33. Andersen R, Gnadt JW. Role of posterior parietal cortex in saccadic eye movements. In: Wurtz R, Goldberg M, eds. *The neurobiology of saccadic eye movements.* Amsterdam: Elsevier, 1989:315–335.

34. Goldberg M, Segraves MA. The visual and frontal cortices. In: Wurtz R, Goldberg M, eds. *The neurobiology of saccadic eye movements.* Amsterdam: Elsevier, 1989: 283–313.

35. Sakata H, Takaoka Y, Kawarasaki A, et al. Somatosensory properties of neurons in the superior parietal cortex (area 5) of the rhesus monkey. *Brain Res* 1973;64: 85–102.

36. Mountcastle VB, Lynch JCGA, Sakata H, et al. Posterior parietal association cortex of the monkey: command functions for operations within extrapersonal space. *J Neurophysiol* 1975;38:871–908.

37. Lacquaniti F, Guigon E, Bianchi L, et al. Representing spatial information for limb movement: role of area 5 in the monkey. *Cereb Cortex* 1995;5:391–409.

38. Pandya DN, Seltzer B. Intrinsic connections and architectonics of posterior parietal cortex in the rhesus monkey. *J Comp Neurol* 1982;204:196–210.

39. Murray EA, Coulter JD. Supplementary sensory area. In: Woolsey CN, eds. *Cortical sensory organization,* vol 1: *Multiple somatic areas.* Clifton, NJ: Humana Press, 1981:167–195.

40. Luppino G, Matelli M, Camarda R, et al. Multiple representations of body movements in mesial area 6 and the adjacent cingulate cortex: an intracortical microstimulation study. *J Comp Neurol* 1991;311:463–482.

41. Wiesendanger M. Recent developments in studies of the supplementary motor area of primates. *Rev Physiol Biochem Pharmacol* 1986;103:1–59.

42. Massion J. Movement, posture, and equilibrium: interaction and coordination. *Progr Neurobiol* 1992;38: 35–56.

43. Matelli M, Govoni P, Galletti C, et al. Superior area 6 afferents from the superior parietal lobule in the macaque monkey. *J Comp Neurol* 1998;402:327–352.

44. Kalaska JF, Cohen DAD, Prud'homme M, et al. Parietal area 5 neuronal activity encodes movement kinematics, not movement dynamics. *Exp Brain Res* 1990;80: 351–364.

45. Colby CL, Duhamel J-R. Heterogeneity of extrastriate visual areas and multiple parietal areas in the macaque monkeys. *Neuropsychologia* 1991;29:517–537.

46. Galletti C, Fattori P, Battaglini PP, et al. Functional demarcation of a border between areas V6 and V6A in the superior parietal gyrus of the macaque monkey. *Eur J Neurosci* 1996;8:30–52.

47. Galletti C, Fattori P, Kutz DF, et al. Arm movement-related neurons in visual area V6A of the macaque superior parietal lobule. *Eur J Neurosci* 1997;9: 410–413.

48. Kurata K. Distribution of neurons with set- and movement-related activity before hand and foot movements in the premotor cortex of rhesus monkey. *Exp Brain Res* 1989;77:245–256.

49. Kurata K, Hoffman DS. Differential effects of muscimol microinjection into dorsal and ventral aspects of the premotor cortex of monkeys. *J Neurophysiol* 1994;71: 1151–1164.

50. Wise SP, Boussaoud D, Johnson PB, et al. Premotor and parietal cortex: corticocortical connectivity and combinatorial computations. *Annu Rev Neurosci* 1997;20: 25–42.

51. Fogassi L, Raos V, Franchi G, et al. Visual responses in the dorsal premotor area F2 of the macaque monkey. *Exp Brain Res* 1999;128:194–199.

52. Jeannerod M. *The neural and behavioral organization of goal-directed movements.* Oxford: Clarendon Press, 1988:283.

Neocortical Epilepsies.
Advances in Neurology, Vol. 84,
edited by P. D. Williamson, A. M. Siegel,
D. W. Roberts, V. M. Thadani, and M. S. Gazzaniga.
Lippincott Williams & Wilkins, Philadelphia © 2000.

6

Sensorimotor Processing in Parietal Neocortex

Hans-Joachim Freund

Department of Neurology, Heinrich Heine University Düsseldorf,
D-40225 Düsseldorf, Germany

The functional anatomy of the parietal lobe as described for the monkey in the chapter by Matelli and Luppino (Chapter 5) has undergone major changes in the human. Figure 6.1 shows the comparison between the Brodmann cytoarchitectonic maps for monkeys and humans. It is in particular the posterior parietal cortex (PPC) that has greatly expanded in the human. The PPC is subdivided by the intraparietal sulcus (IPS) into a superior parietal lobule (SPL) and an inferior parietal lobule (IPL). As shown in Fig. 5.1 in Matelli's chapter in this book, the monkey IPS comprises a variety of different functional modules. Their functional homologies to the human IPS are as unclear as the homologies for Brodmann (BM) areas 5, 7, 39, and 40. In this chapter, the somatosensory, motor, visuomotor and at-

tentional aspects of parietal lobe function are considered on the basis of lesion and activation studies and discussed in relation to monkey data (Fig. 6.1).

ROLE OF PARIETAL LOBE IN SOMATOSENSORY FUNCTIONS

Anterior Parietal Lobe

The well-known concept of a dichotomy of visual information flow into a ventral and a dorsal stream holds that the ventral stream relates to the cognitive aspects of visual information processing, whereas the dorsal stream funnels into parietal processing stages related to action and visuomotor processing (1,2). This concept is supported by lesion studies in pri-

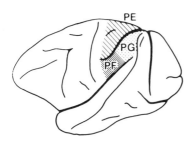 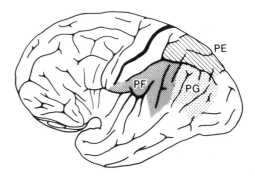

FIG. 6.1. Lateral views of monkey and human cerebral hemispheres showing the major differences particularly for the posterior parietal cortex.

mate and human subjects that revealed that patients with temporal lesions show visual cognitive disturbances, such as the various agnosias, but leave visuomotor processing intact (3).

In contrast to the visual modality, somatosensory information is thoroughly processed in the parietal lobe, including its cognitive aspects. This is particularly obvious for the sophisticated functions of the hand. The employment of the hand for object recognition and manipulation is a prominent feature of hand function. If the projection areas on the postcentral gyrus are damaged, the situation resembles that in deafferentated patients with concomitant breakdown of complex somatosensory functions such as graphesthesia and stereognosis.

The effects of postcentral excisions (4) or lesions (5–7) are classically described as closely resembling the effects of deafferentation with prominent ataxia, dysmetria, and poverty of movement. Foerster (4) reported that surgical excisions of the postcentral gyrus lead initially to complete anaesthesia, areflexia, and hypotonia of the contralateral side and to a disturbance of motility with slightly diminished force and slowing of movement. The execution of accurate movements or the selective muscle activation required for fractionated finger movements becomes impossible. Ataxia becomes prominent, closely resembling that seen after dorsal root section. Excess activation of the agonist and antagonist muscles leads to discontinuous movement patterns. Dystonic posturing is frequently seen, and control of the fine finger movements during prehension and object manipulation or exploration is impaired.

Posterior Parietal Lobe

Lesions of the Superior Posterior Parietal Cortex

Damage of the SPL is associated with impairment of complex somatosensory functions, such as object recognition *(astereognosis)* and identification of materials or textures without deficits of elementary somatosensory functions. On the motor side, the hand is severely compromised so that active touch, object exploration, and manipulation are disturbed (8). Quantitative analysis of hand and finger movements in these patients showed a derangement of the dynamics in the digital palpation of objects, along with a breakdown of the finely tuned scanning process of the fingers, preventing the sequential sampling of mechanoreceptive information. The essence of this disturbance lies in the impairment of the conception and generation of the spatiotemporal movement patterns required to bring those receptor sheets into action that normally would provide the information underlying the identification and manipulation of objects.

The sensory information obtained by the hand comprises two component elements: *exteroceptive* and *proprioceptive*. The combination of these two inputs is the important variable specifying the difference between touching and being touched (9). Active touch can elaborate the unity, stability, plasticity, and shape of phenomenal objects. When a single object is grasped with several fingers, the subject perceives one object only, although several cutaneous receptor sheets are engaged. The complex feature extraction relating spatial information about corners, edges, and straight planes can be distinguished with respect to their interrelationship, even when subjects cannot identify the patterns formed by the various cutaneous pressures. The percept is the object form and not skin form because the movements of the fingers are not continuously perceived. Features like curvatures, planarities, and slant of surface with respect to gravity, parallelity, plane angles, and distances all have to underlie object identification. In patients with lesions around the anterior part of the IPS, there is a disturbance of the ability to engage the hand in the motor performance required to collect that sensory information. As to the shaping of input necessary to gain the information about external objects, this cannot be properly accomplished. The extraction of sensory features relies on the adequacy of the purposive motor acts. Consequently, somatosensory association cortex is not only involved in the processing of somatosensory information but also in the elaboration of the movement concepts adequately matching the object features.

The disturbance of this process leads to a specific unimodal sensorimotor dysfunction, confined to the somatosensory modality, and affecting only the contralesional hand (8, 10–12). In cases with isolated somatomotor deficits, visuomotor performances or the employment of the hand for tasks unrelated to active touch and object manipulation may be well preserved. Clinically, this somatomotor deficit was earlier described by Delay (13), who coined the term *tactile apraxia* as being a loss of the tactile use of objects combined with tactile agnosia. Tactile apraxia represents a unimodal somatomotor apraxia that can be allocated to the SPL, most likely the anterior part of IPS, a possible homologue of area AIP (anterior intraparietal sulcus) in the monkey. This area is known to be involved in the control of grasping (14–16,40). Evidence for a prominent role of AIP in humans comes from combined lesion-activation studies [for review see Schnitzler et al. (17)] showing that the common zone of lesion overlap in patients with tactile apraxia and the activated area during grasping is approximately coextensive (Fig. 6.2).

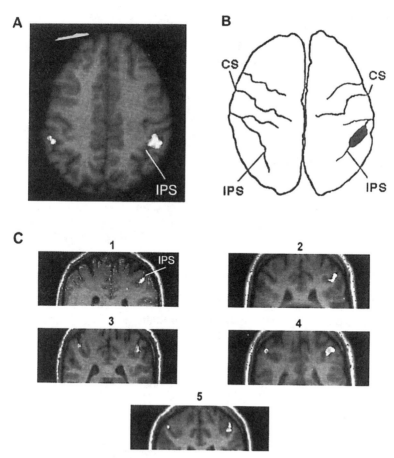

FIG. 6.2. A: fMRI study during grasping compared with pointing shows a significant activation area in the anterior lateral bank of the intraparietal sulcus in a normal subject. **B:** The activated area corresponds to the location of the common zone of overlap in the patients with lesions including anterior IPS and prehension deficits. **C:** The stereotactic coordinates were $x = -45$; $y = -35$; $z = 43$. *CS,* central sulcus. The localization of the activation foci in the coronal sections of the five volunteers is, despite the obvious interindividual variations in sulcal anatomy, consistent across subjects. (From Binkofski F, Dohle C, Posse S, et al. Human anterior intraparietal area subserves prehension: a combined lesion and functional MRI activation study. *Neurology* 1998;50:1253–1259, with permission.)

Damage of the Inferior Posterior Parietal Lobule

The effects of lesions of the IPL depend on the side of the lesion. Damage to the language-dominant hemisphere is associated with ideational or ideomotor apraxia and the Gerstmann syndrome. According to Liepmann's (18,19) definition, ideational apraxia is characterised by a deficiency in the conception of the movement so that the patient does not know what to do or how to organize movement sequences. In ideokinetic (ideomotor) apraxia, the patient does not know how to perform a particular motor act, such as a gesture. The disturbance affects both sides of the body and often is associated with aphasia. On the basis of observations about the apraxias, Liepmann postulated that the left hemisphere is not only dominant for language but also for praxis. The apraxias seen after IPL damage are supramodal in nature. This is compatible with the presumed supramodal organisation proposed for the human IPL.

Unlike language organization, where the minor hemisphere is virtually unable to maintain residual language functions after the age of 10 to 14 years, the right hemisphere is fully able to concert the whole movement repertoire for the opposite side of the body. Damage of the corpus callosum can produce an apraxia of the left hand but only because language information is not available to that hemisphere. The reason a left hemisphere lesion interferes with the otherwise normal control of left-sided motor behavior by the right hemisphere is unclear. Freeman (20) proposed that the principal function of the left hemisphere is instrumentation of a priority of action control.

The plasticity of sensory motor processing is illustrated by observations on deaf-mute patients (21) using American Sign Language (ASL). The fact that a visual–gestural communication system can substitute for the auditory–vocal system, illustrates the capacity of the human nervous system to deal with symbolic and iconic information in a context-specific way, irrespective of the sensory modality or the motor subsystem involved. In patients with left hemisphere damage, the breakdown in the capacity to communicate by ASL affects both comprehension and production. The patients' inability to produce the spatiotemporal trajectories required for ASL stands in contrast to the flawless performance of a range of tasks, including drawing, spatial construction, spatial attention, judgment of line orientation, and spatial discrimination. Conversely, right hemisphere–damaged deaf-mute ASL patients showed gross impairment in the latter tasks but were flawless in ASL.

In terms of motor performance, ASL motor aphasia is also an apraxia. As in the case of the unimodal apraxias such deficiencies are highly specific, as was shown by a series of apraxia tests in the signers with left hemisphere lesions and ASL aphasia. The results showed that the language deficiencies were due to specific linguistic components of sign language rather than to an underlying motor disorder of the capacity to express and comprehend symbols, or of the production and imitation of representational and nonrepresentational movements. This finding demonstrates that, in aphasic and apraxic disturbances, only specific functions are selectively disturbed. This is also the case in agnosias. Furthermore, it raises another interesting point, namely, that sign language aphasia is a special type of apraxia in ASL patients, affecting comprehension and the generation of limb movements that convey linguistic information. This is consistent with Liepmann's interpretation of the disorders of verbal expression as apraxia of the speech muscles.

Lesions affecting the left angular gyrus have been associated with the Gerstmann syndrome, a combination of agraphia, acalculia, finger agnosia, and right–left disturbances. These signs often do not occur together but may occur in any combination.

Lesions of the right IPL frequently are associated with constructional apraxia (22). This deficiency is characterized by difficulty in putting one-dimensional units together to form two- or three-dimensional figures or patterns. It appears in formative activities, such as arranging, building, or drawing, where the specialized part of the task is faulty, although the movement elements are normal. It also has been seen with lesions of the dominant hemisphere but typically is observed with lesions of the nondominant side. Patients with damage of the right parietal lobe also may have an impairment of spatial orientation, route-finding, and topographic memory.

VISUOMOTOR PROCESSING

Lesions in the occipito-parietal area in humans and in the posterior parietal area in primates produce visuomotor ataxia characterized by misreaching and false gaze direction. Visual cognitive functions are less compromised in these patients. The disturbance originally was described as *optic ataxia* (23) and later as *visuomotor ataxia* (24). The movement disturbance affects only the visual domain, representing another unimodal movement disturbance. Again, there is a perceptive, a cognitive, and a motor aspect of the dysfunction: the imperfect perception of distances and spatial relationships paralleled by inadequate target-directed adjustment of the arm and eyes and by a grossly deranged movement pattern. This makes the condition different from purely ataxic disturbances, in which the process of aiming is faulty, but the movement is otherwise executed with a correct kinematic pattern. Therefore, the apraxic motor behavior is distinctly different from that observed in acutely blind patients, who can easily remember target location and perform smooth and accurate movements to remembered targets. In contrast, patients with optic ataxia show grossly deranged trajectories of reaching, aiming, grasping, and hand preshaping. Their ability to learn to reach for targets with known locations cued by proprioceptive or acoustic input is poor. For these reasons, we prefer the term *visuomotor apraxia* to characterize the deficient visual guidance and also the apraxic kinematic features (8,11,27). The location of the common zone of overlap of the lesions reported to be

associated with visuomotor ataxia [for review, see Rondot et al. (24)] is still unclear. Most were bilateral and scattered around the occipito-parietal junction. Since Haaxma and Kuypers (28) observed visuomotor ataxia after transsection of the long occipito-frontal association fibers in the white matter underlying that area, such a deficit could represent a disconnection syndrome. This explanation is difficult to sustain in view of the absence of data on anterior lesions interrupting these long corticocortical tracts. An alternative possibility was suggested by Classen et al. (27), who observed visuomotor ataxia/apraxia after subcortical lesions below the level of the long corticocortical association fibers, but damaging the parietopontine projections conveying visual signals toward the brainstem (29,30). Here the integration with vestibular and proprioceptive information provides the basis for the complex postural and oculomotor orienting behavior (Fig. 6.3).

The problem of the interpretation of lesion studies is always in how far cortical or subcortical fiber damage is causing the resulting deficits. In most cases, this cannot be disentangled, as most `cortical' lesions are both, that is, combined cortical–subcortical destructions. Some purely cortical lesions, however, may be of particular interest for the parietal epilepsies. Figure 6.3 shows a case with selective cortical necrosis as it typically occurs after short-lasting focal ischemia caused by emboli. This lesion type is well known from neuropathology and can be recognized on magnetic resonance imaging scan by the typical cortical lining in contrast-enhanced images. In these cases, the deficits can be attributed to the cortical lesion.

Visuomotor processing has been investigated extensively for the act of reaching and grasping, and a wealth of information is available about the neuronal mechanisms underlying these behaviors in the monkey that can be compared with lesion and activation studies in the human. Experimentally, it has been shown that sensory signals from many modalities—visual, vestibular, auditory and somatosensory—are combined in area 7a lateral intra-

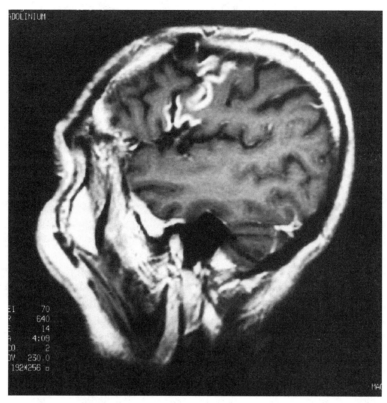

FIG. 6.3. Gadolinium-enhanced MRI scan showing a selectively cortical stroke lesion.

parietal sulcus (LIP) (31) and (medial superior temporal area (MST) to code for the spatial location of goals for movement (32–36). Hereby, the multimodal signals can build a common reference frame but also can concurrently code target locations in multiple coordinate frames required for different behaviors, such as the control of gaze or an arm or of navigation. The central proprioceptive representation of the spatiotemporal pattern of arm movements and postures as signalled by neurones in area 5 is also required for the construction of a body-centered reference frame (37). According to the functional anatomy of these functional modules as described in Chapter 5 by Matelli and Luppino in this book, chemical lesions of single areas lead to selective disturbances, such as those of reaching or grasping (14,38,39).

Although such small focal lesions are rarely seen in human patients, detailed kine-matic analysis of a few cases disclosed similar structure–function relationships. Complementary information was obtained from activation studies in normal subjects, in whom specific grasp-induced activations appeared at the same location, but in the patients, lesions interfered with that behavior (40). An example of such a combined lesion-activation approach was shown in Fig. 6.2: when the common zone of overlap is around the anterior intraparietal sulcus (AIP), the patients' characteristic deficit is a disturbance of grasping, whereas lesions of more posterior parts of the IPS interfere with reaching without affecting grasping.

A specific deficit of visuomotor processing was described as *mirror agnosia* (41–43). This disturbance is characterised by the fact that the patients, when seeing an object through a mirror, believe the object is actually in the mirror and keep grasping there without being able to learn from other cues that the real object is indeed somewhere else. Another group of patients was aware of the real position of the object but could not point to or grasp correctly the objects shown through a mirror. They misreached somewhere between the mirror and the real object with frequent corrections of the movement trajectory. Because of the correct cognitive but ataxic motor behavior, *mirror ataxia* was the term chosen to describe their characteristic disturbance. The lesions in patients with mirror agnosia scattered around the occipito-temporal-parietal Carrefour and the lesions in the patients with mirror ataxia around the intraparietal sulcus (Fig. 6.4).

A typical recording of the movement trajectory is shown in Fig. 6.4; one patient with mirror agnosia performs normal movements toward the mirror without corrections. The velocity profile shows that the trajectory formation is normal. In contrast, the patient with visuomotor ataxia shows a variable and hesitating performance with frequent corrections. The velocity profile is deranged, and the spatial trajectory remains ataxic. Consequently, the lesion site in mirror agnosia is likely to interfere more with cognitive aspects of visual information processing, whereas the lesion site in visuomotor ataxia interferes with visuomotor functions. It is unclear whether the agnostic part results from damage of the IPL or even from subcortical fiber destruction of the SPL, but it is likely to be parietal rather than temporal, because lesion scatter might affect the superior temporal cortex but not the visual ventral route in the inferior temporal lobe.

ATTENTIONAL MECHANISMS

Ample evidence has been found that the parietal lobe, in particular the IPL, plays an important role in regulating attention. Although most functional imaging studies in humans imply a prominent role for SPL in visual attention (44,45), nonhuman primate brain studies (32,46–48) and neuropsychological studies in patients (49) strongly suggest that the inferior parts of the posterior parietal lobe are crucially important for visuospatial attention.

There are several possible reasons for this discrepancy. For example, in covert attention tasks, some of the activations observed in response to visual stimuli seem to lie within and around the IPS. In primates, neural activity has been demonstrated in this region when eye movements are made (50,51). Suppression of eye movements in covert attention tasks may involve this region in a similar way in humans (52). It has been proposed that the PCC may be involved in disengaging attention (53); however, activation of this same area also has been found in a divided-attention task involving global and local processing (54) and in feature-conjunction search (45), suggesting that this area is involved in more than shifts of spatial attention. Activation of the inferior left parietal lobe, in particular Brodmann area 40, was observed in a study in which subjects were required to locate an object in peripheral space or when they had to make a judgment about object-based properties (52). Failure of other functional imaging studies on visuospatial attention to detect activations in this area may be explained by the actual task demands: Human inferior parietal cortex is likely to be involved in visuospatial functions that subserve object manipulation or action in general. Although it is unclear whether attentional effects begin at the level of the IPL, this area is certainly part of a network subserving attentional functions. This network also comprises the anterior cingulum [projecting to the supplementary motor area (SMA), premotor cortex (PMC), and prefrontal cortex (PFC)], with the posterior cingulum controlling the IPL and the intralaminar thalamic nuclei (55,56).

It has already been mentioned that the attentional and eye-movement systems are closely linked (57). According to results of recordings from the superior colliculus in monkeys, attentional shifts during different tasks are closely associated with preparation for eye movement (58). Activation studies in humans also indicate that overt and covert attentional shifts activate the same neural network (52). Whereas we usually move our head

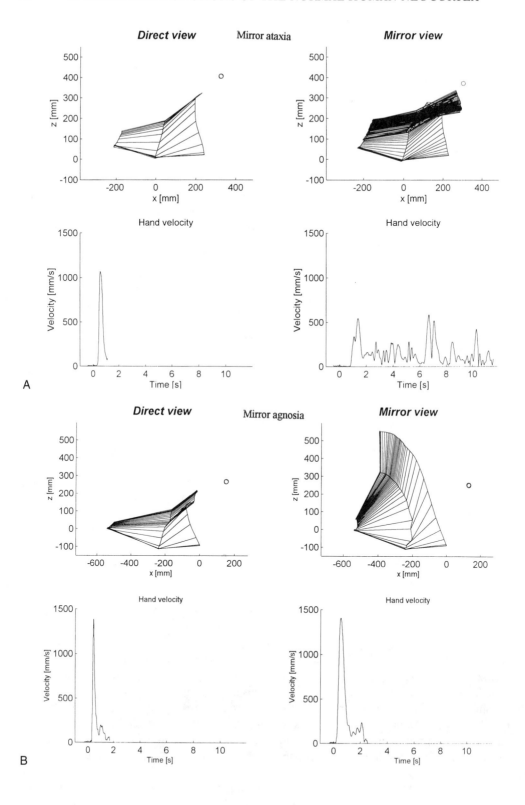

and eyes to fixate on an attention-capturing stimulus, attention can be oriented covertly toward a location in the visual field without moving the head or eyes. It has been proposed that covert shifts of visual attention activate the same neural networks as those programming saccadic eye movements, the only difference being a suppression of the executive decision to perform eye movements; see the premotor theory of attention of Rizzolatti et al. (57,59). Covert shifts of attention enhance the detection of events in the precued space (60) both in terms of speed of performance and reduction of threshold for target detection. Normally, however, attentional shifts lead to eye movements that bring the percept of interest into focus.

To direct orienting eye or body movements toward visual stimuli, visuospatial information must be combined with postural information, such as direction of gaze plus head and body position relative to a target. This requires the comparison of retinal image location with eye and head positions to determine the location of the target relative to the body. Further, world-referenced postural information is required to determine where something lies in the world. In the monkey, neurones in the lateral area of the intraparietal sulcus (LIP) and in area 7a are referenced to the body and to the world, respectively, showing a segregation of spatial information, which is consistent with the information path carrying body information for the control of gaze and the other channel carrying world-referenced information for navigation and other tasks that require an absolute frame of reference (61). According to the premotor theory of attention, visuospatial neglect is regarded as a representational deficit consequent to lesions of neural networks underlying motor-plan organization in which space is coded in non-retinal coordinates.

The neural mechanisms involved in the organization of internal representation of space required for perception and action involve representations composed by various sensory modalities. Rather than representing a unitary system, such multiple representations led to distinctions between perceptual and premotor spatial systems. The abstract representation of space constructed by this multimodal integration can be modified by attentional factors forming gain fields regarded as the foundation of a population code for the neural construct of space (62).

The cortical coding of reaching obviously is not restricted to parietal areas but results from the operation of distributed populations of parietal and frontal neurones. Medial parietal areas (7m) coding for arm posture and movement influence neuronal processes involved in early stages of visuomotor transformation, and the influence is not merely added downstream in frontal motor cortex (63,64). Consequently, coding of reaching does not represent a serial process of coordinate transformation, each performed by a particular area, but as a recursive and parallel process. Against this experimental background, optic ataxia is regarded as a consequence of the breakdown of the operations occurring in the combinatorial domains of the SPL (65). The medial areas 7m showed clusters with cell activity either related to eye or arm position conjointly to combined eye–

FIG. 6.4. Kinematic recordings of reaching movements of the right arms of patients with mirror ataxia *(A)* and mirror agnosia *(B)*. **A:** The stick figures representing the position of the wrist, elbow, and shoulder show the different movement paths toward the object *(o)* under direct visual control and to the mirror when the object is presented through the mirror. The velocity profiles show that both movements were performed with the same peak velocity and with no additional corrections. **B:** The stick figures show that the object was reached under direct view and when presented through the mirror; however, the movement path shows many corrections as can also be seen on the deranged velocity profile with many velocity peaks. (From Binkofski F, Buccino G, Dohle C, et al. Mirror agnosia and mirror ataxia constitute different parietal lobe disorders. *Ann Neurol* 1999;46:51–61, with permission.)

hand actions so that this area is involved in eye–arm coordination (66).

Neglect

The *neglect syndrome* (67) is defined as a behavioral failure to report, respond, or orient to novel or meaningful stimuli presented to the body side contralateral to a brain lesion. This failure cannot be attributed to either sensory or motor defects. The neglect syndrome may affect different modalities appearing either as hemi-inattention, sensory extinction, or motor neglect (akinesia, intentional neglect). Although often accompanied by multimodal neglect, pure motor neglect sometimes is observed in isolation (68,69). Neglect may be caused by lesions of the parietal (7,68) or frontal cortex (68) or by subcortical lesions that damage or functionally suppress a presumed subcorticocortical network (55,70).

Chronic visuospatial neglect, however, is most frequently consequent on lesions whose center is the right inferior parietal (or parietotemporal) cortex. Lesions restricted to right superior parietal cortex do not usually provoke neglect. Rather, they are associated with visual extinction and optic ataxia (71,72). In addition, lesions of superior parietal cortex are implicated in an "extinction-like reaction time pattern" in response to invalid cueing of attentional shifts (53).

In clinical terms, the role of the parietal lobe in spatial cognition is controversial. One hypothesis is that it subserves spatial perception, whereas alternative views favor a primary role in the direction of spatial movement. Mattingley et al. (73) presented evidence showing that patients with right IPL lesions have a specific deficit initiating leftward movements toward visual targets on the left hemispace. This motor impairment was not found in patients with frontal lesions who had a neglect syndrome. These results favor the hypothesis that the IPL operates as a sensorimotor interface rather than subserving a purely perceptual function. A dissociation of sensory attentional from motor intentional neglect also was observed by Na et al. (74),

who reported that some patients with right hemisphere damage and left-sided hemispatial neglect showed motor intentional rather than sensory attentional neglect.

Rosetti et al. (75) showed that the frequent parietal locus of the lesion producing neglect reflects impairment of coordinate transformation used by the nervous system to represent extrapersonal space. Prism adaptation shifting the visual field to the right in such patients improved their body midline as revealed by classic neuropsychological tests. Unlike caloric stimulation and other manipulations used to improve neglect, the improvement lasted several hours after prism removal.

Another proposal is that a spatial reference frame for exploratory behavior is disturbed in patients with neglect (76). According to this view, the failure to explore the contralesional side is interpreted as a consequence of a distorted input transformation, resulting in a rotational rather than translational deviation of egocentric space representation to the ipsilesional side.

The neurobehavioral discussion swings between views stating that neglect may result from a defect of intention (77), from a malfunctioning arousal–attention mechanism, or from a neural representation deficit inducing attentional disturbances as secondary phenomena, with predominant damage to the right cerebral hemisphere (69,78). Bisiach et al. (79) proposed that neglect represents a disorder of left–right space representation, a horizontal anisometry. Mesulam proposed a disruption of a cortical network in hemineglect that is normally sustained in conscious awareness. This network is composed of local components including the parietal association cortex, a limbic component in the cingulate gyrus, a frontal component (premotor cortices including the frontal eye field) and a subcortical component attributed to the mesencephalic reticular formation, the ventrolateral thalamus and the intralaminar thalamic nuclei (55,77). Lesions in only one component of this network yield partial unilateral neglect syndromes. Thus, the multiplicity of neglect-causing lesions does not result from a diffuse cerebral localization of attention but instead reflects the existence of a highly organized multifocal and interconnected network subserving directed attention. Whereas the individual components allow for behavioral specialization, such as sensory represential and motor exploratory function mediated primarily in the parietal lobe, a separate role has been attributed to the anterior and posterior cingulate cortex, possibly reflecting a segregation between attentional and intentional neural mechanisms (73).

REFERENCES

1. Ungerleider LG, Mishkin M. In: Ingle DJ, Goodale MA, Mansfield RJW, eds. *Analysis of visual behavior.* Cambridge, MA: MIT Press, 1982:549–586.
2. Goodale MA, Milner AD. Separate visual pathways for perception and action. *TINS* 1992;15:20–25.
3. Goodale MA, Milner AD, Jakobson LS, et al. A neurological dissociation between perceiving objects and grasping them. *Nature* 1991;349:154–156.
4. Foerster O. Motorische Felder und Bahnen: sensible corticale Felder. In: Bumke H, Foerster O, eds. *Handbuch der Neurologie.* Berlin: Springer-Verlag, 1936:358–448.
5. Déjérine J. A propos de l'agnosie tactile. *Rev Neurol (Paris)* 1907;15:781–784.
6. Head H, Holmes G. Sensory disturbances from cerebral lesions. *Brain* 1911–1912;34:102–254.
7. Critchley M. *The parietal lobes.* New York: Hafner, 1953.
8. Pause M, Kunesch E, Binkofski F, et al. Sensorimotor disturbances in patients with lesions of the parietal cortex. *Brain* 1989;112:1599–1625.
9. Gibson JJ. Observations on active touch. *Psychol Rev* 1962;69:477–491.
10. Freund H-J. Abnormalities of motor behaviour after cortical lesions in humans. In: Plum F, ed. *Handbook of physiology.* Section 1. The nervous system. Vol. V. *Higher functions of the brain.* Part 2. Bethesda, MD: American Physiology Society, 1987:763–810.
11. Freund H-J. The apraxias. In: Asbury AK, McKhann GM, McDonald GI, eds. *Diseases of the nervous system: clinical neurobiology,* vol II. Chichester, UK: John Wiley & Sons, 1992:751–767.
12. Freund H.-J. The apraxias. In: Kennard CH, ed. *Recent advances in clinical neurology.* New York: Churchill Livingstone, 1995:29–49.
13. Delay J. *Les astéréognosies, pathologie du toucher.* Paris: Masson & Cie, 1935.
14. Gallese V, Murata A, Kaseda M, et al. Deficit of hand preshaping after muscimol injection in monkey parietal cortex. *Neuroreport* 1994;5:1525–1529.
15. Binkofski F, Buccino G, Posse S, et al. A fronto-parietal circuit for object manipulation in man: evidence from a fMRI-study. *Eur J Neurosc* 1999;128:210–213.
16. Binkofski F, Buccino G, Stephan KM, et al. A parieto-motor network for object manipulation: evidence from neuroimaging. *Exp Brain Res* 1999;11:3276–3286.
17. Schnitzler A, Seitz RJ, Freund HJ. The somatosensory

system. In: Maziota, Toga, eds. *Brain mapping:* the systems. (In press.)
18. Das Krankheitsbild der Apraxie ("motorische asymbolie"), auf Grund eines Falles von einseitiger Apraxie. *Monatsschrift Psychiatrie und Neurologie* 1900;8: 182–197.
19. Liepmann H. Apraxie. In: *Brugsch's Ergebnisse der Gesamten Medizin.* Berlin: Urban & Schwarzenberg, 1920:518–543.
20. Freeman RB Jr. The apraxias, purposeful motor behavior, and left-hemisphere function. In: Prinz W, Sanders AF, eds. *Cognition and motor processes.* Berlin: Springer-Verlag, 1984:29–50.
21. Bellugi U, Poizner H, Klima ES. Language, modality, and the brain. *Trends Neurosci* 1989;12:380–388.
22. Kleist K. Der Gang und der gegenwärtige Stand der Apraxieforschung. *Ergeb Neurol Psychiatr* 1911;1: 342–452.
23. Balint R. Seelenlähmung des Schauens, optische Ataxie, räumliche Störung der Aufmerksamkeit. *Monatsschrift Psychiatrie und Neurologie* 1909;25:51–81.
24. Rondot P, de Recondo J, Ribadeau Dumas L. Visuomotor apraxia. *Brain* 1977;100:355–376.
25. Jeannerod M. *The neural and behavioural organization of goal-directed movements.* Oxford: Clarendon Press, 1988.
26. Jeannerod M. The hand and the object: the role of posterior parietal cortex in forming motor representations. *Can J Physiol Pharmacol* 1994;72:535–541.
27. Classen J, Kunesch E, Binkofski F, et al. Subcortical origin of visuomotor apraxia. *Brain* 1995;118:1365–1374.
28. Haaxma R, Kuypers HGJM. Intrahemispheric cortical connexions and visual guidance of hand and finger movements in the rhesus monkey. *Brain* 1975;98:239–260.
29. Glickstein M, Cohen JL, Dixon B, et al. Corticopontine visual projections in macaque monkeys. *J Comp Neurol* 1980;190:209–229.
30. Glickstein M, May J, Mercer B. Cortico-pontine projections in the macaque: the distribution of labelled cortical cells after large injections of horseradish peroxidase in the pontine nuclei. *J Comp Neurol* 1985;235:343–359.
31. Mazzoni P, Bracewell RM, Barash S, et al. Motor intention activity in the macaque's lateral intraparietal area. I. Dissociation of motor plan from sensory memory. *J Neurophysiol* 1996;76:1439–56.
32. Andersen RA. Encoding of intention and spatial location in the posterior parietal cortex. *Cereb Cortex* 1995; 5:457–469.
33. Andersen RA. Multimodal integration for the representation of space in the posterior parietal cortex. *Philos Trans R Soc Lond B Biol Sci* 1997;352:1421–1428.
34. Clower DM, Hoffman JM, Votaw JR, et al. Role of posterior parietal cortex in the recalibration of visually guided reaching. *Nature* 1996;383:618–621.
35. Kalaska JF, Crammond DJ. Cerebral cortical mechanisms of reaching movements. *Science* 1992;255:1517–1523.
36. Kalaska JF, Scott SH, Cisek P, et al. Cortical control of reaching movements. *Curr Opin Neurobiol* 1997;7: 849–859.
37. Lacquaniti F, Guigon E, Bianchi L, et al. Representing spatial information for limb movement: role of area 5 in the monkey. *Cereb Cortex* 1995;5:391–409.
38. Jeannerod M, Arbib MA, Rizzolatti G, et al. Grasping objects: the cortical mechanisms of visuomotor transformation. *Trends Neurosci* 1995;18:314–320.
39. Hirosaka O, Tanaka M, Sakamoto M, et al. Deficits in

manipulative behaviors induced by local injection of muscimol in the first somatosensory cortex of the conscious monkey. *Brain Res* 1985;325:375–380.

40. Binkofski F, Dohle C, Posse S, et al. Human anterior intraparietal area subserves prehension: a combined lesion and functional MRI activation study. *Neurology* 1998;50:1253–1259.

41. Ramachandran VS, Altschuler EL, Hillyer S. Mirror agnosia. *Proc R Soc Lond B Biol Sci* 1998;264:645–647.

42. Binkofski F, Dohle C, Hefter H, et al. Deficits in 3D limb coordination in parietal patients with and without apraxia. In: Fetter M, Misslisch H, Tweed D, eds. *Three-dimensional kinematics of eye, head, and limb movements*. 1997:329–336.

43. Binkofski F, Buccino G, Dohle C, et al. Mirror agnosia and mirror ataxia constitute different pariental lobe disorders. *Ann Neurol* 1999;46:51–61.

44. Corbetta M, Miezin FM, Shulman G, et al. A PET study of visuospatial attention. *J Neurosci* 1993;13:1202–1226.

45. Corbetta M, Shulman G, Miezin FM, et al. Superior parietal cortex activation during spatial attention shifts and visual feature conjunction. *Science* 1995;270:802–805.

46. Lynch J, McLaren JW. Deficits in visual attention and saccadic eye movements after lesions of parietooccipital cortex in monkeys. *J Neurophysiol* 1989;61:74–90.

47. Mountcastle VB, Motter BC, Steinmetz MA, et al. Common and differential effects of attentive fixation on the excitability of parietal and prestriate (V4) cortical visual neurons in macaque monkey. *J Neurosci* 1987;7:2239–2255.

48. Steinmetz MA, Constantinidis C. Neurophysiological evidence for a role of posterior parietal cortex in redirecting visual attention. *Cereb Cortex* 1995;5:448–456.

49. Milner AD, Goodale MA. *The visual brain in action.* Oxford: Oxford University Press, 1995.

50. Thier P, Andersen RA. Electrical microstimulation suggests two different forms of representation of head-centered space in the intraparietal sulcus of rhesus monkey. *Proc Natl Acad Sci USA* 1996;93:4962–4967.

51. Thier P, Andersen RA. Multiple parietal "eye fields": insights from electrical microstimulation. In: Thier P, Karnath H-O, eds. *Parietal lobe contributions to orientation in 3D space.* Heidelberg: Springer-Verlag, 1997:95–108.

52. Fink GR, Dolan RJ, Halligan PW, et al. Space-based and object-based visual attention: shared and specific neural domains. *Brain* 1997;120:2013–2028.

53. Posner MI, Walker JA, Friedrich FJ, et al. Effects of parietal injury on covert orienting of attention. *J Neurosci* 1984;4:1863–1874.

54. Fink GR, Halligan PW, Marshall JC, et al. Where in the brain does visual attention select the forest and the trees? *Nature* 1996;382:626–628.

55. Mesulam MM. A cortical network for directed attention and unilateral neglect. *Ann Neurol* 1981;10:309–325.

56. Paillard J. A propos de la négligence motrice. Issues et perspectives. *Rev Neurol* 1990;146:600–611.

57. Rizzolatti G. Mechanisms of selective attention in mammals. In: Ewert JP, Capranica RR, Ingle DJ, eds. *Advances in vertebrate neuroethology.* New York: Plenum Press, 1983:261–297.

58. Kustov AA, Robinson DL. Shared neural control of attentional shifts and eye movements. *Nature* 1996;384:74–77.

59. Rizzolatti G, Riggio L, Dascola I, et al. Reorienting attention across the horizontal and vertical meridians: evidence in favor of a premotor theory of attention. *Neuropsychologia* 1983;25:31–40.

60. Posner MI. Orienting of attention. *Q J Exp Psychol A* 1980;32:3–25.

61. Snyder LH, Grieve KL, Brotchie P, et al. Separate body- and world-referenced representations of visual space in parietal cortex. *Nature* 1998;394:887–891.

62. Andersen RA, Snyder LH, Bradely DC, et al. Multimodal representation of space in the posterior parietal cortex and its use in planning movements. *Annu Rev Neurosci* 1997;20:303–330.

63. Battaglia-Mayer A, Ferraina S, Marconi B, et al. Early motor influences on visuomotor transformations for reaching: a positive image of optic ataxia. *Exp Brain Res* 1998;123:172–189.

64. Ferraina S, Garasto MR, Battaglia-Mayer A, et al. Visual control of hnd-reaching movement: activity in parietal area 7m. *Eur J Neurosci* 1997;9:1090–1095.

65. Johnson PB, Ferraina S, Bianchi L, et al. Cortical networks for visual reaching: physiological and anatomical organization of frontal and parietal lobe arm regions. *Cereb Cortex* 1996;6:102–119.

66. Ferraina S, Johnson PB, Garasto MR, et al. Combination of hand and gaze signals during reaching: activity in parietal area 7m of the monkey. *J Neurophysiol* 77(2):1034–1028.

67. Heilman KM, Bowers D, Valenstein E, et al. Disorders of visual attention. *Baillieres Clin Neurol* 1993;2:389–413.

68. Castaigne P, Laplane D, Degos JD. Trois cas de négligence motrice par lésion frontale pré-rolandique. *Tome* 1972;126:5–15.

69. Laplane D, Degos JD. Motor neglect. *J Neurol Neurosurg Psychiatry* 1983;46:152–158.

70. von Giesen HJ, Schlaug G, Steinmetz H, et al. Cerebral network underlying unilateral motor neglect: evidence from positron emission tomography. *J Neurol Sci* 1994;125:29–38.

71. Milner AD. Neglect, extinction, and the cortical streams of visual processing. In: Thier P, Karnath H-O, eds. *Parietal lobe contributions to orientation in 3D space.* Heidelberg: Springer-Verlag, 1997:3–22.

72. Vallar G. The anatomical basis of spatial hemineglect in humans. In: Robertson IH, Marshall JC, eds. *Unilateral neglect:* clinical and experimental studies. Hove, UK: Lawrence Erlbaum, 1993:27–59.

73. Mattingley JB, Husain M, Rorden C, et al. Motor role of human inferior parietal lobe revealed in unilateral neglect patients. *Nature* 1998;392:179–182.

74. Na DL, Adair JC, Williamson DJG, et al. Dissociation of sensory-attentional from motor-intentional neglect. *J Neurol Neurosurg Psychiatry* 1998;64:331–338.

75. Rosetti Y, Rode G, Pisella L, et al. Prism adaptation to a rightward optical deviation rehabilitates left hemispatial neglect *Nature* 1998;395:166–169.

76. Karnath HO. Spatial orientation and the representation of space with parietal lobe lesions. *Philos Trans R Soc Lond B* 1997;352:1411–1429.

77. Watson RT, Valenstein E, Day A, et al. Posterior neocortical systems subserving awareness and neglect: neglect associated with superior temporal sulcus but not area 7 lesions. *Arch Neurol* 1994;51:1014–1021.

78. Rizzolatti G, Berti A. Neglect as a neural representation deficit. *Rev Neurol (Paris)* 1990;146:626–634.

79. Bisiach E, Pizzamiglio L, Nico D, et al. Beyond unilateral neglect. *Brain* 1996;119:851–857.

Neocortical Epilepsies.
Advances in Neurology, Vol. 84,
edited by P. D. Williamson, A. M. Siegel,
D. W. Roberts, V. M. Thadani, and M. S. Gazzaniga.
Lippincott Williams & Wilkins, Philadelphia © 2000.

7

Occipitotemporal and Occipitoparietal Visual Pathways in the Primate Brain

Melvyn A. Goodale

MRC Group on Action and Perception, Department of Psychology, The University of Western Ontario, London, Ontario, Canada N6A 5C2

It has often been said that our eyes are our "windows to the world," allowing us to experience the rich array of objects beyond our bodies. The use of this metaphor, however, rests on the assumption that the human visual system is nothing more than a passive recipient of the information conveyed by the complex pattern of light falling on the retina. More than a hundred years of research on vision has shown that this assumption is quite incorrect. Our perception of the external world is not a passive reflection of the light striking our eyes, but it is instead a representation that has been constructed by a highly active visual system, a system that not only filters and processes the incoming information in complicated ways but also interprets that information in terms of prior knowledge, both learned and hardwired, about the nature of the world and the objects within it. There is more to the story than this, however. The construction of perceptual representations of the world is only one of the things that vision does for us. Vision also allows us to move through that world and interact with the objects we encounter with remarkable adeptness and skill.

In evolutionary terms, the role of vision in the control of movement predates its role in the construction of perceptual representations, a fact not always appreciated, even by scientists studying vision and the visual sys-

tem. Animals used the signals from differential activation of visual receptors to control their movements long before they used that input to construct perceptual representations of the world. Perceptual representations of the external world did not emerge until animals began to think about and plan their actions and remember the consequences of those actions. In short, perception evolved hand in hand with the emergence of cognitive operations. Even though the visual areas in the cerebral cortex that construct our visual perception of the world are highly evolved in humans, the phylogenetically older subcortical pathways that direct our actions also are elaborated in the cerebral cortex. Although the perception and action networks in the human cerebral cortex operate in close association, the transformations they perform on incoming visual information are fundamentally different. This chapter reviews some of the neurologic evidence for this distinction between vision for perception and vision for action and discusses the possible neural substrates of these two rather different functions of the human visual system.

TWO VISUAL SYSTEMS

Although the retina projects to a number of different nuclei in the primate brain, one of the most prominent projections is to the dorsal part of the lateral geniculate nucleus (LGNd). New projections arise from the LGNd and project, in turn, to primary visual cortex or V1 in the occipital lobe. Beyond V1, visual information is conveyed to a large number of extrastriate areas (1). Despite the complexity of the interconnections between these different areas, two broad "streams" of projections from V1 have been identified in the macaque brain (Fig. 7.1): a *ventral stream* projecting eventually to the inferotemporal cortex and a *dorsal stream* projecting to the posterior parietal cortex (2). Of course, these regions also receive inputs from a number of other subcortical visual structures, such as the superior colliculus, which sends prominent projections to the dorsal stream (via the thalamus). Neuroimaging evidence from a broad range of studies (3–5) suggests that the visual projections from the primary visual cortex to the temporal and parietal lobes in the human brain also are separated into ventral and dorsal streams.

Ungerleider and Mishkin (2) argued that the two streams of visual processing play different but complementary roles in the processing of incoming visual information. According to their original account, the ventral stream plays a critical role in the identification and recognition of objects, and the dorsal stream mediates the localization of those same objects. This distinction in visual processing sometimes is described as one between "what" versus "where." Support for this idea came from work with monkeys. Lesions of the inferotemporal cortex in monkeys produced deficits in their ability to discriminate between objects on the basis of their visual features but did not affect their performance on a spatially demanding "landmark" task (6,7). Conversely, lesions of the posterior parietal cortex produced deficits in performance on the landmark task but did not affect object discrimination learning. (For a detailed critique of these studies, see 8,9.) Although the evidence for the Ungerleider and Mishkin proposal initially seemed quite compelling, recent findings from a broad range of studies in both humans and primates has forced a reinterpretation of the division of labor between the two streams. This reinterpretation, which was put forward by Goodale and

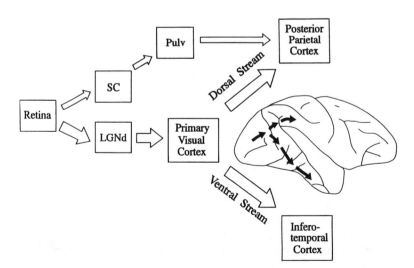

FIG. 7.1. The major routes of visual input into the dorsal and ventral streams. The diagram of the macaque brain on the right of the figure shows the approximate routes of the corticocortical projections from the primary visual cortex to the posterior parietal and the inferotemporal cortex, respectively. LGNd, lateral geniculate nucleus, pars dorsalis; Pulv, pulvinar; SC, superior colliculus. (Adapted from Goodale MA, Meenan JP, Bülthoff HH, et al. Separate neural pathways for the visual analysis of object shape in perception and prehension. *Curr Biol* 1994;4:604–610, with permission.)

Milner (9,10), rather than emphasizing differences in the visual input handled by the two streams (object vision versus spatial vision), focuses instead on the differences in the requirements of the output systems that each stream of processing serves.

According to Goodale and Milner (9,10), the ventral stream plays the major role in constructing the perceptual representation of the world and the objects within it, whereas the dorsal stream mediates the visual control of actions directed at those objects. In other words, processing within the ventral stream allows us to recognize an object, such as a pencil on the desktop, and processing within the dorsal stream provides critical information about the location, orientation, size, and shape of the pencil so that we can reach out and pick it up. This is not a distinction between what and where. In Goodale and Milner's account, the structural and spatial attributes of the goal object are being processed by both streams, but for different purposes. The ventral stream transforms visual information into perceptual representations, which embody the enduring characteristics of objects and their spatial relations. These representations form the foundation for our cognitive life, allowing us to recognize objects and understand their causal relations, to communicate with others about the world beyond our bodies, and to identify goals and plan actions with respect to those goals. The visual transformations carried out in the dorsal stream, which use moment-to-moment information about the disposition of objects within egocentric frames of reference, mediate the control of those goal-directed acts. In short, although there are certainly differences in the distribution of visual inputs to the two streams, the main difference lies in the nature of the transformations that each stream performs on those two sets of inputs.

Effects of Damage to the Dorsal Stream

Some of the most compelling evidence for the idea that "vision for perception" and "vision for action" depend on different neural substrates has come from studies with neurologic patients. For example, patients who have sustained damage to the superior portion of the posterior parietal cortex, the major terminus of the dorsal stream in the human brain, are unable to use visual information to reach out and grasp objects in the hemifield contralateral to the lesion. Clinically, this deficit is called *optic ataxia* (11). Such patients have no difficulty using other sensory information, such as proprioception, to control their reaching; nor do they usually have difficulty recognizing or describing objects that are presented in that part of the visual field (12,13). Thus, their deficit is neither purely visual nor purely motor. They appear instead to have a visuomotor deficit, that is, a deficit in the transformation of visual input into action. This deficit cannot be explained as a disturbance in spatial vision. In fact, in one clear sense, their spatial vision is quite intact because often they are able to describe the relative location of objects in their contralesional field, even though they cannot pick up those objects (12,13).

Work in several laboratories has shown that patients with lesions in the posterior parietal cortex sometimes show deficits in their ability to adjust the orientation of their hand when reaching toward an object (13–15). These same patients, however, have no difficulty describing the orientation of the object they cannot grasp (13). Patients with posterior parietal lesions also can have trouble adjusting their grasp to reflect the size of an object they are asked to pick up, although again their perceptual estimates of object size remain quite accurate (16,17). To pick up an object successfully, however, it is not enough to orient the hand and scale the grip appropriately; the fingers and thumb must be placed at appropriate opposition points on the object's surface. To do this, the visuomotor system must compute the outline shape or boundaries of the object. There is evidence that patients with posterior parietal lesions are unable to carry out this kind of analysis. In a recent experiment, for example, a patient with bilateral lesions of the occipitoparietal region was asked to pick up a series of small, flat, non-symmetric, smoothly contoured objects using a precision grip, which required her to place her index finger and thumb in appropriate positions on either side of each object (18). Despite the fact that the patient could readily distinguish these objects from one another, she often failed to place her fingers on the appropriate opposition points when she attempted to pick up the objects (Fig. 7.2).

This pattern of deficits cannot be explained in terms of a deficit in the "where" system (2). The observations are consistent, however, with Goodale and Milner's (9,10) proposal that the dorsal stream plays a critical role in the visuomotor transformations required for skilled actions, such as visually guided prehension, in which control of an accurate grasp requires information not only about an object's location but also about its orientation, size, and shape. It should be emphasized that

not all patients with damage to the posterior parietal region show the same kind of visuomotor deficit. Some patients have difficulty with hand postures, some with controlling the direction of their grasp, and some with foveating the target (e.g., 14). Indeed, depending on the size and locus of the lesion, a patient can demonstrate any combination of these visuomotor deficits (for review, see 9). Different subregions of the posterior parietal cortex, it appears, support transformations related to the visual control of specific motor outputs (19). Different actions would invoke different combinations of these visuomotor networks.

Effects of Damage to the Human Ventral Stream

Other patients, in whom the brain damage appears to involve ventral rather than dorsal

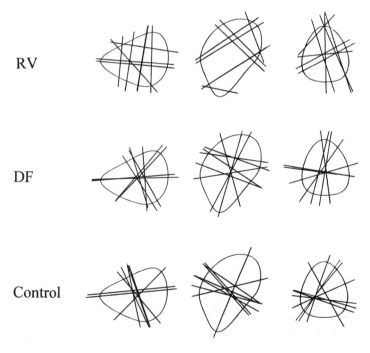

FIG. 7.2. The "grasp lines" (joining points where the index finger and the thumb first made contact with the shape) selected by a patient with optic ataxia *(RV),* a patient with visual form agnosia (D.F.), and the control subject when picking up three of the twelve shapes that were presented to them. The four different orientations in which each shape was presented have been rotated so that they are aligned. No distinction is made between the points of contact for the thumb and finger in these plots. (Adapted from Goodale MA, Meenan JP, Bülthoff HH, et al. Separate neural pathways for the visual analysis of object shape in perception and prehension. *Curr Biol* 1994;4:604–610, with permission.)

stream structures, show the complementary pattern of deficits and spared visual abilities. In other words, these patients can grasp objects quite accurately despite their failure to recognize what it is they are picking up. One such patient is D.F., a young woman who developed a profound *visual form agnosia* (20) following near-asphyxiation by carbon monoxide. Not only is D.F. unable to recognize the faces of her relatives and friends or the visual shape of common objects, but she is also unable to discriminate between simple geometric forms, such as a triangle and a circle. D.F. has no problem identifying people from their voices or identifying objects from how they feel. Her perceptual problems are exclusively visual. Moreover, her deficit seems largely restricted to the form of objects. She can use color and other surface features to identify objects (21–23). What she seems unable to perceive are the contours of objects, no matter how the contours are defined (24). Thus, she cannot identify shapes whose contours are defined by differences in luminance, color, or visual texture or by differences in the

direction of motion or the plane of depth. A selective deficit in form perception with spared color and other surface information is characteristic of the severe visual agnosia that sometimes follows an anoxic episode. Although magnetic resonance imaging (MRI) shows a pattern of diffuse brain damage in D.F. that is consistent with anoxia, most of the damage was evident in the ventrolateral region of the occipital lobe sparing primary visual cortex (Fig. 7.3).

D.F.'s deficit in form perception means she is unable to recognize line drawings of familiar objects. In addition, she is unable to copy them, meaning that her failure to identify drawings, such as those illustrated on the left-hand side of Fig. 7.3, cannot be due simply to a failure of the visual input to invoke the stored representations of the objects. It is a failure instead of perceptual organization, a deficit that Lissauer (25) called *apperceptive agnosia*. Although D.F. cannot copy line drawings, she can draw objects reasonably well from long-term memory (23). In fact, formal tests of her visual imagery shows that it is

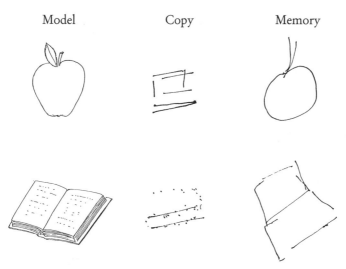

FIG. 7.3. Three samples of drawings made by D.F., a patient with visual form agnosia. The **left-hand column** shows examples of line drawings that were shown to D.F., the **middle column** shows some of D.F.'s drawings of three objects from memory, and the **right-hand column** shows examples of D.F.'s copies of the line drawings shown in the left column. (Adapted from Goodale MA. The cortical organization of visual perception and visuomotor control. In: Kosslyn S, Osherson D, eds. *An invitation to cognitive science,* vol 2. *Visual cognition and action,* 2nd ed. Cambridge, MA: MIT Press, 1995:167–213, with permission.)

remarkably intact, suggesting that it is possible to have a profound deficit in the perceptual processing of form without any deficit in the corresponding visual imagery (26).

D.F.'s deficit in form perception cannot be explained by appealing to disturbances in "low-level" sensory processing. She is able to detect luminance-defined targets out to at least 30 degrees; her flicker detection and fusion rates are normal; and her spatial contrast sensitivity is normal above ten cycles per degree and only moderately impaired at lower spatial frequencies (24). [Of course, even though she could detect the presence of the gratings used to measure her contrast sensitivity, she could not report their orientation (see also 27).]

There is an even more compelling reason to doubt that D.F.'s perceptual deficit is due to a problem in low-level visual processing. Even though D.F. is unable to recognize the shape, size, and orientation of objects, she shows strikingly accurate guidance of hand and finger movements directed at those very same objects (28). Thus, when D.F. was presented with a large slot that could placed in one of a number of different orientations, she showed great difficulty in indicating the orientation of the slot either verbally or even manually by rotating a hand-held card (Fig. 7.4, top). When she was asked simply to reach out and insert the card, she performed as well as normal subjects, rotating her hand in the appropriate direction as soon as she began the movement (Fig. 7.4, bottom). A similar dissociation was seen in D.F.'s responses to the spatial dimensions of objects (28). When presented with a pair of rectangular blocks of the same or different dimensions, she was unable to distinguish between them. Even when she was asked to indicate the width of a single block by means of her index finger and thumb, her matches bore no relationship to the dimensions of the object and showed considerable trial-to-trial variability. In contrast, when she was asked simply to reach out and pick up the block, the aperture between her index finger and thumb changed systematically with the width of the object as the movement unfolded,

as in normal subjects. Finally, as can be seen in Fig. 7.2, even though D.F. could not discriminate between target objects that differed in outline shape, she nevertheless could pick up such objects successfully, placing her index finger and thumb on stable grasp points (18). In other words, the posture of D.F.'s reaching hand was "tuned" to the orientation, size, and shape of the object she was about to pick up, even though she appeared to be unable to perceive those same object attributes.

These spared visuomotor skills are not limited to reaching and grasping movements; D.F. can walk around quite well under visual control. She can walk through a room without bumping into furniture or tripping over the carpet. Formal testing has shown that she is able to step over obstacles as well as control subjects, even though her verbal descriptions of the heights of the obstacles were far from normal (29). These findings are difficult to reconcile with Ungerleider and Mishkin's (2) idea that object vision is the preserve of the ventral stream, for here we have a patient in whom a profound loss of object perception exists alongside a preserved ability to use object features such as size, outline shape, and orientation to guide skilled actions.

Such a dissociation is consistent with Goodale and Milner's (9,10) proposal that there are separate neural pathways for transforming incoming visual information for action and perception. Presumably, it is the latter and not the former that is compromised in D.F. In other words, the brain damage she suffered as a consequence of anoxia appears to have interrupted the normal flow of shape and contour information into her perceptual system without affecting the processing of shape and contour information by the visuomotor modules comprising her action system. If, as Goodale and Milner have suggested, the perception of objects and events is mediated by the ventral stream of visual projections to inferotemporal cortex, then D.F. should show evidence for damage relatively early in this pathway. Certainly, the pattern of damage revealed by MRI is consistent with this interpretation; the major focus of cortical damage

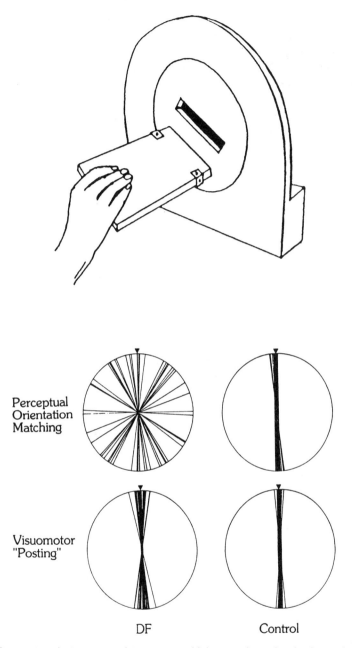

FIG. 7.4. Top: Apparatus that was used to test sensitivity to orientation in the patient D.F. The slot could be placed in any one of a number of orientations around the clock. Subjects were required either to rotate a hand-held card to match the orientation of the slot or to 'post' the card into the slot as shown in this figure. **Bottom:** Polar plots of the orientation of the hand-held card on the perceptual matching task and the visuomotor posting task for D.F. and an age-matched control subject. The correct orientation on each trial has been rotated to vertical. Note that although D.F. was unable to match the orientation of the card to that of the slot in the perceptual matching card, she did rotate the card to the correct orientation as she attempted to insert it into the slot on the posting task. (Adapted from Goodale MA, Milner AD, Jakobson LS, et al. A neurological dissociation between perceiving objects and grasping them. *Nature* 1991;349:154–156, with permission.)

is in the ventrolateral region of the occipital cortex, an area thought to be part of the human homologue of the ventral stream (4,5). Primary visual cortex, which provides input for both the dorsal and ventral streams, appears to be largely intact. Thus, although input from primary visual cortex to the ventral stream may have been compromised in D.F., input from this structure to the dorsal stream appears to be essentially intact. In addition, the projections from the superior colliculus to the dorsal stream (via the pulvinar, a nucleus in the thalamus) also could play a role in mediating some of the residual visuomotor responses in D.F..

It must not be forgotten, however, that D.F.'s problems arose, not from a discrete lesion, but from anoxia. Therefore, the brain damage in D.F., while localized to some extent, is much more diffuse than it would be in a patient with a stroke or tumor. For this reason, any attempt to map the striking dissociation between perceptual and visuomotor abilities in D.F. onto the ventral and dorsal streams of visual processing must be regarded as tentative. The proposal is strengthened, however, by observations in the patients described earlier whose pattern of deficits is complementary to D.F.'s and whose brain damage can be confidently localized to the dorsal stream.

EVIDENCE FROM MONKEYS

The division of labor between the dorsal and ventral streams of processing is also supported by a wealth of anatomic, electrophysiologic, and behavioral studies in the monkey. For example, monkeys with lesions of inferotemporal cortex, who show profound deficits in object recognition, are nevertheless as capable as normal animals at picking up small objects (30), at catching flying insects (31), and at orienting their fingers to extract morsels of food embedded in small slots (32). Like D.F., these monkeys are unable to discriminate between objects on the basis of the same visual features that they apparently use to direct their grasping movements. In addition to the lesion studies, there is a long his-

tory of electrophysiologic work showing that cells in inferotemporal cortex and neighbouring regions of the superior temporal sulcus are tuned to specific objects and object features; some maintain their selectivity irrespective of viewpoint, retinal image size, and even color (for review, see 9). Feature-specific cells in the inferotemporal region also appear to be organized in a columnar fashion, similar to the ocular dominance and orientation columns in primary visual cortex (33). Moreover, the responses of these cells are not affected by the animal's motor behavior. It does not appear to matter whether the animal is moving its eyes or limbs. The cells are sensitive, however, to the reinforcement history and significance of the visual stimuli that drive them. It has been suggested that cells in this region might play a role in comparing current visual inputs with internal representations of recalled images (e.g., 34), which themselves presumably are stored in other regions, such as neighboring regions of the medial temporal lobe and related limbic areas (35,36). In fact, sensitivity to particular objects can be created in ensembles of cells in inferotemporal cortex simply by training the animals to discriminate between different objects (37). There is also evidence to suggest that activity of cells in inferotemporal cortex is related to what the monkey actually *perceives,* not just to what is falling on the retina (38). These and other studies too numerous to cite here lend considerable support to the suggestion that the object-based descriptions provided by the ventral stream form the basic raw material for recognition memory and other long-term representations of the visual world. In short, the ventral stream and associated regions have the characteristics one would expect to see in a system dedicated to providing the perceptual foundation for the monkey's (and presumably our) cognitive life.

In sharp contrast to the activity of cells in the ventral stream, the responses of cells in the dorsal stream are greatly dependent on the concurrent motor behavior of the animal. Thus, separate subsets of visual cells in the posterior parietal cortex, the major terminal zone for the dorsal stream, have been shown to be implicated in visual fixation, pursuit and saccadic eye movements, visually guided reaching, and the manipulation of objects (39,40). In reviewing these studies, Andersen (41) pointed out that most neurons in these areas "exhibit both sensory-related and move-ment-related activity." Moreover, the motor modulation is quite specific. Recent work in Andersen's laboratory, for example, showed that visual cells in the posterior parietal cortex that code the location of a target for a saccadic eye movement are in a separate but neighbor-ing region from those that code the location for a manual aiming movement to the same target (42). In other experiments (43,44), cells in the posterior parietal region that fire when the monkey manipulates an object also have been shown to be sensitive to the intrinsic object features, such as size and orientation, that determine the posture of the hand and fin-gers during a grasping movement. Lesions in this region of the posterior parietal cortex pro-duce deficits in the visual control of reaching and grasping similar in many respects to those seen in humans following damage to the homologous region (e.g., 45,46). The posterior parietal cortex is also intimately linked with premotor cortex, the superior colliculus, and pontine nuclei, brain areas that also have been implicated in various aspects of the visual con-trol of eye, limb, and body movements. In short, the networks in the dorsal stream have the functional properties and interconnections that one might expect to see in a system con-cerned with the moment-to-moment control of visually guided actions.

Evidence from Human Functional Neuroimaging

As mentioned earlier, neuroimaging studies revealed an organization of visual areas in the human cerebral cortex that is remarkably simi-lar to that seen in the macaque (4,5). Although clear differences in the topography of these areas emerges as one moves from monkey to human, the functional separation into a ventral occipitotemporal and a dorsal occipitoparietal

pathway appears to be preserved. Thus, areas in the occipitotemporal region appear to be specialized for the processing of color, texture, and form differences of objects (47–52). In contrast, regions in the posterior parietal cor-tex have been found that are activated when subjects engage in visually guided move-ments, such as saccades, reaching movements, and grasping (53).

The specialization that exists within the dorsal and ventral streams of the monkey is also evident in the human occipitotemporal and occipitoparietal visual pathways. Activa-tion studies have identified regions in the human ventral stream for the processing of faces that are distinct from those involved in the processing of other objects (54–56). Sim-ilarly, there is evidence that different areas in and around the intraparietal sulcus are acti-vated when subjects make saccadic eye move-ments as opposed to manual pointing move-ments toward visual targets (57). A region in the human brain that appears to correspond to that part of the monkey posterior parietal region where visually sensitive manipulation cells have been localized, shows selective ac-tivation during visually guided grasping (14). Finally, a recent study of prism adaptation showed that selective activation of the poste-rior parietal cortex occurs during the remap-ping of visual and proprioceptive representa-tions of hand position (58).

Thus, as this brief review of the rapidly growing neuroimaging literature indicates, many of the findings are consistent with the idea that there are two visual streams in the human cerebral cortex, just as there are in the monkey. In addition, the results of several studies suggested that areas in the posterior parietal cortex of the human brain are involved in the visual control of action, whereas areas in the occipitotemporal region appear to play a role in object recognition.

Evidence from Studies of Normal Observers

Neuropsychologic studies in brain-dam-aged patients, anatomic and electrophysiologic studies in the monkey, and recent brain-imaging experiments all provide support for the idea of separate visual systems for perception and action. There is other less direct, but equally compelling, evidence for this division of labor that comes from experiments with normal observers. For example, it has long been known that our perception of the position of a small dot is affected to a large degree by the position of the frame surrounding the dot. Thus, when the frame is moved unexpectedly to the left, we typically see the frame as stationary and the dot as moving to the right—the so-called *Duncker illusion* (59). Nevertheless, our visuomotor systems are rarely fooled, and when we are asked to point to the dot, our pointing movements are not influenced by changes in the position of the frame, and typically we continue to point in the correct direction (60,61). Similar dissociations have been observed with respect to object size. Thus, the scaling of grasping movements is unaffected by typical size-contrast illusions that have a profound affect on perceptual judgments of size (62–64). Such paradoxes show that what we think we "see" is not always what guides our actions and therefore provides powerful evidence for the parallel operation, within our everyday life, of two types of visual processing, each apparently designed to serve quite different purposes, and each characterized by quite different properties.

INTERACTIONS BETWEEN THE TWO STREAMS

Throughout this chapter, I have been developing the idea that the ventral perception system and the dorsal action system are two independent and decidedly different visual systems within the primate brain. It should not be forgotten, however, that the two systems evolved together in the primate line and play complementary roles in the control of behavior. Indeed, one might argue that the limitations of one system are the strengths of the other. Thus, although the ventral stream delivers a rich and detailed representation of the world and one that is quite long lasting, the metrics of the world with respect to the organism are not well specified in this representation. In contrast, the dorsal stream delivers accurate metric information in the required egocentric coordinates for a particular action but these computations are sharply focused on the goal object and are relatively short lived.

Successful and adaptive behavior requires that these two systems work in a closely integrated fashion. Although it is true that the execution of a goal-directed act depends on dedicated visual control systems in the dorsal stream, the selection of appropriate goal objects and actions depends in large measure on the perceptual machinery of the ventral stream. Future research and theory must focus on how the two streams interact both with each other and with other brain regions in the production of purposive behavior. Some ideas about how these interactions might take place are now beginning to be developed (3,65,66).

ACKNOWLEDGMENTS

Much of the research described in this chapter was supported by a grant to the author from the Medical Research Council of Canada.

REFERENCES

1. Zeki S. *A vision of the brain*. Oxford: Blackwell Scientific Publications, 1993.
2. Ungerleider LG, Mishkin M. Two cortical visual systems. In: Ingle DJ, Goodale MA, Mansfield RJW, eds. *Analysis of visual behavior*. Cambridge, MA: MIT Press, 1982:549–586.
3. Goodale MA, Humphrey GK. The objects of action and perception. *Cognition* 1998;67:181–207.
4. Tootell RBH, Dale AM, Sereno MI, et al. New images from human visual cortex. *Trends Neurosci* 1996;19:481–489.
5. Tootell RBH, Hadjikhani NK, Mendola JD, et al. From retinotopy to recognition: fMRI in human visual cortex. *Trends in Cognitive Sciences* 1998;2:174–183.
6. Pohl W. Dissociation of spatial discrimination deficits following frontal and parietal lesions in monkeys. *J Comp Physiol Psychol* 1973;82:227–239.
7. Ungerleider LG, Brody BA. Extrapersonal spatial orientation: the role of posterior parietal, anterior frontal, and inferotemporal cortex. *Exp Neurol* 1977;56:265–280.
8. Goodale MA. The cortical organization of visual perception and visuomotor control. In: Kosslyn S, Osherson D, eds. *An invitation to cognitive science*, vol 2. *Visual*

cognition and action, 2nd ed. Cambridge, MA: MIT Press, 1995:167–213.

9. Milner AD, Goodale MA. *The visual brain in action.* Oxford: Oxford University Press, 1995.

10. Goodale MA, Milner AD. Separate visual pathways for perception and action. *Trends Neurosci* 1992;15:20–25.

11. Bálint R. Seelenlämung des 'Schauens', optische Ataxie, räumliche Störung der Aufmerksamkeit. *Monatschrift für Psychiatrie und Neurologie* 1909;25:51–81.

12. Jeannerod M. *The neural and behavioural organization of goal-directed movements.* Oxford: Oxford University Press, 1988.

13. Perenin M-T, Vighetto A. Optic ataxia: a specific disruption in visuomotor mechanisms. I. Different aspects of the deficit in reaching for objects. *Brain* 1988;111:643–674.

14. Binkofski F, Dohle C, Posse S, et al. Human anterior intraparietal area subserves prehension. *Neurology* 1998;50:1253–1259.

15. Jeannerod M, Decety J, Michel F. Impairment of grasping movements following a bilateral posterior parietal lesion. *Neuropsychologia* 1994;32:369–380.

16. Goodale MA, Murphy KJ, Meenan JP, et al. Spared object perception but poor object-calibrated grasping in a patient with optic ataxia. *Society for Neuroscience Abstracts* 1993;19:775.

17. Jakobson LS, Archibald YM, Carey DP, et al. A kinematic analysis of reaching and grasping movements in a patient recovering from optic ataxia. *Neuropsychologia* 1991;29:803–809.

18. Goodale MA, Meenan JP, Bülthoff HH, et al. Separate neural pathways for the visual analysis of object shape in perception and prehension. *Curr Biol* 1994;4:604–610.

19. Rizzolatti G, Luppino G, Matelli M. The organization of the cortical motor system: new concepts. *Electroencephal Clin Neurophysiol* 1998;106:283–296.

20. Benson DF, Greenberg JP. Visual form agnosia: a specific deficit in visual discrimination. *Arch Neurol* 1969;20:82–89.

21. Humphrey GK, Goodale MA, Jakobson LS, et al. The role of surface information in object recognition: studies of a visual form agnosic and normal subjects. *Perception* 1994;23:1457–1481.

22. Humphrey GK, Symons LA, Herbert AM, et al. A neurological dissociation between shape from shading and shape from edges. *Behav Brain Res* 1996;76:117–125.

23. Servos P, Goodale MA, Humphrey GK. The drawing of objects by a visual form agnosic: contribution of surface properties and memorial representations. *Neuropsychologia* 1993;31:251–259.

24. Milner AD, Perrett DI, Johnston RS, et al. Perception and action in visual form agnosia. *Brain* 1991;114:405–428.

25. Lissauer H. Ein Fall von Seelenblindheit nebst einem Beitrage zur Theorie derselben. *Arch Psychiatr Nervenkrank* 1890;21:222–270.

26. Servos P, Goodale MA. Preserved visual imagery in visual form agnosia. *Neuropsychologia* 1995;33:1383–1394.

27. Humphrey GK, Goodale MA, Gurnsey R. Orientation discrimination in a visual form agnosic: evidence from the McCollough effect. *Psychol Sci* 1991;2:331–335.

28. Goodale MA, Milner AD, Jakobson LS, et al. A neurological dissociation between perceiving objects and grasping them. *Nature* 1991;349:154–156.

29. Patla AE, Goodale MA. Obstacle avoidance during locomotion is unaffected in a patient with visual form agnosia. *Neuroreport* 1996;8:165–168.

30. Klüver H, Bucy PC. Preliminary analysis of functions of the temporal lobes of monkeys. *Arch Neurol Psychiatr* 1939;42:979–1000.

31. Pribram KH. Memory and the organization of attention. In: Lindsley DB, Lumsdaine AA, eds. *Brain function,* vol IV. *UCLA forum in medical sciences.* Berkeley: University of California Press, 1967:79–112.

32. Glickstein M, Buchbinder S, May JL III. Visual control of the arm, the wrist, and the fingers: pathways through the brain. *Neuropsychologia* 1998;36:981–1001.

33. Tanaka K. Inferotemporal cortex and object vision. *Ann Rev Neurosci* 1996;19:109–139.

34. Eskandar EM, Richmond BJ, Optican LM. Role of inferior temporal neurons in visual memory. I. Temporal encoding of information about visual images, recalled images, and behavioral context. *J Neurophysiol* 1992;68:1277–1295.

35. Fahy FL, Riches IP, Brown MW. Neuronal signals of importance to the performance of visual recognition memory tasks: evidence from recordings of single neurones in the medial thalamus of primates. In: Hicks TP, Molotchnikoff S, Ono T, eds. *The visually responsive neuron: from basic neurophysiology to behavior. Progress in brain research,* vol 95. Amsterdam: Elsevier, 1993:401–416.

36. Nishijo HT, Ono T, Tamura R, et al. Amygdalar and hippocampal neuron responses related to recognition and memory in monkey In: Hicks TP, Molotchnikoff S, Ono T, eds. *The visually responsive neuron: from basic neurophysiology to behavior: progress in brain research,* vol 95. Amsterdam: Elsevier, 1993:339–358.

37. Logothetis NK, Pauls J, Poggio T. Shape representation in the inferior temporal cortex of monkeys. *Curr Biol* 1995;5:552–563.

38. Logothetis NK. Object vision and visual awareness. *Curr Opin Neurobiol* 1998;8:536–544.

39. Hyvärinen J, Poranen A. Function of the parietal associative area 7 as revealed from cellular discharges in alert monkeys. *Brain* 1974;97:673–692.

40. Mountcastle VB, Lynch JC, Georgopoulos A, et al. Posterior parietal association cortex of the monkey: command functions for operations within extrapersonal space. *J Neurophysiol* 1975;38:871–908.

41. Andersen RA. Inferior parietal lobule function in spatial perception and visuomotor integration. In: Mountcastle VB, Plum F, Geiger SR, eds. *Handbook of physiology,* section 1: *The nervous system,* vol V. *Higher functions of the brain,* Part 2. Bethesda, MD: American Physiological Association, 1987:483–518.

42. Snyder LH, Batista AP, Andersen RA. Coding of intention in the posterior parietal cortex. *Nature* 1997;386:167–170.

43. Taira M, Mine S, Georgopoulos AP, et al. Parietal cortex neurons of the monkey related to the visual guidance of hand movement. *Exp Brain Res* 1990;83:29–36.

44. Sakata H, Taira M. Parietal control of hand action. *Curr Opin Neurobiol* 1994;4:847–856.

45. Ettlinger G. Parietal cortex in visual orientation. In: Rose FC, ed. *Physiological aspects of clinical neurology.* Oxford: Blackwell Scientific Publications 1977:93–100.

46. Gallese V, Murata A, Kaseda M, et al. Deficit of hand preshaping after muscimol injection in monkey parietal cortex. *Neuroreport* 1994;5:1525–1529.

47. Kanwisher N, Chun MM, McDermott J, et al. Functional imaging of human visual recognition. *Cognitive Brain Research* 1996;5:55–67.
48. Kiyosawa M, Inoue C, Kawasaki T, et al. Functional neuroanatomy of visual object naming: a PET study. *Graefes Arch Clin Exp Ophthalmol* 1996;234:110–115.
49. Malach R, Reppas JB, Benson RR, et al. Object-related activity revealed by functional magnetic resonance imaging in human occipital cortex. *Proc Natl Acad Sci USA* 1995;92:8135–8139.
50. Price CJ, Moore CJ, Humphreys GW, et al. The neural regions subserving object recognition and naming. *Proc R Soc Lond B* 1996;263:1501–1507.
51. Puce A, Allison T, Asgari M, et al. Differential sensitivity of human visual cortex to faces, letterstrings, and textures: a functional magnetic resonance imaging study. *J Neurosci* 1996;16:5205–5215.
52. Vanni S, Revonsuo A, Saarinin J, et al. Visual awareness of objects correlates with activity of right occipital cortex. *Neuroreport* 1996;8:183–186.
53. Matsumura M, Kawashima R, Naito E, et al. Changes in rCBF during grasing in humans examined by PET. *Neuroreport* 1996;7:749–752.
54. Kanwisher N, McDermott J, Chun MM. The fusiform face area: a module in human extrastriate cortex specialized for face perception. *J Neurosci* 1997;17:4302–4311.
55. McCarthy G, Puce A, Gore JC, et al. Face specific processing in the human fusiform gyrus. *J Cognitive Neuroscience* 1997;9:605–610.
56. Sams M, Hietanen JK, Hari R, et al. Face-specific responses from the human inferior occipito-temporal cortex. *Neuroscience* 1997;77:49–55.
57. Kawashima R, Naitoh E, Matsumura M, et al. Topographic representation in human intraparietal sulcus of reaching and saccade. *Neuroreport* 1996;7:1253–1256.
58. Clower DM, Hoffman JM, Votaw JR, et al. Role of posterior parietal cortex in the calibration of visually guided reaching. *Nature* 1996;383:618–621.
59. Duncker K. Induced motion. In: Ellis WD, ed. *A source book of Gestalt psychology*. New York: Humanities Press, 1928/1938:161–172.
60. Wong E, Mack A. Saccadic programming and perceived location. *Acta Psychol* 1981;48:123–131.
61. Bridgeman B, Kirch M, Sperling A. Segregation of cognitive and motor aspects of visual function using induced motion. *Percept Psychophysics* 1981;29:336–342.
62. Aglioti S, DeSouza JFX, Goodale MA. Size-contrast illusions deceive the eye but not the hand. *Curr Biol* 1995;5:679–685.
63. Brenner E, Smeets JBJ. Size illusion influences how we lift but not how we grasp an object. *Exp Brain Res* 1996;111:473–476.
64. Haffenden A, Goodale MA. The effect of pictorial illusion on prehension and perception. *J Cog Neurosci* 1998;10:122–136.
65. Andersen RA. Multimodal integration for the representation of space in the posterior parietal cortex. *Philos Trans R Soc Lond B* 1997;352:1421–142.
66. Goodale MA. Visuomotor control: where does vision end and action begin? *Curr Biol* 1998;8:R489–R491.

Neocortical Epilepsies.
Advances in Neurology, Vol. 84,
edited by P. D. Williamson, A. M. Siegel,
D. W. Roberts, V. M. Thadani, and M. S. Gazzaniga.
Lippincott Williams & Wilkins, Philadelphia © 2000.

8

Complementary Roles of Prefrontal Cortical Regions in Cognition, Memory, and Emotion in Primates

Helen Barbas

Department of Health Sciences, Boston University, Boston, Massachusetts 02215

OVERVIEW

The frontal cortex in primates encompasses a region extending from the central sulcus to the frontal pole. This large cortical expanse is roughly divided into two functionally distinct but interconnected regions: a *posterior region,* which includes the motor and premotor cortices, and an *anterior region,* which includes the prefrontal cortex (Fig. 8.1). The motor cortex, or Brodmann's (1) area 4, is situated anterior to the central sulcus and extends into its rostral bank. The premotor cortex is found immediately in front of the motor cortex. In nonhuman primates, the rostral border of the premotor cortex on the lateral surface is marked by the posterior bank of the arcuate sulcus. The premotor cortex is roughly coextensive with Brodmann's area 6, which was later subdivided into several subsectors on the basis of its architecture and connections (e.g., 2–6). The supplementary motor area (SMA or MII) lies on the dorsomedial border of the premotor cortex. Recent studies mapped additional premotor areas on the medial surface within area 24 (e.g., 4,7,8; for review, see 9).

The anterior half of the frontal cortex is the *prefrontal cortex,* a name introduced to distinguish it from the neighboring premotor cortices with which it shares a border. In addition to areas on the medial and lateral surfaces (Fig. 8.1A,B,D,E), the prefrontal cortex includes the orbitofrontal cortex on the basal surface (Fig. 8.1C). Caudally, the orbitofrontal cortex is bordered by the olfactory areas and the anterior insula, and rostrally it extends to the frontal pole.

The prefrontal cortex has been associated with central executive functions, an idea upheld by its special connectional relationship with the neighboring premotor cortices, which, in turn, are connected with the motor cortex. The premotor as well as the motor cortices give rise to robust descending pathways that lead to the final common pathway for action, the motoneurons in the spinal cord (e.g., 7,10,11). In addition to this relatively direct access to descending motor pathways, the prefrontal cortex is unique among association cortices as the recipient of input from the basal ganglia through the thalamus, a feature it shares with the premotor and motor cortices (for reviews, 12–14). Through its rich interconnections with motor control systems, the prefrontal cortex is in a unique position to initiate motor responses in behavioral settings.

The prefrontal areas commonly associated with central executive functions are the lateral areas, particularly the caudal areas (caudal part of areas 46, 8, 9, and 12), which have

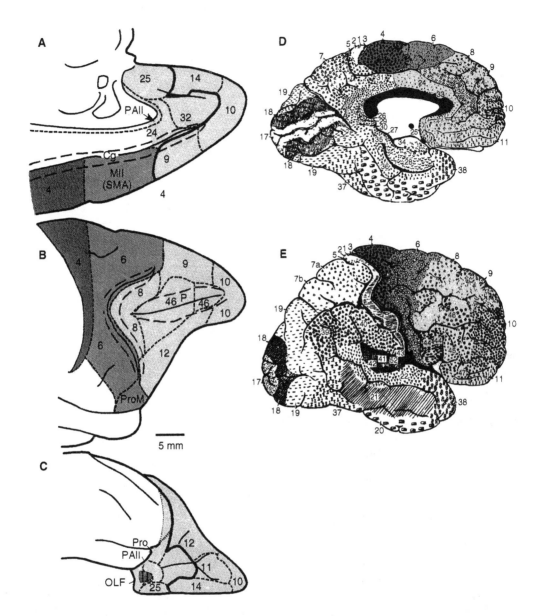

FIG. 8.1. The major subdivisions of the frontal cortex composed of the primary motor (area 4), pre-motor (areas 6 and MII), and the rostrally adjacent prefrontal cortices in the rhesus monkey shown on the medial **(A)**, lateral **(B)**, and orbital **(C)** surfaces and in the human, as shown on the map of Brodmann (31) on the medial **(D)** and lateral **(E)** surfaces. Additional motor areas have been identified with area 24 in primates (for review, see 159). The heavy lines in A and C delineate the agranular and dysgranular (limbic) cortices posteriorly, from the eulaminate prefrontal areas, anteriorly. The *fine dotted line* posterolaterally in C shows the part of area Pro that is normally hidden by the overlying temporal pole. The map of the prefrontal cortex in the rhesus monkey is according to reference 55, and the scale applies only for A–C. A, arcuate sulcus; Cg, cingulate sulcus; OLF, olfactory areas; P, principal sulcus; PAll, periallocortex; Pro, proisocortex; ProM, pro-motor area.

received the most experimental attention. Functionally, these areas are known for their role in cognitive tasks requiring the selection, retrieval, and holding of information in working memory long enough to accomplish a task with several sequential parts (for reviews, 15–17). The prefrontal cortex, however, has additional components on the medial and orbitofrontal surfaces (Fig. 8.1A,C, and D). The posterior parts of medial and orbitofrontal cortices belong to the cortical component of the limbic system by virtue of their architecture and connections, which were first demonstrated in classic studies (18–21). The most prominent and enduring deficits observed after damage to the prefrontal limbic areas lie in the realm of emotional behavior and social interactions in both human and nonhuman primates (for reviews, see 22–24). The limbic components of the prefrontal cortex have strong connections with the rest of the prefrontal cortex, providing the anatomic basis for the synthesis of cognitive and emotional processes in the cortex (for discussion, see 25). The strong linkage of areas associated with emotion and cognition underscores the biologic importance of this interaction (23). In fact, when areas associated with cognition and emotion are disconnected, both processes are disrupted, with profound effects on behavior, as evidenced in several psychiatric and neurologic diseases (for review, see 23).

From the perspective of its connections and functional characteristics, the prefrontal cortex may be viewed as a global executive decision and command center, using information from structures associated with sensory perception, memory, and emotion specific to a behavioral task. Distinct domains of the prefrontal cortex have specific but interrelated roles in behavior. Here evidence is presented that different regions of the prefrontal cortex have a set of functionally distinct cortical and subcortical connections that underlie their distinct roles in cognitive, mnemonic, and emotional processes and their capacity to activate different motor control channels for action. Ultimately, the roles of different prefrontal sectors are complementary and inextricably linked in executive functions in complex behavioral settings.

Sensory Input to Prefrontal Cortices

Sensory information is necessary for evaluating the environment for action. The prefrontal cortex is neither purely sensory nor motor but may be viewed as a region that acts on sensory information in a behavioral setting. One of the most impressive features of the prefrontal cortex is its robust linkage with sensory association cortices. Most sensory association cortices issue projections to prefrontal cortices, with the notable exception of the primary koniocortices, including visual area V1, somatosensory area 3b and auditory area A1. The primary cortices do not appear to interact monosynaptically with cortices outside their specific modality (for review, see 26). All other sensory association cortices, however, project to prefrontal cortices with some degree of specificity. For example, within the lateral prefrontal cortex, input from visual association cortices targets heavily the cortex within the anterior bank of the concavity of the arcuate sulcus and its inferior limb (area 8) and the caudal extent of the principal sulcus (areas 46 and 12) (27–37). Input from auditory cortices reaches several sites within the lateral prefrontal cortex but targets most heavily the frontal polar cortex (area 10), several sites of the dorsal bank of the principal sulcus (area 46), and the rostral part of the upper limb of the arcuate sulcus (area 8) (27–29,31). Somatosensory cortices project heavily to the central portion of the principal sulcus (ventral area 46) and the adjoining area 12 situated on the ventrolateral convexity of the prefrontal cortex (27,29,31,34,38).

Sensory input reaches medial and orbitofrontal cortices as well. Medial prefrontal areas receive projections from auditory cortices (27,39–41). Projections from visual and somatosensory cortices to medial prefrontal cortices, although present, are sporadic. This information suggests that outside the auditory modality medial cortices do not rely on direct

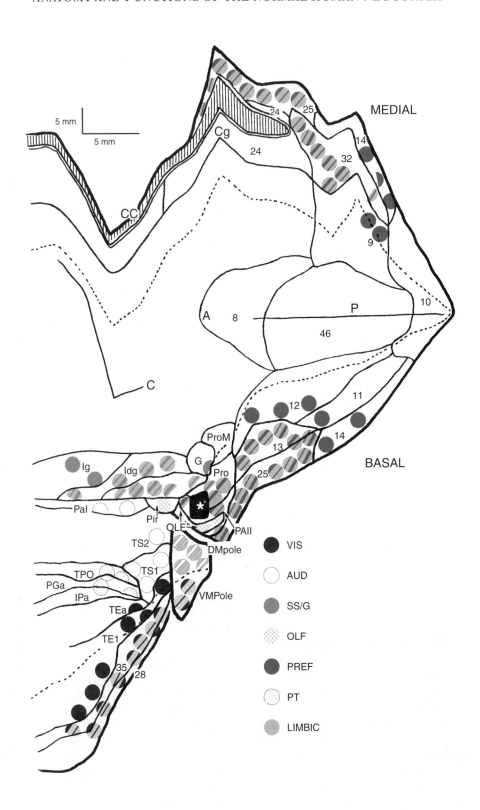

sensory information from the cortex. In sharp contrast, direct and robust projections from all unimodal sensory cortices reach the orbitofrontal cortices (Fig. 8.2). Distinguished initially for their association with the primary olfactory cortices (for review, see 42), there is now evidence that orbitofrontal areas receive robust projections from visual, auditory, and somatosensory cortices as well (43–45). This portion of the prefrontal cortex is truly polymodal, comparable, in extent and diversity, perhaps only to the rhinal regions in the temporal lobe (46–49).

Functional Specificity of Sensory Input to Prefrontal Cortices

The preceding discussion indicates that all sectors of the prefrontal cortex receive sensory input, albeit to differing extents. One of the ways to gain insight about the role of sensory input to the prefrontal cortex is to examine the nature of the input reaching each site. One way to infer the nature of input is to examine the topography of connections. There is evidence that sensory information in the cortex, particularly within the visual domain, is processed in parallel pathways (50). Moreover, the flow of information retains a certain degree of segregation all the way to the prefrontal cortex in primates (27,51), including humans (52). Thus, in rhesus monkeys, ventral occipital and inferior temporal visual cortices associated with feature analysis and their memory project primarily to ventrolateral and orbitofrontal cortices (Fig. 8.3, triangles, squares). In contrast, dorsomedial occipital and parietal visual cortices associated with visual spatial analysis project mostly to dorsolateral and medial prefrontal cortices (27) (Fig. 8.3, dots).

There is evidence that a comparable degree of segregation occurs in the somatosensory projections to prefrontal cortices as well, at least with regard to topography. For example, projections emanating from the medial bank of the intraparietal sulcus and the adjacent medial parietal cortex (area PE of Bonin and Bailey, 53) reach the upper bank of the principal sulcus (54). In contrast, the central portion of ventral area 46 and the ventrally adjacent area 12 receive projections from lateral somatosensory areas PF, 1, 2, and SII (27,29).

It should be noted, however, that the segregation of presumably functionally specific visual and somatosensory pathways to prefrontal cortices is only partial (27). Moreover, because there are connections between mediodorsal and basoventral prefrontal cortices (55) and between dorsal and ventral visual and somatosensory pathways, there is opportunity for considerable interaction between functionally distinct pathways (for reviews, see 26,56). What the topography of connections suggests is that there may be a bias for specific types of processing within a series of functionally related cortices rather than functional segregation. Damage to an area within the series may

FIG. 8.2. Diverse cortical input to orbitofrontal limbic cortex. An unfolded map of the frontal and temporal cortices shows the major sources of projections directed to orbitofrontal area PAll/Pro *(black area with white asterisk)*, originating in olfactory *(OLF)*, visual *(VIS)*, auditory *(AUD)*, somatosensory/gustatory *(SS/G)*, and parietotemporal *(PT)* association cortices. *Dark gray* shows projections from eulaminate prefrontal cortices, which have six layers; *light gray* shows projections from all limbic cortices, which have fewer than six layers. *Patterns over gray* identify limbic areas by the cortical system to which they are adjacent. *A*, arcuate sulcus; *AUD*, auditory cortices; *C*, central sulcus; *CC*, corpus callosum; *Cg*, cingulate sulcus; *DMpole*, dorsomedial temporal pole; *G*, gustatory area; *Ia*, agranular insula; *Idg*, dysgranular insula; *Ig*, granular insula; *OLF*, olfactory areas; *Pal*, parainsula; *Pir*, piriform (olfactory) cortex; *PREM*, premotor areas; *PT*, parietotemporal polymodal association areas (areas PGa, IPa, and TPO situated in the depths of the superior temporal sulcus); *SS*, somatosensory association areas; *TRANS*, transitional (limbic) areas; *TS1*, *TS2*, auditory association areas in the anterior superior temporal gyrus; *VIS*, visual association areas. (Adapted from Barbas H. Organization of cortical afferent input to orbitofrontal areas in the rhesus monkey. *Neuroscience* 1993;56:841–864, with permission.)

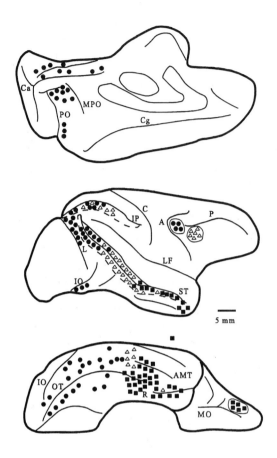

FIG. 8.3. Summary of projections from visual cortices to some lateral and orbitofrontal cortices. Projections directed to lateral prefrontal area 8 *(black dots)* in the concavity of the arcuate sulcus (A, *circled dotted area*) originate in posterior visual association cortices *(dots)*, those directed to the posterior periprincipalis area 46 *(circled triangles)* originate in posterior inferior temporal cortices *(triangles)*, and those directed to orbitofrontal area 11 *(circled squares)* originate in anterior inferior temporal cortices *(squares)*. *A*, arcuate sulcus, *AMT*, anterior middle temporal dimple; *C*, central sulcus; *Ca*, calcarine fissure; *Cg*, cingulate sulcus; *IO*, inferior occipital sulcus; *IP*, intraparietal sulcus; *LF*, lateral fissure; *MO*, medial orbital sulcus; *MPO*, medial parietooccipital sulcus; *P*, principal sulcus; *PO*, parietooccipital sulcus.

result in deficits with a bias of the principal functions of the damaged pathway.

Sensory input to prefrontal cortices varies in a significant way along the rostrocaudal dimension as well, where sensory processing varies serially with regard to the size of the receptive fields and specific features necessary to activate neurons. For example, within the visual cortical system, there are differences in the sensory processing of cortices associated with feature analysis along the anteroposterior dimension. Moreover, there are differences in the projections of these visual cortices to the prefrontal cortex (Fig. 8.3). For example, caudal periarcuate areas receive robust projections from caudal visual areas, including areas V2, V3, V4, and the posterior part of the inferior temporal cortex, including area TEO (27,28, 36,37,57) (Fig. 8.3). In contrast, orbitofrontal cortices receive projections from anterior inferior temporal cortices (e.g., 43), including a

substantial input from ventral temporal polar regions (Fig. 8.2), which are polymodal in nature (58). The significance of this organization lies in the functional attributes of the visual areas that project to prefrontal cortices along the rostrocaudal axis. Thus, periarcuate areas receive information from areas representing relatively early stages of visual processing, comparable to what other unimodal visual areas receive. Projections to periarcuate cortices, therefore, may contain relatively detailed information about specific aspects of the visual environment. In contrast, orbitofrontal cortices receive projections from anterior inferior temporal and ventral temporal polar cortices (27,43), where the visual receptive fields are global (58,59).

A comparable rostrocaudal organization can be seen in the projections from auditory areas to prefrontal cortices. For example, periarcuate (area 8) and the caudal principalis area

(area 46) receive projections from caudal areas in the superior temporal gyrus (27–29,40,60). In contrast, orbitofrontal and medial areas receive projections from the anterior superior temporal gyrus (39,43; for review, see 26). Thus, input to caudal lateral areas emanates from auditory areas that are closer to the primary auditory areas and auditory periphery, whereas projections to orbitofrontal and medial prefrontal cortices originate from areas that are comparatively far from the primary auditory areas.

Emotional Processing in the Prefrontal Cortices

The preceding discussion indicates that sensory input reaches the prefrontal cortex with some degree of specificity. An intriguing question concerns the role of sensory input to nonsensory areas, such as the prefrontal cortex. An important dimension of the sensory environment is its emotional significance, conveyed through the sensory modalities, such as the visual, in the form of a disturbing or joy-ful scene, or through the auditory modality at the sound of happy or sad news. The prefrontal cortex may use emotionally relevant sensory signals for action.

Information about the emotional undertones of events may be conveyed to the prefrontal cortices from the amygdala, a structure with a key role in emotions (for reviews, see 23,61,62). The prefrontal limbic cortices, in general, and their orbitofrontal component, in particular, are distinguished as recipient of heavy projections from the amygdala (45,63–66), originating from a diverse set of amygdaloid nuclei, including the basolateral, basomedial (also known as accessory basal), the lateral and the cortical, suggesting that prefrontal limbic cortices participate in a network associated with emotions. In fact, the orbitofrontal limbic cortices and the amygdala in primates have several features in common. For example, the orbitofrontal cortex and the amygdala are strikingly similar as recipients of robust projections from all sensory cortices (43–45,67,68) (Fig. 8.4). Moreover, sensory input to both structures is qualitatively similar,

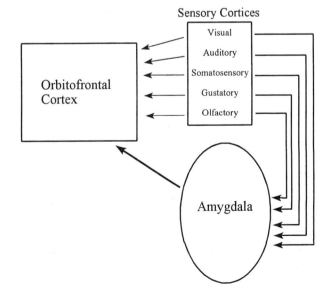

FIG. 8.4. Direct and possible indirect projections from sensory cortices to orbitofrontal cortices. Orbitofrontal areas receive projections from olfactory, gustatory, somatosensory, auditory, and visual association cortices. Like the orbitofrontal cortex, the amygdala receives projections from cortices associated with each of the sensory modalities. In turn, the amygdala projects to orbitofrontal cortex, providing a potential indirect pathway for sensory information to reach the orbitofrontal cortex.

originating in areas where the emphasis on processing appears to be in the significance of features of stimuli and their memory (for review, see 25). Monkeys with damage to the orbitofrontal cortex or the amygdala do not exhibit appropriate emotional responses necessary for maintaining normal social interactions (for review, see 69). This point has been exemplified for humans in the neurologic archives, including the famous case of Phineas Gage, who sustained a massive injury to the orbitofrontal cortex and exhibited marked changes in personality (for review, see 24).

Notwithstanding the connectional and functional similarities of the amygdala and the orbitofrontal cortex, their contribution to emotions may be distinct. Recent findings indicate that the amygdala increases its activity during viewing of masked fearful faces, when there is no conscious awareness of the event (70). Moreover, a short subcortical loop connecting the amygdala with the thalamus can support fear conditioning (71). The amygdala thus receives signals concerned with the internal environment and issues efferent signals directly or indirectly to hypothalamic and brainstem autonomic structures (for review, see 72), suggesting that it may be likened to an elaborate central reflex structure for the internal milieu.

Because the experience of specific emotions is conscious, however, the question arises as to which pathway mediates this process. Classic studies indicate that the cortex is an essential component for the conscious perception of emotion (73). The amygdala is associated with emotion and projects robustly to orbitofrontal cortices (63–66; for reviews, see 23,25); therefore, this pathway may be essential for emotional awareness. The orbitofrontal cortex appears to represent a different level of processing of emotional information, distinguished as the recipient not only of massive sensory input from the cortex directly but also indirectly through the amygdala (Fig. 8.4). The rich direct and indirect sensory input to orbitofrontal limbic cortices may underlie the process through which events acquire emotional significance and awareness.

Although orbitofrontal cortices receive the heaviest projections from the amygdala, medial prefrontal cortices receive a substantial projection from the amygdala as well (e.g., 64,65). Unlike the multimodal orbitofrontal limbic cortices, however, the medial prefrontal cortices seem to receive preferential input from auditory cortices (27,39–41,74,75). Auditory input to medial prefrontal cortices originates in the parabelt and the anterior part of the superior temporal gyrus (39), where neurons do not respond to pure auditory tones but rather are broadly tuned (76) and respond best to complex species-specific vocalizations in monkeys (77,78). In fact, cingulate areas situated around the rostrum of the corpus callosum have a role in vocalization (79–83; for reviews, see 84,85), which depend on a special relationship with auditory association areas (86,87). In monkeys, anterior cingulate areas seem to be specialized for emotional communication, such as distress calls emitted by infants when separated from their mothers (88).

In humans, there appears to be a functional distinction in the activity of medial prefrontal and auditory cortices during monitoring of actual versus inner speech; moreover, these relationships are altered in schizophrenic patients who hallucinate (89–91). This evidence suggests that medial prefrontal and auditory cortices function in concert to monitor inner speech and to distinguish external auditory stimuli from internal auditory representations. In addition to input from unimodal auditory cortices, medial prefrontal cortices receive robust projections from dorsal superior temporal polar cortices, which are considered limbic and may encode the emotional significance of auditory stimuli. The commonly experienced emotional undertones of auditory hallucinations by schizophrenic patients (for review, see 92) may be explained by the strong projections from temporal polar cortices to medial prefrontal cortices (39).

The preceding discussion suggests that although caudal orbitofrontal and medial prefrontal cortices have a role in emotion, they may have specialized roles within this domain. Whereas the orbitofrontal cortex seems to have a role in the appreciation of the emotional significance of events, in general, the medial prefrontal cortices seem to have a role in emotional vocalization and species-specific communication.

In contrast to both orbitofrontal and medial prefrontal cortices, lateral prefrontal cortices receive few, and topographically restricted projections from the amygdala (64). The question arises as to whether the lateral prefrontal cortices have a role in emotion. Lateral prefrontal cortices are connected with the prefrontal limbic areas (55) and thus may have indirect access to information from the amygdala. As the recipient of input from relatively early sensory processing cortices and from parietal visuomotor regions (e.g., 27,28,32, 93,94), the role of lateral prefrontal cortices may be in discriminating and sampling sensory input (17,95) and in evaluating whether a specific set of actions is necessary in emotional situations. On the basis of their connections, lateral prefrontal cortices may be construed as having a role in the cognitive component of emotions.

The preceding discussion suggests that lateral and limbic prefrontal cortices have complementary roles in emotions. The differential role of distinct prefrontal cortices in emotions may be illustrated with an example. A noise in the path during a walk in the forest initially may suggest that a snake is lurking in the brush. Activation of pathways linking the amygdala with prefrontal limbic cortices is likely to mediate the conscious perception of fear. Lateral prefrontal cortices, on the other hand, may be responsible for discriminating and evaluating what action is necessary. Directed attention toward the noise is necessary for deciding whether the situation is threatening. If the noise agent is a squirrel, no immediate action is necessary. On the other hand, if the noise agent is indeed a snake, purposive action is necessary to run from danger in the opposite direction. The robust connections of lateral prefrontal cortices with early sensory cortices (for review, see 25), as well as their strong connections with premotor cortices in macaque monkeys (e.g., 2,96–98), pro-

vide the anatomic basis for the discriminatory component as well as the executive response for this task.

Mnemonic Processing in the Prefrontal Cortices

Lateral Prefrontal Cortices and Working Memory

The rich variety of input to prefrontal cortices has an important function in the selection of stimuli and monitoring of responses while performing a task. As described, the strong connections of lateral prefrontal cortices with relatively early processing sensory cortices (Fig. 8.3) may endow them with the capability of interpreting the sensory environment for action. In the periarcuate area, visual and auditory input may be involved in directing the eyes and head to behaviorally relevant stimuli in the environment. This idea is supported by the robust and preferential projections from visuomotor areas in the lateral bank of the caudal intraparietal sulcus to periarcuate and caudal periprincipalis areas in macaque monkeys (27–29,54,93,99) (Fig. 8.3). Damage to the periarcuate cortex or the lateral parietal cortex leads to inattention to stimuli on the contralateral side of the lesion (for review, see 100). In the frontal eye fields, neurons that respond to visual stimuli increase their response when the monkey orients to the stimulus or uses the information to guide behavior (101,102).

Lateral prefrontal cortices generally have been ascribed a role in sequential tasks involving orientation and selection of behaviorally relevant stimuli and monitoring self-generated responses to perform a task (for reviews, see 15–17). There is evidence that cognitive tasks with different demands engage different prefrontal cortices (e.g., 17,95,103–106), although generally they are considered under the rubric of *working memory* because all require monitoring external stimuli or self-initiated responses. The task may involve looking at a map and remembering the route long enough while driving to get to the airport in a strange city. One of the essential elements of such a task is the ability to hold information temporarily in memory. Classic studies indicated that damage to lateral prefrontal cortices, in particular an area around the principal sulcus, impairs the ability of monkeys to remember after a few seconds' delay where a food reward was hidden (107; for reviews, see 16,108,109). Physiologic data indicate that there is a set of neurons that fire during the delay period (104,110–114) and may represent the neural correlate of holding events temporarily in mind.

Orbitofrontal and Medial Prefrontal Cortices and Long-term Memory

In contrast to lateral prefrontal cortices, the orbitofrontal and medial cortices appear to tap into qualitatively different sources of mnemonic information by virtue of their principal connections. Unlike area 8 or caudal area 46, there is no evidence that orbitofrontal and medial cortices are connected with parietal visuomotor regions. Sensory input reaches the orbitofrontal and medial prefrontal cortices from sensory cortices which are at a considerable distance from the sensory periphery (Figs. 8.2 and 8.3). In addition to more global processing of the visual environment, neurons in increasingly anterior inferior temporal visual cortices show increased responses to mnemonic information within the visual domain (115,116). The same pattern is seen in the projections from auditory cortices (for reviews, see 25,26). Thus, both orbitofrontal and medial prefrontal cortices receive projections from anterior auditory association regions, which are not only globally tuned but appear to encode the significance of auditory stimuli, as discussed previously.

Several connectional features of orbitofrontal and medial prefrontal cortices suggest that their role in mnemonic processing is distinct from that of lateral prefrontal cortices. Posterior medial and orbitofrontal cortices are distinguished by their connections with cortical and subcortical structures implicated in remembering information on a long-term basis, including the perirhinal region (areas 35 and 36), the entorhinal cortex (area 28),

and the parahippocampal cortex (areas TF and TH) (27,46,47,117,118) (Fig. 8.5). In addition, the hippocampus sends robust projections to prefrontal limbic cortices as well, particularly to caudal medial, but also to orbitofrontal cortices (45,65,119,120). Damage to medial temporal and hippocampal areas in humans and nonhuman primates results in an inability to remember events occurring after the damage (for reviews, see 121–124). On the basis of their robust connections with the medial temporal cortices, caudal medial and orbitofrontal limbic cortices (Fig. 8.1A,C) appear to be aligned with medial temporal cortices in networks concerned with long-term memory.

In marked contrast to the orbitofrontal and medial cortices, lateral prefrontal cortices do

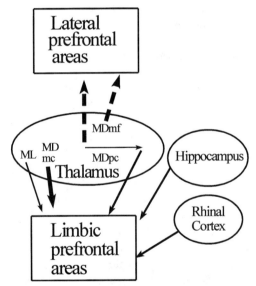

FIG. 8.5. The differential projection from structures associated with mnemonic processes to prefrontal cortices. Input from structures associated with long-term memory, including the hippocampus, the rhinal cortex (areas 28, 35, 36), the thalamic MDmc, the posterior part of MDpc and midline nuclei *(ML)* project preferentially to limbic prefrontal cortices. In contrast, lateral prefrontal cortices receive thalamic projections mostly from the rostral part of MDpc and from the multiform division of MD *(MDmf)*. Arrow above MDpc shows the rostrocaudal dimension of this subdivision of MD.

not have significant connections with rhinal cortices or the hippocampus. Instead, the only significant monosynaptic interaction of lateral prefrontal cortices with limbic cortices appears to be through their connection with posterior cingulate areas associated with attentional processes and eye movement (100,125,126). These connections, coupled with a strong projection from parietal visuomotor regions (for review, see 127), reinforce the idea that lateral prefrontal cortices have a role in attentional processes.

Qualitative Matching of Thalamic and Cortical Input in Functionally Distinct Prefrontal Cortices

Mnemonic Processing: Lateral Prefrontal Cortices

In the sensory systems, the thalamus conveys signals from the sensory periphery to the respective sensory cortices. The thalamus, however, is a major relay for all parts of the cortex (for review, see 128), raising the intriguing question of the role of thalamic input to association cortices, such as the prefrontal. In all systems, the thalamus receives input from subcortical and cortical structures and thus is not just a relay but an important processing center. In the sensory systems, thalamic processing is specific to each modality. By analogy with sensory cortices, projections from the thalamus to functionally distinct prefrontal cortices may reinforce signals associated with their specific cognitive, mnemonic, and emotional processing.

The idea that thalamocortical interactions may support specific prefrontal functions is supported by different sets of thalamic projections directed to functionally distinct prefrontal cortices. For example, area 8 (which includes the frontal eye fields (FEF), receives robust projections from the lateral portion of the mediodorsal nucleus (MDpc), its multiform division (MDmf), the suprageniculate, and limitans nuclei (28,129). These thalamic nuclei, in turn, receive projections from the superior colliculus and the lateral part of the

substantia nigra, both of which have been implicated in eye movement (130–138). In addition, area 8 receives input from the upper parts of the central lateral and paracentral thalamic nuclei (28,129), which have visual and visuomotor properties (139,140). In quantitative analyses in the same animals, we found that when the majority of cortical projection neurons originate in visual and visuomotor areas, most of the thalamic projection neurons originate in nuclei with visual and visuomotor properties as well (28,129) (Fig. 8.6).

The FEF has been implicated in searching the environment in behavioral tasks through accurate timing of eye movements (141). Moreover, there appears to be specificity in this function within subsectors of area 8. For example, electric microstimulation of rostral area 8, at the tip of the upper limb of the arcuate sulcus, elicits large saccadic eye movements (142) within an area that receives input from auditory cortices and from visual cortices representing peripheral visual fields (28). In contrast, electric stimulation of caudal area 8 at the junction of the upper and lower limbs of the arcuate sulcus elicits small and medium-sized saccades (142,143), coinciding with an area that receives robust projections from visual cortices, including substantial input from areas representing central visual fields (27,28). Thus, as the recipient of projections from visual, visuomotor, and auditory cortices, area 8 appears to be well suited for scanning central parts of the visual field using small saccades or orienting to peripheral visual and auditory stimuli using large saccades and head movement. Moreover, the thalamic connections of area 8 appear to be in functional register with its cortical connections.

An important function associated with lateral prefrontal cortices, particularly caudal area 46, is remembering information over a short delay (for reviews, see 15,16,108,109). Functional studies in humans demonstrated the involvement of lateral prefrontal cortices in a variety of tasks requiring holding information in memory on a temporary basis (e.g., 52,144–153). Most thalamic neurons projecting to areas 46 and 9 are found in MD, partic-

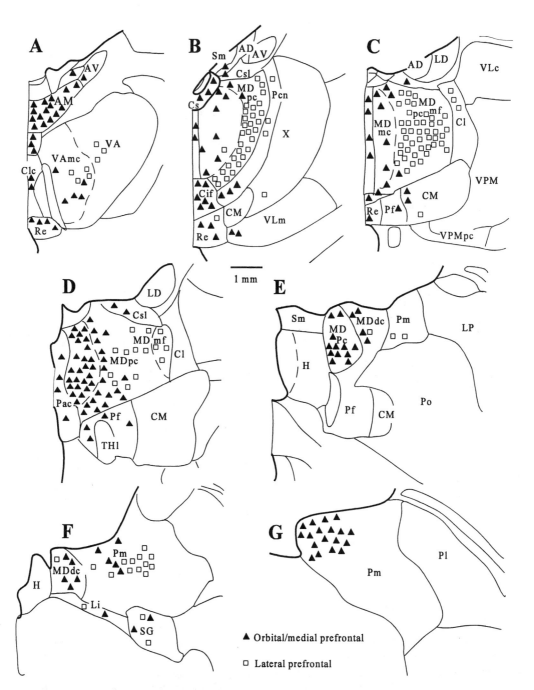

FIG. 8.6. Summary of the major projections from the thalamus to prefrontal areas. **A–G** represent anterior to posterior thalamic levels. *Triangles* represent neurons directed to some orbitofrontal and medial cortices, and *squares* depict neurons projecting to lateral cortices (areas 46 and 8). *AD*, anterior dorsal; *AM*, anterior medial; *AV*, anterior ventral; *Cl*, central lateral; *Clc*, central latocellular; *CM*, centromedian; *H*, habenula; *LD*, lateral dorsal; *Li*, limitans; *LP*, lateral posterior; *MD* (mediodorsal, with the following subdivisions: *dc*, densocellular; *mc*, magnocellular; *mf*, multiform; *pc*, parvicellular); *Pac*, paraventricular, caudal; *Pcn*, paracentral; *Pf*, parafascicular; *Pl*, pulvinar lateralis; *Pm*, pulvinar medialis; *Po*, pulvinar oralis; *Re*, reuniens; *SG*, suprageniculate; *VA* (ventral anterior; *mc*, magnocellular subdivision); *VL*, ventrolateral, *VLc*, ventral lateral caudal; *VLm*, ventral lateral medial; *VPM*, ventral posterior medial; *THl*, habenulo-interpeduncular tract. (Adapted from Barbas H, Henion TH, Dermon CR. Diverse thalamic projections to the prefrontal cortex in the rhesus monkey. *J Comp Neurol* 1991;313:65–94, with permission.)

ularly its parvicellular component (129,154). Physiologic studies indicate that in MD, like in lateral prefrontal cortices, neurons are active when animals must hold information temporarily in memory in delayed response tasks (155). Thus, the visual, visuomotor and working memory tasks associated with lateral areas 8 and 46 are matched by their thalamic connections with nuclei associated with these functions (Fig. 8.6).

Mnemonic Processing: Medial and Orbitofrontal Limbic Cortices

In contrast, prefrontal limbic cortices receive projections from a different set of thalamic nuclei, including the midline, the magnocellular sector of the mediodorsal nucleus (MDmc), and the caudal part of parvicellular MD (MDpc) (45,129,154,156,157) (Fig. 8.5). All these thalamic nuclei have been implicated in long-term memory, and their damage leads to the classic amnesic syndrome (158,159; for review, see 160). Even though MDpc projects to a certain extent to all prefrontal cortices, the projections originate from functionally distinct sectors. Thus, the caudal part of MDpc, which has been implicated in long-term memory in both humans and monkeys (159,161,162), projects preferentially to orbitofrontal and medial prefrontal cortices. In contrast, lateral prefrontal cortices receive projections from the anterior part of MDpc (Figs. 8.5 and 8.6). The thalamic connections of limbic and lateral prefrontal cortices, therefore, are consistent with the nature of signals conveyed to these cortices from functionally distinct cortices.

Emotional Processing

In a previous section, it was shown that the amygdala, which has a pivotal role in emotions, sends robust projections to prefrontal limbic cortices, particularly the orbitofrontal. In addition, the amygdala targets heavily MDmc (66,163,164), which, in turn, provides robust projections to prefrontal limbic cortices, particularly the caudal orbitofrontal (129,154,156,157,165,166). This circuitry

provides yet another example in which sensory signals, in this case concerning the emotional environment, reach the orbitofrontal cortices directly from the amygdala and indirectly through MDmc. Finally, midline thalamic nuclei associated with the affective aspect of pain (for review, see 167) project preferentially to prefrontal limbic cortices (129,154).

Moreover, our quantitative analyses indicate that whereas MDmc and the midline nuclei most heavily target prefrontal limbic cortices on the caudal orbitofrontal and medial surfaces, they do so in opposite directions. Thus, MDmc issues a higher proportion of the thalamic neurons directed to orbitofrontal cortices than to medial cortices, whereas the opposite is observed for projections from midline nuclei (154). The differential projection from MDmc and midline nuclei suggests that orbitofrontal and medial prefrontal cortices may have distinct roles in emotional processes, as suggested on the basis of their cortical connections. The preferential projection from MDmc aligns the orbitofrontal cortices with the amygdala, which issues robust projections to both MDmc and orbitofrontal cortices (66). The preferential projection from midline nuclei to caudal medial prefrontal cortices suggests that they may have a role in the affective significance of pain (for review, see 84), including aspects of psychic pain, such as distress and the sense of suffering experienced by patients in several psychiatric diseases.

In summary, based on the linkages of the specific thalamic nuclei that project to the prefrontal cortex, the thalamus may be construed as providing information about the internal environment. In the case of lateral prefrontal cortices, this information may be used to focus attention on behaviorally relevant events and to hold information in working memory. In the case of prefrontal limbic cortices, information from the thalamus appears to be concerned with retrieval of information from long-term memory stores and signals concerning the emotional environment. Moreover, the thalamic connections of lateral and limbic prefrontal cortices match well the rest of the cortical and subcortical connections of these areas with structures associated with cognitive, mnemonic, and emotional processes.

Access of Functionally Specific Prefrontal Cortices to Distinct Motor Control Systems

Basal Ganglia

Prefrontal cortices with executive functions must be linked with motor control systems. The prefrontal cortices, including lateral, medial, and orbitofrontal cortices, are a major target of the basal ganglia. The striatum, a major component of the basal ganglia, receives a wealth of information from all cortical areas but targets selectively the frontal cortex, which includes the posterior cortical motor system and the prefrontal cortex, shown in Fig. 8.1 (for reviews, see 12,14, 168). Unlike the direct projections from the cortex to the striatum, the ascending influences from the basal ganglia to the cortex occur indirectly through the thalamus (Fig. 8.6A). In the case of the prefrontal cortex, projections from the basal ganglia are relayed through the thalamic MD and ventral anterior (VA) nuclei (for review, see 168). As demonstrated in classic and recent studies, prefrontal cortices are distinguished by their robust projections from MD (for review, see 128); however, nuclei besides MD project to prefrontal cortices as well (e.g., 169). One of these is the VA complex (VA and VAmc), which contributes anywhere from about 2% to a quarter of all projection neurons from the thalamus directed to lateral, orbitofrontal, and medial prefrontal cortices (129,154) (Fig. 8.6A). Moreover, functionally distinct prefrontal areas are influenced by the basal ganglia via largely parallel pathways (12), suggesting that they have specific roles in motor behavior.

The segregation of pathways through the basal ganglia to prefrontal cortices appears to be relative rather than absolute (168). Evidence based on connections suggests that the pathway from lateral prefrontal cortices through the basal ganglia is directed not only to the lateral cortices of origin but also to the premotor cortices. Similarly, the motor path-

way projects not only to the motor cortices and the supplementary motor area (SMA) but also to the lateral prefrontal cortices (168). This evidence suggests that lateral prefrontal cortices have multiple interactions with premotor cortices for action.

Lateral Prefrontal Cortices Are Linked with Specialized Brainstem and Cortical Premotor Systems

Additional access to specialized motor control systems is seen for lateral cortices. For example, the FEF projects to the superior colliculus and brainstem oculomotor control systems necessary for eye movements (for review, see 170). In addition, lateral prefrontal cortices, including areas 8, 46, and 9, have rich direct interconnections with premotor cortices (Fig. 8.7B) situated in the posterior bank of the arcuate sulcus and in the cingulate region (2,4,34,96,98,171–176) and thus have access to areas for limb and body movement. The preceding discussion suggests that lateral prefrontal cortices have direct corticocortical connections with premotor cortices and brainstem oculomotor structures as well as rich indirect connections with motor control systems through the basal ganglia.

Prefrontal Limbic Cortices and Motor Access for Emotions

The association of prefrontal limbic cortices with the striatum is with its ventral component, also known as the *limbic striatum* because of its connections with subcortical limbic structures, including the amygdala and the hippocampus (177,178). The limbic striatum projects through a relay in the ventral pallidum to MDmc, which then projects back to prefrontal limbic cortices (for review, see 168). In addition, the limbic striatum projects to the substantia nigra pars reticulata, which projects via other sectors of MD to lateral prefrontal cortices. As indicated, lateral prefrontal cortices have direct access to premotor cortices for action. These pathways may be considered multisynaptic pathways through which emotion can influence motor behavior.

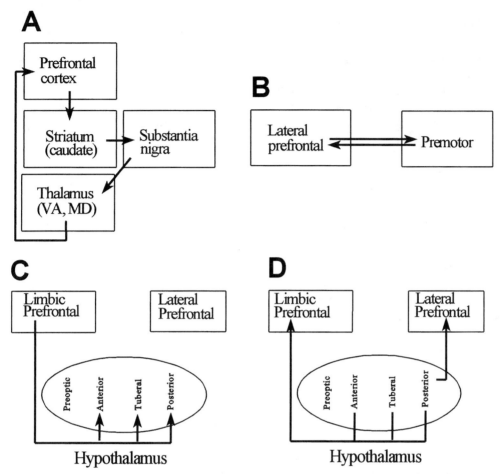

FIG. 8.7. Summary of some of the pathways linking prefrontal cortices with motor control systems. **A:** All prefrontal cortices project to the caudate nucleus of the basal ganglia and are, in turn, influenced by the basal ganglia indirectly through multisynaptic pathways conveyed to the thalamic VA and MD nuclei and back to prefrontal cortices. **B:** Lateral prefrontal cortices are connected bidirectionally with premotor cortices. **C:** Specialized descending projections from the prefrontal limbic cortices to hypothalamic autonomic centers provide a possible pathway for the expression of emotions. **D:** Lateral prefrontal cortices, like the limbic, receive projections from the hypothalamus, but they do not issue projections to the hypothalamus (see 179).

In the case of the prefrontal limbic cortices, there is an additional motor control pathway involving the autonomic effector structures recruited for the expression of emotions. Recent findings indicate that there is a robust and selective descending projection from prefrontal limbic cortices to hypothalamic autonomic centers in rhesus monkeys (179) (Fig. 8.7C). This indicates that prefrontal limbic cortices not only receive ascending projections from the amygdala, but they also issue robust descending projections to hypothalamic autonomic centers and thus are capable of changing cardiac and respiratory responses in emotional situations. These findings are consistent with evidence that damage to the orbitofrontal cortex in humans impairs their ability to respond autonomically in emotional situations (180,181). Although they retain cognitive function, such patients make poor decisions, suggesting that cognitive processes become dissociated from an emotionally driven autonomic response. This behavior may be attributed to a disconnection of prefrontal limbic cortices from autonomic effector centers that innervate peripheral autonomic organs normally engaged in emotional situations. Medial prefrontal cortices appear to have a specific role in emotional vocalization, effected through an additional projection to brainstem structures that innervate laryngeal muscles necessary for phonation (for reviews, see 85,182).

In contrast to orbitofrontal and medial limbic cortices, lateral prefrontal cortices receive only ascending input from the hypothalamus (Fig. 8.7D), comparable to the widespread projections seen from neurotransmitter specific brainstem and basal forebrain structures to all cortical areas (e.g., 183,184). The preceding discussion suggests that the executive functions of distinct prefrontal cortices depend on functionally specific motor control systems that match well their regional specialization in cognitive and emotional processes.

Significance of Feedback Systems for Neural Function

Corticosubcortical Interactions

An important principle in the organization of the nervous system is that connections are more often than not reciprocal, suggesting that neural systems function as closed-loop systems through feedforward and feedback communication. The significance of bidirectional circuits has become increasingly apparent in recent years in functionally diverse neural systems. For example, in the visual system, activation of a feedback pathway between the primary visual cortex and the lateral geniculate nucleus increases the efficacy of feature specific input to the visual cortex (185). The initiation of motor action is thought to depend on bidirectional activation of multisynaptic pathways from the cortex through the striatum and back to the frontal cortex and is greatly impaired when part of this loop is disrupted in Parkinson's disease (for review, see 14).

The functions of prefrontal cortices appear to depend on bidirectional connections with

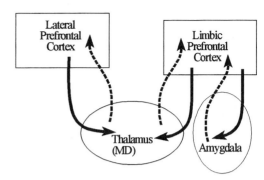

FIG. 8.8. Bidirectional activation of a pathway connecting lateral and limbic prefrontal cortices with distinct parts of MD may reinforce their respective roles in working memory and long-term memory. Bidirectional pathways linking the prefrontal limbic cortices with the amygdala may underlie perceptual awareness of emotion. In the corticosubcortical pathways, information is relayed to the cortex and back to the thalamus from different layers.

specific subcortical structures as well. For example, in the lateral prefrontal cortex as well as in MD, neurons fire in association with delayed response tasks (51,113,186, 187), and when the lateral prefrontal cortex is incapacitated by cooling, neuronal responses in MD associated with working memory are seriously disrupted (186). This evidence suggests that bidirectional interactions between the prefrontal cortex and MD are intricately involved in a specific task that requires mnemonic processing. Moreover, the topographically distinct connections of MD with prefrontal limbic and lateral areas may reinforce their respective role in long-term memory and working memory (Fig. 8.8). The additional bidirectional connections between the amygdala and prefrontal limbic cortices (Fig. 8.8) may be the structural basis for the conscious perception of emotion. Disruption of this interaction is likely to disconnect emotional processes from cognitive processes with detrimental effects on behavior (23).

Corticocortical Interactions

Cerebral cortices are connected through bidirectional pathways in a consistent manner

(188). With regard to the prefrontal cortex, we previously showed that cortical structure can be used to predict whether one area will send projections predominantly from its deep layers or from its upper layers (189). *Structure* in this context refers to broad laminar features of areas, based on the number of identifiable layers and the relative distinction of the layers. Limbic areas differ from other prefrontal cortices in their connections, and they also differ in their structure. Limbic areas have three or four identifiable layers, whereas all other prefrontal areas have six layers and are called *eulaminate areas,* although they, too, vary in the definition of their layers (55). When a cortex with more layers or higher laminar definition is connected with a cortex with fewer layers or lower laminar definition, projection neurons originate mostly in the upper layers (2–3), and their axons terminate in the deep layers (4–6). Connections proceeding in the opposite direction originate predominantly in the deep layers (5–6), and their axons terminate mostly in the upper layers (1–3,189). Thus, when lateral prefrontal areas, which are eulaminate, project to limbic areas, most projection neurons originate in the upper layers. Conversely, when limbic areas project to eulaminate areas, most projection neurons originate in the deep layers (188). This rule applies to all limbic cortices in primates (for review, see 25). Projection neurons from deep layers in sensory systems have been ascribed a feedback role (e.g., 190–193). By analogy, limbic cortices may provide feedback to the entire cortex as well as to subcortical structures.

Clinical Implications of Differences in Structure and the Pattern of Connections

The above discussion suggests that connections follow specific rules based on the structure of the interconnected cortices. This finding raises several questions. For example, how does such a specific pattern of connections arise? What are the functional and clinical implications of these connections? In the rhesus monkey connections of prefrontal cortices are established prenatally (194) and their pat-

tern is likely to depend on a variety of developmental factors (for reviews see 195,196). It is possible that prefrontal cortices with different structure develop at separate times or rate and thus are subject to distinct developmental constraints, as suggested by the following observations. Recent evidence indicates that prefrontal limbic areas have a lower density of neurons than the eulaminate areas (197). Moreover, prefrontal limbic cortices, in comparison with the eulaminate, have a higher density of neurons that are positive for nitric oxide synthase (198), an enzyme that is expressed early in cortical development (199). The preceding observations are consistent with differences in the temporal sequence of development of limbic and eulaminate cortices because the onset or duration of neurogenesis affects neural density (e.g., 200). Earlier completion of development would coincide with a time when fewer neurons leave the cell cycle and migrate to their final cortical destination, and would result in a lower density of neurons in the cortex. Temporal differences in development also may account for differences in the neurochemical profile and the pattern of connections of areas, based on the specific developmental constraints at distinct ontogenetic periods.

Prefrontal limbic cortices are preferentially vulnerable in several neurologic and psychiatric diseases, including epilepsy and Alzheimer's disease (201–210). Differences in cortical structure and neurochemical characteristics may underlie the preferential vulnerability of limbic areas in these diseases. Experimentally induced epileptiform activity in the hippocampus abolishes parvalbumin immunoreactivity in a subset of inhibitory basket cells, suggesting either diminished synthesis of the protein or the selective loss of a subpopulation of basket cells (211). In this context, it is intriguing that in normal monkeys prefrontal limbic areas have a lower density of the calcium-binding protein parvalbumin than eulaminate areas (197). This, and a number of other neurochemical features that distinguish prefrontal limbic and eulaminate areas, may contribute to the predilection of limbic areas to epileptiform activity.

Limbic cortices are found at the bottom of cortical structural hierarchies and thus may function as a feedback system to the neuraxis. The idea that prefrontal limbic areas are a model feedback system has several clinical implications in view of their preferential involvement in several neurologic and psychiatric diseases, including epilepsy, Alzheimer's disease, schizophrenia, obsessive compulsive disorder, and Tourette's syndrome (212–214; for reviews, see 210,215). The pattern of connections implies that disruption of limbic cortices in these diseases is likely to affect preferentially a major feedback communication system with specific functions. For example, the mnemonic deficits in Alzheimer's disease may be explained, in part, by the preferential involvement of limbic areas, in general, and the prevalence of degeneration in the deep layers (216), in particular. The degenerative process in this case is likely to disrupt feedback projections emanating from the deep layers of prefrontal limbic cortices to MDmc and the posterior part of MDpc, both of which have a role in long-term memory, as discussed already.

Preferential involvement of limbic areas in psychiatric diseases, such as schizophrenia, is likely to affect a feedback system from prefrontal limbic cortices to lateral prefrontal and other cortices and dissociate the interaction of circuits underlying cognitive and emotional processes. Reduced activation of pathways connecting the amygdala with prefrontal limbic cortices (Fig. 8.8) is likely to disrupt a circuit associated with attaching the appropriate emotion to an event and may account for the flattening of emotions and inappropriate affect in several diseases, including schizophrenia, psychopathic personality, or autistic behavior. This idea is consistent with observations that activity in prefrontal limbic cortices is reduced in some of these disorders and is exemplified by inappropriate affect when orbitofrontal cortices are damaged (e.g., 23,181).

Conversely, excessive and persistent bidirectional activation of the amygdala and limbic prefrontal cortices may occur in mental diseases, such as obsessive compulsive disorder accompanied by anxiety. The increased activation of the orbitofrontal cortex in this disorder is well documented, although the striatum also has been implicated (215), possibly for translating thoughts into action, such as washing the hands.

CONCLUSION

In summary, specialized sectors of the prefrontal cortex appear to have distinct and complementary roles in cognition, memory, and emotion. This idea is supported by the complex but functionally related connections of distinct prefrontal cortices. In each prefrontal sector, cortical input is complemented by connections with functionally related subcortical structures, and each sector has access to specialized motor control systems that appear to be engaged synergistically in executive functions. Reciprocity of connections appears to be a common feature in neural systems and is fundamental to normal function. Damage to one part of a bidirectional circuit may effectively change a closed-loop system to an open-loop system, with detrimental effects on neural function. In their participation in bidirectional circuits, limbic areas appear to function as a model feedback system to the neuraxis. Prefrontal limbic cortices are preferentially involved in several neurologic and psychiatric diseases, suggesting that disconnection of feedback systems associated with cognitive, mnemonic, and emotional processes is a common thread in these diseases.

ACKNOWLEDGMENTS

I thank Troy Ghashghaei and Joshua Kolonick for help with graphics. This work was supported by National Institutes of Health (NIH) grants NS24760 (NINDS) and NS57414 (NIMH).

REFERENCES

1. Brodmann K. Beitrage zur histologischen localisation der Grosshirnrinde. III. Mitteilung: die Rindenfelder der niederen Affen. *J Psychol Neurol* 1905;4:177–266.

2. Barbas H, Pandya DN. Architecture and frontal cortical connections of the premotor cortex (area 6) in the rhesus monkey. *J Comp Neurol* 1987;256:211–218.

3. Dum RP, Strick PL. Medial wall motor areas and skeletomotor control. *Curr Opin Neurobiol* 1992;2: 836–839.

4. He S-Q, Dunn RP, Strick PL. Topographic organization of corticospinal projections from the frontal lobe: motor areas on the medial surface of the hemisphere. *J Neurosci* 1995;15:3284–3306.

5. Luppino G, Matelli M, Camarda RM, et al. Multiple representations of body movements in mesial area 6 and the adjacent cingulate cortex: an intracortical microstimulation study in the macaque monkey. *J Comp Neurol* 1991;311:463–482.

6. Matelli M, Luppino G, Rizzolatti G. Architecture of superior and mesial area 6 and the adjacent cingulate cortex in the macaque monkey. *J Comp Neurol* 1991; 311:445–462.

7. Galea MP, Darian-Smith I. Multiple corticospinal neuron populations in the macaque monkey are specified by their unique cortical origins, spinal terminations, and connections. *Cereb Cortex* 1994;4:166–194.

8. Matsuzaka Y, Aizawa H, Tanji J. A motor area rostral to the supplementary motor area (presupplementary motor area) in the monkey: neuronal activity during a learned motor task. *J Neurophysiol* 1992;68:653–662.

9. Picard N, Strick PL. Motor areas of the medial wall: a review of their location and functional activation. *Cereb Cortex* 1996;6:342–353.

10. Dum RP, Strick PL. The origin of corticospinal projections from the premotor areas in the frontal lobe. *J Neurosci* 1991;11:667–689.

11. Hutchins KD, Martino AM, Strick PL. Corticospinal projections from the medial wall of the hemisphere. *Exp Brain Res* 1988;71:667–672.

12. Alexander GE, Delong MR, Strick PL. Parallel organization of functionally segregated circuits linking basal ganglia and cortex. *Annu Rev Neurosci* 1986;9: 357–381.

13. Alheid GF, Heimer L, Switzer RC III. Basal ganglia. In: Paxinos G, ed. *The human nervous system.* San Diego: Academic Press, 1990:483–582.

14. Graybiel AM, Aosaki T, Flaherty AW, et al. The basal ganglia and adaptive motor control. *Science* 1994;265: 1826–1831.

15. Fuster JM. Frontal lobes. *Curr Opin Neurobiol* 1993; 3:160–165.

16. Goldman-Rakic PS. Topography of cognition: parallel distributed networks in primate association cortex. *Annu Rev Neurosci* 1988;11:137–156.

17. Petrides M. Lateral frontal cortical contribution to memory. *Seminars in the Neurosciences* 1996;8: 57–63.

18. Broca P. Anatomie compareé des enconvolutions cérébrales: Le grand lobe limbique et la scissure limbique dans la serie des mammifères. *Rev Anthrop* 1878;1: 385–498.

19. Nauta WJH. Expanding borders of the limbic system concept. In: Rasmussenand T, Marino R, eds. *Functional neurosurgery.* New York: Raven Press, 1979: 7–23.

20. Papez JW. A proposed mechanism of emotion. *AMA Arch Neurol Psychiatry* 1937;38:725–743.

21. Yakovlev PI. Motility, behavior, and the brain: stereo-dynamic organization and neurocoordinates of behavior. *J Nerv Ment Dis* 1948;107:313–335.

22. Barbas H. Two prefrontal limbic systems: their common and unique features. In: Sakata H, Mikamiand A, Fuster JM, eds. *The association cortex: structure and function.* Amsterdam: Harwood Academic, 1997: 99–115.

23. Damasio AR. *Descartes' error: emotion, reason, and the human brain.* New York: Putnam, 1994.

24. Damasio H, Grabowski T, Frank R, et al. The return of Phineas Gage: clues about the brain from the skull of a famous patient. *Science* 1994;264:1102–1105.

25. Barbas H. Anatomic basis of cognitive–emotional interactions in the primate prefrontal cortex. *Neurosci Behav Rev* 1995;19:499–510.

26. Pandya DN, Seltzer B, Barbas H. Input-output organization of the primate cerebral cortex. In: Steklisand HD, Erwin J, eds. *Comparative primate biology,* vol 4. *Neurosciences.* New York: Alan R. Liss, 1988:39–80.

27. Barbas H. Anatomic organization of basoventral and mediodorsal visual recipient prefrontal regions in the rhesus monkey. *J Comp Neurol* 1988;276:313–342.

28. Barbas H, Mesulam M-M. Organization of afferent input to subdivisions of area 8 in the rhesus monkey. *J Comp Neurol* 1981;200:407–431.

29. Barbas H, Mesulam M-M. Cortical afferent input to the principalis region of the rhesus monkey. *Neuroscience* 1985;15:619–637.

30. Boussaoud D, Ungerleider LG, Desimone R. Pathways for motion analysis: cortical connections of the medial superior temporal and fundus of the superior temporal visual areas in the macaque. *J Comp Neurol* 1990;296: 462–495.

31. Chavis DA, Pandya DN. Further observations on corticofrontal connections in the rhesus monkey. *Brain Res* 1976;117:369–386.

32. Huerta MF, Krubitzer LA, Kaas JH. Frontal eye field as defined by intracortical microstimulation in squirrel monkeys, owl monkeys, and Macaque monkeys. II. Cortical connections. *J Comp Neurol* 1987;265: 332–361.

33. Jacobson S, Trojanowski JQ. Prefrontal granular cortex of the rhesus monkey. I. Intrahemispheric cortical afferents. *Brain Res* 1977;132:209–233.

34. Jones EG, Powell TPS. An anatomical study of converging sensory pathways within the cerebral cortex. *Brain* 1970;93:793–820.

35. Maioli MG, Squatrito S, Galletti C, et al. Cortico–cortical connections from the visual region of the superior temporal sulcus to frontal eye field in the macaque. *Brain Res* 1983;265:294–299.

36. Schall JD, Morel A, King DJ, et al. Topography of visual cortex connections with frontal eye field in macaque: convergence and segregation of processing streams. *J Neurosci* 1995;15:4464–4487.

37. Webster MJ, Bachevalier J, Ungerleider LG. Connections of inferior temporal areas TEO and TE with parietal and frontal cortex in macaque monkeys. *Cereb Cortex* 1994;4:470–483.

38. Preuss TM, Goldman-Rakic PS. Connections of the ventral granular frontal cortex of macaques with perisylvian premotor and somatosensory areas: anatomical evidence for somatic representation in primate frontal association cortex. *J Comp Neurol* 1989;282:293–316.

39. Barbas H, Ghashghaei H, Dombrowski SM, et al.

Medial prefrontal cortices are unified by common connections with superior temporal cortices and distinguished by input from memory-related areas in the rhesus monkey. *J Comp Neurol* 1999;410:343–367.

40. Petrides M, Pandya DN. Association fiber pathways to the frontal cortex from the superior temporal region in the rhesus monkey. *J Comp Neurol* 1988;273:52–66.

41. Vogt BA, Pandya DN. Cingulate cortex of the rhesus monkey: II. Cortical afferents. *J Comp Neurol* 1987; 262:271–289.

42. Takagi SF. Studies on the olfactory nervous system of the old world monkey. *Prog Neurobiol* 1986;27: 195–250.

43. Barbas H. Organization of cortical afferent input to orbitofrontal areas in the rhesus monkey. *Neuroscience* 1993;56:841–864.

44. Carmichael ST, Price JL. Sensory and premotor connections of the orbital and medial prefrontal cortex of macaque monkeys. *J Comp Neurol* 1995;363:642–664.

45. Morecraft RJ, Geula C, Mesulam M-M. Cytoarchitecture and neural afferents of orbitofrontal cortex in the brain of the monkey. *J Comp Neurol* 1992;323: 341–358.

46. Insausti R, Amaral DG, Cowan WM. The entorhinal cortex of the monkey: II. Cortical afferents. *J Comp Neurol* 1987;264:356–395.

47. Suzuki WA, Amaral DG. Perirhinal and parahippocampal cortices of the macaque monkey: cortical afferents. *J Comp Neurol* 1994;350:497–533.

48. Van Hoesen GW. Some connections of the entorhinal (area 28) and perirhinal (area 35) cortices of the rhesus monkey. I. Temporal lobe afferents. *Brain Res* 1975; 95:1–24.

49. Van Hoesen GW, Pandya DN, Butters N. Cortical afferents to the entorhinal cortex of the rhesus monkey. *Science* 1972;175:1471–1473.

50. Ungerleider L, Mishkin M. Two cortical visual systems. In: Ingle DJ, Goodaleand MA, Mansfield RJW, eds. *Analysis of visual behavior*. Cambridge, MA: MIT Press, 1982:549–586.

51. Wilson FA, Scalaidhe SP, Goldman-Rakic PS. Dissociation of object and spatial processing domains in primate prefrontal cortex. *Science* 1993;260:1955–1958.

52. Courtney SM, Ungerleider LG, Keil K, et al. Object and spatial visual working memory activate separate neural systems in human cortex. *Cereb Cortex* 1996;6: 39–49.

53. Von Bonin G, Bailey P. *The Neocortex of* Macaca mulatta. Urbana, IL: The University of Illinois Press, 1947.

54. Petrides M, Pandya DN. Projections to the frontal cortex from the posterior parietal region in the rhesus monkey. *J Comp Neurol* 1984;228:105–116.

55. Barbas H, Pandya DN. Architecture and intrinsic connections of the prefrontal cortex in the rhesus monkey. *J Comp Neurol* 1989;286:353–375.

56. Merigan WH, Maunsell JHR. How parallel are the primate visual pathways? *Annu Rev Neurosci* 1993;16: 369–402.

57. Distler C, Boussaoud D, Desimone R, et al. Cortical connections of inferior temporal area TEO in macaque monkeys. *J Comp Neurol* 1993;334:125–150.

58. Desimone R, Gross CG. Visual areas in the temporal cortex of the macaque. *Brain Res* 1979;178:363–380.

59. Gross CG, Bender DB, Rocha-Miranda CE. Visual receptive fields of neurons in inferotemporal cortex of the monkey. *Science* 1969;166:1303–1306.

60. Romanski LM, Bates JF, Goldman-Rakic PS. Auditory belt and parabelt projections to the prefrontal cortex in the rhesus monkey. *J Comp Neurol* 1999;403:141–157.

61. Davis M. The role of the amygdala in fear and anxiety. *Annu Rev Neurosci* 1992;15:353–375.

62. LeDoux JE. Emotion, memory, and the brain. *Sci Am* 1994;270:50–57.

63. Amaral DG, Price JL. Amygdalo–cortical projections in the monkey (*Macaca fascicularis*). *J Comp Neurol* 1984;230:465–496.

64. Barbas H, De Olmos J. Projections from the amygdala to basoventral and mediodorsal prefrontal regions in the rhesus monkey. *J Comp Neurol* 1990;301:1–23.

65. Carmichael ST, Price JL. Limbic connections of the orbital and medial prefrontal cortex in macaque monkeys. *J Comp Neurol* 1995;363:615–641.

66. Porrino LJ, Crane AM, Goldman-Rakic PS. Direct and indirect pathways from the amygdala to the frontal lobe in rhesus monkeys. *J Comp Neurol* 1981;198: 121–136.

67. Herzog AG, Van Hoesen GW. Temporal neocortical afferent connections to the amygdala in the rhesus monkey. *Brain Res* 1976;115:57–69.

68. Turner BH, Mishkin M, Knapp M. Organization of the amygdalopetal projections from modality-specific cortical association areas in the monkey. *J Comp Neurol* 1980;191:515–543.

69. Kling A, Steklis HD. A neural substrate for affiliative behavior in nonhuman primates. *Brain Behav Evol* 1976;13:216–238.

70. Whalen PJ, Rauch SL, Etcoff NL, et al. Masked presentations of emotional facial expressions modulate amygdala activity without explicit knowledge. *J Neurosci* 1998;18:411–418.

71. Romanski LM, LeDoux JE. Equipotentiality of thalamo-amygdala and thalamo-cortico-amygdala circuits in auditory fear conditioning. *J Neurosci* 1992;12: 4501–4509.

72. Price JL, Russchen FT, Amaral DG. The limbic region. II. The amygdaloid complex. In: Björklund A, Hökfeltand T, Swanson LW, eds. *Handbook of chemical neuroanatomy*, vol 5. Integrated systems of the CNS, Part I. Amsterdam: Elsevier, 1987:279–381.

73. Kennard MA. Focal autonomic representation in the cortex and its relation to sham rage. *J Neuropathol Exp Neurol* 1945;4:295–304.

74. Jones EG. Interrelationships of parieto-temporal and frontal cortex in the rhesus monkey. *Brain Res* 1969; 13:412–415.

75. Müller-Preuss JD, Newman JD, Jürgens U. Anatomical and physiological evidence for a relationship between the cingular vocalization area and the auditory cortex in the squirrel monkey. *Brain Res* 1980;202:307–315.

76. Kosaki H, Hashikawa T, He J, et al. Tonotopic organization of auditory cortical fields delineated by parvalbumin immunoreactivity in macaque monkeys. *J Comp Neurol* 1997;386:304–316.

77. Rauschecker JP. Parallel processing in the auditory cortex of primates. *Audiology and Neurootology* 1998; 3:86–103.

78. Rauschecker JP, Tian B, Hauser M. Processing of complex sounds in the macaque nonprimary auditory cortex. *Science* 1995;268:111–114.

79. Jürgens U. Projections from the cortical larynx area in the squirrel monkey. *Exp Brain Res* 1976;25:401–411.
80. Müller-Preuss P, Jürgens U. Projections from the 'cingular' vocalization area in the squirrel monkey. *Brain Res* 1976;103:29–43.
81. Smith WK. The functional significance of the rostral cingular cortex as revealed by its responses to electrical excitation. *J Neurophysiol* 1945;8:241–255.
82. Sutton D, Larson C, Lindeman RC. Neocortical and limbic lesion effects on primate phonation. *Brain Res* 1974;71:61–75.
83. Sutton D, Trachy RE, Lindeman RC. Discriminative phonation in macaques: effects of anterior mesial cortex damage. *Exp Brain Res* 1985;59:410–413.
84. Devinsky O, Morrell MJ, Vogt BA. Contributions of anterior cingulate cortex to behaviour. *Brain* 1995;118:279–306.
85. Vogt BA, Barbas H. Structure and connections of the cingulate vocalization region in the rhesus monkey. In: Newman JD, ed. *The physiological control of mammalian vocalization*. New York: Plenum Press, 1988:203–225.
86. Dolan RJ, Fletcher P, Frith CD, et al. Dopaminergic modulation of impaired cognitive activation in the anterior cingulate cortex in schizophrenia. *Nature* 1995;378:180–182.
87. Frith C, Dolan R. The role of the prefrontal cortex in higher cognitive functions. *Cognitive Brain Research* 1996;5:175–181.
88. MacLean PD. Brain evolution relating to family, play, and the separation call. *Arch Gen Psychiatry* 1985;42:405–417.
89. Frith C, Dolan RJ. Brain mechanisms associated with top-down processes in perception. *Philos Trans R Soc Lond B* 1997;352:1221–1230.
90. McGuire PK, Silbersweig DA, Wright I, et al. Abnormal monitoring of inner speech: a physiological basis for auditory hallucinations. *Lancet* 1995;346:596–600.
91. McGuire PK, Silbersweig DA, Wright I, et al. The neural correlates of inner speech and auditory verbal imagery in schizophrenia: relationship to auditory verbal hallucinations. *Br J Psychiatry* 1996;169:148–159.
92. Frith C. The role of the prefrontal cortex in self-consciousness: the case of auditory hallucinations. *Philos Trans R Soc Lond B* 1996;351:1505–1512.
93. Andersen RA, Asanuma C, Essick G, et al. Corticocortical connections of anatomically and physiologically defined subdivisions within the inferior parietal lobe. *J Comp Neurol* 1990;296:65–113.
94. Schwartz ML, Goldman-Rakic PS. Callosal and intrahemispheric connectivity of the prefrontal association cortex in rhesus monkey: relation between intraparietal and principal sulcal cortex. *J Comp Neurol* 1984;226:403–420.
95. Petrides M. Specialized systems for the processing of mnemonic information within the primate frontal cortex. *Philos Trans R Soc Lond B* 1996;351:1455–1462.
96. Arikuni T, Watanabe K, Kubota K. Connections of area 8 with area 6 in the brain of the macaque monkey. *J Comp Neurol* 1988;277:21–40.
97. Matelli M, Camarda R, Glickstein M, et al. Afferent and efferent projections of the inferior area 6 in the Macaque monkey. *J Comp Neurol* 1986;251:281–298.
98. McGuire PK, Bates JF, Goldman-Rakic PS. Interhemispheric integration: I. Symmetry and convergence of the corticocortical connections of the left and the right principal sulcus (PS) and the left and the right supplementary motor area (SMA) in the rhesus monkey. *Cereb Cortex* 1991;1:390–407.
99. Cavada C, Goldman-Rakic PS. Posterior parietal cortex in rhesus monkey. II. Evidence for segregated corticocortical networks linking sensory and limbic areas with the frontal lobe. *J Comp Neurol* 1989;287:422–445.
100. Mesulam M-M. A cortical network for directed attention and unilateral neglect. *Ann Neurol* 1981;10:309–325.
101. Goldberg ME, Bushnell MC. Behavioral enhancement of visual responses in monkey cerebral cortex. II. Modulation in frontal eye fields specifically related to saccades. *J Neurophysiol* 1981;46:773–787.
102. Wurtz RH, Mohler CW. Enhancement of visual responses in monkey striate cortex and frontal eye fields. *J Neurophysiol* 1976;39:766–772.
103. Funahashi S, Bruce CJ, Goldman-Rakic PS. Mnemonic coding of visual space in the monkey's dorsolateral prefrontal cortex. *J Neurophysiol* 1989;61:331–349.
104. Funahashi S, Bruce CJ, Goldman-Rakic PS. Dorsolateral prefrontal lesions and occulomotor delayed-response performance: evidence for mnemonic "scotomas." *J Neurosci* 1993;13:1479–1497.
105. Koechlin E, Basso G, Pietrini P, et al. The role of the anterior prefrontal cortex in human cognition. *Nature* 1999;399:148–151.
106. Petrides M, Alivisatos B, Evans AC. Functional activation of the human ventrolateral frontal cortex during mnemonic retrieval of verbal information. *Proc Natl Acad Sci USA* 1995;92:5803–5807.
107. Jacobsen CF. Studies of cerebral function in primates. I. The functions of the frontal association area in monkeys. *Comp Psychol Monogr* 1936;13:3–60.
108. Fuster JM. *The prefrontal cortex*. New York: Raven Press, 1989.
109. Goldman-Rakic PS. Cellular basis of working memory. *Neuron* 1995;14:477–485.
110. Fuster J M. Unit activity in prefrontal cortex during delayed-response performance: neuronal correlates of transient memory. *J Neurophysiol* 1973;36:61–78.
111. Joseph JP, Barone P. Prefrontal unit activity during a delayed oculomotor task in the monkey. *Exp Brain Res* 1987;67:460–468.
112. Kubota K, Niki H. Prefrontal cortical unit activity and delayed alternation performance in monkeys. *J Neurophysiol* 1990;34:337–347.
113. Kubota K, Tonoike M, Mikami A. Neuronal activity in the monkey dorsolateral prefrontal cortex during a discrimination task with delay. *Brain Res* 1980;183:29–42.
114. Watanabe M. Prefrontal unit activity during delayed conditional discriminations in the monkey. *Brain Res* 1981;225:51–65.
115. Fuster JM, Bauer RH, Jervey JP. Effects of cooling inferotemporal cortex on performance of visual memory tasks. *Exp Neurol* 1981;71:398–409.
116. Miller EK, Li L, Desimone R. Activity of neurons in anterior inferior temporal cortex during a short-term memory task. *J Neurosci* 1993;13:1460–1478.
117. Bachevalier J, Meunier M, Lu MX, et al. Thalamic and temporal cortex input to medial prefrontal cortex in rhesus monkeys. *Exp Brain Res* 1997;115:430–444.
118. Van Hoesen GW, Pandya DN, Butters N. Some connections of the entorhinal (area 28) and perirhinal (area 35)

cortices of the rhesus monkey. II. Frontal lobe afferents. *Brain Res* 1975;95:25–38.

119. Barbas H, Blatt GJ. Topographically specific hippocampal projections target functionally distinct prefrontal areas in the rhesus monkey. *Hippocampus* 1995;5:511–533.

120. Rosene DL, Van Hoesen GW. Hippocampal efferents reach widespread areas of cerebral cortex and amygdala in the rhesus monkey. *Science* 1977;198:315–317.

121. Amaral DG, Insausti R, Zola-Morgan S, et al. The perirhinal and parahippocampal cortices and medial temporal lobe memory function. In: *Vision, memory, and the temporal lobe.* New York: Elsevier, 1990: 149–161.

122. Squire LR. Memory and the hippocampus: a synthesis from findings with rats, monkeys, and humans. *Psychol Rev* 1992;99:195–231.

123. Squire LR, Zola-Morgan S. Memory: brain systems and behavior. *Trends Neurosci* 1988;11:170–175.

124. Zola-Morgan S, Squire LR. Neuroanatomy of memory. *Annu Rev Neurosci* 1993;16:547–563.

125. Mesulam M-M. Large-scale neurocognitive networks and distributed processing for attention, language, and memory. *Ann Neurol* 1990;28:597–613.

126. Vogt BA, Finch DM, Olson CR. Functional heterogeneity in cingulate cortex: the anterior executive and posterior evaluative regions. *Cereb Cortex* 1992;2: 435–443.

127. Barbas H. Architecture and cortical connections of the prefrontal cortex in the rhesus monkey. In: Chauvel P, Delgado-Escueta AV, Halgren E, Bancaud J, eds. *Frontal lobe seizures and epilepsies. Advances in neurology,* vol 57. New York: Raven Press, 1992:91–115.

128. Jones EG. *The thalamus.* New York: Plenum Press, 1985.

129. Barbas H, Henion TH, Dermon CR. Diverse thalamic projections to the prefrontal cortex in the rhesus monkey. *J Comp Neurol* 1991;313:65–94.

130. Benevento LA, Fallon JH. The ascending projections of the superior colliculus in the rhesus monkey *(Macaca mulatta). J Comp Neurol* 1975;160:339–362.

131. Hikosaka O, Wurtz RH. Visual and oculomotor functions of monkey substantia nigra pars reticulata. I. Relation of visual and auditory responses to saccades. *J Neurophysiol* 1983;49:1230–1253.

132. Hikosaka O, Wurtz RH. Visual and oculomotor functions of monkey substantia nigra pars reticulata. II. Visual responses related to fixation of gaze. *J Neurophysiol* 1983;49:1254–1267.

133. Hikosaka O, Wurtz RH. Visual and oculomotor functions of monkey substantia nigra pars reticulata. III. Memory-contingent visual and saccade responses. *J Neurophysiol* 1983;49:1268–1284.

134. Hikosaka O, Wurtz RH. Visual and oculomotor functions of monkey substantia nigra pars reticulata. IV. Relation of substantia nigra to superior colliculus. *J Neurophysiol* 1983;49:1285–1301.

135. Ilinsky IA, Jouandet ML, Goldman-Rakic PS. Organization of the nigrothalamocortical system in the rhesus monkey. *J Comp Neurol* 1985;236:315–330.

136. Ilinsky IA, Kultas-Ilinsky K. Sagittal cytoarchitectonic maps of the *Macaca mulatta* thalamus with a revised nomenclature of the motor-related nuclei validated by observations on their connectivity. *J Comp Neurol* 1987;262:331–364.

137. Lynch JC, Hoover JE, Strick PL. Input to the primate frontal eye field from the substantia nigra, superior colliculus, and dentate nucleus demonstrated by transneuronal transport. *Exp Brain Res* 1994;100(Suppl): 181–186.

138. Wurtz RH, Albano JE. Visual-motor function of the primate superior colliculus. *Annu Rev Neurosci* 1980; 3:189–226.

139. Schlag J, Schlag-Rey M. Visuomotor functions of central thalamus in monkey. II. Unit activity related to visual events, targeting, and fixation. *J Neurophysiol* 1984;51:1175–1195.

140. Schlag-Rey M, Schlag J. Visuomotor functions of central thalamus in monkey. I. Unit activity related to spontaneous eye movements. *J Neurophysiol* 1984;51: 1149–1174.

141. Schiller PH, Chou I-H. The effects of frontal eye field and dorsomedial frontal cortex lesions on visually guided eye movements. *Nature Neuroscience* 1998; 1:248–253.

142. Robinson DA, Fuchs AF. Eye movements evoked by stimulation of the frontal eye fields. *J Neurophysiol* 1969;32:637–648.

143. Bruce CJ, Goldberg ME, Bushnell MC, et al. Primate frontal eye fields. II. Physiological and anatomical correlates of electrically evoked eye movements. *J Neurophysiol* 1985;54:714–734.

144. Bechara A, Damasio H, Tranel D, et al. Dissociation of working memory from decision making within the human prefrontal cortex. *J Neurosci* 1998;18: 428–437.

145. Braver TS, Cohen JD, Nystrom LE, et al. A parametric study of prefrontal cortex involvement in human working memory. *Neuroimage* 1997;5:49–62.

146. Chao LL, Knight RT. Contribution of human prefrontal cortex to delay performance. *J Cogn Neurosci* 1998;10:167–177.

147. Cohen JD, Perlstein WM, Braver TS, et al. Temporal dynamics of brain activation during a working memory task. *Nature* 1997;386:604–608.

148. Courtney SM, Petit L, Maisog JM, et al. An area specialized for spatial working memory in human frontal cortex. *Science* 1998;279:1347–1351.

149. D'Esposito M, Detre JA, Alsop DC, et al. The neural basis of the central executive system of working memory. *Nature* 1995;378:279–281.

150. McCarthy G, Puce A, Constable RT, et al. Activation of human prefrontal cortex during spatial and nonspatial working memory tasks measured by functional MRI. *Cereb Cortex* 1996;6:600–611.

151. Owen AM. The functional organization of working memory processes within human lateral frontal cortex: the contribution of functioal neuroimaging. *Eur J Neurosci* 1997;9:1329–1339.

152. Owen AM, Evans AC, Petrides M. Evidence for a two-stage model of spatial working memory processing within the lateral frontal cortex: a positron emission tomography study. *Cereb Cortex* 1996;6:31–38.

153. Swartz BE, Halgren E, Fuster JM, et al. Cortical metabolic activation in humans during a visual memory task. *Cereb Cortex* 1995;5:205–214.

154. Dermon CR, Barbas H. Contralateral thalamic projections predominantly reach transitional cortices in the rhesus monkey. *J Comp Neurol* 1994;344:508–531.

155. Fuster JM, Alexander GE. Firing changes in cells of

the nucleus medialis dorsalis associated with delayed response behavior. *Brain Res* 1973;61:79–91.

156. Goldman-Rakic PS, Porrino LJ. The primate mediodorsal (MD) nucleus and its projection to the frontal lobe. *J Comp Neurol* 1985;242:535–560.

157. Ray JP, Price JL. The organization of projections from the mediodorsal nucleus of the thalamus to orbital and medial prefrontal cortex in macaque monkeys. *J Comp Neurol* 1993;337:1–31.

158. Aggleton JP, Mishkin M. Visual recognition impairment following medial thalamic lesions in monkeys. *Neuropsychologia* 1983;21:189–197.

159. Isseroff A, Rosvold HE, Galkin TW, et al. Spatial memory impairments following damage to the mediodorsal nucleus of the thalamus in rhesus monkeys. *Brain Res* 1982;232:97–113.

160. Markowitsch HJ. Thalamic mediodorsal nucleus and memory: a critical evaluation of studies in animals and man. *Neurosci Biobehav Rev* 1982;6:351–380.

161. Victor M, Adams RD, Collins GH. *The Wernicke–Korsakoff syndrome*. Philadelphia: FA Davis, 1971.

162. Zola-Morgan S, Squire LR. Amnesia in monkeys after lesions of the mediodorsal nucleus of the thalamus. *Ann Neurol* 1985;17:558–564.

163. Aggleton JP, Mishkin M. Projections of the amygdala to the thalamus in the cynomolgus monkey. *J Comp Neurol* 1984;222:56–68.

164. Russchen FT, Amaral DG, Price JL. The afferent input to the magnocellular division of the mediodorsal thalamic nucleus in the monkey, Macaca fascicularis. *J Comp Neurol* 1987;256:175–210.

165. Giguere M, Goldman-Rakic PS. Mediodorsal nucleus: areal, laminar, and tangential distribution of afferents and efferents in the frontal lobe of rhesus monkeys. *J Comp Neurol* 1988;277:195–213.

166. Tobias TJ. Afferents to prefrontal cortex from the thalamic mediodorsal nucleus in the rhesus monkey. *Brain Res* 1975;83:191–212.

167. Vogt BA, Sikes RW, Vogt LJ. Anterior cingulate cortex and the medial pain system. In: Vogtand BA, Gabriel M, eds. *Neurobiology of cingulate cortex and limbic thalamus: a comprehensive handbook*. Boston: Birkhauser, 1993:313–344.

168. Joel D, Weiner I. The organization of the basal ganglia-thalamocortical circuits: open interconnected rather than closed segregated. *Neuroscience* 1994;63:363–379.

169. Kievit J, Kuypers HGJM. Organization of the thalamo-cortical connexions to the frontal lobe in the rhesus monkey. *Exp Brain Res* 1977;29:299–322.

170. Schiller PH. The neural control of visually guided eye movements. In: Richards JE, ed. *Cognitive neuroscience of attention*. Mahwah, NJ: Lawrence Erlbaum Associates, 1998:3–50.

171. Bates JF, Goldman-Rakic PS. Prefrontal connections of medial motor areas in the rhesus monkey. *J Comp Neurol* 1993;336:211–228.

172. Pandya DN, Dye P, Butters N. Efferent cortico-cortical projections of the prefrontal cortex in the rhesus monkey. *Brain Res* 1971;31:35–46.

173. Pandya DN, Kuypers HGJM. Cortico-cortical connections in the rhesus monkey. *Brain Res* 1969;13:13–36.

174. Pandya DN, Van Hoesen GW, Mesulam M-M. Efferent connections of the cingulate gyrus in the rhesus monkey. *Exp Brain Res* 1981;42:319–330.

175. Pandya DN, Vignolo LA. Intra- and interhemispheric projections of the precentral, premotor, and arcuate areas in the rhesus monkey. *Brain Res* 1971;26:217–233.

176. Selemon LD, Goldman-Rakic PS. Common cortical and subcortical targets of the dorsolateral prefrontal and posterior parietal cortices in the rhesus monkey: evidence for a distributed neural network subserving spatially guided behavior. *J Neurosci* 1988;8:4049–4068.

177. Haber SN, Kunishio K, Mizobuchi M, et al. The orbital and medial prefrontal circuit through the primate basal ganglia. *J Neurosci* 1995;15:4851–4867.

178. Nauta WJH. Limbic innervation of the striatum. *Neuroscience* 1982;35:41–47.

179. Rempel-Clower N, Barbas H. Topographic organization of connections between the hypothalamus and prefrontal cortex in the rhesus monkey. *J Comp Neurol* 1998;398:393–419.

180. Bechara A, Tranel D, Damasio H, et al. Failure to respond autonomically to anticipated future outcomes following damage to prefrontal cortex. *Cereb Cortex* 1996;6:215–225.

181. Damasio AR, Tranel D, Damasio H. Individuals with sociopathic behavior caused by frontal damage fail to respond autonomically to social stimuli. *Behav Brain Res* 1990;41:81–94.

182. Jürgens U. The role of the periaqueductal grey in vocal behaviour. *Behav Brain Res* 1994;62:107–117.

183. Foote SL, Morrison JH. Extrathalamic modulation of cortical function. *Annu Rev Neurosci* 1987;10:67–95.

184. Mesulam MM, Mufson EJ, Levey AI, et al. Cholinergic innervation of cortex by the basal forebrain: cytochemistry and cortical connections of the septal area, diagonal band nuclei, nuclei, nucleus basalis (Substantia Innominata), and hypothalamus in the rhesus monkey. *J Comp Neurol* 1983;214:170–197.

185. Sillito AM, Jones HE, Gerstein GL, et al. Feature-linked synchronization of thalamic relay cell firing induced by feedback from the visual cortex. *Nature* 1994;369:479–482.

186. Alexander GE, Fuster JM. Effects of cooling prefrontal cortex on cell firing in the nucleus medialis dorsalis. *Brain Res* 1973;61:93–105.

187. Kubota K, Niki H, Goto A. Thalamic unit activity and delayed alternation performance in the monkey. *Acta Neurobiol Exp* 1972;32:177–192.

188. Barbas H. Pattern in the laminar origin of corticocortical connections. *J Comp Neurol* 1986;252:415–422.

189. Barbas H, Rempel-Clower N. Cortical structure predicts the pattern of corticocortical connections. *Cereb Cortex* 1997;7:635–646.

190. Friedman DP, Murray EA, O'Neill JB, et al. Cortical connections of the somatosensory fields of the lateral sulcus of macaques: evidence for a corticolimbic pathway for touch. *J Comp Neurol* 1986;252:323–347.

191. Maunsell JHR, Van Essen DC. The connections of the middle temporal visual area (MT) and their relationship to a cortical hierarchy in the macaque monkey. *J Neurosci* 1983;3:2563–2586.

192. Rockland KS, Pandya DN. Laminar origins and terminations of cortical connections of the occipital lobe in the rhesus monkey. *Brain Res* 1979;179:3–20.

193. Rockland KS, Van Hoesen GW. Direct temporal-occipital feedback connections to striate cortex (V1) in the macaque monkey. *Cereb Cortex* 1994;4:300–313.

194. Schwartz ML, Rakic P, Goldman-Rakic PS. Early phenotype expression of cortical neurons—evidence that a subclass of migrating neurons have callosal axons. *Proc Natl Acad Sci USA* 1991;88:1354–1358.

195. O'Leary DD, Schlaggar BL, Tuttle R. Specification of neocortical areas and thalamocortical connections. *Annu Rev Neurosci* 1994;17:419–439.

196. Sur M, Cowey A. Cerebral cortex: function and development. *Neuron* 1995;15:497–505.

197. Dombrowski SM, Barbas H. Distinction of prefrontal architectonic areas using stereologic procedures. *Neurosci Abstr* 1998;24:1163.

198. Dombrowski SM, Barbas H. Differential expression of NADPH diaphorase in functionally distinct prefrontal cortices in the rhesus monkey. *Neuroscience* 1996;72:49–62.

199. Bredt DS, Snyder SH. Transient nitric oxide synthase neurons in embryonic cerebral cortical plate, sensory ganglia, and olfactory epithelium. *Neuron* 1994;13:301–313.

200. Caviness VS Jr, Takahashi T, Nowakowski RS. Numbers, time, and neocortical neuronogenesis: a general developmental and evolutionary model. *Trends Neurosci* 1995;18:379–383.

201. Braak H, Braak E. Alzheimer's disease affects limbic nuclei of the thalamus. *Acta Neuropathol* 1991;81:261–268.

202. Gloor P, Olivier A, Quesney LF, et al. The role of the limbic system in experiential phenomena of temporal lobe epilepsy. *Ann Neurol* 1982;12:129–144.

203. Hooper MW, Vogel FS. The limbic system in Alzheimer's disease. *Am J Pathol* 1976;85:1–20.

204. Hyman BT, Van Hoesen GW, Damasio AR, et al. Alzheimer's disease: cell-specific pathology isolates the hippocampal formation. *Science* 1984;225:1168–1170.

205. Kromer Vogt LJ, Van Hoesen GW, Hyman BT, et al. Pathological alterations in the amygdala in Alzheimer's disease. *Neuroscience* 1990;37:377–385.

206. Penfield W, Jasper H. *Epilepsy and the functional anatomy of the human brain.* Boston: Little, Brown, 1954.

207. Reynolds JP. Beyond the dopamine hypothesis: the neurochemical pathology of schizophrenia. *Br J Psychiatry* 1989;155:305–316.

208. Roberts GW, Ferrier IN, Lee Y, et al. Peptides, the limbic lobe, and schizophrenia. *Brain Res* 1983;288:199–211.

209. Vogt BA, Van Hoesen GW, Vogt LJ. Laminar distribution of neuron degeneration in posterior cingulate cortex in Alzheimer's disease. *Acta Neuropathol (Berl)* 1990;80:581–589.

210. Weinberger DR. Schizophrenia and the frontal lobe. *Trends Neurosci* 1988;11:367–370.

211. Sloviter RS. Permanently altered hippocampal structure, excitability, and inhibition after experimental status epilepticus in the rat: the "Dormant basket cell" hypothesis and its possible relevance to temporal lobe epilepsy. *Hippocampus* 1991;1:41–66.

212. Abbruzzese M, Bellodi L, Ferri S, et al. Frontal lobe dysfunction in schizophrenia and obsessive-compulsive disorder: a neuropsychological study. *Brain Cogn* 1995;27:202–212.

213. Breiter HC, Rauch SL, Kwong KK, et al. Functional magnetic resonance imaging of symptom provocation in obsessive-compulsive disorder. *Arch Gen Psychiatry* 1996;53:595–606.

214. Weeks RA, Turjanski N, Brooks DJ. Tourette's syndrome: a disorder of cingulate and orbitofrontal function? *QJM* 1996;89:401–408.

215. Rapoport JL, Fiske A. The new biology of obsessive-compulsive disorder: implications for evolutionary psychology. *Perspect Biol Med* 1998;41:159–175.

216. Chu C-C, Tranel D, Damasio AR, et al. The autonomic-related cortex: pathology in Alzheimer's disease. *Cereb Cortex* 1997;7:86–95.

Neocortical Epilepsies.
Advances in Neurology, Vol. 84,
edited by P. D. Williamson, A. M. Siegel,
D. W. Roberts, V. M. Thadani, and M. S. Gazzaniga.
Lippincott Williams & Wilkins, Philadelphia © 2000.

9

Impairments in Working Memory After Frontal Cortical Excisions

Michael Petrides

Departments of Neurology and Neurosurgery, Montreal Neurological Institute,
McGill University, Montreal, Quebec, Canada H3A 2B4

Patients with cortical excisions of the dorso-lateral frontal cortex perform well on standard tests of recognition memory and on various tests of short-term memory, such as story recall or the digit span (1). Performance on such tests can be normal even when the lesions are bilateral, as shown by several studies of patients who had undergone frontal lobotomies (1–3). Damage to the dorsolateral frontal cortex, however, can yield impairments on memory tasks when successful performance requires certain executive processes (1). During the past 20 years, we have tried to elucidate the essential nature of the specific contribution of the lateral prefrontal cortex to mnemonic processing using a variety of approaches, such as studies of patients with frontal cortical excisions, analyses of the effects of selective lesions in monkeys, and functional neuroimaging work with normal human subjects.

The frontal cortex comprises several architectonic areas that differ markedly in terms of their connections with other cortical and subcortical areas (4–7); therefore, elucidating the contribution of the frontal cortex to mnemonic processing will depend ultimately on understanding the nature of the specific functional interactions between the different frontal cortical areas and the other brain areas with which they are connected. It has become clear that different parts of the lateral pre-frontal cortex make distinct contributions to mnemonic performance.

This chapter focuses on the contribution of the mid-dorsolateral part of the frontal cortex (i.e., areas 46 and 9) to working memory (Fig. 9.1). We first observed that patients with excisions limited to the lateral prefrontal cortex were severely impaired on a novel working memory task, the self-ordered task, although they could perform well on several other tests of short-term memory (8). Successful performance on the self-ordered task required that the subjects carefully monitor their recent selections from a set of stimuli. In other words, this task attempted to combine short-term memory with one aspect of executive processing, namely monitoring (8).

In the self-ordered task, the subjects are presented with different arrangements of the same set of stimuli and have to select a different stimulus on each trial until all the stimuli are selected (Fig. 9.2). Thus, from the moment they start responding, the subjects must constantly compare the responses they have already made with those still remaining. In other words, each selection must be marked in the subject's mind and simultaneously considered in relation to the others that remain to be selected. This is what we termed *monitoring of events within working memory* (9,10).

In work in monkeys where lesions can be placed with great precision, it was shown that

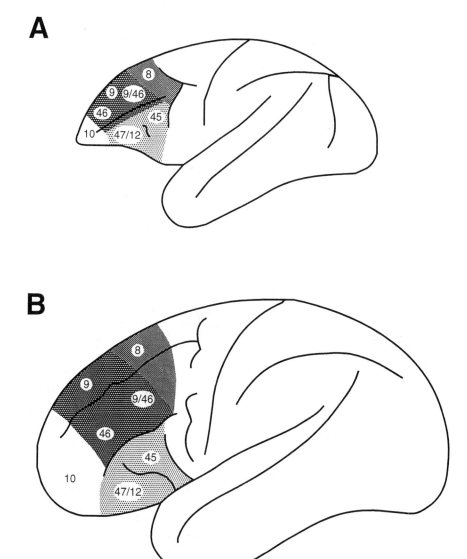

FIG. 9.1. Schematic drawing of the lateral surface of the macaque monkey brain **(A)** and that of the human brain **(B)** to indicate the location of the mid-dorsolateral frontal region (areas 46, 9, and 9/46). The term mid-dorsolateral frontal cortex is used to distinguish this region from the frontopolar cortex (area 10) and the posterior dorsolateral frontal cortex (area 8 and rostral area 6). In the human brain, the mid-dorsolateral frontal cortex occupies the midsection of the middle and superior frontal gyri. The mid-ventrolateral frontal region occupies the pars triangularis (area 45) and pars orbitalis (area 47/12) of the inferior frontal gyrus.

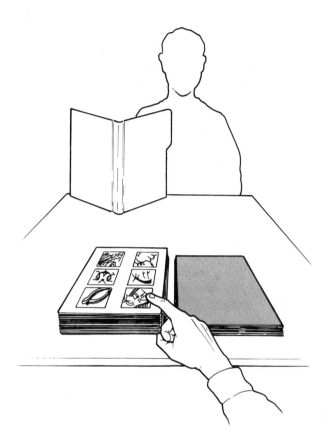

FIG. 9.2. Schematic diagram of the experimental arrangement in the self-ordered task. Each card has the same stimuli depicted but in a different arrangement. The stimuli can be abstract designs (illustrated), words, or representational drawings.

excisions limited to the mid-dorsal part of the lateral frontal cortex (i.e., areas 46, 9/46, and 9) (Fig. 9.1) impair performance on these and other similar tasks, such as the externally ordered tasks that require monitoring of the occurrence of stimuli from an expected set (11,12). Analysis of the impairment of monkeys with mid-dorsolateral frontal lesions on the self-ordered and externally ordered working memory tasks is consistent with the results obtained in studies with patients. Monkeys with such lesions can remember stimuli, as demonstrated by normal performance on recognition memory tests and on other short-term memory tasks (e.g., object delayed alternation in which they must be constantly switching between two recurring stimuli) (12). The fundamental problem of these animals in the self-ordered and on the externally ordered working memory tasks has been shown to stem from the monitoring requirements of these tasks,

that is, the number of stimuli that must be kept in mind and considered as the responses are being made (12). The mid-dorsolateral part of the frontal cortex therefore appears to be a specialized area of the cerebral cortex in which information can be held online for monitoring (in the sense described above) and for the manipulation of stimuli. Note that the manipulation of stimuli implies the simultaneous consideration of several stimuli together and thus ultimately depends on monitoring. A detailed description of a model outlining this concept of the role of the frontal cortex in mnemonic processing has been published elsewhere (9,10).

The critical importance of the functional interaction between the lateral frontal cortex and the limbic region of the medial temporal lobe, and in particular the hippocampal region, for performance of the self-ordered working memory tasks became evident from the first study we conducted with patients (8). In that study, we found that patients with anterior temporal lobe excisions that included the anterior temporal neocortex, the amygdala, and its surrounding cortex were not impaired on these tasks (Fig. 9.3). By contrast, patients with similar anterior temporal lobe excisions that extended posteriorly to include a sizable portion of the hippocampus and the surrounding parahippocampal cortex exhibited an impairment as severe as that observed in patients with frontal lesions. These findings suggested that the lateral frontal cortex and the hippocampal region of the medial temporal lobe are in close functional interaction during performance of these working memory tasks.

Bilateral lesions of the limbic region of the medial temporal lobe, namely the amygdala, hippocampus, and the cortex surrounding these structures (i.e., the entorhinal, the peri-rhinal, and the posterior parahippocampal cortex), give rise to a severe amnesic syndrome that is characterized by an inability to store new information about facts and events (13–15). In patients, unilateral temporal lobe lesions, invading to a varying extent these limbic structures, yield a material-specific memory impairment (13). Patients with left temporal lobe excisions exhibit a verbal memory impairment, whereas those with right temporal lobe excisions exhibit a memory impairment for spatial information and other information that cannot be coded easily in verbal terms (13,16–18). Patients with damage restricted to the limbic region of the medial temporal lobe have no difficulty perceiving and interpreting new information and maintaining it within immediate short-term memory. Thus, perception and immediate short-term memory, which depend on pro-

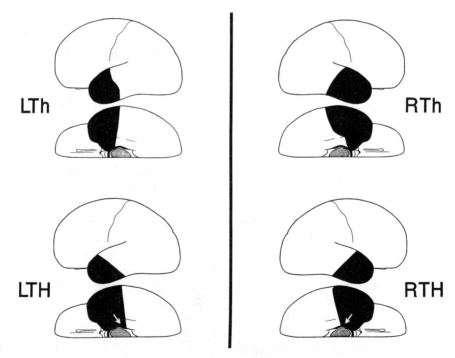

FIG. 9.3. Diagrams illustrating temporal lobe excisions in four patients. *LTh* and *RTh* refer to patients with left or right temporal excisions involving the anterior temporal neocortex, the amygdala, and its surrounding cortex, but with little damage to the hippocampal system. *LTH* and *RTH* refer to patients with left or right temporal excisions that involve the same areas as in the LTh and RTh patients, but with additional extensive damage, on the medial surface, of the parahippocampal cortex and the hippocampus. *Arrows* indicate the location of the additional damage in these cases.

cessing within posterior association cortical regions, are unaffected by damage to the medial temporal lobe. The limbic region of the medial temporal lobe, however, is critical if information that has been encoded is to be maintained on a long-term basis when attention is shifted to new information or when the capacity of short-term memory is exceeded.

One proposal of the role of the hippocampal system posits that its critical function lies in working memory (19). This view was based on work demonstrating that lesions of the hippocampus and related structures in the rat yield severe impairments on the radial maze, a spatial test of working memory (19). It has been argued, however, that the limbic region of the medial temporal lobe, of which the hippocampus is a major component, participates in working memory by virtue of its more general involvement in the maintenance of information about facts and events when the short-term memory capacity is exceeded and when attention shifts from one piece of processed information to another (9). In other words, the impairment in working memory after hippocampal system lesions can be seen as secondary to a primary mnemonic disorder; therefore, the fundamental function of the hippocampal system cannot be described as working memory (9).

Working memory depends on a neural circuit that includes the posterior association cortex, where information is encoded and maintained for short-term periods, and the lateral frontal cortex, where executive processes such as monitoring and manipulation of this information are being carried out (9). These cortical association areas are dependent on the medial temporal lobe memory system when the capacity of short-term memory is exceeded.

The findings reviewed above demonstrate the close functional interaction between the dorsolateral frontal cortex and the hippocampal system for the performance of certain working memory tasks. What are the anatomic pathways on which this functional interaction may be based? Earlier studies showed the existence of connections between

the dorsolateral frontal cortex and the hippocampal system via projections to the retrosplenial region (20,21). We recently conducted an extensive reexamination of the origin and termination of connections linking the frontal cortex with the hippocampal system (22). This work demonstrated that a major fiber system originates in the mid-dorsolateral frontal cortex, courses as part of the cingulum bundle, and terminates along the way within the posterior cingulate cortex, the adjacent retrosplenial cortex, and finally the caudal presubicular component of the hippocampal complex (Fig. 9.4). This association fiber system is probably the one subserving the functional interactions between the mid-dorsolateral frontal cortex and the hippocampal system that are critical for normal working memory processing. The posterior cingulate region, in turn, is strongly connected with the presubicular field of the hippocampal system (23).

The importance of the mid-dorsolateral prefrontal cortex together with the posterior cingulate cortical region and retrosplenial area for the mnemonic processing underlying working memory was highlighted in a recent functional neuroimaging study (24). In this study, local cerebral blood flow was measured with positron emission tomography in normal human subjects while they performed a visual self-ordered working memory task, a visual matching control task, and a visual conditional task (24). The same eight visual stimuli (abstract designs) were used in all three tasks, and these stimuli were presented in a different random arrangement on each trial. The subjects were required to indicate their response by pointing to particular stimuli. Thus, the only difference between the three tasks lay in their cognitive requirements. In the self-ordered task, which was directly analogous to those we previously used with patients (8) and monkeys (11,12), the subjects were required to select a different stimulus on each trial until all had been selected. The subjects were therefore required to consider actively (i.e., monitor) their earlier selections as they were preparing their next response. In the matching

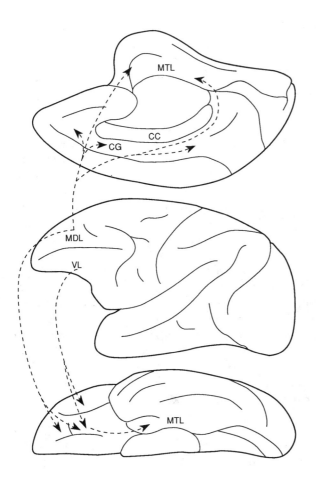

FIG. 9.4. Diagrammatic representation of the linkages of the mid-dorsolateral *(MDL)* prefrontal region with the posterior cingulate cortex, the retrosplenial region, and the presubiculum. *VL,* ventrolateral prefrontal region; *CG,* cingulate gyrus; *CC,* corpus callosum; *MTL,* medial temporal region.

control task, the subjects had to search and find the same stimulus on each trial. The control task involved the same visual stimuli and searching behavior as the self-ordered task, but it did not require that the subjects consider their earlier responses in relation to the current one. In the conditional task, the subjects had learned, prior to scanning, specific associations between the abstract designs and the color stimuli. During scanning, they were required to select the abstract design that was appropriate for the color presented. Thus, the searching among the stimuli was the same as in the self-ordered task, but because the stimulus to be selected on each trial was determined completely by the color cue presented, no monitoring within working memory of prior selections was required.

Performance of the self-ordered task, in comparison with either the matching control or the conditional task, resulted in significantly greater activity within the mid-dorsolateral frontal cortex (areas 46 and 9/46), particularly within the right hemisphere (Fig. 9.5). There was no activation in this region when cerebral blood flow in the conditional task was compared with that of the control task, although there was now significant activity within the posterior dorsolateral frontal cortex in area 8, a region known to be critical for visual conditional learning (25). These results are in agreement with work in the monkey demonstrating a functional difference between the mid-dorsolateral and the posterior dorsolateral frontal cortex. In addition, during performance of both the self-ordered and the conditional task, there was activation of the posterior cingulate region and the adjacent ventral part of the medial posterior parietal cortex. This activation is consistent with the

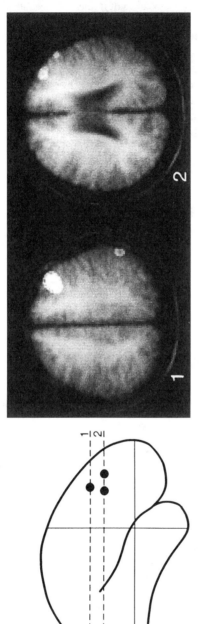

FIG. 9.5. Horizontal sections (1, 2) through the brain to show increased activity within the mid-dorsolateral prefrontal cortex during the monitoring of abstract designs in the context of a self-ordered working memory task.

suggestion that, for the type of mnemonic processing discussed in this article, critical functional interactions between the dorsolateral frontal cortex and the hippocampal system may be occurring through this posterior cingulate/medial parietal region and the adjacent posterior parahippocampal region. Several subsequent studies confirmed these early findings demonstrating that whenever monitoring of information in working memory is required, the mid-dorsolateral prefrontal region of the human cerebral cortex exhibits an increase in activity (for reviews, see 26,27).

ACKNOWLEDGMENTS

This research was supported by grants from the Medical Research Council and the Natural Sciences and Engineering Research Council of Canada.

REFERENCES

1. Petrides M. Frontal lobes and memory. In: Boller F, Grafman J, eds. *Handbook of neuropsychology*. Amsterdam: Elsevier, 1989;3:75–90.
2. Jus A, Jus K, Villeneuve A, et al. Studies on dream recall in chronic schizophrenic patients after prefrontal lobotomy. *Biol Psychiatry* 1973;6:275–293.
3. Stuss DT, Kaplan EF, Benson DF, et al. Evidence for the involvement of orbitofrontal cortex in memory functions: an interference effect. *J Comp Physiol Psychol* 1982;96:913–925.
4. Petrides M, Pandya DN. Dorsolateral prefrontal cortex: comparative cytoarchitectonic analysis in the human and the macaque brain and corticocortical connection patterns. *Eur J Neurosci* 1999;11:1011–1036.
5. Barbas H. Anatomic organization of basoventral and mediodorsal visual recipient prefrontal regions in the rhesus monkey. *J Comp Neurol* 1988;276:313–342.
6. Barbas H, Pandya DN. Architecture and intrinsic connections of the prefrontal cortex in the rhesus monkey. *J Comp Neurol* 1989;286:353–375.
7. Carmichael ST, Price JL. Limbic connections of the orbital and the medial prefrontal cortex in macaque monkeys. *J Comp Neurol* 1995;363:615–641.
8. Petrides M, Milner B. Deficits on subject-ordered tasks after frontal- and temporal-lobe lesions in man. *Neuropsychologia* 1982;20:249–262.
9. Petrides M. Frontal lobes and working memory: evidence from investigations of the effects of cortical exci-
sions in nonhuman primates. In: Boller F, Grafman J, eds. *Handbook of neuropsychology*. Amsterdam: Elsevier, 1994;9:59–82.
10. Petrides M. Specialized systems for the processing of mnemonic information within the primate frontal cortex. *Philos Trans R Soc Lond B* 1996;351:1455–1462.
11. Petrides M. Monitoring of selections of visual stimuli and the primate frontal cortex. *Proc R Soc Lond B Bio Sci* 1991;246:293–298.
12. Petrides M. Impairments on nonspatial self-ordered and externally ordered working memory tasks after lesions of the mid-dorsal part of the lateral frontal cortex in the monkey. *J Neurosci* 1995;15:359–375.
13. Milner B. Disorders of learning and memory after temporal lobe lesions in man. *Clin Neurosurg* 1972;19:421–446.
14. Mishkin M. A memory system in the monkey. *Philos Trans R Soc Lond B* 1982;298:85–95.
15. Squire LR, Zola-Morgan S. The medial temporal lobe memory system. *Science* 1991;253:1380–1386.
16. Corkin S. Tactually-guided maze learning in man: effects of unilateral cortical excisions and bilateral hippocampal lesions. *Neuropsychologia* 1965;3:339–351.
17. Milner B. Visually guided maze learning in man: effects of bilateral hippocampal, bilateral frontal, and unilateral cerebral lesions. *Neuropsychologia* 1965;3:317–338.
18. Smith ML, Milner B. The role of the right hippocampus in the recall of spatial location. *Neuropsychologia* 1981; 19:781–793.
19. Olton DS. Memory functions and the hippocampus. In: Seifert W, ed. *Neurobiology of the hippocampus*. London: Academic Press, 1983:335–373.
20. Adey WR, Meyer M. An experimental study of hippocampal afferent pathways from prefrontal and cingulate areas in the monkey. *J Anat* 1952;86:58–75.
21. Goldman-Rakic PS, Selemon LD, Schwartz ML. Dual pathways connecting the dorsolateral prefrontal cortex with the hippocampal formation and parahippocampal cortex in the rhesus monkey. *Neuroscience* 1984;12: 719–743.
22. Morris R, Pandya DN, Petrides M. Fiber system linking the mid-dorsolateral frontal cortex with the retrosplenial/presubicular region in the rhesus monkey. *J Comp Neurol* 1999;407:183–192.
23. Pandya DN, Van Hoesen GW, Mesulam M-M. Efferent connections of the cingulate gyrus in the rhesus monkey. *Exp Brain Res* 1981;42:319–330.
24. Petrides M, Alivisatos B, Evans AC, et al. Dissociation of human mid-dorsolateral frontal cortex in memory processing. *Proc Natl Acad Sci USA* 1993;90:873–877.
25. Petrides M. Conditional learning and the primate frontal cortex. In: Perecman E, ed. *The frontal lobes revisited*. New York: IRBN Press, 1987:91–108.
26. Owen AM. The functional organization of working memory processes within the human lateral frontal cortex: the contribution of functional neuroimaging. *Eur J Neurosci* 1997;9:1329–1339.
27. Petrides M. Mapping prefrontal cortical systems for the control of cognition. In: Toga AW, Mazziota JC, eds. *Brain mapping: the systems*. San Diego: Academic Press (in press).

Neocortical Epilepsies.
Advances in Neurology, Vol. 84,
edited by P. D. Williamson, A. M. Siegel,
D. W. Roberts, V. M. Thadani, and M. S. Gazzaniga.
Lippincott Williams & Wilkins, Philadelphia © 2000.

10

International Classification: Implications for Neocortical Epilepsies

Jerome Engel, Jr.

Departments of Neurology and Neurobiology, UCLA School of Medicine,
Los Angeles, California 90095

The International League Against Epilepsy (ILAE) accepts two international classifications. The International Classifications of Epileptic Seizures (ICES) (Table 10.1) (1) was last revised in 1981, and the International Classification of Epilepsies and Epileptic Syndromes (ICEES) (Table 10.2) (2) was last revised in 1989. It is essential to keep the concept of epilepsies, which implies a continuous disturbance in brain structure or function, separate from the concept of epileptic seizures, which are the intermittent electroclinical manifestations of these underlying disorders; a given epileptic syndrome or disease may be associated with multiple seizure types, whereas epileptic seizures often occur in patients for whom no syndrome or disease diagnosis can be made. The two international classifications have been widely accepted, and their almost universal use in the literature has greatly enhanced the exchange of clinical information and research. Some criticism has been leveled at these classifications, however, and some aspects of each have become outdated in the past decade or so as a result of new insights into fundamental mechanisms and anatomic substrates, as well as technologic advances that enhance our ability to noninvasively identify specific pathophysiologic conditions in individual patients. Consequently, the ILAE is now considering a

TABLE 10.1. *International classification of epileptic seizures*

I. Partial (focal, local) seizures
  A. Simple partial seizures
    1. With motor signs
    2. With somatosensory or special sensory symptoms
    3. With autonomic symptoms or signs
    4. With psychic symptoms
  B. Complex partial seizures
    1. Simple partial onset followed by impairment of consciousness
    2. Impairment of consciousness at onset
  C. Partial seizures evolving to secondarily generalized seizures
    1. Simple partial seizures evolving to generalized seizures
    2. Complex partial seizures evolving to generalized seizures
    3. Simple partial seizures evolving to complex partial seizures evolving to generalized seizures
II. Generalized seizures (convulsive or nonconvulsive)
  A. Absence seizures
    1. Typical absences
    2. Atypical absences
  B. Myoclonic Seizures
  C. Clonic seizures
  D. Tonic seizures
  E. Tonic–clonic seizures
  F. Atonic seizures (astatic seizures)
III. Unclassified epileptic seizures

From the Commission on Classification and Terminology of the International League Against Epilepsy: proposal for revised clinical and electroencephalographic classification of epileptic seizures. *Epilepsia* 1981;22:489–501, with permission.

TABLE 10.2. *International classification of epilepsies, epileptic syndromes, and related seizure disorders*

1. Localization related (focal, local, partial)
 1.1 Idiopathic (primary)
  Benign childhood epilepsy with centrotemporal spikes
  Childhood epilepsy with occipital paroxysms
  Primary reading epilepsy
 1.2 Symptomatic (secondary)
  Temporal lobe epilepsies
  Frontal lobe epilepsies
  Parietal lobe epilepsies
  Occipital lobe epilepsies
  Chronic progressive epilepsia partialis continua of childhood
  Syndromes characterized by seizures with specific modes of precipitation
 1.3 Cryptogenic, defined by:
  Seizure type
  Clinical features
  Etiology
  Anatomic localization
2. Generalized
 2.1 Idiopathic (primary)
  Benign neonatal familial convulsions
  Benign neonatal convulsions
  Benign myoclonic epilepsy in infancy
  Childhood absence epilepsy (pyknolepsy)
  Juvenile absence epilepsy
  Juvenile myoclonic epilepsy (impulsive petit mal)
  Epilepsies with grand mal seizures (GTCS) on awakening
  Other generalized idiopathic epilepsies
   Epilepsies with seizures precipitated by specific modes of activation
 2.2 Cryptogenic and symptomatic
  West syndrome (infantile spasms, Blitz–Nick–Salaam Krämpfe)
  Lennox–Gastaut syndrome
  Epilepsy with myoclonic–astatic seizures
  Epilepsy with myoclonic absences
 2.3 Symptomatic (secondary)
  2.3.1 Nonspecific etiology
   Early myoclonic encephalopathy
   Early infantile epileptic encephalopathy with suppression bursts
   Other symptomatic generalized epilepsies
  2.3.2 Specific syndromes
   Epileptic seizures may complicate many disease states
3. Undetermined epilepsies
 3.1 With both generalized and focal seizures
  Neonatal seizures
  Severe myoclonic epilepsy in infancy
  Epilepsy with continuous spike waves during slow wave sleep
  Acquired epileptic aphasia (Landau–Kleffner syndrome)
  Other undetermined epilepsies
 3.2 Without unequivocal generalized or focal features
4. Special syndromes
 4.1 Situation-related seizures (Gelegenheitsanfälle)
  Febrile convulsions
  Isolated seizures or isolated status epilepticus
  Seizures occurring only when there is an acute or toxic event caused by factors such as alcohol, drugs, eclampsia, nonketotic hyperglycemia

From Commission on Classification and Terminology of the International League Against Epilepsy: proposal for revised classification of epilepsies and epileptic syndromes. *Epilepsia* 1989;30:389–399, with permission.

TABLE 10.3. *Uses of a classification system for epilesy*

Personal conceptualization
Teaching
Communication between physicians
  Primary care physicians and other health workers
  Neurologists and epileptologists
Presurgical evaluation
Clinical pharmacology trials
Epidemiological studies
Prognosis
Pathophysiological implications
Etiology

major revision in these classifications (3). Because there are many different uses for classification systems (Table 10.3), multiple classifications or variations of classifications may need to be constructed to address each of these specific uses.

NEW CLASSIFICATION SCHEME

It is anticipated that the new international classification will consist of four parts. The first will be a glossary for describing the phenomenology of epileptic events, which will provide a standardized way for physicians to document ictal behavior. This will be based in part on the suggestions of Lüders (4) and will be recommended for clinical use, creating databases, and in research publications when presenting the component parts of specific ictal events before any presumptions of underlying etiology are made. This system also may give rise to the development of uniform protocols for long-term monitoring reports.

The next part will be a classification of epileptic seizures based on presumed pathophysiologic and anatomic substrates, which will replace the current, largely phenomenologic, ICES. In contrast to the glossary, which can be used to describe purely phenomenologic information about ictal events, the new classification of epileptic seizures, in effect, will be a *diagnosis* derived from all available clinical and laboratory information, and it will have implications for etiology, therapy, and prognosis. This classification will com-

plement the classification of syndromes and diseases because therapy and prognosis can be based on a seizure diagnosis when a syndrome or disease diagnosis cannot be made.

The third part will be a classification of epileptic syndromes and diseases based largely on the present ICEES; however, it will distinguish between epileptic syndromes, epileptic diseases, and diseases associated with epilepsy. Epileptic syndromes have either unknown or multiple etiologies, whereas epileptic diseases have a unique etiology. Epileptic seizures are the essential and invariant manifestations of epileptic diseases, whereas diseases associated with epilepsy give rise to epileptic seizures as one common, but not obligatory, manifestation of a pathological process that also causes other characteristic signs and symptoms.

The field of molecular genetics is expanding rapidly, and an exponential rise in the identification of "epilepsy genes" will greatly impact any attempt to classify epileptic syndromes and diseases. When an idiopathic epileptic syndrome is found to be the unique result of a single gene, it becomes a disease. It now appears likely, however, that often more than one gene will have the capability to give rise to the same phenotypic epileptic disorder, in which case the disorder would remain a syndrome with multiple causes. Each of the individual genetic disturbances could be considered an epileptic disease, however, if the essential and invariant clinical manifestation is epilepsy. On the other hand, it is also becoming common to find that a single genetic abnormality causes different family members to have different idiopathic epileptic syndromes. In this case, the single gene disturbance could be considered an epileptic disease, with multiple manifestations. Therefore, any new classification of epileptic syndromes and diseases will need to be extremely flexible to accommodate the advances in gene discovery that inevitably will continue to occur.

An important concept for the new classification of epileptic syndromes and diseases is that there will be no attempt to make it comprehensive. It will consist only of identified disorders, with the understanding that a syndromic or disease diagnosis will not be possible in many patients with epilepsy. For these patients, a seizure diagnosis will suffice, and there will be no reason to force patients inappropriately into specific syndrome or disease categories.

In contrast to the current ICEES, the new classification will be divided into conditions that are generally accepted and those that are still controversial or uncertain. They also will be organized first by the age of onset, which is most useful for differential diagnosis, and distinction between localization-related and generalized epilepsies will be deemphasized in view of the difficulty in distinguishing between these two groups for many epileptic conditions.

The fourth part will be a classification of functional disability caused by epilepsy and epileptic seizures. This classification will be based on the classification of the World Health Organization on the impact of diseases, modified to take into account disabilities caused by the intermittent nature of epileptic seizures (5).

Current understanding of neocortical epilepsies, the topic of this volume, will have a major impact on new classifications of epileptic seizures and of epileptic syndromes and diseases, and deserve some further discussion here.

CLASSIFICATION OF NEOCORTICAL SEIZURES

The current ICES is intended to be phenomenologic, without reference to pathophysiologic mechanisms or anatomic substrates. Consequently, there is no distinction between ictal events generated in neocortex and those generated in limbic structures. The new classification of epileptic seizures will not only recognize that limbic and neocortical seizures represent different diagnostic entities but also will attempt to define various types of neocortical seizures based on multiple pathophysiologic and anatomic criteria, not on a single diagnostic feature such as lobe of origin.

It will be important to define ictal signs and symptoms that can indicate involvement of specific cortical areas, but these will be used in conjunction with other clinical information to derive the seizure diagnosis and never will be used alone. Previous classifications have referred to frontal, temporal, parietal, and occipital lobe seizures. It is now recognized, however, that not only are there different functional cortical areas within a single lobe, giving rise, for instance, to more than one characteristic type of frontal lobe seizure, but also that some multilobar areas must be considered functional units because they give rise to the same ictal manifestations, for example, the perirolandic area, the temporal parietal occipital junction, and, to a certain extent, the frontal, parietal, and temporal operculum (6).

There may be distinctive characteristic features that warrant separating seizures based on specific types of structural abnormalities, such as developmental lesions versus alien tissue lesions versus the effects of localized trauma or infection. In this regard, an important challenge for future research is to identify the pathophysiologic basis of seizures resulting from what is now referred to as *cryptogenic epilepsy,* that form of symptomatic epilepsy for which no magnetic resonance imaging or historical evidence for a specific lesion exists. The epileptogenic zone for most, if not all, patients with cryptogenic epilepsies who are evaluated with invasive electrophysiologic studies for surgery turn out to be neocortical. Perhaps some of these epileptogenic abnormalities are due to cell loss and neuronal reorganization in neocortex resembling that now believed to underlie mesial temporal lobe epilepsy (MTLE) with hippocampal sclerosis, or to other localized epileptogenic disturbances *unique* to neocortex (7).

Age is another factor that influences the epileptic seizure diagnosis. Neonatal seizures and infantile spasms are examples of specific diagnostic seizure entities that are age specific, are not recognized as a syndrome or disease category, and invariably are replaced by other types of ictal events or disappear when the susceptible age is exceeded.

Finally, neuropharmacologic criteria can be used to dissect apart epileptic seizures that are due to different mechanisms. Although responsivity to currently available antiepileptic drugs might be helpful for distinguishing among and categorizing seizures with specific pathophysiologic substrates, the fact is that partial neocortical seizures as a group are more often medically refractory than generalized convulsions or absences (8), perhaps because virtually all new compounds to be tested for antiepileptic potential are screened against animal models of generalized convulsions (electroconvulsive shock) or absences (subcutaneous pentylenetetrazol) for economic reasons (9). Consequently, drugs that might be effective against partial neocortical seizures never reach clinical trials if they lack anticonvulsant or antiabsence properties. Therefore, another major challenge for the future for those interested in neocortical seizures will be to create appropriate experimental animal models of various neocortical ictal phenomena. Such animal models might not only enhance research into basic mechanisms but also may lead to more cost-effective ways to screen drugs for antiepileptic effects against neocortical seizures.

CLASSIFICATION OF NEOCORTICAL EPILEPSIES

The current ICEES recognizes three localization-related idiopathic epilepsies: benign childhood epilepsy with centrotemporal spikes, childhood epilepsy with occipital paroxysms, and primary reading epilepsy. Since acceptance of this classification, two separate varieties of idiopathic occipital epilepsy have been described. The more common form, early onset benign childhood occipital seizures (10), is associated with only a few ictal events during a specific period of development, whereas the less common form, which was the one originally described, is not necessarily so benign and might now be referred to as *late-onset occipital epilepsy* (11). All four of these disorders most likely belong to a family of idiopathic localization-related epilepsies, including conditions with focal interictal spikes located in other neocortical areas, such as the parietal lobe, and with other symptoms (12).

Recently, the condition of autosomal-dominant familial frontal lobe epilepsy has been accepted (13), and a gene has been localized (14). The product of this genetic defect is an abnormal acetylcholine nicotinic receptor (15). If this is the only gene causing this condition, it might be considered an epileptic disease. A syndrome of familial TLE also has been described (16). Although localization of the epileptogenic region in all these disorders is only assumed from electroclinical correlations, the most common primary site of pathophysiologic disturbance is likely to be the neocortex. As specific genetic defects are found that give rise to disturbances in neurotransmitter receptor function and channel opathies, it will be of great interest to determine how defects that ought to have a profound generalized impact on nervous system function can manifest as a localization-related neocortical epilepsy.

Perhaps most people with epilepsy suffer from what is now categorized as *symptomatic localization-related epilepsies;* however, only two syndromes are generally accepted. *MTLE*, that form of temporal lobe epilepsy associated with hippocampal sclerosis, is by far the most common, and the pathophysiology is now sufficiently well understood that it might even be considered an epileptic disease (17). *Epilepsia partialis continua* is usually neocortical and has been subdivided into two forms. One, *Rasmussen's encephalitis,* is more diffuse and recently was shown to be caused by an antibody to a glutamate receptor subunit, GluR3 (18). The other is more localized and usually due to a structural lesion in neocortex (19). The current ICEES does not distinguish between MTLE and TLE of neocortical origin and also inappropriately denotes other anatomic syndromes based only on lobe of origin: frontal, parietal, and occipital lobe epilepsies. Furthermore, these are described as types of seizures, not syndromes, and should not be included in a classification of the epilepsies.

A major task for those constructing the new international classification will be to identify and categorize discrete symptomatic localization-related neocortical epileptic disorders as either syndromes or diseases. Despite extensive use of the most advanced noninvasive and invasive diagnostic techniques in the course of presurgical evaluation for medically refractory partial neocortical seizures (20), this remains the major terra incognita of epileptology. Consequently, this volume, and the conference from which it is derived, is most timely and should mark the beginning of a concerted effort to understand more fully this important area of clinical epilepsy.

ACKNOWLEDGMENTS

Original research reported by the author was supported in part by Grants NS-02808, NS-15654, NS-33310, and GM-24839 from the National Institutes of Health and Contract DE-AC03-76-SF00012 from the Department of Energy.

REFERENCES

1. Commission on Classification and Terminology of the International League Against Epilepsy. Proposal for revised clinical and electroencephalographic classification of epileptic seizures. *Epilepsia* 1981;22:489–501.
2. Commission on Classification and Terminology of the International League Against Epilepsy. Proposal for revised classification of epilepsies and epileptic syndromes. *Epilepsia* 1989;30:389–399.
3. Engel J Jr. Classifications of the International League Against Epilepsy: time for reappraisal. *Epilepsia* 1998; 39:1014–1017.
4. Lüders HO, Acharya J, Baumgartner C, et al. Semiological seizure classification. *Epilepsia* 1998;39:1006–1013.
5. ICIDH-2 Beta-1 Draft for Field Trials. International classification of impairments, activities, and participation: a manual of dimensions of disablement and functioning. Geneva: World Health Organization, 1997.
6. Williamson PD, Engel J Jr, Munari C. Anatomic classification of localization-related epilepsies. In: Engel J Jr,

Pedley TA, eds. *Epilepsy: a comprehensive textbook.* Philadelphia: Lippincott–Raven, 1998:2405–2416.
7. Engel J Jr, Dichter MA, Schwartzkroin PA. Basic mechanisms of human epilepsy. In: Engel J Jr, Pedley TA, eds. *Epilepsy: a comprehensive textbook.* Philadelphia: Lippincott–Raven, 1998:499–512.
8. Hauser WA, Hesdorffer DH. *Epilepsy: frequency, causes, and consequences.* New York: Demos Press, 1990.
9. Kupferberg HJ, Schmutz M. Screening of new compounds and the role of the pharmaceutical industry. In: Engel J Jr, Pedley TA, eds. *Epilepsy: a comprehensive textbook.* Philadelphia: Lippincott–Raven, 1998: 1417–1434.
10. Panayiotopolous CP. Benign childhood epilepsy with occipital paroxysms: a 15-year prospective study. *Ann Neurol* 1989;26:51–56.
11. Gastaut H, Zifkin BG. Benign epilepsy of childhood with occipital spike and wave complexes. In: Andermann F, Lugaresi E, eds. *Migraine and epilepsy.* Boston: Butterworths, 1987:47–81.
12. Gobbi G, Guerrini R. Childhood epilepsy with occipital spikes and other benign localization-related epilepsies. In: Engel J Jr, Pedley TA, eds. *Epilepsy: a comprehensive textbook.* Philadelphia: Lippincott–Raven, 1998: 2315–2326.
13. Scheffer IE, Bhatia KP, Lopes-Cendes I, et al. Autosomal dominant nocturnal frontal lobe epilepsy: a distinctive clinical disorder. *Brain* 1995;118:61–73.
14. Phillips HA, Scheffer IE, Berkovic SF, et al. Localization of a gene for autosomal dominant nocturnal frontal lobe epilepsy. *Nat Genet* 1995;10:117–118.
15. Steinlein OK, Mulley JC, Propping P, et al. A missense mutation in the neuronal nicotinic acetylcholine receptor of $\alpha4$ subunit is associated with autosomal dominant nocturnal frontal lobe epilepsy. *Nat Genet* 1995;11: 201–203.
16. Tassinari CA, Michelucci R. Familial frontal and temporal lobe epilepsies. In: Engel J Jr, Pedley TA, eds. *Epilepsy: a comprehensive textbook.* Philadelphia: Lippincott–Raven, 1998:2427–2431.
17. Engel J Jr, Williamson PD, Wieser H-G. Mesial temporal lobe epilepsy. In: Engel J Jr, Pedley TA, eds. *Epilepsy: a comprehensive textbook.* Philadelphia: Lippincott–Raven, 1998:2417–2426.
18. So NK, Andermann F. Rasmussen's syndrome. In: Engel J Jr, Pedley TA, eds. *Epilepsy: a comprehensive textbook.* Philadelphia: Lippincott–Raven, 1998:2379–2388.
19. Biraben A, Chauvel P. Epilepsia partialis continua. In: Engel J Jr, Pedley TA, eds. *Epilepsy: a comprehensive textbook.* Philadelphia: Lippincott–Raven, 1998: 2447–2453.
20. Arroyo S, Lesser RP, Awad IA, et al. Subdural and epidural grids and strips. In: Engel J Jr, ed. *Surgical treatment of the epilepsies,* 2nd ed. New York: Raven Press, 1993:377–386.

Neocortical Epilepsies.
Advances in Neurology, Vol. 84,
edited by P. D. Williamson, A. M. Siegel,
D. W. Roberts, V. M. Thadani, and M. S. Gazzaniga.
Lippincott Williams & Wilkins, Philadelphia © 2000.

11

Classification of Neocortical Epilepsies

Masakazu Seino, *Peter D. Williamson, Yushi Inoue, Tadahiro Mihara,
Kazumi Matsuda, and Takayasu Tottori

*National Epilepsy Center, Shizuoka Higashi Hospital, Shizuoka 420-8688, Japan;
*Section of Neurology, Dartmouth–Hitchcock Medical Center,
Lebanon, New Hampshire 03756*

An *epileptic syndrome* is defined as an epileptic disorder characterized by a cluster of signs and symptoms customarily occurring together. The signs and symptoms may be clinical (e.g., case history, seizure type, modes of seizure occurrence, neurological and psychological findings) or findings detected by ancillary studies, such as electroencephalography (EEG), computed tomography, and nuclear magnetic resonance (1). According to this definition, among a variety of symptomatic localization-related epilepsies, only mesial temporal lobe epilepsy deserves a syndromic entity in terms of demographics, risk factors, natural history, clinical seizure characteristics, scalp and intracranial EEG expressions, findings of neuroimaging, neuropsychological testing, and results of pathological examination (2). The other categories correspond to neocortical epilepsies and comprise epilepsies of great variability; these categories are based on seizure types and other clinical features as well as anatomic location. The neocortical epilepsies have been classified according to the anatomic substrate from which the seizure originates. None of the temporal, frontal, parietal or occipital lobes represent functionally homogeneous or unique regions, however (3).

Neocortical epilepsies are thus clinically synonymous with extratemporal epilepsies if lateral (neocortical) temporal epilepsy is separable from temporal lobe epilepsy. The neocortical epilepsies do not conform to epilepsies or epileptic syndromes but consist of a mixture of a variety of simple and complex partial seizures. It has been well accepted that the clinical characteristics of complex partial seizures, accompanying impairment of consciousness by definition (4), have no anatomic localization value, whereas simple phases of partial seizures often denote cortical localization, provided that the area of seizure origin on the cortex is associated with a known and recognized function. Many clinical seizure manifestations are a reflection of propagation from the region of origin, and unlike mesial temporal lobe seizures, the spread patterns of neocortical onset seizures may vary among patients and among seizures in the same patient (3). This chapter proposes an anatomic classification of neocortical epilepsies that has been found clinically useful and provides "pure culture" cases typical of each category of neocortical epilepsy.

A pure culture case of frontal lobe epilepsy was defined by Rasmussen as "patients with epileptogenic lesions who have undergone excision of portions of the frontal lobe for the relief of medically refractory focal seizures, and who have subsequently become and remained seizure free. It seems logical to assume that, in these patients, the essential seizure-producing mechanisms were contained in the excised portions of the frontal lobe, and such patients thus represent a pure culture of frontal lobe epilepsy" (5). The epileptogenic lesion in this definition corresponds in the current concept and terminology to epileptogenic zone rather than lesion (6).

NEOCORTICAL TEMPORAL LOBE EPILESPY

Lateral Temporal or Neocortical Temporal Lobe Seizures

There is very little information about lateral (neocortical) temporal lobe epilepsy. Several reviews do not attempt to differentiate seizures of medial from lateral temporal lobe origin (7,8). It has been stated that distinguishing characteristics of seizures of neocortical temporal lobe origin do not exist, or, if they do exist, pure cases are rare (9). Extensive connections between lateral temporal neocortex and mesial structures would explain why clinical features of seizures would be similar in both regions (10). Some features, however, may help to identify lateral temporal seizures. Auditory, vertiginous, and complex visual hallucinations have been equated with lateral temporal origin (11). The revised International League Against Epilepsies classification of epileptic syndromes notes that simple seizures characterized by auditory hallucinations, illusions, dreamy states, visual misperceptions, or language disorders in case of language-dominant hemisphere focus, may occur in lateral temporal seizures. They may progress to complex partial seizures if propagation to mesial temporal or extratemporal structures occurs (12). On one hand, the analyses of magnetic resonance imaging (MRI) scans after temporal lobe neocorticectomy showed unexpected and extensive encroachment on medial structures in most patients who had undergone surgery (13); on the other hand, we have experienced several "pure culture" patients with lateral temporal lobe seizures, all having detectable lesions on MRI.

Case Report

This 39-year-old woman was right-handed and left-speech dominant. She had temporal lobe epilepsy–lateral temporal seizures. She developed seizure events consisting of motionless stare with dystonic posturing of the right hand, followed by automatisms of smacking and fumbling at age 25. Emitting meaningless utterances 20 to 30 seconds prior to the outset of the automatisms was the initial sign of her seizures. An MRI T2 elongation lesion in the left first temporal gyrus was found. In intracranial EEG/video studies, flattening of EEG activities over the left lateral temporal cortex corresponded to the occurrence of the jargonophasia, followed by spreading of spike discharges bilaterally to the mesial and basal temporal regions that corresponded to the occurrence of automatisms (Figs. 11.1 and 11.2) (14). Postictal disorientation, anomia, an inability to comprehend speech, and long-lasting amnesia ensued postictally.

Left neocorticectomy was performed with the medial structures spared, which was confirmed by postsurgical MRI. She has been seizure free for 5 years after the surgery. In the resection specimen, focal cortical dysplasia was confirmed.

FRONTAL LOBE EPILEPSIES

In the 1985 ILAE classification of epileptic syndromes, frontal lobe epilepsies were divided into seven subtypes: supplementary motor seizures, cingulate seizures, anterior frontopolar region seizures, orbitofrontal seizures, dorsolateral seizures, opercular seizures, and motor cortex seizures, including Kojewnikow's syndrome and perirolandic seizures. In the preamble of the proposal, it was stated that "these are preliminary descriptions of syndromes related to sometimes unusually precise localization. The basis for these descriptions includes data collected by contributors working with depth electrodes. It is fully recognized that patients thus studied represent a highly selected minority, and that these descriptions are extraction because fre-

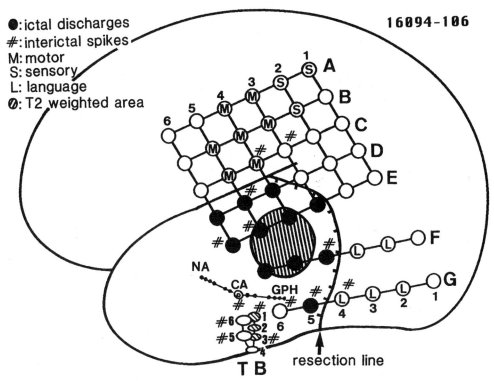

FIG. 11.1. Placement of subdural (A to G, and TB) and intracerebral electrodes (NA, CA, and GPH). *NA*, amygdaloid body; *CA*, hippocampus; *GPH*, parahippocampal gyrus; *TB*, temporal base. (Inoue Y, Mihara T, Fukao K, et al. Ictal paraphasia induced by language activity. *Epilepsy Research* 1999;35:69–79, with permission.)

quently discharging lesions are not confined to such closely circumscribed foci" (1). In the 1989 revised classification, general characteristics of frontal lobe epilepsies were described as (a) generally short seizures; (b) complex partial seizures, often with minimal or no postictal confusion; (c) rapid generalization; (d) prominent motor manifestations, which are either tonic or postural; (e) complex gestural automatisms, frequently at the onset; and (f) frequent falling when the discharge is bilateral (12).

During the 1990s, interest in frontal lobe epilepsy and seizures heightened, as reflected in the publications from two symposia specifically concerning classified topographic distribution of frontal lobe seizures based on findings of stereo EEG (SEEG) exploration. Most commonly, those arose from areas 4 and 6 and the medial intermediate frontal region

anterior to the supplementary motor area. Less commonly, seizures originated from the dorsolateral intermediate region anterior to area 6, including the frontal eye fields, and the operculoinsular region. Seizures in which the discharge initially affected the posterior portion of the inferior frontal gyrus, the frontopolar cortex, and the orbitofrontal region were least common (14).

Williamson and co-workers proposed in 1997 a classification of frontal lobe epilepsies into three broad categories: *focal clonic motor seizures, asymmetric tonic seizures,* and *frontal lobe complex partial (psychomotor) seizures,* recognizing that there can be considerable admixture among the three groups (3) (Table 11.1). Coincidentally, Mihara and coworkers proposed a classification also into three groups, but in different terminology, based on ictal symptomatology: *supplementary motor*

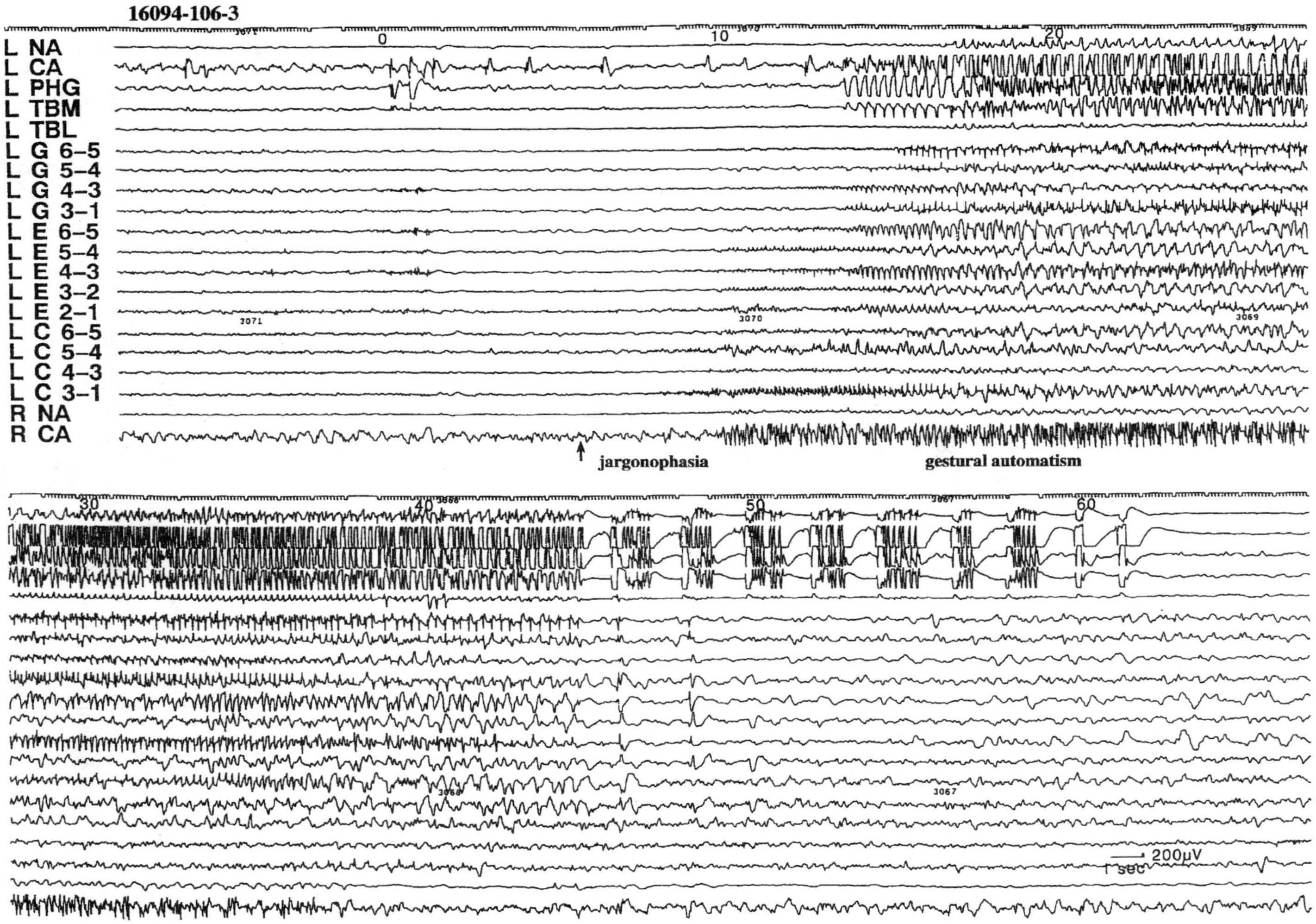

FIG. 11.2. Intracranial seizure discharges. For abbreviations, see Fig. 11.1. (Reproduced from Inoue Y, Mihara T, Fukao K, et al. Ictal paraphasia induced by language activity. *Epilepsy Research* 1999;35:69–79, with permission.)

TABLE 11.1. *Classification of neocortical epilepsies (3)*

Temporal lobe epilepsy
  Lateral (Neocortical) temporal lobe epilepsy
Frontal lobe epilepsy
Focal clonic motor seizures
Asymmetrical tonic seizures
Frontal lobe complex partial seizures
Occipital lobe epilepsy
Parietal lobe epilepsy

seizures with tonic posturing and with consciousness retained, *focal motor seizures* with elementary clonic or tonic symptoms, also with consciousness retained; and *psychomotor seizures* with automatisms usually accompanied by impairment of consciousness (15). In both the focal motor seizure group and the supplementary motor seizure group, the epileptogenic zones were restricted to the poste-

rior one third of the frontal lobe, whereas in the psychomotor group, they were largely localized in the anterior two thirds of the frontal lobe. These findings were confirmed by the postsurgical outcome of 18 pure culture patients (15) (Fig. 11.3). A recent report supports the three-part classification of frontal lobe seizures into those with supplementary motor seizures, those with focal motor seizures, and those with complex partial seizures as a result of metanalyses of clusters of seizure manifestations of patients with frontal lobe epilepsy (16).

Focal Clonic Motor Seizures

Focal clonic motor seizures are simple partial seizures caused by seizure activity in the primary motor area when they occur in isolation. Focal motor clonic seizures are often

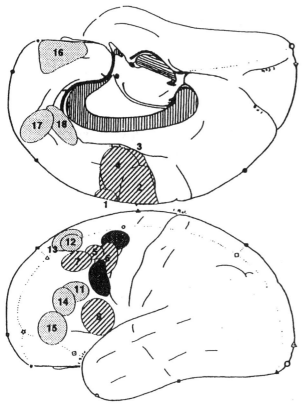

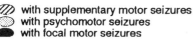
with supplementary motor seizures
with psychomotor seizures
with focal motor seizures

FIG. 11.3. Location of lesions in three patient groups. Arabic numerals indicate patient number. (Reproduced from Mihara T, Tottori T, Matsuda K, et al. Analysis of seizure manifestations of "Pure" frontal lobe origin. *Epilepsia* 1997(Suppl 6):42–47, with permission.)

part of other frontal or extrafrontal activation of primary motor cortex (3). In the 1989 revised ILAE classification of epileptic syndromes, motor cortex seizures are characterized mainly by simple partial seizures, and their localization depends on the side and topography of the area involved. In the case of the lower perirolandic area, there may be speech arrest, vocalization or dysphasia, tonic-clonic movements of the face on the contralateral side, or swallowing. Generalization frequently occurs. In the rolandic area, partial motor seizures with or without Jacksonian march occur, particularly beginning in the contralateral upper extremities. In the case of seizures involving the paracentral lobule, tonic movements of the ipsilateral foot may occur as well as the expected leg movements. Postictal Todd's paralysis is frequent (12).

Case Report

A 27-year-old right-handed man, left speech dominant, had frontal lobe epilepsy—focal clonic motor seizures. At age 15, he had developed convulsive episodes that were characterized by indiscernible auras followed by unilateral facial spasms several times a day. In video EEG monitoring, seizures began with a feeling of stiffness around the mouth, jerky hemifacial spasms on the right, progressing to head and eye turning toward the right and then clonic and tonic elevation of the right arm. The seizures ceased within several seconds, with consciousness fully retained. Todd's paresis followed. He could hardly speak, but he could recall what happened during the seizure. Ictal single-photon emission computed tomography (SPECT) revealed a hyperperfusion lesion in the left frontoparietal area. Electric stimulation at a prerolandic site elicited habitual seizures. He has been completely seizure free after corticectomy for the past 5 years.

Asymmetric Tonic Seizures

Supplementary motor area (SMA) seizures are the classic type of asymmetric tonic seizures (17). Seizures have subjective symp-

toms, such as somatosensory sensations of numbness or tingling. A general feeling of constriction or tightness may precede tonic posturing of extremities. Motor manifestations in well-documented examples of SMA seizures include asymmetric tonic or dystonic posturing of both upper and lower extremities; unilateral rigid, straight tonic upper-extremity posturing; abducted, flexed posturing of the upper extremity with the fist clenched; flailing, thrashing movements of the ipsilateral arm; kicking and stepping activity of the lower extremities; tonic/dystonic posturing of the contralateral lower extremity; and athetoid dystonic movements of the contralateral hand, arm, leg, or both (3). These seizures can secondarily generalize into tonic–clonic seizures. Even in the case of generalization, the postictal clinical and EEG suppression is surprisingly short. The SMA seizures stop as suddenly as they start and may occur in clusters. These electroclinical features make it possible to differentiate asymmetric tonic seizures of focal origin from the axial or axorhythmelic tonic states of generalized seizures. The manifestations are the exception, and there are many variations among different patients, although usually they are stereotyped for a given patient (18). Seizures originating outside the SMA can have asymmetric tonic posturing closely resembling SMA seizures. These include seizures beginning entirely outside the frontal lobe (19,20).

Mihara and co-workers described surgical strategies for five patients with SMA seizures (21). The cardinal manifestations of SMA seizures were complex postural synergies involving the trunk and proximal extremities. Postural movements showed a tendency to be bilateral. It was observed in all patients that bilateral tonic facial contractions, or downward retraction of mouth corners, appeared prior to or concomitant with the postural motor signs (Fig. 11.4). In patients in whom the seizure discharges were confined to the SMA, the clinical signs consisted exclusively of the bilateral facial constrictions or downward retraction of mouth corners. This sign was induced by electric stimulation on SMA,

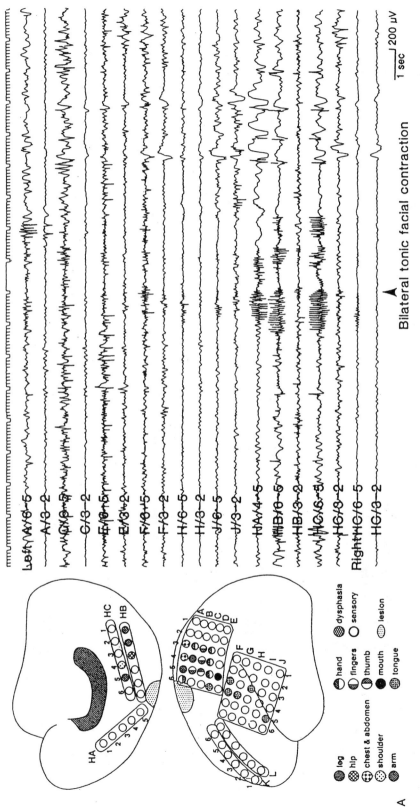

FIG. 11.4. Electroclinical correlation of bilateral tonic facial contraction. (Reproduced from Mihara T, Tottori T, Inoue Y, et al. Surgical strategies for patients with supplementary sensorimotor area epilepsy: the Japanese experience. In: Lüders HO, ed. *Supplementary sensorimotor area. Advances in Neurology*, vol 70. Philadelphia: Lippincott-Raven, 1996:405–414, with permission.)

and the facial contractions appeared unilaterally accompanying a run of afterdischarges. This suggests that bilateral facial contraction or downward retraction of mouth corners might be related to activation of contralateral SMA or other cortical areas connected with SMA (21).

Case Report

An 18-year-old right-handed woman had frontal lobe epilepsy–asymmetric tonic seizures. She had rubella encephalitis at age 6 and developed initial seizures at the age of 14 years, presenting with brief and asymmetric tonic convulsions followed by paresis of the right arm. The attacks were diurnal and repeated more than ten times a day. The seizures were stereotypic: cephalic aura followed by head and eyes turning toward the right, mimicking a fencing posture with the right arm extended upward. They lasted about 30 seconds, often accompanied by urinary incontinence. No secondarily generalized seizures ensued. Consciousness was not impaired, and complex gestural automatisms often were observed during the later phase of seizures. In both MRI and ictal SPECT, a circumscribed lesion was demonstrated in the left supplementary motor area where cortical dysplasia was found in a surgery specimen. Seizure discharges originated from an area within or adjacent to the lesion from where habitual seizures were provoked by electric stimulation. The patient has been completely free from seizures after corticectomy for 4 years (Fig. 11.5).

Frontal Lobe Complex Partial Seizures

Frontal lobe complex partial seizures (FLCPS) usually occur frequently, often in clusters day and night. The seizures are brief, lasting at longest 1 minute, with little or no postictal confusion. Motor automatisms are complex, beginning suddenly with violent or agitated appearance. Vocalization commonly occurs, varying from simple humming to shouting (3,18,22–25). As with other types of frontal lobe seizures, there can be a transition between FLCPS and asymmetric tonic seizures, in some patients exhibiting seizure components of both. FLCPS have been described with seizures of orbitofrontal ori-

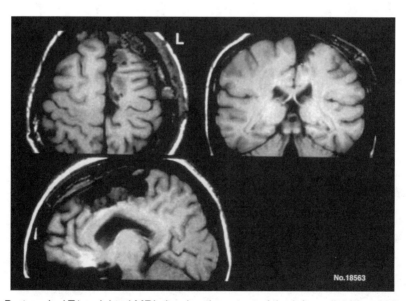

FIG. 11.5. Postsurgical T1-weighted MRI showing the extent of the left medial frontal lobe resection including SMA.

gin (26,27), with seizures of mesial frontal origin (28), and with seizures of frontal polar and dorsal convexity (29). Seizure features such as pelvic thrusting, side-to-side head movements, kicking, pedaling, nocturnal preponderance, short duration, younger age at seizure onset, and prone position during seizures are characteristic of FLCPS (3). Interictal and even ictal EEGs are often unrevealing in patients with FLCPS. This problem, coupled with the bizarre atypical appearance of seizures, frequently leads to erroneous diagnosis of hysteric or psychogenic, nonepileptic seizures (27,30). The clinical characteristics of FLCPS were described in a title by Wada as predominantly nocturnal recurrence of intensely affective vocal and facial expression associated with powerful bimanual, bipedal, and axial activity as ictal manifestations of mesial frontal lobe epilepsy (28).

Case Report

This 30-year-old right-handed woman had frontal lobe epilepsy–complex partial seizures. At the age of 5 years, she had an episode of fear, occurring later in clusters, more than ten times a day, with nocturnal preponderance. A lesion was found by computed tomography (CT)/MRI in the left anterior cingulate cortex. In intracranial EEG studies, ictal discharges originated from the left anteromesial portion and spread to the ipsilateral dorsolateral portion and contralateral mesial frontal cortex. Coincidentally, she uttered loudly the words "fearful, disgustful, help me, pardon me, ouch and heated" while pounding the rail of the bed or reciprocally swinging her extremities and hips. Urinary incontinence often followed. She seemed to remember all the events occurring during the seizures, although it was difficult for her to describe them clearly. She sensed a kind of fear coming from her back, but it was indiscernible. The ictal discharges were confined to the mesial and dorsolateral portion of the left frontal lobe during the seizure and never spread to the temporal lobe (Fig. 11.6). An ex-

tensive medial frontal corticectomy was performed. The histologic diagnosis of the surgical specimen was cortical dysplasia (Fig. 11.7). She has been free from seizures for the past 4 years (21).

Case Report

This 34-year-old right-handed woman was diagnosed as having frontal lobe epilepsy–frontal-lobe complex partial seizures. She developed brief spells at age 18 years; these spells occurred several times a day, and after 26 years a series of complex gestural automatisms had developed. The automatisms repeated day and night some 70 times, eventually culminating in a fracture of her left femur. The seizures were stereotypic and began with a gesture of grasping something with her hand. Shaking her legs from side to side, she groaned loudly and then writhed violently. These actions were accompanied by vigorous movements of the legs as if kicking, of the arms as if swimming, and of the hips thrusting. Such seizures lasted about 40 seconds or longer each and gradually subsided, often with urinary incontinence. She was totally amnestic for any events during the seizure. An MRI lesion was found adjacent to the right cingulate cortex near the genu of the corpus callosum. When the medial portion of the contralateral frontal lobe was involved, the behavioral seizures burst out. Electric stimulation at an electrode adjacent to the lesion elicited habitual seizures. The seizure discharges originated from the vicinity of the lesion and spread to the opposite side. An extensive medial frontal corticectomy was performed (Fig. 11.8). The histologic diagnosis of the surgical specimen was cortical dysplasia. For 6 years, was completely seizure free and is now working as a school teacher (15).

Case Report

This 28-year-old right-handed woman was diagnosed as having frontal lobe epilepsy–frontal-lobe complex partial seizures. She had her first major convulsion at the age of 17 years and developed complex gestural auto-

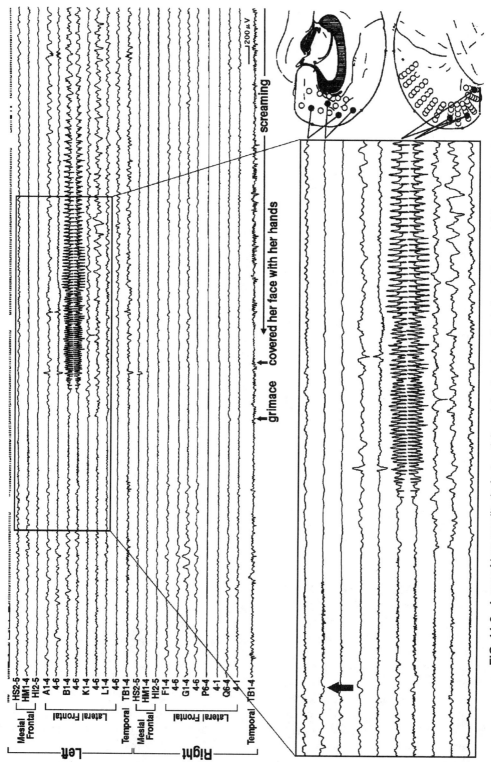

FIG. 11.6. A run of low-amplitude fast activity originating from the left anterior mesial frontal lobe, followed by a gradual buildup of high amplitude spikes on the ipsilateral anterior dorsolateral frontal lobe corresponding to the onset of automatisms.

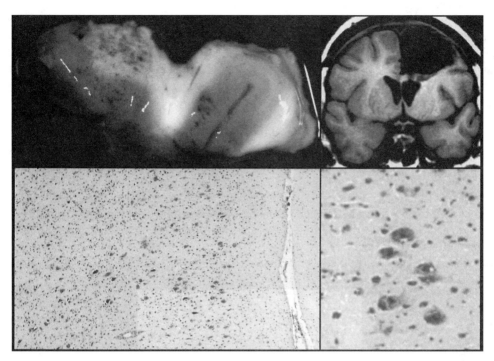

FIG. 11.7. Post-surgical specimen and MRI. The boundaries between the gray and white matter are blurred **(upper left)**, disorganized cortical layer formation of the cortex **(lower left)**, dysplastic giant neurons in magnification **(lower right)**, and MRI **(upper right)**.

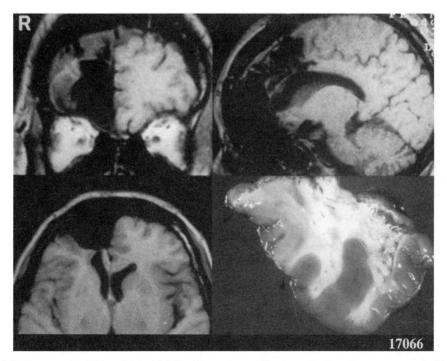

FIG. 11.8. Postsurgical T-1 weighted MRI and specimen. The boundaries of cortex toward white matter are not well defined, indicated by *arrows* **(lower right)**.

matisms consisting of bimanual rhythmic movements and tachypnea after the age of 20 years, and they occurred several times a month. A lesion was found by MRI in the right mesial orbitofrontal region. The ictal discharges originated from the vicinity of the lesion and spread to the surroundings. About 35 seconds after onset of the seizure, rhythmic discharges appeared from the ipsilateral temporal base. Immediately after the appearance of the new rhythm, she seemed to lose contact with persons nearby and repeatedly continued semipurposeful gestures or actions that she had been exhibiting immediately before the onset; these actions were associated with rhythmic smacking and munching along with tachypnea or pallor. A long confusion ensued postictally. She was amnesic for the events during the seizure. Ictal onset zone was right mesial orbitofrontal cortex; complex partial seizures emerged after they spread to the ipsilateral temporal base. As a result of extensive corticectomy of anterior mesial frontal lobe, she has been completely seizure free for 6 years. The histologic diagnosis of the surgery specimen was desembryoplastic neuroepitherial tumor.

Occipital Lobe Epilepsy

Occipital lobe epilepsy is characterized by simple partial seizures and secondarily generalized seizures. Complex partial seizures may occur with spread beyond the occipital lobe (20,31). Elementary visual seizures are characterized by fleeting visual manifestations that may be either negative (scotoma, hemianopia, amaurosis) or positive (sparks or flashes, phosphenes). Perceptive illusions, in which objects appear to be distorted, may occur. A change in size (macropsia or micropsia) or in distance, an inclination of objects and distortion of objects, or a sudden change in shape (metamorphopsia) can occur. In some cases, the scene is distorted or made smaller. Such visual illusions and hallucinations involve epileptic discharge in the temporoparieto-occipital junction (32). The initial signs also may include tonic or clonic contra-

version of eyes, palpebral jerks, and forced closure of eyelids (20,33). The discharge may spread to the temporal lobe, producing seizure manifestations of either lateral posterior temporal or amygdalohippocampal seizures indistinguishable from those seen in temporal lobe epilepsy (20,31,34). When the primary focus is located in the supracalcaline area, the discharge can spread forward to the suprasylvian convexity or the mesial surface, mimicking those of parietal or frontal lobe seizures (20,35,36). Spread to contralateral occipital lobe may be rapid. Occasionally, the seizure tends to become secondarily generalized (10).

Case Report

This right-handed 18-year-old woman who was left speech dominant had occipital lobe epilepsy–visual seizures evolving to verbal automatisms. She developed visual seizures at the age of 9 years and complained of a strange sensation in the eyes along with blurring of vision or phosphenes, dizziness, forced blinking that evolved to head and eye turning toward the right as if pursuing something, and verbal automatisms emitting incomprehensible words. Postictally, difficulties of naming and ambulatory automatisms were often observed. An MRI revealed a T2 elongation lesion in the left temporo-occipital region (Fig. 11.9). Seizure discharges originated from the left lateral occipital region corresponding to deviation of the head and eyes toward the right, and they spread to the right mesial occipital lobe and subsequently forward to the right mesial temporal structures corresponding with dysphasia.

Parietal Lobe Epilepsy

Most seizures arising in the parietal lobe remain simple partial seizures, but complex partial seizures may arise with spread beyond the parietal lobe. Simple partial seizures are predominantly sensory. Positive phenomena consist of tingling and a feeling of electricity, which may be confined or may spread in a Jacksonian manner (19,37). There may be a desire to move a part of the body or a sensa-

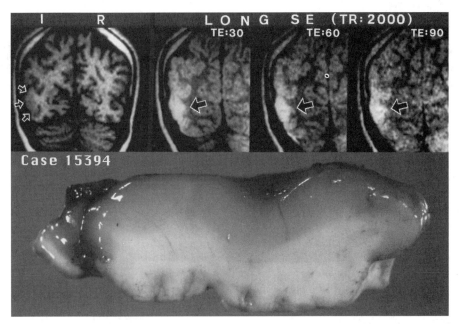

FIG. 11.9. Presurgical MRI images **(upper row)**. Pachygyic changes on the left lateral occipital lobe in inversion recovery MRI **(upper left)**, high signal areas in prolonged T2 (three frames, **upper right**), and postsurgical specimen showing blurred boundaries between the gray and white matter **(lower)**.

tion of part of the body being moved. The parts most frequently involved are those with the largest cortical representation (e.g., the hand, arm, face). There may be sensations of crawling on the tongue, stiffness, or coldness. Facial sensory phenomena may occur bilaterally. Occasionally, an intraabdominal sensation of sinking, choking, or nausea may occur, particularly in cases of inferior and lateral parietal lobe involvement (32,37). Rarely, there may be a painful sensation (3). Metamorphopsia with distortion, foreshortenings, and elongation may occur frequently in cases involving the non–speech-dominant hemisphere. Negative phenomena include numbness and a feeling that a body part is absent known as asomatognosia. Severe vertigo or disorientation in space may be indicative of inferior parietal lobe seizures (32). Seizures in the dominant parietal lobe result in a variety of receptive or conductive language disturbances. Some well-localized genital sensations may occur with paracentral involvement. Seizures of the paracentral lobule have a tendency to become secondarily generalized (38).

Case Report

This 24-year-old man was diagnosed as being shifted sinister and having parietal lobe epilepsy, with somatosensory seizures evolving to postural seizures. Since age 10 years, he had experienced a feeling of tingling or numbness on the right arm moving down to the fingers that often progressed to vocalization, hemifacial spasms on the right, tonic elevation of the right arm, head and eye turning toward the right, and eventually generalized convulsions. There was a nocturnal preponderance. Independent of these seizures, clonic movements of the right hand and arm lasting continuously when awake resulted in a weakness and inability to use the right hand. The epilepsia partialis continua (EPC) ceased after sleep and never secondarily generalized. There was mild right-sided hemiparesis but no hypaesthesia. In CT, MRI, and SPECT, no lesions were found. Seizure discharge originated from the left superior postrolandic cortex, when the patient felt a tingling sensation in his right hand and arm and shouted "attack is coming," immediately followed by asymmetric posturing. There was no one-to-one correlation between the twitches of EPC and intracranial EEG activities. Surgery has not been carried out.

OTHER NEOCORTICAL EPILEPSIES

The neocortical epilepsies aforementioned are, in the International Epilepsy Classification, all included in the category of symptomatic or cryptogenic localization-related epilepsies. These epilepsies are non–age-related in terms of seizure onset. To the contrary, chronic progressive EPC of childhood has been recognized as an independent syndrome in children, also known as *Rasmussen's syndrome* (39). In comparing symptomatic and idiopathic localization-related epilepsies, the epileptogenic lesions can be traced to one part of one cerebral hemisphere in most symptomatic localization-related epilepsies, but in idiopathic age-related epilepsies with focal seizures, corresponding regions of both hemispheres may be functionally involved (12).

Idiopathic localization-related epilepsies are childhood epilepsies with partial seizures and focal EEG abnormalities. They are age related, without demonstrable anatomic lesions, and subject to spontaneous remission. Clinically, patients have neither neurologic or intellectual deficit nor a history of antecedent illness, but they frequently have a family history of benign epilepsy. In the 1989 international classification, three syndromes were recognized: benign childhood epilepsy with centrotemporal spikes, childhood epilepsy with occipital paroxysms, and primary reading epilepsy. During the past decade, several syndromes of idiopathic localization-related epilepsies have been proposed: autosomal-dominant nocturnal frontal lobe epilepsy (40), familial temporal lobe epilepsy (41), idiopathic photosensitive occipital lobe epilepsy (42), and benign partial epilepsy of infancy with complex partial seizures (43).

REFERENCES

1. Commission on Classification and Terminology of the International League Against Epilepsy. Proposal for classification of epilepsies and epileptic syndromes. *Epilepsia* 1985;26(Suppl 3):268–278.
2. Engel J Jr, Williamson PD, Wieser HG. Mesial temporal lobe epilepsy. In: Engel J Jr, Pedley TA, eds. *Epilepsy: a comprehensive textbook.* Philadelphia: Lippincott–Raven, 1997:2417–2426.
3. Williamson PD, Engel J Jr, Munari C. Anatomic classification of localization-related epilepsies. In: Engel J Jr, Pedley YA, eds. *Epilepsy: a comprehensive textbook.* Philadelphia: Lippincott–Raven, 1997:2405–2416.
4. Commission on Classification and Terminology of the International League Against Epilepsy. Proposal for revised clinical and electroencepahlographic classification of epileptic seizures. *Epilepsia* 1981;22:489–501.
5. Rasmussen T. Characteristics of a pure culture of frontal lobe epilepsy. *Epilepsia* 1983;24:482–493.
6. Lüders HO, Engel J Jr, Munari C. General principles. In: Engel J Jr, ed. *Surgical treatment of the epilepsies,* 2nd ed. New York: Raven Press, 1993:137–153.
7. Kotagal P. Seizure symptomatology of temporal lobe origin. In: Lüders HO, ed. *Epilepsy surgery.* New York: Raven Press, 1991:143–155.
8. Wieser HG, Engel J Jr, Williamson PD, et al. Surgically remediable temporal lobe syndromes. In: Engel J Jr, ed. *Surgical treatment of the epilepsies,* 2nd ed. New York: Raven Press, 1993:49–63.
9. Walczak TS. Neocortical temporal lobe epilepsy: characterizing the syndrome. *Epilepsia* 1995;36:633–635.
10. Blume WR, Girvin JP, Stenerson P. Temporal neocortical role in ictal experiential phenomena. *Ann Neurol* 1993;33:105–107.
11. Williamson PD, Wieser HG, Delgado-Escueta AV. Clinical characteristics of partial seizures. In: Engel J Jr, ed. *Surgical treatment of the epilepsies.* New York: Raven Press, 1987:101–120.
12. Commission on Classification and Terminology of the International League Against Epilepsy. Proposal for revised classification of epilepsies and epileptic syndromes. *Epilepsia* 1989;30:389–399.
13. Jones-Gotman M, Zatorre RJ, Olivier A, et al. Learning and retention of words and designs following excision from medial or lateral temporal lobe structures. *Neuropsychologia* 1997;35:963–973.
14. Bancaud J, Talairach J. Clinical semiology of frontal lobe seizures. In: Chauvel P, Delgado-Escueta AV, Halgren E, Bancaud J, eds. *Frontal lobe seizures and epilepsies. Advances in Neurology,* vol 57. New York: Raven Press, 1992:3–58.
14a. Inoue Y, Mihara T, Fukao K, et al. Ictal paraphresia induced by language activity. *Epilepsy Research* 1999;35:69–79.
15. Mihara T, Tottori T, Matsuda K, et al. Analysis of seizure manifestations of "Pure" frontal lobe origin. *Epilepsia* 1997;(Suppl 6);42–47.
16. Salanova V, Morris HH, Van Ness P, et al. Frontal lobe seizures: electroclinical syndromes. *Epilepsia* 1995;36:16–24.
17. Penfield W, Jasper H. *Epilepsy and the functional anatomy of the human brain.* Boston: Little, Brown, 1954:373–377.

18. Williamson PD. Frontal lobe epilepsy: some clinical characteristics. In: Jasper HH, Riggio S, Goldman-Rakic PS, eds. *Epilepsy and the functional anatomy of the frontal lobe.* New York: Raven Press, 1995:127–152.
19. Williamson PD, Boon PA, Thadani VM, et al. Parietal lobe epilepsy: diagnostic considerations and results of surgery. *Ann Neurol* 1992;31:193–201.
20. Williamson PD, Thadani VM, Darcey TM, et al. Occipital lobe epilepsy: clinical characteristics, seizure pread patterns, and results of surgery. *Ann Neurol* 1992;31:3–13.
21. Mihara T, Tottori T, Inoue Y, et al. Surgical strategies for patients with supplementary sensorimotor area epilepsy: the Japanese experience. In: Lüders HO, ed. *Supplementary sensory motor area. Advances in Neurology,* vol 70. Philadelphia: Lippincott–Raven, 1996:405–414.
22. Bancoud J, Talairach J. Clinical semiology of frontal lobe seizures. In: Chauvel P, Delgado-Escueta AV, Halgren E, Bancaud J, eds. *Frontal lobe seizures and epilepsies. Advances in Neurology,* vol 57. New York: Raven Press, 1992:3–58.
23. Delgado-Escueta AV, Swartz B, Maldonado H, et al. Complex partial seizures of frontal lobe origin. In: Wieser G, Elger CE, eds. *Presurgical evaluation of epileptics: basics, techniques, implications.* New York: Springer-Verlag, 1987:268–299.
24. Waterman K, Purves SJ, Kosaka B, et al. An epileptic syndrome caused by mesial frontal lobe foci. *Neurology* 1987;37:77–582.
25. Williamson PD. Frontal lobe seizures: problems of diagnosis and classification. In: Chauvel P, Delgado-Escueta AV, Halgren E, Bancaud J, eds. *Frontal lobe seizures and epilepsies. Advances in Neurology,* vol 57. New York: Raven Press, 1992:289–309.
26. Tharp BR. Orbital frontal seizures: a unique elcctroencephalographic and clinical syndrome. *Epilepsia* 1972;13:627–642.
27. Williamson PD, Spencer DD, Spencer SS, et al. Complex partial seizures of frontal lobe origin. *Ann Neurol* 1985;18:497–504.
28. Wada JA. Predominantly nocturnal recurrence of intensively affective vocal and facial expression associated with powerful bimanual, bipedal, and axial activity as ictal manifestations of mesial frontal lobe epilepsy. *Advances in epileptology.* New York: Raven Press, 1989:261–267.
29. Quesney LF, Constain M, Rasmussen T. Seizures from the dorsolateral frontal lobe. In: Chauvel P, Delgado-Escueta AV, Halgren E, Bancaud J, eds. *Frontal lobe seizures and epilepsies. Advances in Neurology,* vol 57. New York: Raven Press, 1992:233–244.
30. Saygi S, Katz A, Marks DA, et al. Frontal lobe partial seizures and psychogenic seizures: comparison of clinical and ictal characteristics. *Neurology* 1992;42:1274–1277.
31. Salanova V, Andermann F, Olivier A, et al. Occipital lobe epilepsy: electroclinical manifestations, electrocorticography, cortical stimulation, and outcome in 42 patients treated between 1930 and 1991. *Brain* 1992;115:1655–1680.
32. Sveinbjornsdottir S, Duncan JS. Parietal and occipital lobe epilepsy: a review. *Epilepsia* 1993;34(3):493–521.
33. Olivier A, Gloor P, Andermann F, et al. Occipitotemporal epilepsy studied with stereotaxically implanted depth electrodes and successfully treated by temporal resection. *Ann Neurol* 1982;11:428–432.
34. Palmini A, Andermann F, Dubeau F, et al. Occipitotemporal epilepsies: evaluation of selected patients requiring depth electrodes studies and rationale for surgical approaches. *Epilepsia* 1993;34:84–96.
35. Ajmone-Marsan C, Ralston BL. *The epileptic seizure: its functional morphology and diagnostic significance.* Springfield, IL: Charles C. Thomas, 1957:211–215.
36. Blume WT. Occipital lobe epilepsies. In: Lüders HO, ed. *Epilepsy surgery.* New York: Raven Press, 1991:167–171.
37. Cascino GD, Hulihan JF, Sharbrough FW, et al. Parietal lobe lesional epilepsy: electroclinical correlation and operative outcome. *Epilepsia* 1993;34:522–527.
38. Ho SS, Berkovic SF, Newton MI, et al. Parietal lobe epilepsy: clinical features and seizure localization by ictal SPECT. *Neurology* 1994;44:2277–2284.
39. Rasmussen T, Olszewski J, Lloyd-Smith DL. Focal seizures due to chronic localized encephalitis. *Neurology* 1958;8:435–455.
40. Sheffer IE, Bhatia KP, Lopes-Cendes I, et al. Autosomal dominant nocturnal frontal lobe epilepsy: a disitnctive clinical disorder. *Brain* 1995;118:61–73.
41. Berkovic SF, Howell RA, Hopper JL. Familial temporal lobe epilepsy: a new syndrome with adolescent/adult onset and a benign course. In: Wolf P, ed. *Epileptic seizures and syndromes.* London: John Libby, 1994:257–263.
42. Guerrini R, Dravet CH, Genton P, et al. Idiopathic photosensitive occipital lobe epilepsy. *Epilepsia* 1995;36:883–891.
43. Watanabe K, Yamamoto N, Aso K, et al. Benign complex partial epilepsy in infancy. *Pediatr Neurol* 1987;3:208–211.

Neocortical Epilepsies.
Advances in Neurology, Vol. 84,
edited by P. D. Williamson, A. M. Siegel,
D. W. Roberts, V. M. Thadani, and M. S. Gazzaniga.
Lippincott Williams & Wilkins, Philadelphia © 2000.

12

Dynamic Properties of Cells, Synapses, Circuits, and Seizures in Neocortex

Barry W. Connors and *Albert E. Telfeian

Department of Neuroscience, Brown University, Providence, Rhode Island 02912;
*Department of Neurosurgery, School of Medicine, University of Pennsylvania,
Philadelphia, Pennsylvania 19104

TIME AND SPACE IN THE NEOCORTEX

Timing is a critical feature of normal neural activity, although we are far from understanding how the brain uses timing (1,2). Timing is also important to the initiation, propagation, continuation, and termination of seizures. Seizure activity encompasses a wide time scale, from the scant milliseconds between action and synaptic potentials to the months separating some ictal events. Seizure discharges are defined in part by their timing, whether measured by the spiking activity of a single neuron or the patterns of an electroencephalogram. The timing of neural activity can determine the spatial progress of a seizure; certain temporal patterns favor the devastating spread of a epileptiform activity from a small focus of neurons into a large expanse of cortex. Timing of neural activity in the short term may influence seizures in the long term; when neural activity occurs in particular frequencies or patterns, it can induce alterations of neural circuits that influence their future patterns of activity, both normal and abnormal. Clearly, understanding the role of timing in the behavior of neurons is critical to a full appreciation of seizure mechanisms.

The individual cellular elements of the brain are exquisitely sensitive to timing. Each neuron has a restricted temporal repertoire of intrinsic spiking behavior. Each synapse varies its strength in a particular way when it is activated repetitively; however, there are few general rules for the temporal behavior of neurons. The spiking dynamics of different types of neurons vary widely. When activated at moderate frequencies, the synapses of some pathways tend to depress strongly, whereas synapses of other pathways facilitate. Moreover, a variety of neuromodulators can alter the dynamics of both neurons and synapses, also in ways specific to cell and synapse type. Finally, when neurons are interconnected by synapses, new dynamics can emerge from the properties of the resulting circuit. Slight rewiring of a circuit, without changing its constituent cellular elements, can produce an entirely different set of dynamics.

This chapter reviews some of the biologic forces in the neocortex that regulate the timing of its neural activity and discusses the relevance of timing to the genesis of seizures. We briefly describe, in turn, the dynamic properties of neurons, synapses, and circuits in the neocortex, illustrating some relevant examples of epileptiform activity along the way.

DYNAMICS OF SINGLE NEURONS

A cortical neuron collects information from the thousands of synapses that terminate on its soma and dendrites. It transforms this information into a code that is defined entirely by the timing of the action potentials coursing out along its axon. The character of the transformation depends critically on the intrinsic membrane properties of the neuron. In neocortex, indeed across the central nervous system, different types of neurons can have distinctly different types of intrinsic membrane properties (3). Thus, each neuron imposes its own idiosyncratic influence on the information flowing through it.

Pyramidal cells are the principal type of neuron in the neocortex. The synapses they make are glutamatergic and excitatory, they are highly interconnected with one another, and they are the sole source of cortical output (4). These features make them the likely generators of most seizure activity. There are many subtypes of pyramidal cells that can be distinguished by the laminar locations of their soma, the patterns of their dendrites, the destinations of their axon, and the intrinsic firing properties of their membranes. The latter can be characterized quickly by observing a cell's response to prolonged pulses of injected current. Current injection is more controllable than natural synaptic stimuli; synapses have dynamic characteristics of their own that can confuse the issue, as described in the following section.

Most pyramidal neurons, conventionally termed *regular-spiking cells,* respond to a strong current stimulus with a brief period of high spiking frequency, followed by strong adaptation to a much lower steady-state level. Among regular-spiking neurons, the rates and degrees of adaptation vary widely (5,6). Much less common than regular-spiking cells are *intrinsically bursting pyramidal cells,* usually found in layer 5 of the rodent cortex (7) but occasionally observed in other layers in various species (8). The singular feature of the intrinsically bursting cell is its tendency to respond to stimuli with clusters (i.e., *bursts*) of

spikes rather than with monotonic temporal patterns (Fig. 12.1). Again, there is diversity between cells; some yield a single burst at the onset of a stimulus, followed by single spiking, whereas others can sustain repetitive bursting indefinitely under certain conditions (9,10). Among the repetitively bursting neurons, one group in layer 5 generates relatively slow-burst rhythms of 5 to 10 Hz (11), whereas another group in the upper layers can "chatter" along at 20 to 80 Hz (12).

The inhibitory interneurons of the neocortex are a much more diverse lot than the pyramidal cells (13), and their intrinsic physiologies are equally varied. A significant proportion of inhibitory cells have "fast-spiking" properties. Their action potentials are exceptionally brief, and they can fire at high frequencies, with little or no adaptation (7). Other subtypes of inhibitory cells in neocortex have intrinsic spiking properties akin to those of certain pyramidal cells, including regular-spiking and burstlike temporal patterns. In some cases, the physiologic properties of cells have been correlated with the expression of particular neuroactive peptides and calcium-binding proteins and with their somadendritic and axonal patterns (14). Nevertheless, classifying the myriad inhibitory cells of the cerebral cortex continues to be a challenge.

The importance of a neuron's intrinsic physiology is that it can alter the patterns of activity that flow through the cell. Regular-spiking cells perform a type of high-pass filtering such that the cell responds more robustly to rapidly changing features of its input but cannot sustain its interest when the input continues. Fast-spiking cells more faithfully report both transient and sustained features of their inputs. Intrinsically bursting cells seem to be the most domineering of neurons, amplifying some inputs (those just reaching threshold), ignoring others (those arriving during the long refractory period after a burst), and sometimes imposing their own rhythmicity (during weak but steady inputs that keep them near threshold). Bursting may help to enhance the strength of a cell's otherwise weak synapses (15), serve as

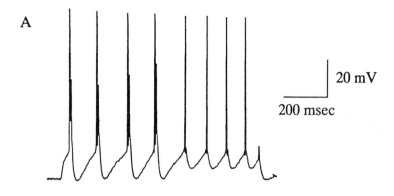

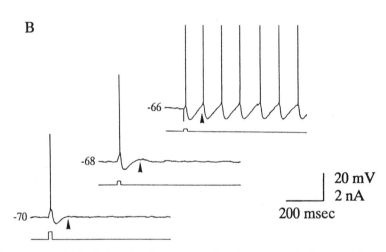

FIG. 12.1. A: Rhythmic intrinsic bursting in response to a long current stimulus; intracellular recording from a pyramidal cell in layer 5 of rat somatosensory cortex in vitro. **B:** Bistable, oscillatory spiking in a different layer 5 pyramidal cell. Small current pulses triggered single spikes when membrane potential was held at −70 or −68 mV, but when applied at −66 mV, the stimulus triggered repetitive firing that far outlasted the pulse. (L.R. Silva and B.W. Connors, unpublished.)

a pacemaker in the service of a rhythm-generating circuit (12), or in some cases usurp the functions of a circuit by initiating seizure activity.

The first direct evidence that intrinsically bursting cells could mediate epileptiform activity was provided by Miles and Wong, working in the CA3 area of the disinhibited hippocampus (16). Early research on models of seizure generation in neocortex suggested that there is something uniquely epileptogenic

about the circuitry of the middle cortical layers (17–19). In disinhibited rodent neocortex, layer 5 is the onset site of epileptiform activity (20); its neurons can uniquely sustain epileptiform activity, even when detached from other layers; and it is the layer most sensitive to some locally applied convulsant drugs. Layer 5 is also the site of the large intrinsically bursting pyramidal neurons, and several lines of evidence implicate these cells in initiating seizure discharges. Recordings of

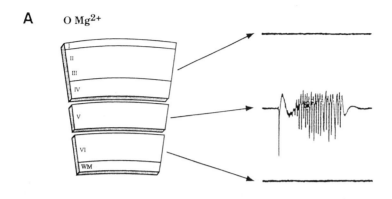

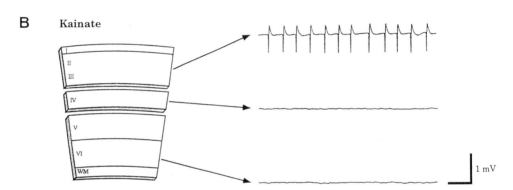

FIG. 12.2. Layer-specific initiation of experimental seizure activity. **A:** Neocortical slices bathed in solutions with nominally zero (Mg^{2+}) spontaneously generate short, seizure-like epochs. When slices are dissected with horizontal cuts, only fragments containing layer 5 sustain epileptiform activity (traces shown to the right). **B:** Slices bathed in kainic acid-containing solutions generate a different form of epileptiform activity. When slices are dissected, only superficial layers are necessary and sufficient. (Adapted from Flint AC, Connors BW. Two types of network oscillations in neocortex mediated by distinct glutamate receptor subtypes and neuronal populations. *J Neurophysiol* 1996;75:951–956, with permission.)

synaptic activity during disinhibtion-induced experimental seizures implied that bursting cells were the only major neuronal subtype strongly participating in the discharge (21); in synchrony with the phasic excitation of bursting cells, regular-spiking neurons were most often dominated by inhibition. Flint et al. (22) showed that the emergence of neurons with intrinsic bursting behavior through development correlates well with the onset of epileptiform activity mediated by NMDA receptors (11). Temporal similarities between rhythmically bursting cells and rhythmic NMDA receptor-mediated seizures are also sugges-

tive. Both the natural interburst frequency of single neurons and the ongoing oscillations of epileptiform population events are about 5 to 12 Hz (Fig. 12.2A). Further, kainate-induced epileptiform activity, which depends only on regular-spiking cells of the upper cortical layers but not on the bursting cells of layer 5 (23), has much more phasic and lower frequency discharges (Fig. 12.2B).

DYNAMICS OF SINGLE SYNAPSES

The basic molecular mechanisms of chemical synapses are highly conserved (24), and yet synapses have evolved a wide range of functional characteristics. Release probability, quantal content, plasticity, presynaptic modulation, postsynaptic receptors, and, of course, transmitter type are highly variable and specific for different synapses (25,26). As an example, we describe variations in short- and long-term plasticity in synapses of the thalamocortical system.

The efficacy of a chemical synapse changes with activity and time (27); unfortunately, the nomenclature of synapse dynamics is abstruse. Some changes are long-term, lasting for hours or longer, and either potentiate or depress synaptic efficacy. Long-term changes may be limited to only certain synapse types, but it is likely that all synapses display short-term (milliseconds to minutes) changes in efficacy–facilitation, depression, augmentation, and potentiation. All short-term forms seem to involve presynaptic mechanisms (28,29), although postsynaptic processes sometimes may contribute. Facilitation apparently depends on a small, residual increase in presynaptic internal (Ca^{2+}) following activation (30). Synapses with an inherently low probability of release tend to display large facilitation because it is more likely that the second of a stimulus pair will evoke release. In contrast, synapses with an inherently high probability of release tend to display depression, presumably because the pool of available vesicles for release becomes depleted (31,32). A different source of short-term synaptic depression can come from neuromodulators that are released by stimuli. These can act presynaptically, usually to reduce release probability (33), but sometimes to enhance it (34). A crucial point is that the functional properties of synapses vary widely, but that function certainly cannot be determined from structure alone. There is, however, some evidence that the strength of a synapse may correlate with its size (35,36).

The short-term plasticity of cerebral cortical synapses varies widely. For example, hippocampal pathways often show strong facilitation, whereas neocortical synapses more often depress (37,38) (Fig. 12.3). Posttetanic

potentiation has not been described in neocortex, but is quite potent in the hippocampus pathway (39). The few published studies of the dynamics of neocortical synapses have focused on intracortical or unidentified synapses. Interestingly, synapses from layer 5 pyramidal cells ending on other pyramidal cells usually show depression (along with a high probability of release to the first stimulus; 40,41), whereas pyramidal cell synapses ending on certain types of inhibitory interneurons show dramatic facilitation (and low probability of first release). This implies that presynaptic function might be developmentally determined by the postsynaptic neuron, although this cannot be universally true (26). In visual and somatosensory cortex, differences of dynamics sometimes correlate with the presynaptic neuron type (34,42). Markram and Tsodyks (43) found that the rates of short-term depression seen at synapses between layer 5 pyramidal cells changed after pairing-induced, long-term potentiation (LTP); this was not a simple change in synaptic "gain" but involved a more complex temporal "redistribution" of synaptic efficacy. We recently observed a similar change in short-term depression of neocortical synapses following several days of innocuous sensory deprivation (clipping of the large facial whiskers in rats); the changes were consistent with increases in synaptic strength in pathways near the border of deprived and spared cortex (44).

Theoretic work suggests broad implications for short-term synaptic dynamics. Depression may serve to enhance the information capacity of intracortical synapses (45). Experimentally, the degree and rate of depression vary widely across pyramidal cell pairs; when depression is relatively fast, postsynaptic responses reflect the temporal coherence of presynaptic firing. Slower rates of depression provide dynamic gain control, equalizing the postsynaptic responses to equal percentage changes in presynaptic firing frequency.

An additional consequence of a synapse's short-term dynamics may be its propensity to generate long-term alterations following certain patterns of activation. We tested this

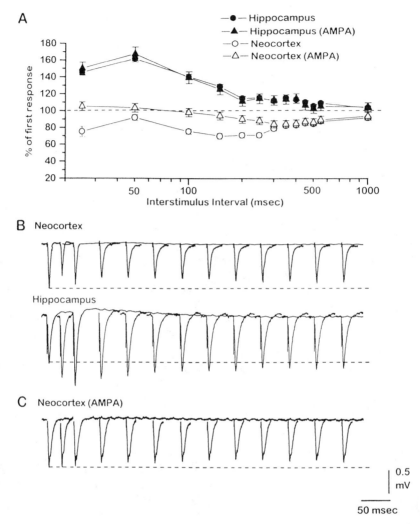

FIG. 12.3. Comparison of the short-term dynamics in excitatory pathways of hippocampus and neo-cortex. Paired stimuli were applied to the Schaffer collateral pathway of the hippocampal CA1 region or to the layer 4 to layer 2/3 pathway in neocortex while field potentials were measured. **A:** Graph of the size of the second response as a function of the first, versus interval, shows that the hippocampal synapses generated facilitation while the neocortical synapses usually were depressed. Blockade of NMDA receptors with APV (AMPA responses) did not change this difference. **B,C:** Raw, superimposed field potential records from experiment shown in A. (Adapted from Castro-Alamancos MA, Connors BW. Short-term synaptic enhancement predicts long-term potentiation in neocortex. *Proc Natl Acad Sci USA* 1996;93:1335–1339, with permission.)

notion in two adjacent areas of the rat neocortex, the primary somatosensory (SI) and motor (MI) areas (46). All measurements were carried out simultaneously, but the differences were striking. Patterned tetanic stimuli delivered to an ascending pathway generated LTP in the SI cortex, but similar stimuli failed to

induce LTP in MI. MI was capable only of generating LTP after it had been slightly disinhibited with the GABA$_A$ receptor antagonist bicuculline. Standard presynaptic and postsynaptic pairing protocols also produce LTP in MI neurons. Thus, the tested synapses in MI have the potential to generate LTP. Why do the

SI and MI pathways differ so dramatically in their ability to express LTP? We found that synaptic pathways in SI produced a strong short-term enhancement during LTP-producing theta-burst stimuli, whereas the response in motor cortex was stable and nonenhancing (47). The amount of short-term enhancement predicted well the magnitude of LTP ultimately generated by any theta-burst series. These experiments demonstrate that short-term synaptic dynamics can strongly influence long-term synaptic plasticity.

The importance of short-term synaptic dynamics on seizure activity has not been studied explicitly in the neocortex; however, consider the time course of seizure-related activity. Spike frequencies during interictal and ictal events can rise briefly to many hundreds of Hertz, which would rapidly cause transmission across strongly depressing synapses to fail. Interburst frequencies during seizures range from 1 to 20 Hz; this is similar to the patterned theta-burst stimuli that optimally generate short-term forms of enhancement (46) and ultimately LTP. The physiological and pharmacological similarities between LTP and kindling models of epilepsy have often been noted (48). Lower frequency, sustained stimuli are now known to generate LTD in various areas of neocortex (46,49). In general, long-term synaptic plasticity is most likely to occur following synchronous, prolonged, moderate to rapid repetitive activity. It is probably no coincidence that this kind of activity is also characteristic of seizures.

DYNAMICS OF NEOCORTICAL CIRCUITS

Although it is good to know the specific dynamic properties of each type of neuron and synapse in the neocortex, seizures by definition occur only in assemblies of neurons, and the behavior of neuronal assemblies is almost never as simple as that of its cellular constituents. A circuit of neurons is much more complex, variable, and flexible than the activity of its individual neurons imply. The novel behavior of the circuit "emerges" from the interac-

tions of its parts. Explaining, not to mention predicting, the behavior of a neural circuit goes beyond the capabilities of informed intuition and hand waving. Formal theoretic approaches have been reasonably successful in explaining relatively simple aspects of circuit behaviors, such as locomotor pattern generation (50) and the interictal discharge of the hippocampus (51); however, neocortex is both more complex and less well understood than these systems. We describe one simple network phenomenon of the normal neocortex that we have studied in some detail. It has features relevant to cell and circuit dynamics, the spread of synchronous behavior, and rapid neural regulation. Attempting to understand it required us to consider the interactive roles of basic synaptic physiology, intrinsic membrane properties, circuit anatomy, kinetics of inhibition, and behavioral modulation.

Two thalamocortical pathways partially converge onto frontoparietal cortex, and these pathways behave distinctively: The motor-related ventral–lateral (VL) thalamic nucleus induces a progressively increasing cortical response when stimulated at 7 to 14 Hz; in contrast, responses evoked from the somatosensory ventral–posterior–lateral (VPL) nucleus show depression when stimulated at greater than 5 Hz (52) (Fig. 12.4A). The enhanced VL-evoked response is identical to the classical "augmenting response," first described in the 1940s by Dempsey and Morison (53); the depressing response of the VPL pathway we termed the *decrementing response* (Fig. 12.4B). We found that the augmenting response is a cortical phenomenon that does not depend on the thalamus; that it entails wide, horizontal intracortical spread of activity; and that it occurs in both anesthetized and in freely moving, unanesthetized animals in area MI but not area SI.

The cellular mechanisms of the augmenting response have been debated since its discovery, and no consensus emerged. Our studies led us to a novel hypothesis (54): augmenting from VL input originates with neurons of layer 5 and includes a sequence of synaptic (thalamocortical) excitation onto layer 5 cells, feed-

A

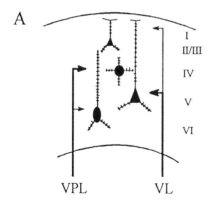

VPL   VL

B

Decremental Response   Augmenting Response

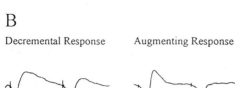

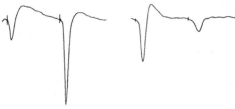

FIG. 12.4. A: Schematic diagram of the thalamocortical connections from the VPL and VL nuclei to sensorimotor cortex in rats. **B:** Responses recorded extracellularly in sensorimotor cortex following paired stimuli (100 msec intervals) applied to the VL nucleus (**left**: "augmenting response") or the VPL nucleus (**right**: "decrementing response"). (M.A. Castro-Alamancos and B.W. Connors, unpublished.)

forward inhibition, and rebound excitation due to activation of intrinsic low-threshold currents in subsets of layer 5 cells, followed by network amplification via recurrent intracortical excitatory circuits. A central role is played by $GABA_A$ receptor-mediated inhibition within the cortex, which hyperpolarizes membranes and deinactivates membrane currents that, on termination of inhibition, cause rebound spiking and augmentation.

The augmenting response provides an easily measured window onto some of the mechanisms that modulate the excitability of the cortex during awake behavior. The response is simple to assess with field potentials, and yet it is a sensitive indicator of thalamocorti-

cal function. In awake, unrestrained animals, the augmenting response is prominent when animals are immobile and resting (but nevertheless awake), and it promptly inactivates during active exploration of the environment or performance of a skilled motor task (55). The behavioral modulation is specific; during exploration, the primary (first) thalamocortical response is unaltered, but subsequent responses at optimal stimulus intervals are not augmented. This implies that the frequency–selectivity of the VL-to-cortex pathway is modulated moment-by-moment during behavior.

Our hypothesis is that behavioral modulation arises from a change in the activity of some diffuse neuromodulatory system associated with arousal or attention. Preliminary experiments with cortically implanted microdialysis probes suggest that noradrenergic systems may mediate the behavioral modulation of the augmenting response because infusion of norepinephrine or receptor agonists mimics the specific effect of behavioral modulation, whereas cholinergic agonists do not (56).

The horizontal propagation of epileptiform activity is quite a different example of an emergent behavior of neocortical circuits. We studied the phenomenology and mechanisms of propagation, and its dependence on temporal and spatial dynamics are beginning to be understood. When slices of cortex are disinhibited slightly, neural activity progresses from a contained, local process to a fragile but more frankly epileptiform phenomenon that propagates large distances (57). If disinhibition is strong, propagation is robust and reliable; however, propagation velocity usually varies widely, often periodically, as it moves across the cortex (58,59). Propagation patterns depend on anatomic and physiologic considerations, including the strength or density of horizontal connections (60). The pathway taken by propagating seizures is not arbitrary. In both disinhibition and NMDA receptor-dependent models, axons and neurons in layer 5 seem to be critical for propagation (61). Finally, the velocity of propagation may depend strongly on the types of postsynaptic receptors mediating it. Propagation relying on AMPA-type glutamate receptors moves at five times the speed of propagation using only NMDA-type receptors (Fig. 12.5) (62). Thus, seizure propagation velocity and pattern depend on numerous dynamic features of the cortical circuit, including presynaptic and postsynaptic properties, intrinsic firing behavior, and cell-to-cell connectivity.

DYNAMICS IN HUMAN NEOCORTICAL EPILEPSY

Intraoperative electrocorticography (ECoG) routinely is performed during epilepsy surgery to define epileptogenic zones. The presence of interictal spikes on intraoperative ECoG is believed to represent synchronized neuronal activity in discrete cortical regions and has been used to guide resections for the surgical treatment of patients with intractable epilepsy associated with a neocortical lesion. Although ECoG routinely is performed during epilepsy surgery, there is little evidence that it is a useful guide to tailoring resections (63,64).

Intracellular recordings from in vitro slices prepared from neocortex resected from epileptic patients have not revealed striking abnormalities in either the intrinsic firing patterns or passive membrane properties of neurons (65,66). Synaptic bursts associated with diminished inhibitory postsynaptic potentials (IPSPs) (67–69), and an absence of such responses in cortex from nonepileptic patients (70) has been reported, however, by a number of laboratories. These findings suggest, but far from prove, that an imbalance of synaptic excitation and inhibition may mediate the generation of human seizures. Recent results indicated that synaptic bursting is a general characteristic of neocortex resected from patients with symptomatic epilepsy and is not localized specifically to regions that generate interictal spikes (71). If synaptic bursting is peculiar to epileptic tissue, it may be distributed more generally rather than restricted to spiking regions. In studies of electrographically quiet neocortex from patients with hippocampal sclerosis, no synaptic bursting was observed (72), suggesting that synaptic bursting may, indeed, be a sign of an intrinsic rather than projected pathological entity.

It is worth noting that intrinsically bursting neurons have not been reported for human neocortex. This is in contrast to rodent neocortex, where intrinsic bursts are seen in approximately 30% of layer 5 pyramidal cells (3,7). Foehring et al. (73) and Tasker et al. (74) described brief clusters of action potentials in response to depolarizing current injections in a subpopulation of epileptic human neocortical cells, but they did not observe more classically defined intrinsically bursting cells. These data raise the possibility that subtle differences exist in the functional organization of human and rodent neocortex that are relevant for seizure mechanisms. Unfortunately, the paucity of cellular mechanistic studies in primate neocortex precludes detailed comparisons.

The spatial progress of a seizure must depend on the patterns of neurons and their connections across the cortex. Multiple subpial transection (MST) was conceived as a treatment of partial epilepsies that encroach on eloquent cortex; its mechanism of action, in principle, depends on the interruption of horizontal connections that are critical to the propagation of epileptiform activity while sparing the vertically oriented "functional columns" of cortical architecture and their vascular supply (75). One study of the depth variability of lesions made in human MST cases concluded that most transections sever only as deep as the midlevel horizontal fibers (deep layer 3 and layer 4) (76). If the lower cortical layers contain a critical pathway for seizure propagation in humans, as they do for some rodent models (61), then refinements to the current MST methods might reduce the number of necessary transections, allow superficial layers to be spared, and be more clinically effective.

Better understanding of cortical dynamics might allow more dynamic therapies for seizures. Seizure prevention would be aided greatly by seizure prediction. In some studies, clinical seizures have been anticipated by many minutes by using intracranial record-

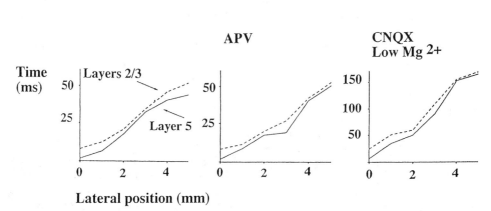

FIG. 12.5. Propagation patterns of three types of experimental epileptiform discharges. Neocortical slices were treated with the GABA$_A$ receptor antagonist **(A)**, picrotoxin plus the NMDA receptor antagonist APV **(B)**, or with zero (Mg^{2+}) plus the AMPA receptor antagonist CNQX **(C)**. Discharge propagation time was measured in either layer 5 *(solid)* or layer 2/3 *(dashed)* and plotted as a function of position across the cortex. The data demonstrate that discharges appear slightly earlier in layer 5, regardless of whether they are mediated by AMPA receptors (A,B) or NMDA receptors (C). However, the former propagate about five times faster than the latter. (Adapted from Telfeian AE, Connors BW. Epileptiform propagation patterns mediated by NMDA and nonNMDA receptors in neocortex. *Epilepsia* 1999;40:1580–1586.)

ings and nonlinear indicators to characterize the extended spatiotemporal nature of the pre-ictal recruitment process (77,78). With practical methods of prediction, it might be possible to use appropriate electrical stimulation to prevent seizures, as studies of epileptogenic rat hippocampal slices have suggested (79).

The dynamics of local circuits largely determine the organization, timing, and route of neocortical seizures. Understanding the biologic forces that regulate the dynamics of neurons, synapses, and circuits in neocortex can be an important step toward designing new treatments for human epilepsy.

ACKNOWLEDGMENTS

We thank Yael Amitai, Michael Beierlein, Manuel Castro-Alamancos, Gerald Finnerty, Jay Gibson, Ziv Gil, and Carole Landisman for their contributions to the work described here. The authors' research was supported by the National Institutes of Health and the American Epilepsy Society.

REFERENCES

1. Rieke F, Warland D, de Ruyter van Steveninck R, et al. *Spikes.* Cambridge, MA: MIT Press, 1997.
2. Shadlen MN, Newsome WT. Noise, neural codes, and cortical organization. *Curr Opin Neurobiol* 1994;4: 569–79.
3. Connors BW, Gutnick MJ. Intrinsic firing patterns of diverse neocortical neurons. *Trends Neurosci* 1990;13: 99–104.
4. White EL. *Cortical circuits: synaptic organization of the cerebral cortex—structure, function, and theory.* Boston: Birkhauser, 1989.
5. Agmon A, Connors BW. Correlation between intrinsic firing patterns and thalamocortical responses of mouse barrel cortex neurons. *J Neurosci* 1992;12:319–330.
6. Stafstrom CE, Schwindt PC, Crill WE. Repetitive firing in layer V neurons from cat neocortex in vitro. *J Neurophysiol* 1984;52:264–277.
7. McCormick DA, Connors BW, Lighthall JW, et al. Comparative electrophysiology of pyramidal and sparsely spiny stellate neurons of the neocortex. *J Neurophysiol* 1985;54:782–806.
8. Nunez A, Amzica F, Steriade M. Electrophysiology of cat association cortical cells in vivo: intrinsic properties and synaptic responses. *J Neurophysiol* 1993;70: 418–30.
9. Agmon A, Connors BW. Repetitive burst-firing neurons in the deep layers of mouse somatosensory cortex. *Neurosci Lett* 1989;99:137–141.
10. Wang Z, McCormick DA. Control of firing mode of corticotectal and corticopontine layer V burst-generating

neurons by norepinephrine, acetylcholine, and 1S,3R-ACPD. *J Neurosci* 1993;13:2199–2216.

11. Silva LR, Amitai Y, Connors BW. Intrinsic oscillations of neocortex generated by layer 5 pyramidal neurons. *Science* 1991;251:432–435.

12. Gray CM, McCormick DA. Chattering cells: superficial pyramidal neurons contributing to the generation of synchronous oscillations in the visual cortex. *Science* 1996;274:109–113.

13. Jones EG. GABAergic neurons and their role in cortical plasticity in primates. *Cereb Cortex* 1993;3:361–72.

14. Kawaguchi Y, Kubota Y. GABAergic cell subtypes and their synaptic connections in rat frontal cortex. *Cereb Cortex* 1997;7:476–486.

15. Lisman JE. Bursts as a unit of neural information: making unreliable synapses reliable. *Trends Neurosci* 1997; 20:38–43.

16. Miles R, Wong RKS. Single neurones can initiate synchronized population discharge in the hippocampus. *Nature* 1983;306:371–373.

17. Chatt AB, Ebersole JS. The laminar sensitivity of cat striate cortex to penicillin induced epileptogenesis. *Brain Res* 1982;241:382–387.

18. Connors BW. Initiation of synchronized neuronal bursting in neocortex. *Nature* 1984;310:685–687.

19. Connors BW, Amitai Y. Functions of local circuits in neocortex: synchrony and laminae. In: Mody I, Gutnick MJ, eds. *The cortical neuron.* New York: Cambridge Press, 1995:123–141.

20. Telfeian AE, Connors BW. Layer-specific pathways for the horizontal propagation of epileptiform discharges in neocortex. *Epilepsia* 1998;39:700–708.

21. Chagnac-Amitai Y, Connors BW. Synchronized excitation and inhibition driven by intrinsically bursting neurons in neocortex. *J Neurophysiol* 1989;62:1149–1162.

22. Flint AC, Maisch US, Kriegstein AR. Postnatal development of low (Mg^{2+}) oscillations in neocortex. *J Neurophysiol* 1997;78:1990–1996.

23. Flint AC, Connors BW. Two types of network oscillations in neocortex mediated by distinct glutamate receptor subtypes and neuronal populations. *J Neurophysiol* 1996;75:951–956.

24. Ferro-Novick S, Jahn R. Vesicle fusion from yeast to man. *Nature* 1994;370:191–193.

25. Zucker RS. Short-term synaptic plasticity. *Ann Rev Neurosci* 1989;12:13–31

26. Davis GW, Murphey RK. Long-term regulation of short-term transmitter release properties: retrograde signalling and synaptic development. *Trends Neurosci* 1994;17:9–13.

27. Magleby KL. Short-term changes in synaptic efficacy. In: Edelman GM, Gall VE, Cowan KM, eds. *Synaptic function.* New York: John Wiley & Sons, 1987:21–56.

28. Kamiya H, Zucker RS. Residual Ca^{2+} and short-term synaptic plasticity. *Nature* 1994;371:603–606.

29. Zengel JE, Magleby KL, Horn JP, et al. Facilitation, augmentation, and potentiation of synaptic transmission at the superior cervical ganglion of the rabbit. *J Gen Physiol* 1980;76:213–231.

30. Regehr WG, Delaney KR, Tank DW. The role of presynaptic calcium in short-term enhancement at the hippocampal mossy fiber synapse. *J Neurosci* 1994;14: 523–537.

31. Stevens CF, Wang Y. Facilitation and depression at single central synapses. *Neuron* 1995;14:795–802.

32. Debanne D, Guérineau N, Gähwiler BH, et al. Paired-pulse facilitation and depression at unitary synapses in rat hippocampus: quantal fluctuation affects subsequent release. *J Physiol (Lond)* 1996;491:163–176.

33. Rosenmund C, Clements JD, Westbrook GL. Non-uniform probability of glutamate release at a hippocampal synapse. *Science* 1993;262:754–757.

34. Gil Z, Connors BW, Amitai Y. Differential regulation of neocortical synapses by neuromodulators and activity. *Neuron* 1997;19:679–686.

35. Pierce JP, Lewin GR. An ultrastructural size principle. *Neuroscience* 1994;58:441–446.

36. Schikorski T, Stevens CF. Quantitative ultrastructural analysis of hippocampal excitatory synapses. *J Neurosci* 1997;17:5858–5867.

37. Thomson AM, West DC. Fluctuations in pyramid-pyramid excitatory postsynaptic potentials modified by presynaptic firing pattern and postsynaptic membrane potential using paired intracellular recordings in rat neocortex. *Neuroci* 1993;54:329–346.

38. Castro-Alamancos MA, Connors BW. Distinct forms of short-term plasticity at excitatory synapses of hippocampus and neocortex. *Proc Natl Acad Sci USA* 1997; 94:4161–4166.

39. Malenka RC. Synaptic plasticity in the neocortex and hippocampus: a comparison. In: Mody I, Gutnick MJ, eds. *The cortical neuron.* New York: Cambridge Press, 1995:98–110.

40. Thomson AM, Deuchars J. Temporal and spatial properties of local circuits in neocortex. *Trends Neurosci* 1994;17:119–126.

41. Tsodyks MV, Markram H. The neural code between neocortical pyramidal neurons depends on neurotransmitter release probability. *Proc Natl Acad Sci USA* 1997;94:719–723.

42. Stratford KJ, Tarczy-Hornoch K, Martin KAC, et al. Excitatory synaptic inputs to spiny stellate cells in cat visual cortex. *Nature* 1996;382:258–261.

43. Markram H, Tsodyks M. Redistribution of synaptic efficacy between neocortical pyramidal cells. *Nature* 1996;382:807–810.

44. Finnerty GT, Roberts LS, Connors BW. Sensory experience modifies short-term dynamics of neocortical synapses. *Nature* 1999;400:367–371.

45. Abbott LF, Varela JA, Sen K, et al. Synaptic depression and cortical gain control. *Science* 1997;275:220–224.

46. Castro-Alamancos MA, Donoghue JP, Connors BW. Different forms of synaptic plasticity in somatosensory and motor areas of the neocortex. *J Neurosci* 195;15: 5324–5333.

47. Castro-Alamancos MA, Connors BW. Short-term synaptic enhancement predicts long-term potentiation in neocortex. *Proc Natl Acad Sci USA* 1996;93:1335–1339.

48. McNamara JO. Cellular and molecular basis of epilepsy. *J Neurosci* 1994;14:3413–3425.

49. Kirkwood A, Dudek SM, Gold JT, et al. Common forms of synaptic plasticity in the hippocampus and neocortex in vitro. *Science* 1993;260:1518–1521.

50. Grillner S, Georgopoulos AP. Neural control. *Curr Opin Neurobiol* 1996;6:741–743.

51. Miles R, Traub RD. *Neuronal networks in the hippocampus.* Cambridge: Cambridge University Press, 1991.

52. Castro-Alamancos MA, Connors BW. Spatiotemporal properties of short-term plasticity in sensorimotor thal-

amocortical pathways of the rat. *J Neurosci* 1996;16: 2767–2779.

53. Dempsey EW, Morison RS. The electrical activity of a thalamocortical relay system. *Am J Physiol* 1943;138: 283–296.

54. Castro-Alamancos MA, Connors BW. Cellular mechanisms of the augmenting response: short-term plasticity in a thalamocortical pathway. *J Neurosci* 1996;16: 7742–7756.

55. Castro-Alamancos MA, Connors BW. Behavioral state dynamically modulates short-term plasticity of a thalamocortical pathway. *Science* 1996;272:274–277.

56. Castro-Alamancos MA, Connors BW. Noradrenergic and cholinergic modulation of augmenting responses in thalamocortical pathways. *Soc Neurosci Abst* 1996;22: 18.

57. Chagnac-Amitai Y, Connors BW. Horizontal spread of synchronized activity in neocortex, and its control by GABA-mediated inhibition. *J Neurophysiol* 1989;61: 747–757.

58. Chervin RD, Pierce PA, Connors BW. Periodicity and directionality in the propagation of epileptiform discharges across neocortex. *J Neurophysiol* 1988;60: 1695–1713.

59. Tsau Y, Guan L, Wu JY. Initiation of spontaneous epileptiform activity in the neocortical slice. *J Neurophysiol* 1998;80:978–982.

60. Golomb D, Amitai Y. Propagating neuronal discharges in neocortical slices: computational and experimental study. *J Neurophysiol* 1997;78:1199–1211.

61. Telfeian AE, Connors BW. Layer-specific pathways for the horizontal propagation of epileptiform discharges in neocortex. *Epilepsia* 1998;39:700–708.

62. Telfeian AE, Connors BW. Epileptiform propagation patterns mediated by NMDA and nonNMDA receptors in neocortex. *Epilepsia* 1999;40:1580–1586.

63. Schwartz TH, Bazil CW, Walczak TS, et al. The predictive value of intraoperative electrocorticography in resections for limbic epilepsy associated with mesial temporal sclerosis. *Neurosurgery* 1994;40:302–309.

64. Lombardi D, Marsh R, de Tribolet N. Low grade glioma in intractable epilepsy: lesionectomy versus epilepsy surgery. *Acta Neurochir Suppl (Wien)* 1997; 68:70–74.

65. Foehring RC, Lorenzon NM, Herron P, et al. Correlation of physiologically and morphologically identified neuronal types in human association cortex in vitro. *J Neurophysiol* 1991;66:1825–1837.

66. Avoli M, Olivier A. Electrophysiological properties and synaptic responses in the deep layers of the human epileptogenic neocortex in vitro. *J Neurophysiol* 1989; 61:589–606.

67. Schwartzkroin P, Haglund MM. Spontaneous rhythmic synchronous activity in epileptic human and normal monkey temporal lobe. *Epilepsia* 1986;27:523–533.

68. Hwa GG, Avoli M. Excitatory synaptic transmission mediated by NMDA and non-NMDA receptors in the superficial/middle layers of the epileptogenic human neocortex maintained in vitro. *Neurosci Lett* 1992;143: 83–86.

69. Strowbridge BW, Masukawa LM, Spencer DD, et al. Hyperexcitability associated with localizable lesions in epileptic patients. *Brain Res* 1992;587:158–163.

70. Prince DA, Wong RKS. Human epileptic neurons studied in vitro. *Brain Res* 1981;210:323–333.

71. Telfeian AE, Spencer DD, Williamson A. Lack of correlation between neuronal hyperexcitability and electrocorticographic responsiveness in epileptogenic human neocortex. *J Neurosurg* 1999;90:939–945.

72. Strowbridge BW, Masukawa LM, Spencer DD, et al. Hyperexcitability associated with localizable lesions in epileptic patients. *Brain Res* 1992;587:158–163.

73. Foehring RC, Lorenzon NM, Herron P, et al. Correlation of physiologically and morphologically identified neuronal types in human association cortex in vitro. *J Neurophysiol* 1991;66:1825–1837.

74. Tasker JG, Hoffman NW, Kim YI, et al. Electrical properties of neocortical neurons in slices from children with intractable epilepsy. *J Neurophysiol* 1996;75: 931–939.

75. Morrell F. Multiple subpial transections and other interventions. In: Engel J Jr, Pedley TA, eds. *Epilepsy: a comprehensive textbook.* Philadephia: Lippincott–Raven, 1998:1877–1890.

76. Kaufmann WE, Krauss GL, Uematsu S, et al. Treatment of epilepsy with multiple subpial transections: an acute histologic analysis in human subjects. *Epilepsia* 1996; 37:342–352.

77. Martinerie J, Adam C, Le Van Quyen M, et al. Epileptic seizures can be anticipated by non-linear analysis. *Nat Med* 1998;4:1173–1176.

78. Elger CE, Lehnertz K. Seizure prediction by non-linear time series analysis of brain electrical activity. *Eur J Neurosci* 1998;10:786–789.

79. Schiff SJ, Jerger K, Duong DH, et al. Controlling chaos in the brain. *Nature* 1994;370:615–620.

Neocortical Epilepsies.
Advances in Neurology, Vol. 84,
edited by P. D. Williamson, A. M. Siegel,
D. W. Roberts, V. M. Thadani, and M. S. Gazzaniga.
Lippincott Williams & Wilkins, Philadelphia © 2000.

13

Perinatal Brain Damage, Cortical Reorganization (Acquired Cortical Dysplasias), and Epilepsy

Miguel Marín-Padilla

Molecular Neuroscience Program, Mayo Clinic, Rochester, Minnesota 55906

Neonatal encephalopathies constitute a heterogeneous group of congenital or acquired brain disorders characterized by variable distribution, severity, unsolved pathogenesis, and often, a poor clinical outcome. Despite excellent clinical, pathological, and radiologic (imaging) reviews of these disorders, their impact on the subsequent maturation of the infant brain remain inadequately studied. This chapter describes the evolving neuropathology and developmental impact of selected encephalopathies as investigated in infants who survived perinatal brain damage. Acquired neonatal encephalopathies are associated with prematurity, respiratory difficulties (neonatal asphyxia), circulatory disturbances, monozygous twining (fetal transfusion syndrome), infections, trauma, and labor complications (1–15).

In acquired neonatal encephalopathies, the spared cortex adjacent to the damage site undergoes postinjury reorganization. Previous studies showed that this spared cortex undergoes cytoarchitectural alterations compatible with acquired cortical dysplasia that could influence the subsequent maturation of the infant brain (17–20). Moreover, infants who survive acquired neonatal encephalopathies eventually could develop a variety of neurologic disorders, including epilepsy, cerebral palsy, dyslexia, mental (cognitive and behavioral) impairment, poor school performance,

and minimal brain damage (4,10,12,13, 15–22). The pathogenesis of these neurologic sequelae and their relationship to the acquired cortical dysplasia remain poorly understood and inadequately studied. The postinjury reorganization of the spared cortex (acquired cortical dysplasia) rather than the original brain lesion has been considered the main underlying mechanism in the pathogenesis of the ensuing neurologic sequelae (17–20). This chapter explores, in selected encephalopathies, some aspects of the postinjury reorganization of the spared cortex and evaluates their impact on the subsequent maturation of the infant brain.

MATERIAL AND METHODS

From the Pediatric Autopsy Service of Dartmouth–Hitchcock Medical Center, 36 cases of infants who survived a variety of perinatally acquired encephalopathies were selected. In all cases, perinatal brain damage was documented; the infants' birth age ranged from 21 weeks' gestation to term, and their survival ranged from a few hours to days, weeks, or months, to several years (Table 13.1). Eventually, all infants died, of a variety of unrelated reasons; complete postmortem studies were carried out. The neuropathology and subsequent impact of the following perinatal brain lesions were studied: subpial hemorrhages

TABLE 13.1. *Perinatal neocortical damage: clinical and pathological data*

Case	Born	Lived	Clinical findings	Stains	Autopsy findings (neocortex)
I. Acute stages					
1 9368	21 wg PCD	1 h	Cardiac Ebstein's malformation	HE	PVH, PH, focal WMH & GMH
2 8941	26 wg PCD	2 h	RDS	HE & Golgi, Bodian	PVH, focal WMH
3 8442	22 wg PCD	2 h	Aspiration meconium	HE & Golgi	Early multifocal PVH; PH
4 9379	24 wg PCD	3 h	RDS	HE, Bodian	Early multifocal PVH focal WMH, PH
5 8460	27 wg PCD	4 h	RDS	HE & Golgi	PVH, IVH
6 9548	24 wg PCD	17 h	Fetal transfusion syndrome	HE	Anemic twin, early WMD; Pletoric twin, severe WMD PVH & IVH
7 8937	30 wg PCD	1 day	RDS	HE & Golgi, Bodian	Early PVH, IVH, PH; focal WMD and GMD
8 804493	26 wg PCD	1 day	RDS	HE & Golgi	PVH, focal PVL, GMD
9 9353	25 wg PCD	3 days	RDS, early BPD	HE, Bodian	Early PVH, PH, IVH; focal WMH & GMH
II. Subacute (healing) stages					
10 9478	32 wg PCD	4 days	Pletoric twin, fetal transfusion, prenatal WM damage	HE, GFAP, neurofilament	Multicystic encephalopathy, healed WMD, surviving GM neocortical dysplasia
11 91135	33 wg PCD	5 days	RDS, aspiration meconium	HE	Multicystic encephalopathy PVL, WMD, mild hydrocephalus
12 8845	28 wg PCD	5 days	RDS, prenatal WM damage	HE & Golgi, myclin, Bodian	LMH, focal PH, necrosis WM; multicystic encephalopathy, acute hydrocephalus
13 89129	26 wg PCD	9 days	RDS, BPD	HE, Bodian	PVH, cerebral edema, WMD necrosis WM axons
14 804720	28 wg PCD	10 days	Enterocolitis peritonitis	HE & Golgi	PVH, early PVL
15 9054	38 wg PCD	12 days	RDS, BPD; prenatal WM damage	HE & Golgi	Multicystic encephalopathy, WMD, early PVL, focal LMH surviving GM
16 90108	28 wg PCD	15 days	BPD	HE & Golgi	WMD, cerebral edema, PH, GMH, IVH
17 9045	26 wg PCD	16 days	RDS, pneumonia hyperthermia	HE & Golgi	WMD, Subpial edema, PH, early PVL, hydrocephalus
18 8971	29 wg PCD	17 days	RDS, early BPD	HE & Golgi	Recent MH, early PVL
19 794170	34 wg PCD	18 days	RDS, microcephaly, retarded growth, prenatal WM damage	HE & Golgi	Multicystic encephalopathy, extensive LMH, microgyria

Case	wg PCD	Age	Clinical history	Stains	Pathology
20 722143	35 wg PCD	26 days	GI atresia surgically treated, BPD	HE & Golgi	Focal WMD & GMD
21 83273	31 wg PCD	26 days	RDS, BPD	HE, myelin	Focal WMD and edema GMD

III. Chronic (repaired) stages

Case	wg PCD	Age	Clinical history	Stains	Pathology
22 9449	30 wg PCD	32 days	Prenatal WM damage	HE & Golgi, neurofilament	Multicystic encephalopathy; healed WMD, surviving GM
23 9210	39 wg PCD	5 wk	Prenatal WM damage, pneumonia, BPD	HE, GFAP	Focal microgyria, PVL, WMD, multicystic encephalopathy WHD, hydrocephalus ex vacuo
24 907	28 mg PCD	3 mo	Perinatal WM damage, developmental delay, BPD	HE & Golgi, myelin, GFAP, neurofilament	WMD, PVL, surviving GM; hydrocephalus ex vacuo, LMHs; neocortical dysplasia
25 9832	27 wg PCD	4 mo	Perinatal brain damage, severe BPD	HE & Golgi, neurofilament, GFAP	Multicystic encephalopathy, extensive WMD, LMHs, focal neocortical dysplasia
26 96137	26 wg PCD	7 mo	Perinatal brain damage, developmental delay, BPD, seizures	HE & GFAP, neurofilament	Multicystic encephalopathy, ulegyria, WMD, GMD, neocortical dysplasia
27 8615	26 wg PCD	8 mo	Perinatal brain damage, developmental delay, BPD	HE & Golgi, Bodian	Multicystic encephalopathy, focal microgyria, PVL hydrocephalus ex vacuo, neocortical dysplasia, HN
28 88272	24 wg PCD	8 mo	Perinatal brain damage, developmental delay, BPD, Seizures	HE & Golgi, GFAP, myelin, neurofilament	GMD & WMD, PVL, LMH multicystic encephalopathy microgyria, hydrocephalus neocortical dysplasia, HN
29 93209	28 wg PCD	2.5 yr	Developmental dalay, Status epilepticus	HE & Golgi, GFAP, neurofilament	WMD, focal ulegyria, ex vacuo hydranencephaly; neocortical dysplasia, HN
30 8511067	32 wg PCD	5 yr Alive	BPD, cerebral palsy, Epilepsy, Mental retardation	HE & Golgi, myelin, GFAP	Frontal lobe Bx. (2.5 yr) GMD, LMHs neocortical dysplasia, HN
31 98147	Term Shaken 11 days PCD	7 yr	Postnatal brain damage; cerebral palsy, blindness, epilepsy, mental retardation	HE, myelin, GFAP, bodian, synaptophysin, neurofilament	Frontotemporal porencephaly; hydrocephalus ex vacuo, ulegyria, PVL, focal LMHs, neocortical dysplasia, HN
32 88175	35 wg PCD	8 yr	Drowning, prenatal WM damage, mental retardation, epilepsy	Myelin, HE, neurofilament, bodian, HE, GFAP	Parietooccipital porencephaly; surviving GM, PVL extensive LMHs, focal ulegyria neocortical dysplasia, HN
33 9517048	Term PCD	10 yr Alive	Postnatal brain damage, left frontal trauma, lobectomy, epilepsy	HE, Golgi, neurofilament	Left frontal GMD and WMD; surviving GM, multicystic encephalopathy, porencephaly neocortical dysplasia HN
34 9381	37 wg	11 years	Postnatal brain damage cerebral palsy, epilepsy mental retardation	HE, GFAP, myelin, neurofilament	Parietooccipital porencephaly PVL, LMHs, surviving GM neocortical dysplasia, HN
35 97173	Term PCD	11 yr	Peritonitis, cerebral palsy, mental retardation, epilepsy	HE, GFAP, neurofilament	Left parieto-temporo-occipital porencephaly, surviving GM atrophy corpus callosum
36 93343	Term	16 yr Alive	Postnatal brain damage, epilepsy, lobectomy	HE, Golgi, GFAP, neurofilament	Right occipital porencephaly, neocortical dysplasia, HN, focal ulegyria

wg, week gestation; PCD, perinatal cortical damage; RDS, respiratory distress syndrome; BPD, bronchopulmonary dysplasia; HE, hematoxylin and eosin; PVL, periventricular leukomalacia; PVH, periventricular hemorrhage; IVH, intraventricular hemorrhage; PH, pial hemorrhages; WMH and GMH, white and gray matter hemorrhage; WMD and GMD, white and gray matter damage; WM and GM, white and gray matter; HN, hypertrophic neurons; LMH, leptomeningeal heterotopia; GFAP, glial fibrillary acidic proteins stain; GI, gastrointestinal.

From Marin-Padilla M. Three-dimensional structural organization of layer I of the human cerebral cortex: a Golgi study. *J Comp Neurol* 1990;229:89–105, with permission.

(four cases), periventricular hemorrhages (eight cases), leptomeningeal heterotopias (seven cases), microgyrias (seven cases), ulegyrias (five cases), multicystic encephalopathies (eleven cases), porencephalies (six cases), hydranencephalies (one case), and various combinations of these disorders (Table 13.1). Various neurohistologic stains were used: (a) routine stains (hematoxylin and eosin, Nissl, Bodian, and luxol–fast blue; (b) immunohistochemical stains (glial fibrillary acidic proteins, anti-human nonphosphorylated neurofilament proteins, palvalbumin, and synaptophysin); and (c) the rapid Golgi method.

RESULTS

In all cases, the spared cortical gray matter (GM) around the original lesion survived and underwent postinjury reorganization resulting in acquired cortical dysplasia. The following aspects were investigated: (a) the direct impact of the lesion on the affected cortex; (b) neuropathologic evolution of each lesion through its acute, subacute (healing), and chronic (repaired) stages; (c) postinjury reorganization of undamaged regions adjacent to the damaged site; (d) repercussion on the subsequent maturation of the infant brain; and (e) the possible role of the acquired cortical dysplasia in the pathogenesis of ensuing neurologic sequelae. The postinjury reorganization (acquired cortical dysplasia) of the spared GM have been explored in the following lesions: (a) the spared GM underlying leptomeningeal heterotopias; (b) the spared GM overlying white matter (WM) lesions; and (c) the residual GM in severe cortical lesions. These cases share similar dysplastic changes involving neurons, interconnecting fibers, synaptic profiles, glial cells, and blood vessels. Regardless of the type of original brain injury, the similarity among the dysplastic changes found in evolving neonatal encephalopathies is a reflection of common repair mechanisms used by the developing cortex.

Leptomeningeal Heterotopias

The external glia limiting membrane (EGLM) is an essential component of the central nervous system (CNS); it demarcates the nervous from the surrounding meningeal tissue. It is composed of closely apposed glial end feet united by tight junctions and covered by the basal lamina (BL) material manufactured by them. Early in development, the EGLM is essentially composed and maintained by the end feet of radial glial (17,18,23). After completion of neuronal migration, the reabsorbing end feet of degenerating radial glial fibers are replaced by those of layer I astrocytes (23,24). During postnatal life, the layer I astrocytes become the essential components of the EGLM, but some fibrous astrocytes also coparticipate in its maintenance. The number of layer I astrocytes increases (layer I gliosis) in some pathologic conditions, including epilepsy (5,10,13).

During vascularization of the neocortex, the EGLM is progressively perforated by meningeal vessels. During this vascular perforation, the BL of the EGLM and that of the perforating vessel fuse at the site of entry restoring the CNS anatomic integrity and permitting the perforating vessel to enter into the nervous tissue (25–31). This BL fusion forms a pial funnel or space between them, thus establishing a perivascular compartment (Virchow–Robin space) around the perforating vessel (32). This perivascular space accompanies the vessels into the CNS and remains open to the leptomeningeal space, thus allowing meningeal (mesodermal) elements to enter through it to and contribute muscle cells to the growing vessel (26,29,30). Inflammatory cells also enter and exit the CNS through this perivascular space. Throughout the CNS terminal capillary plexus, this perivascular space disappears by fusion of both laminae into a single one, which is thereafter manufactured and maintained by the end feet of fibrous or protoplasmic astrocytes (24). Fusion between the BL of the CNS and that of Schwann cells also occurs at the entrance and exit of nerves (27,28,31).

About 15% of hemorrhagic lesions affecting the infant neocortex are subpial hemorrhages (10). These hemorrhages are invariably associated with EGLM damage, which must be repaired promptly to reestablish the neocor-

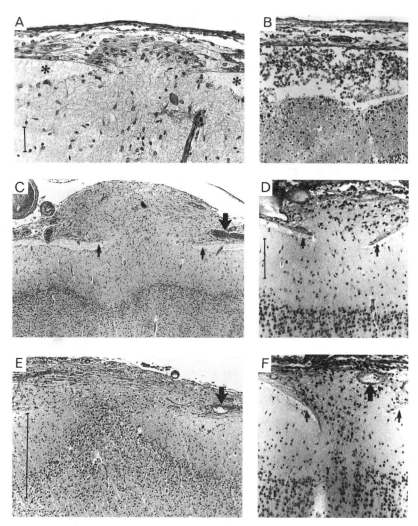

FIG. 13.1. Composite figure showing various pathological stages of subpial (layer I) hemorrhages with EGLM disruption and repair, formation of superficial heterotopias *(LMH)*, and postinjury reorganization of the underlying cortex. Repair **(A)** of small EGLM disruption with a microscopic LMH composed of glial elements, probably without clinical significance and marked edema *(asterisks)* of adjacent glial endfeet (case 14). Recent **(B)** subpial hemorrhage with rupture of perforating vessels, EGLM disruption, and layer I damage (case 1). Verrucous LMH **(C)** with adjacent glial endfeet edema *(small arrows)*, extensive postinjury cytoarchitectural alterations of both layer I and the underlying gray matter, pial vessels buried *(large arrow)* by heterotopia, and partial obliteration (acquired marginal heterotopia) of layer I (case 14). Small LMH **(D)** with disruption of the EGLM persistent glial end-feet edema *(small arrows)* and an absence of obvious postinjury alterations in the underlying cortex (case 18). Extensive LMH **(E)** showing the EGLM disruption, displacement of cellular elements into the leptomeningeal space, and extensive postinjury alterations in both layer I (obliteration) and underlying gray matter (case 26). Large LMH **(F)** showing the EGLM disruption site with adjacent glial endfeet edema *(small arrow)*, columnar displacement of the cellular elements of the underlying gray matter, and a pial vessel buried by the lesion (case 24). Scales = 100 μm. (Reproduced from Marín-Padilla M. Developmental neuropathology and impact of perinatal brain damage. I. Hemorrhagic lesions of neocortex. *J Neuropath Exp Neurol* 1996;55:758–773, with permission.)

tex's anatomic integrity (Fig. 13.1B). Small disruptions are repaired promptly by the end feet of local astrocytes and leave no residual lesion. The repair of large disruptions involves major changes and may result in permanent dysplastic lesions (10,17,33,34). The repair of large EGLM disruptions implies proliferation of local astrocytes, cytoarchitectural alterations in both layer I and the underlying GM, survival and transformation of partially damage neurons, eventual EGLM reparation often occurring within the leptomeningeal space, and formation of residual dysplastic lesion (Fig. 13.1A,C–F).

These superficial dysplastic lesions have been described in the literature with a variety of terms, such as *brain warts, marginal heterotopias, sulci fusion,* and some types of *focal microgyria, agyria,* and *pachygyria* (10,17,20, 24,33–35). I prefer the term *leptomeningeal heterotopia* (LMH) because these lesions are the result of EGLM damage and subsequent reparation, which often occur within the leptomeningeal space (17). The size of these superficial dysplasias varies from microscopic lesions without dysplastic changes (Fig. 13.1A,D) to extensive superficial dysplasias with postinjury alterations of the underlying GM (Fig. 13.1C,E,F). LMHs are recognized by their protrusion above the surrounding cortex, their avascular verrucous surface, and the abrupt disappearance of pial capillaries (covered by the lesion) at the edge of the lesion (Fig. 13.1C–F thick arrows). An LMH is composed of a disorganized admixture of blood vessels, glial cells, displaced neurons, diffused gliosis, the tortuous terminals of axonic and glial fibers, and degenerating elements (Fig. 13.2). LMHs also are characterized by fibrosis and collagen manufactured by local meningeal fibroblasts (Fig. 13.2).

Beneath a large LMH, the cytoarchitecture of layer I and the underlying GM may be permanently altered (17–19,35). The original subpial hemorrhage damages some elements of layer I. Within layer I, the terminal dendritic bouquets of pyramidal neurons, axonic terminals, and radial glial fibers may be destroyed by the hemorrhage. Most of these

elements may be able to survive; eventually, some may regenerate (Fig. 13.3). Surviving dendrotomyzed pyramidal neurons postinjury are transformed into stellate neurons (Fig. 13.3). Some axonic and glial fibers terminals also regenerate and penetrate into the LMH (Figs. 13.2 and 13.3). The horizontal axons of Cajal–Retzius cells are only bent toward the disruption, but they do not penetrate into the LMH (Fig. 13.2). The horizontal pathway of these axons is established within layer I early in development and certainly before the EGLM injury. Therefore, the C–R horizontal axons remain unaffected by the lesion (Fig. 13.2). The postinjury development of the GM under the LMH is also altered. Postinjury alterations of this GM include neuronal disorganization and displacement; fibrillar, glial, and vascular disorganization; alterations of the intrinsic circuitry; and the presence of both atrophic and hypertrophic neurons and of bundles of myelinated fibers. Displaced neurons change their intrinsic circuitry and their morphology may be secondarily altered. Following dendritic pruning, some affected pyramidal cell (layers II and III) are transformed into stellate neurons, thus changing their synaptic profiles and connectivity. Whereas some GM neurons become atrophic with short dendrites and a few spines, others become hypertrophic with long, complex dendrites covered by countless spines and an axon that often arises from one of its dendrites and is locally distributed (Fig. 13.2, white stars). Some of these hypertrophic neurons may represent basket cells with several long horizontal axonic collaterals with numerous pericellular baskets (Fig. 13.2, black arrow). Hypertrophic cells are believed to be postinjury transformed local-circuit neurons. These hypertrophic neurons are strongly positive in neurofilament preparations. Some of these GM alterations may be indistinguishable from those described in neuronal migration anomalies (22).

The LMHs have been described in a variety of neurologic disorders, including dyslexia, cerebral palsy, epilepsy, and fetal alcohol syndrome (9,17,18,22,33,34–40). In principle,

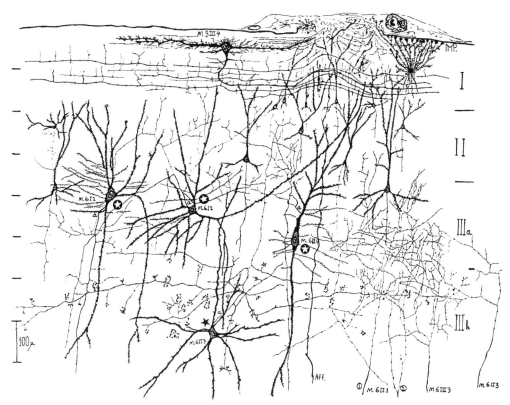

FIG. 13.2. Mosaic of camera lucida drawings from rapid Golgi preparations (case # 18) showing some of the postinjury cytoarchitectural alterations of the cortical GM underlying a LMH caused by a subpial hemorrhagic lesion with EGLM disruption and subsequent repair. The EGLM disruption site and the residual dysplastic lesion formed within the leptomeningeal space (LMH) are illustrated. The LMH contains an admixture of displaced neuronal, fibrillar, glial, and vascular elements. The horizontal axons of Cajal–Retzius neurons bend toward the defect but do not penetrate into the LMH. Below the LMH, several large hypertrophic neurons *(white arrows)* with long dendrites (some reaching into the LMH) covered with numerous spines and axons arising from one of the dendrites are illustrated. The complex intrinsic neurophil formed by several fibers within layer III is also illustrated. Also illustrated are a few atrophic and displaced neurons as well as some normal pyramidal neurons of layer II–III for comparison purposes. Some of these postinjury dysplastic alterations may persist and play a role in the pathogenesis of subsequent neurologic sequelae. Scale = 100 μm. (Reproduced by permission of the publishers from Marín-Padilla M. Pathogenesis of late-acquired leptomeningeal heterotopias and secondary cortical alterations: a Golgi study. In: Galaburda AM, Kemper TL, eds. *Dyslexia and development: neurobiological aspects of extraordinary brains.* Cambridge, MA: Harvard University Press. Copyright © 1993, 64–88, with permission.)

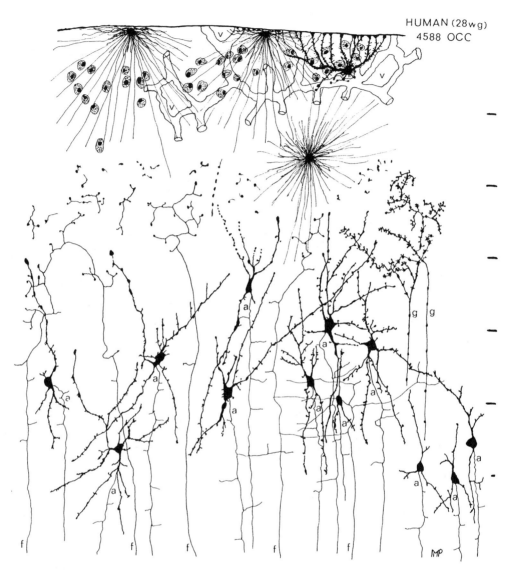

FIG. 13.3. Composite figure of camera lucida drawings from rapid Golgi preparations showing the essential glial and neuronal alterations observed during the subacute or healing stages of subpial (layer I) hemorrhages. Details of the healing stage of layer I (subpial) hemorrhagic injury showing the terminal dendritic pruning of pyramidal neurons damaged (severed) by the hemorrhage and their subsequent postinjury transformation into stellate neurons. Also illustrated are the terminal regeneration of radial glial *(g)* and afferent *(f)* fibers damaged (severed) by the hemorrhage, scattered fragments of degenerating neuronal and glial elements, local proliferation of layer I and fibrous astrocytes, hemosiderin-laden macrophages, and postinjury revascularization *(v)* of the region. Some of these postinjury transformed neurons may persist within the affected cortex (acquired cortical dysplasia) resulting in alterations of the cytoarchitecture and intrinsic circuitry of the affected cortex, which could cause cortical dysfunction and play a role in the pathogenesis of ensuing neurological sequelae. Scales = 100 μm. (Reproduced from Marín-Padilla M. Developmental neuropathology and impact of perinatal brain damage. I. Hemorrhagic lesions of neocortex. *J Neuropath Exp Neurol* 1996;55:758–773, with permission.)

any large LMH could cause local cortical dysfunction and play a role in the pathogenesis of ensuing neurological sequelae.

Acquired Dysplasia of the Spared GM Overlying WM Lesions

The developing WM is particularly vulnerable to perinatal asphyxia, hypoxia, ischemia, circulatory disturbances, and trauma. Its vulnerability may be due to its rapid growth, active metabolic rate, and increasing distance from new perforating vessels by the expansion of the overlying GM (2,5,32). The extent of fiber destruction in WM lesions as well as that of fiber reduction (ex vacuo hydrocephalus) throughout distant cortical regions can be demonstrated by using neurofilament and Golgi preparations. Fiber reduction away from the original lesion is caused by the degeneration (anterograde and retrograde) of corticipetal, corticofugal, and association fibers damaged (severed) by the WM injury.

The developing WM is vascularized by an expanding short-linked anastomotic capillary plexus formed between adjacent perforating vessels (19,24,30,32,41–45). The capillaries of this plexus undergo continuous remodeling by both capillary angiogenesis and reabsorption adjusting to the structural and functional needs of the growing cortex. During neocortical development, the distance between perforating vessels is maintained relatively constant, ranging from 150 to 300 µm. Consequently, the number of entering and exiting vessels of the neocortex increases progressively, paralleling its predevelopmental and postdevelopmental expansions (32).

Vascularization of the GM is a late developmental process that starts after completion of neuronal migration and progresses from lower to upper regions, paralleling its ascending maturation. It is also composed by a plexus arteriovenous capillary loop established between new perforating vessels and preexisting ones (30,32,42,43). The GM, which represents the neocortex's neuronal anlage, is more directly (new perforators), better (new arteriovenous capillary loops), and more profusely (additional perforators) vascularized than the underlying WM. The GM may be better equipped than the underlying WM to endure temporary hypoxia, ischemia, and circulatory disturbances. Moreover, because of its unique developmental features, the vascular destruction that characterizes WM lesions does not necessarily affect the arteriovenous capillary loops of the overlying GM; these remain essentially unaffected, permitting the circulation of blood.

The repair of WM lesions evolves through a series of rapidly succeeding events, including edema, necrosis, liquefaction, removal of debris by macrophages, minimal reactive gliosis, and eventual cavitation. Irregular spaces start to appear within the damaged WM, which may be empty or filled with fluid and inflammatory cells. In surviving infants, the size of these spaces increases, some coalesce into larger ones, and some eventually are transformed into cystic cavities separated by gliovascular and fiber-carrying trabeculi. If the ependymal epithelium also was damaged, these cavities are connected with the ventricular system (e.g., porencephalies). Connected and unconnected cavities may develop concomitantly. The repaired stages of perinatally acquired WM lesions are represented by three distinct clinical neonatal encephalopathies: multicystic encephalopathy (Fig. 13.4A,C), porencephaly (Fig. 13.4B), ex vacuo hydrocephaly (Fig. 13.4D), and hydranencephaly (Fig. 13.4E) or combinations of these disorders (10,14,15,19).

In multicystic encephalopathies, porencephalies, and hydranencephalies, the overlying GM often is spared, it retains its intrinsic vasculature, and undergoes postinjury cytoarchitectural reorganization (acquired cortical dysplasia). This overlying GM, despite partial isolation from sensory inputs (corticipetal fibers destruction) and an inability to reach distant functional targets (corticofugal fiber destruction) survives and is able to continue its —albeit altered—postinjury maturation. This partially isolated GM continues to develop, reorganizing its neuronal, fibrillar, vascular, and glial elements weeks, months, and even years after the original brain damage. The use

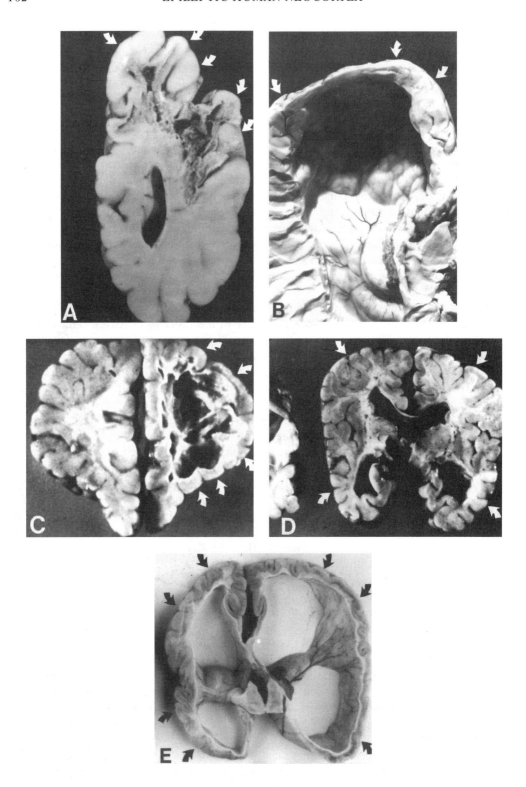

of special neurohistologic methods (neurofilament and Golgi stains) disclosed a variety of postinjury cytoarchitectural alterations. Damaged (severed) corticofugal fibers undergo retrograde (as well as anterograde) degeneration up to the origin of their collaterals, which survive as well as the parent neuron. Some axotomized neurons survive, and their axonic collaterals continue to grow within the GM, their number may increase, and their intracortical distribution assumes new patterns (Fig. 13.5). Some deep-sited axotomyzed pyramidal neurons develop long, horizontal axonic collaterals; these expand, paralleling the border of the necrotic zone (Fig. 13.5A). Eventually, some of these long, horizontal collaterals become incorporated into the residual WM, perhaps retransforming the original cell back to a projective neuron with new and different functional targets. The axonic collaterals of other axotomized pyramidal neurons arch upwardly, bifurcate several times, and ascend vertically for a long distance (Fig. 13.5). These ascending collaterals, which may be quite numerous, are extremely fine and finely beaded, suggesting active growth (Fig. 13.5B). These axotomized pyramidal neurons with long ascending axonic collaterals has been found several months (case 25) after the original brain injury. The axonic collaterals of other axotomized cells are short, irregular, and coarsely beaded, suggesting regressive changes. Another feature of this partially isolated GM is the hypertrophy of some of its intrinsic neurons, including basket cells with long, horizontal axonic collaterals and numerous baskets (Fig. 13.5C). Possibly, the deprivation of afferent terminals stimulates the expansion of the intrinsic circuitry of this spared GM. Synaptic sites vacated by the destruction of afferent fibers may be reused by the terminals of intrinsic neurons, which may become hypertrophic. Throughout this spared GM, the number of intrinsic fibers and the overall intrinsic circuitry increase significantly (Fig. 13.5). The postinjury rewiring of cortical neurons by their own intrinsic fibers may contribute to the long survival of the GM overlying WM lesions.

Neurofilament preparations of the spared GM confirmed the complexity of its intrinsic circuitry as well as the presence of large, hypertrophic, and strongly positive stellate intrinsic neurons (Fig. 13.6). Large hypertrophic stellate neurons are particularly prominent in layers II and III (Fig. 13.6). The strong neurofilament staining of these hypertrophic

---

FIG. 13.4. Composite figure illustrating the essential pathologic features of subacute and chronic WM lesions with the spearing of the overlying GM. **A:** Details of the healing stage of a subacute multicystic encephalopathy (case 14) showing extensive WM necrosis, tissue disintegration, and early cavitation. Although most of the overlying GM survived *(white arrows)*, some areas were damaged (infarcted) by the primary insult. **B:** View of a unilateral occipital lobe porencephaly (case 32) resulting from an extensive WM lesion showing the cystic enlargement of the connected ventricle, the marked reduction of WM, and the survival of the overlying GM *(white arrows)*. **C:** Details of a unilateral multicystic encephalopathy (case 27) showing several WM cavities separated by gliovascular trabeculi and unconnected to the ventricular system as well as the survival of the overlying GM *(white arrows)*. The left frontal lobe was unaffected. **D:** Details of hydrocephalus ex vacuo (case 24) showing universal attenuation of WM tissue, marked atrophy of the corpus callosum, generalized dilatation of the ventricular system, and survival of the overlying GM *(white arrows)*. **E:** Details of hydranencephaly (case 29) showing severe universal hydrocephalus ex vacuo, generalized attenuation of WM tissue, severe atrophy of the corpus callosum, and near universal survival of the overlying GM *(black arrows)*. In all cases, the gyral patterns of the spared GM have evolved within normal limits *(white and black arrows)*. Despite the extent and severity of the original WM lesion, the overlying GM retained its independent blood supply and intrinsic anastomotic microvasculature and has been capable of continuing its postinjury, albeit altered, maturation. The clinical manifestation of epilepsy did occur in cases 27, 29, and 32. (Reproduced from Marín-Padilla M. Developmental neuropathology and impact of perinatal brain damage. II. White matter lesions of the neocortex. *J Neuropath Exp Neurol* 1997;56:219–235, with permission.)

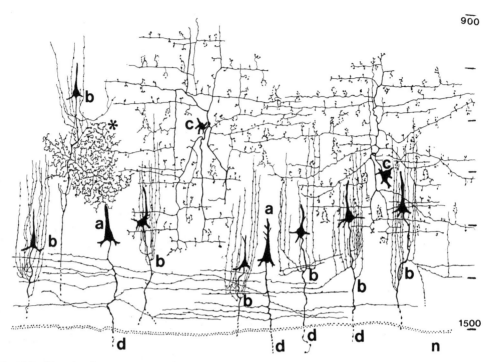

FIG. 13.5. Mosaic of camera lucida drawings from rapid Golgi preparations (case 14) showing some of the postinjury cytoarchitectural alterations observed in the spared GM overlying a subacute WM lesion (Fig. 13.4A). The following GM elements are illustrated: the axonic profiles of two axotomyzed pyramidal neurons *(a)* characterized by long horizontal collaterals bordering the necrotic zone *(n)*; the axonic profiles of seven axotomized pyramidal neurons *(b)* with long ascending (arcuate) collaterals; the axonic profiles of two large (hypertrophic) basket cells *(c)* with long horizontal collaterals and numerous terminal pericellular baskets; and the complex intrinsic neuropil (*) formed by the axonic terminals of unidentified local-circuit neurons. Within the necrotic zone *(N)*, the retrograde degeneration (fragmentation) of some efferent fibers *(d)* progresses up to the origin of axonic collaterals, transforming some projective pyramidal cells into intrinsic local-circuit neurons. The upper border of the necrotic *(N)* zone has been marked with an india ink line. The location (depth) of the necrotic zone is about 1,500 μm from the pial surface, roughly at the border between layers V and VI. Scale = 100 μm. (Reproduced from Marín-Padilla M. Developmental neuropathology and impact of perinatal brain damage. II. White matter lesions of the neocortex. *J Neuropathol Exp Neurol* 1997;56: 219–235, with permission.)

neurons is considered to reflect an actual increase in the number of intrinsic neurofilaments throughout their enlarged soma and long dendrites. Hypertrophic neurons may participate in the postinjury synaptic reorganization of the spared GM, reconnecting synaptic sites vacated by the degenerating afferent fibers destroyed by the WM lesion. Some of these hypertrophic neurons are considered to represent hypertrophic basket cells. Neurofilament preparations also showed the rare presence of some strongly positive Cajal–Retzius cells (Fig. 13.6, CR). Another finding is the presence of bundles of myelinated and neurofilament positive fibers throughout the spared GM. These bundles of fibers cross the cortex in different directions; some are found near or within layer I, and many reach the residual band of WM. These myelinated fibers may be able of carrying normal as well as epileptic impulses from the postinjury transformed GM overlying WM lesions.

Rapid Golgi preparations of the spared GM in some cases (case # 30) showed the

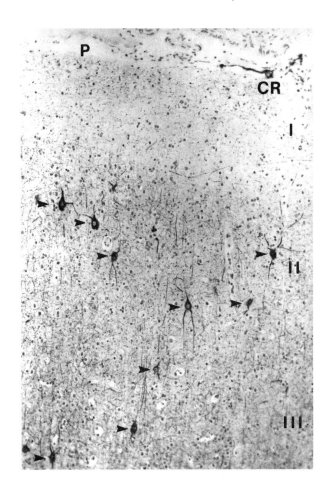

FIG. 13.6. Photomicrograph of the surviving GM overlying a parieto-occipital porencephalic cyst (case 34) showing dysplastic alterations involving layers I, II, and III (from neurofilament preparations). Several strongly positive hypertrophic stellate neurons *(arrows)* in layer II and III and Cajal–Retzius cells (C–R) in layer I are illustrated. These neuron-strong neurofilament reactions are considered to be caused by an increase in the number of neurofilaments and to reflect functional hypertrophy. Although not clearly recognized in this section, this overlying GM is also characterized by layer I gliosis, complex intrinsic neuropil, and cellular disorganization, including columnar arrangements. All these neuropathologic features are consistent with a postinjury acquired cortical dysplasia. These acquired dysplatic changes already were associated with epilepsy in this 11-year-old child.

presence of large neurons with long, spiny dendrites and an intracortical distribution of their axon (Fig. 13.7). The axon of some of these large neurons arises from one of the dendrites at a significant distance from the soma. These large neurons are considered intrinsic neurons that have undergone postinjury structural and functional hypertrophy. Some of these hypertrophic neurons show bizarre dendritic profiles with irregular bends and terminals tufts (Fig. 13.7). Others have dendritic collaterals that grow only from one side of the main apical dendrite, with few or no collaterals arising from the opposite side (Fig. 13.7). Large polymorphous neurons with long spiny dendrites also are found at the GM/WM border. Local disorientation of neurons, neuronal atrophy, and degenerative dendritic changes, and increase in the number of

intrinsic fibers have been also found in the spared GM.

Epilepsy has been reported in surviving children with multicystic encephalopathies, porencephalies, and hydranencephaly. Moreover, the postinjury cytoarchitectural alterations described herein already were associated with the clinical manifestations of epilepsy (cases 28–36).

Acquired Dysplasia of Residual Gray Matter in Severe Cortical Lesions

In some perinatally acquired encephalopathies, the GM is severely damaged and may be reduced to a thin gliotic membrane (Fig. 13.8). This type of severe GM damage often is found in some multicystic encephalopathies, porencephalies (cases 33 and 36), and hydranen-

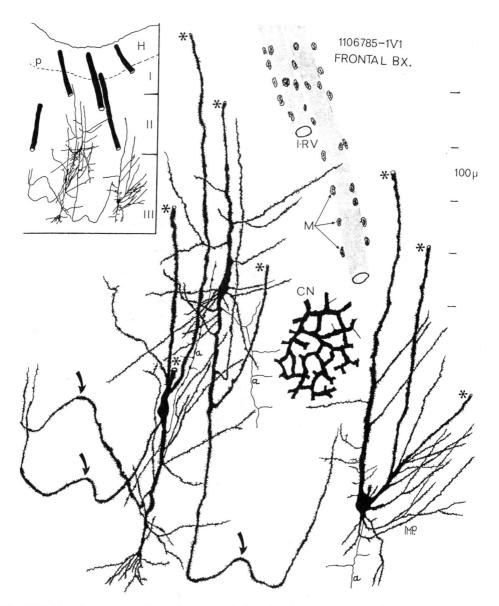

FIG. 13.7. Mosaic reconstruction of camera lucida drawings from rapid Golgi preparations of a frontal lobe biopsy (case 30) showing three postinjury transformed hypertrophic neurons of layers II–III with bizarre dendritic arborizations. Two of these neurons have long ascending and descending dendrites characterized by irregular distribution, numerous spines, anomalous bends *(arrows)*, and terminal tufts. The dendritic collaterals of the third neuron are also numerous and seem to arise predominately from one side of the apical dendrite, with a few or none arriving from the opposite side. These neurons seem to have responded only to imputs arriving from the right side. The axon of these neurons is distributed intracortically. These hypertrophic cells are considered to represent postinjury transformed intrinsic neurons that have responded to anomalies of the cortex intrinsic neuropil resulting from the original brain damage. Also illustrated are views of the cortical microvasculature and of two larger postinflammatory vessels *(IRV)* surrounded my macrophages *(M)* for comparison. The *asterisk* at the end of some dendrites marked its visible end within the section. **Inset:** Location of these three hypertrophic neurons between layers II and III and their relationship to small superficial LMH located above the pial surface *(P)*. Scale = 100 µm. (Reproduced from Marín-Padilla M. Developmental neuropathology and impact of perinatal brain damage. III. Gray matter lesions of the neocortex. *J Neuropathol Exp Neurol* 1999;58:407–429, with permission.)

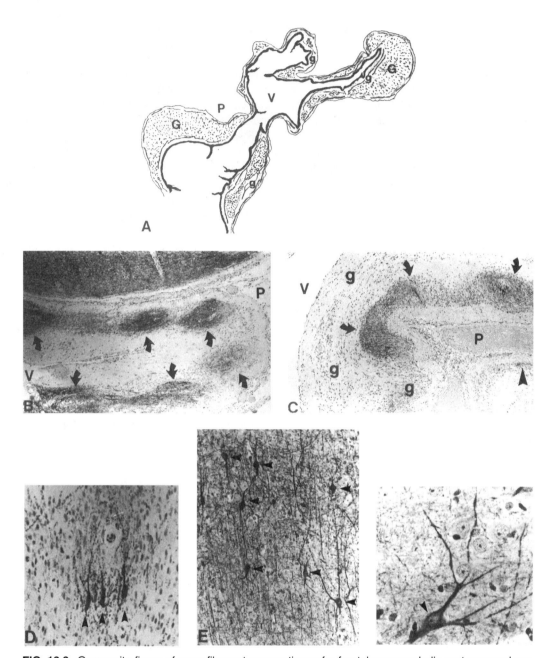

FIG. 13.8. Composite figure of neurofilament preparations of a frontal porencephalic cyst removed surgically for the treatment of intractable epilepsy (case 33). **A:** Schematic drawing of part of the removed cyst showing small islands of surviving gray matter tissue *(G)*, marked gliosis *(g)*, collapsed residual white matter cavity *(V)* with fiber-carrying trabeculi *(T)*, and the pial *(P)* surface. **B:** View of the surgically removed specimen showing a portion of the better preserved cortex separated by the meninges of an intervening sulcus from the more severely damaged cortex reduced to membrane with areas of surviving GM tissue *(arrows)* and diffused gliosis. **C:** High-power view of the severely damaged residual cortex showing small islands of surviving GM *(arrows)* with a few surviving intrinsic neurons embedded within a complex intrinsic neuropil of neurofilament positive, diffused gliosis *(g)*, a few surviving intrinsic fibers of layer I *(arrowhead)*, a few residual white matter fibers, the residual white matter cavity *(V)*, and the pial *(P)* surface. **D:** Detail of a small island of surviving gray matter tissue composed of neurofilament-positive intrinsic fibers and a few intrinsic hypertrophic neurons *(arrowheads)*. **E:** Detail of the better preserved cortex showing a few neurofilament-positive intrinsic hypertrophic neurons *(arrowheads)* embedded within a complex intrinsic neuropil. **F:** Details of a large and strongly neurofilament positive hypertrophic neuron *(arrowhead)* from the better preserved cortex. Bars: B, C = 250 μm; D–F = 100 μm. (Reproduced from Marín-Padilla M. Developmental neuropathology and impact of perinatal brain damage. III. Gray matter lesions of the neocortex. *J Neuropath Exp Neurol* 1999;58:407–429, with permission.)

cephalies. The original necrotic process affecting the WM advances upwardly, involving the cortex, which may be reduced to a few islands of surviving GM tissue (Fig. 13.8).

The surviving WM is reduced to a few gliovascular and fiber-carrying trabeculi and a thin periventricular gliotic band (Fig. 13.8). This band is composed of tightly packed reactive astrocytes with glial filaments running parallel to the ventricular wall, with a few scattered foci of ependymal cells. The ventricular system is invariably expanded (ex vacuo hydrocephalus) by the massive WM fiber destruction and subsequent degeneration.

The surviving cortex is reduced to a thin gliotic membrane with islands of GM tissue (Fig. 13.8B,C). This gliotic cortex is covered by meninges, vascularized by leptomeningeal vessels, and may have a few attached WM fiber-carrying trabeculi (Fig. 13.8). The surviving islands of GM tissue are composed of a few neurofilament positive intrinsic neurons embedded within a rich intrinsic neuropil and surrounded by reactive gliosis (Fig. 13.8B–D). Despite the extensive damage and gliosis, neurofilament and Golgi preparations demonstrated the survival of the intrinsic fibers of layer I and of a few WM fibers throughout this residual cortex (Fig. 13.8C). Some C–R cells also survived in this gliotic cortex. Undoubtedly, preservation of these functional interconnections and the proximity of the leptomeningeal vasculature contribute to the survival of this residual GM tissue, such as permitting its subsequent postinjury reorganization (acquired cortical dysplasia).

Neurofilament and Golgi preparations of the better preserved GM at the edges of the gliotic cortex also have shown dysplastic changes that are more pronounced at its border with the gliotic cortex. These postinjury alterations include cellular and fibrillar disorganization, laminar obliteration, focal obliteration of layer I, complex intrinsic neuropil, diffused cortical gliosis, layer I gliosis, and the presence of atrophic and hypertrophic intrinsic neurons. Atrophic neurons are characterized by a few short dendrites and an axon distributed intracortically. Hypertrophic neurons are characterized by their large size, several long and irregular spiny dendrites, an ascending or descending axon that often arises from one of the main dendrites and branches intracortically, and by their strong neurofilament reaction. Isolated hypertrophic neurons are found at all cortical levels, but they are more prominent in upper layers, where they contrast with these regions small neuronal size.

Some hypertrophic neurons are parvalbumin positive, which gives support to the idea that they may represent postinjury transformed inhibitory neurons. The stellate morphology and long dendrites of some hypertrophic neurons resemble those of the basket cells. Moreover, neurofilament and Golgi preparations demonstrated the presence of prominent axosomatic synapses around the body of some pyramidal cells of the better preserved GM at the lesion edges. Similar types of alterations involving inhibitory basket cells were recently described (46–49). Hypertrophic cells are considered intrinsic (possibly inhibitory) neurons, which have responded to alterations of the intrinsic circuitry of the affected region by structural and functional hypertrophy (46,50–52). The large size and strong neurofilament reaction of these hypertrophic neurons give support to this idea. The possibility of that secondary hypertrophy of some basket cells could be induced by the need to control the excessive (epileptic) firing of projective pyramidal cells should be investigated.

In some cases, neurofilament and Golgi preparations also demonstrated the presence of abnormal bundles of myelinated and strongly neurofilament positive fibers running through the better preserved GM at the lesion edges (cases 32, 33, and 36). These fiber bundles cross the dysplastic cortex vertically or horizontally, often in the proximity of layer I, run within anteroposterior fascicles and may be composed of both corticipetal and corticofugal fibers. These fibers may be capable of interconnecting the dysplastic cortex with other cortical or subcortical regions and of carrying both normal as well as abnormal (epileptic) impulses from it. These islands of GM tissue have become interconnected between them as well as with the better preserved areas of the cortex by the survival of interconnecting fibers, including the intrinsic fibers of layer I and a few residual WM fibers. It is important to emphasize that the neuronal and fibrillar elements of these islands of GM have been able to survive for several years and have become associated with epilepsy (case 33). The altered functional activity of these dysplastic islands of GM tissue may be channels to the better preserved GM at the lesion edge by surviving interconnecting fibers, contribute to cortical dysfunction, and play a role in the pathogenesis of ensuing neurological sequelae.

CONCLUSION

In acquired neonatal encephalopathies, spared regions of GM, despite their functional isolation, survive, retain their blood supply, and continue their postinjury maturation. The postinjury reorganization of this spared GM results in cytoarchitectural alterations compatible with acquired cortical dysplasia. The number of possible alterations that can evolve during the postinjury maturation of this spared GM is extraordinary and difficult to evaluate adequately. Those described herein are but a few of the most prominent alterations. These postinjury alterations are not static processes; rather, they are ongoing processes that started after the injury and continue to evolve throughout weeks, months, and years after the original brain injury. During the postinjury maturation of this spared GM, additional structural and functional changes might evolve from preexisting ones, making it difficult to distinguish original from superimposed alterations. Moreover, the cerebral cortex of an infant who eventually develops epilepsy (or other neurologic sequelae) might undergo further secondary alterations caused by the seizures themselves.

In subpial hemorrhages, dendrotomyized pyramidal cells survive the pruning of terminal dendrites, are transformed into stellate neurons, and undergo modifications of their intrinsic synaptic organization. Axotomized pyramidal neurons of the GM overlying WM lesions survive, are transformed from long-projective into local-circuit neurons, and also modify their synaptic profiles and functional targets. The retrograde degeneration of their damaged (severed) axon progresses up to the origin of axonic collaterals, which continue to evolve, and the parent pyramidal cell survives. In some axotomized neurons, the number of collaterals arising from the proximal axonic stump increases, and they assume new intracortical connections. Although partially deprived of sensory inputs and unable to reach distant targets, these axotomized neurons survive and continue to modify their structure, synaptic profiles, and intrinsic connectivity. Cajal (53) described similar neuronal transformations in the developing neocortex and cerebellum of young kittens. Pyramidal and Purkinje cells recently axotomized by surgical ablation of the underlying WM are transformed from long-projective into local-circuit neurons, expand their axonic collaterals, and assume new patterns of axonic distribution.

Local-circuit intrinsic neurons also survive, develop long spiny dendrites, and participate in the postinjury reorganization of the GM intrinsic neuropil. Some local-circuit neurons develop large bodies with an enlarged nucleus, long dendrites covered with numerous dendritic spines, and an expanded axonic territory (17–20). These large neurons are heavily stained in neurofilament preparations (21,54). In my opinion, and that of others, the increasing number of neurofilaments of these neurons possibly reflect postinjury acquired structural and functional hypertrophy (36,55–59). Destruction of afferent fibers by the underlying WM lesion results in a marked reduction of extrinsic fiber terminals, which will vacate many synaptic sites throughout the spared GM. These vacated synaptic sites may be reused functionally by the terminals of intrinsic fibers. Local-circuit neurons with appropriate receptors may develop additional presynaptic terminals reconnecting these vacated synaptic sites undergoing both structural and functional hypertrophy (17,19,20,55,56,58,

60,61). Nuclear polyploidy has been suspected in some of these large neurons, which further support their postinjury functional hypertrophy (56). It was recently proposed that neurons (like cardiac muscle cells) may be capable of responding to functional demands (physiologic as well as pathological) with nuclear polyploidy and, therefore, with structural and functional hypertrophy (20). The possibility of partial nuclear DNA or RNA reduplication (endomytotic reduplication) by neurons in response to functional demands may explain the DNA replication described in some neurons in the adult animal brain; therefore, it may not be an indication of actual neuron regeneration as has been claimed (62, 63).

Ten of the infants studied developed epilepsy (cases 26, 28–36), two developed cerebral palsy (cases 34 and 35), and several were neurologically and mentally impaired (Table 13.1). These neurologic sequelae are considered consequences of the postinjury structural and functional reorganization of the spared GM rather than a direct consequence of the original brain damage. Each case represents a distinct and unique clinical entity that reflects the particular postinjury reorganization of its spared cortical GM. The literature concerning the association between epilepsy and cortical dysplasia is vast, complex, unclear, and in need of delineation and standardization (21). Epilepsy has been reported in many different conditions, including congenital encephalopathies, metabolic disorders, anomalies of neuronal migration, sequelae of perinatal brain damage, tumors, infections, pachygyria–agyria syndromes, megalencephalic syndromes, trauma, and other disorders. It might be impossible to establish a common denominator from such an heterogeneous group of epileptic disorders; however, most of these disorders could cause, directly and/or indirectly, cytoarchitectural alterations of the developing neocortex resulting from either a genetic or an acquired cortical dysplasia. The different types of epileptic disorders, rather than being the direct consequence of each particular condition, could be the outcome of the postinjury reorganization of the affected

neocortex and, in this sense, share a common pathogenesis.

The infant's brain represents an evolving entity characterized by the progressive and unique organization of its neurons, blood vessels, glial elements, defensive elements, and eventual functional connectivity. Moreover, a neuron is an independent entity characterized by unique features, including (a) unique spatial location and orientation; (b) unique three-dimensional distribution of its dendritic and axonic arborizations; (c) unique distribution and organization of its synapses; and (d) a unique array of axonic connections with many other neurons. Throughout a person's life, these four features evolve and modify progressively from the interplay of each neuron's genetic makeup, unique environment, and unique interneuronal connectivity (64,65). Any lesion (congenital or acquired) affecting the developing infant neocortex could have repercussions on the subsequent structural and functional maturation of its neurons, and result in cytoarchitectural modifications throughout its evolving intrinsic neuropil. Whereas some of these postinjury modifications may be clinically silent, others may be compensated, and still others may be manifested via cortical dysfunction, such as mental retardation, dyslexia, cerebral palsy, epilepsy, cognitive impairment, poor school performance, blindness, speech impairment, various developmental delays, as well as other behavioral and cognitive disturbances. The altered functional activity of a postinjury transformed neocortex may be blocked at motor centers and thus failing to reach lower centers (e.g., cerebral palsy), they may be discharged through abnormal motor activity (e.g., epilepsy), they may result in visual errors (e.g., dyslexia), or they may result in various types of cognitive and behavioral disorders. Concerning perinatal brain damage, the following facts should be emphasized: (a) neurons and intrinsic circuitry of spared GM regions are progressively transformed; (b) the postinjury reorganization of this spared GM results in a variable degree of acquired cortical dysplasias with corresponding cortical dysfunction; and (c) these evolving postinjury cytoarchitectural alterations, rather than the original brain lesion, are the underlying mechanism in the pathogenesis of ensuing neurologic sequelae.

ACKNOWLEDGMENTS

This work was supported by a Jacob Javits Neuroscientist Investigator Award, National Institutes of Health NIH grant NS-22897.

REFERENCES

1. Schwartz P. *Birth injuries of the newborn:* morphology, *pathogenesis, clinical pathology, and prevention.* New York: Hafner, 1961:70–90.
2. Banker BQ, Larroche J-C. Periventricular leukomalacia of infants: a form of neonatal anoxic encephalopathy. *Arch Neurol* 1962;7:386–410.
3. Larroche J-C. *Developmental pathology of the neonate.* Amsterdam: Excepta Medica, 1877:399–446.
4. Larroche J-C. Fetal and perinatal brain damage. In: Wigglesworth JS, Singer DB, eds. *Textbook of fetal and perinatal pathology.* Boston: Blackwell Scientific Publications, 1991:807–838.
5. Rorke JB. *Pathology of perinatal brain injury.* New York: Raven Press, 1992:45–130.
6. Armstrong D, Norman MG. Periventricular leukomalacia in neonates: complications and sequelae. *Arch Dis Child* 1974;49:367–375.
7. Kissane JM. *Pathology of infancy and childhood.* St. Louis: CV Mosby, 1975:117–148.
8. Volpe JJ. *Neurology of the newborn.* Philadelphia: WB Saunders, 1987:160–181.
9. Evrard P, Saint-Geoges D, Kadhim HJ, et al. Pathology of prenatal encephalopathies. In: French JH, ed. *Child neurology and developmental disabilities. Proceedings of the fourth international child neurology congress.* Baltimore: Brooks, 1989:153–176.
10. Friede RL. *Developmental neuropathology.* Berlin: Springer-Verlag, 1989:27–97.
11. Takashima S, Mito T, Ando Y. Pathogenesis of periventricular white matter hemorrhages in preterm infant. *Brain Dev* 1989;8:25–30.
12. Reed GB, Claireaux AE. *Diseases of the fetus and newborn:* pathology, *imaging, genetics, and management.* London: Chapman & Hall Medical, 1989:432–437.
13. Sarnat HB. *Cerebral dysgenesis: embryology and clinical expression.* Oxford: Oxford University Press, 1992: 89–134.
14. Ravavi-Encha F. Fetal neuropathology. In: Ducket S, ed. *Pediatric neuropathology.* Baltimore: Williams & Wilkins, 1995:108–122.
15. Armstrong D. Neonatal encephalopathies. In: Ducket S, ed. *Pediatric neuropathology.* Baltimore: Williams & Wilkins, 1995:334–351.
16. Robertson CMT, Finer NN, Grace MGA. School performance of survival of neonatal encephalopathy associated with asphixia at term. *J Pediatr* 1989;114:753–760.
17. Marín-Padilla M. Pathogenesis of late-acquired leptomeningeal heterotopias and secondary cortical alterations: a Golgi study. In: Galaburda AM, Kemper TL, eds. *Dyslexia and development: neurobiological aspects of extra-ordinary brains.* Cambridge, MA: Harvard University Press, 1993:64–88.
18. Marín-Padilla M. Developmental neuropathology and impact of perinatal brain damage. I. Hemorrhagic lesions of neocortex. *J Neuropathol Exp Neurol* 1996; 55:758–773.
19. Marín-Padilla M. Developmental neuropathology and impact of perinatal brain damage. II. White matter lesions of the neocortex. *J Neuropathol Exp Neurol* 1997;56:219–235.
20. Marín-Padilla M. Developmental neuropathology and impact of perinatal brain damage. III. Gray matter lesions of the neocortex. *J Neuropathol Exp Neurol* 1999;58:407–429.
21. Vinter HV, De Rosa MJ, Farrel MA. Neuropathologic study of resected cerebral tissue from patients with infantile spasms. *Epilepsia* 1993;34:772–779.
22. Mischel PS, Nguyen LP, Vinters HV. Cerebral cortical dysplasia associated with pediatric epilepsy: review of neuropathologic featurs and proposal for a grading system. *J Neuropathol Exp Neurol* 1995;54:137–153.
23. Marín-Padilla M. Three-dimensional structural organization of layer I of the human cerebral cortex: a Golgi study. *J Comp Neurol* 1990;229:89–105.
24. Marín-Padilla M. Prenatal development of fibrous (white matter), protoplasmic (gray matter), and layer I astrocytes in the human cerebral cortex: a Golgi study. *J Comp Neurol* 1995;357:554–572.
25. Andres KH. Über die Feinstruktur der Arachnoidea und Dura mater von Mammalian. *Z Zellforch* 1967;79: 272–295.
26. Casley-Smith E, Földi-Börcsök E, Földi M. The prelymphatic pathway of the brain as revealed by cervical lymphatic obstruction and the passage of particles. *Br J Exp Pathol* 1976;57:179–188.
27. Krisch B, Leonhardt H, Oksche A. The meningeal compartment of the median eminence of the cortex: a comparative analysis in the rat. *Cell Tissue Res* 1982;228: 597–640.
28. Krisch B, Leonhardt H, Oksche A. Compartments and vascular arrangement of the meninges cove M. G. ring the cerebral cortex of the rat. *Cell Tissue Res* 1983;238: 459–474.
29. Pile-Spellman JM, McKusic KA, Strauss HW, et al. Experimental in vivo imaging of the cranial perineural lymphatic pathway. *Am J Neuroradiol* 1984;5: 539–545.
30. Marín-Padilla M. Embryonic vascularization of the mammalian cerebral cortex. In: Peters A, Jones EC, eds. *Cerebral cortex,* vol 7. *Development and maturation of cerebral cortex.* New York: Plenum Press, 1988:479–509.
31. Marín-Padilla M, Amieva MR. Early neurogenesis of the mouse olfactory nerve: Golgi and electron microscopic studies. *J Comp Neurol* 1989;288:339–352.
32. Marín-Padilla M. Embryogenesis of the early vascularization of the central nervous system. In: Yasargil MG, ed. *Microneurosurgery,* vol III. *Clinical considerations and microsurgery of racemous angiomas.* Stuttgart: Thieme-Verlag, 1987:23–47.
33. Brun A. Marginal glioneuronal heterotopias of the central nervous system. *Acta Pathol Microbiol Scand* 1965; 65:221–233.

34. Brun A. The subpial granular layer of the foetal cerebral cortex. *Acta Pathol Microbiol Scand* 1965;79(Suppl 179):1–89.

35. Morgan JT, Marín-Padilla M. Cortical repair and reorganization following traumatic microinjury in the developing rat neocortex (Abstract). *Soc Neurosc* 1992; 18:601.

36. Taylor DC, Falconer MA, Bruton CJ, et al. Focal dysplasia of the cerebral cortex in epilepsy. *J Neurol Neurosurg Psychiatry* 1971;34:369–387.

37. Clarren SK, Smith DW. The fetal alcohol syndrome. *N Engl J Med* 1978;298:1063–1068.

38. Galaburda AM, Kemper TL. Cytoarchitectonic abnormalities in developmental dyslexia: a case study. *Ann Neurol* 1979;6:94–100.

39. Wisniewski K, Dambska M, Sher JH, et al. A clinical neuropathological study of fetal alcohol syndrome. *Neuropediat* 1983;4:197–201.

40. Galaburda AM, Sherman GF, Rosen GD, et al. Developmental dyslexia: four consecutive patients with cortical anomaslies. *Ann Neurol* 1985;18:222–233.

41. Wolff JR, Bär TH, Güldner FH. Common morphogenetic aspects of various organotypic microvascular patterns. *Microvasc Res* 1975;10:373–395.

42. Duvernoy HM, Delon S, Vannson JL. Cortical blood vessels of the human brain. *Brain Res Bull* 1981;7: 519–579.

43. Marín-Padilla M. Early vascularization of the embryonic cetebral cortex: a Golgi and electron microscopic study. *J Comp Neurol* 1985;241:237–249.

44. Akina M, Nonaka H, Kagesawa M, et al. A study on the microvasculature of the cerebral cortex: fundamental architecture and its senile changes in the frontal cortex. *Lab Invest* 1986;55:482–489.

45. Nakamura Y, Okudera T, Hashimoto T. Vascular architecture in white matter of neonates: its relationship to perventricular leukomalacia. *J Neuropathol Exp Neurol* 1994;53:582–589.

46. Spreafico R, Battaglia G, Arcelli P, et al. Cortical dysplasia: an immunocytochemical study of three patients. *Am Acad Neurol* 1998;50:27–36.

47. Moreland DB, Glasauer FE, Egnatchik JG, et al. Focal cortical dysplasia: case report. *J Neurosurg* 1988;68: 487–490.

48. Hanaway J, Lee SI, Netsky MG. Pachygyria: relation findings to modern embryologic concepts. *Neurology* 1968;18:791–799.

49. Meencke HJ, Veith G. Migration disturbances in epilepsy. In: Engel J Jr, Wasterlain C, Cavalheiro EA, et al., eds. *Molecular neurobiology of epilepsy*. Amsterdam: Elsevier, 1992:31–40.

50. Lee WM-Y, Otvos L, Carden MJ, et al. Identification of the mayor multiphosphorilated site in mammalian neurofilaments. *Proc Natl Acad Sci USA* 1988;85: 1998–2002.

51. Yashnis AT, Rocke LB, Lee VM-Y, et al. Expression of neuronal and glial polypeptides during histogenesis of the human cerebellar cortex, including observations on the dentate nucleus. *J Comp Neurol* 1993;334:356–369.

52. Buch MS, Gordon-Weeks PR. Distribution and expression of developmentally regulated phosphorylation epitopes on MAP 1B and neurofilament proteins in the developing rat spinal cord. *J Neurocytol* 1994;23: 682–698.

53. Cajal SR. *Degeneration and regeneration of the nervous system* [translated from the 1928 Spanish edition by May RM]. London: Hafner, 1968:617–677.

54. Adams C, Hwang PA, Gilday DL, et al. Comparison of SPECT, EEG, CT, MRI, and pathology in partial epilepsy. *Pediatr Neurol* 1992;8:97–103.

55. Bignami A, Palladini G, Zappella M. Unilateral megalencephaly with nerve hypertrophy: an anatomical and quatitative study. *Brain Res* 1968;9:103–114.

56. Manz HJ, Phillips TM, Towden G, et al. Unilateral megalencephaly, cerebral cortex dysplasia, neuronal hypertrophy, and heterotopia: cytomorphometric, fluorimetric cytochemical, and biochemical analyses. *Acta Neuropathol* 1979;45:97–103.

57. De Rosa MJ, Ferrel MA, Burke MM, et al. An assesment of the proliferative potential of 'balloon cells' in focal cortical resection performed for childhood epilepsy. *Neuropathol Appl Neurobiol* 1992;18:566–574.

58. Doung T, De Rosa MJ, Poukens V, et al. Neuronal cytoskeletal abnormalities in human cerebral cortical dysplasia. *Acta Neuropathol* 1994;87:493–503.

59. De Felipe J, Sola RG, Marco P. Changes in excitatory and inhibitory synaptic circuits in the human epileptic cortex. In: Conti F, Hicks TP, eds. *Excitatory amino acids and the cerebral cortex*. Cambridge, MA: MIT Press, 1996:299–312.

60. Ferrer I, Pineda M, Tallada M, et al. Abnormal local-circuit neurons in epilepsia partiallis continua associated with cortical dysplasia. *Acta Neuropathol* 1992;83: 647–652.

61. Armstrong DD. The neuropathology of temporal lobe epilepsy. *J Neuropath Exp Neurol* 1993;52:433–443.

62. Nottebohm F. Neuronal replacement in the adulthood. *Ann NY Acad Sci* 1985;457:143–161.

63. Erikson PS, Perfilieva E, Njörk-Erikson T, et al. Neurogenesis in the adult hippocampus. *Nat Med* 1998;4: 1313–1317.

64. Cajal SR. *Histologie du Système Nerveux de l'Homme et des Vertébrés*. Madrid: Consejo Superior Investigaciones Cientificas, 1972:520–532, 836–846.

65. Higgins D, Burack M, Lein P, et al. Mechanisms of neuronal polarity. *Curr Opin Neurobiol* 1997;7:599–604.

Neocortical Epilepsies.
Advances in Neurology, Vol. 84,
edited by P. D. Williamson, A. M. Siegel,
D. W. Roberts, V. M. Thadani, and M. S. Gazzaniga.
Lippincott Williams & Wilkins, Philadelphia © 2000.

14

Occipital Lobe Epilepsies

Warren T. Blume and Samuel Wiebe

London Health Sciences Centre, University Campus, The University of Western Ontario, London, Ontario, Canada N6A 5A5

The several components of the human visual system contrive to effect the possible multiple manifestations of occipital lobe seizures. This principle derives not only from the complex visual processing within the occipital lobe itself, but also from the multiple possible propagation pathways that occipital seizures commonly employ. This chapter reviews the manifestations of seizures occurring within the occipital lobe and those consequent to spread; included are physiologic data relative to these phenomena. A survey of etiologies and differential diagnoses conclude the chapter.

SYMPTOMS OF OCCIPITAL EPILEPTIC DISCHARGE

Sensory Phenomena

Several lines of evidence have indicated that visual input is principally received and processed by the occipital lobe in higher mammals. First, as the cortex develops in parallel with ascension in the mammalian phylogenetic scale, so does its proportion devoted to vision. Although vision constitutes a minimal cortical function in early mammals, the visual cortex, situated posteriorly, becomes progressively larger in higher primates (1).

Correlations between lesion locations and visual-field deficits constitute the second component of such evidence. Gennari, in 1782 (2), was the first to recognize that the human cerebral cortex is not homogeneous throughout its extent. He did this by identifying a thin

whitish strip within the cortex and running parallel to its surface. Gennari (2) recognized the greater prominence of this band posteriorly, but he did not determine its function. This *line of Gennari,* which is abundant in myelinated fibers, appears most elaborately in the calcarine area, hence its name *striate cortex.* A century later, Munk (3) removed one occipital lobe of a monkey and reported a contralateral hemianopia. Within a decade, Henschen (4), a Swedish neuropathologist, was the first to relate hemianopia with occipital lobe lesions in humans. Inouye (5), a Japanese ophthalmologist, ingeniously devised a stereotaxic instrument—called by him a craniocoordinometer—to locate precisely, in three dimensions, the entry and exit points of bullets in skulls of soldiers surviving the Russo–Japanese war of 1905. Having studied the spatial relationship between skull features and major cortical features, Inouye was able to estimate the bullet pathways through the occipital lobe and to correlate these with visual-field defects. Such correlations revealed that macular vision disproportionately occupies the posterior half of the calcarine area and increasingly peripheral visual-field points are represented in progressively anterior and smaller striate locations. Seven years later, Holmes and Lister (6) obtained similar relationships in their studies of World War I veterans.

Stimulation studies have further refined our understanding of visual processing. Hubel and Wiesel (7,8) studied responses of neurons in the cat and monkey visual cortex to white light stimuli of several contours directed to different points of the retina. Such studies demonstrated that small spots of light evoked responses only in occipital cortical layer 4C. Except for the "blob" regions of superficial visual cortical areas, cells in all other cortical layers respond only to stimuli with linear properties. Hubel and Wiesel (7,8) were able to catergorize cells outside the blobs into two major groups: simple and complex, based on their responses to linear stimuli. See Mason and Kandel (9) for further review.

Conversely, stimulation of the occipital lobe cortex in humans usually elicits elementary visual phenomena (10–12), whereas only occipital lobe stimulation produces such visual symptoms (12). Sparks, flickering lights, colors, bright lights, stars, wheels, colored disks, whirling balls, radiating gray spots, lines, and shadows were phenomena described to Penfield and Jasper (12). These and similar phenomena are termed *unformed*. Striate cortex stimulation usually produces these phenomena in that part of the visual field corresponding to its striate projection: central features in the posterior half, peripheral phenomena more anteriorly (10,13). Unformed visual phenomena occurred when either the calcarine or extracalcarine occipital cortex was stimulated by Foerster and by Penfield (10,12). Ebersole and Chatt (14) found layer 4 of the striate cortex to be highly epileptogenic, and so striatopetal spread from extrastriate cortex may underlie this commonality of symptoms. Similarly, Cain (15) readily produced kindling by electric stimulation of the deep layers of occipital cortex in rats, but stimulation of superficial layers usually failed to evoke kindling.

Congruent with the foregoing, unformed visual phenomena were the most common symptoms of occipital lobe seizures in all series, appearing in 47%–100% of cases (16–19) (Table 14.1). These authors described phenomena similar to those elicited by stimulation: flashing or steady white or colored lights, stars, and wheels as "positive" symptoms. A variety of colors has been described.

Straight or zigzag lines, dots, dust particles, and various shapes are other components. These objects may remain stationary or move in any direction, centripetally or centrifugally. A twinkling or pulsating quality of visual figures, to Penfield and Jasper (20), were suggestive of an origin or involvement of the lateral occipital convexity. Patients commonly describe visual blurring as the only symptom suggestive of an occipital origin.

Negative visual phenomena may appear separately or in close conjunction with the aforementioned "positive" ones. Dimming of vision and ictal blindness constituted the second most common symptom of two series (18,19). Williamson et al. (19) found "blackouts" to be more common than "whiteouts." The intensity of positive and negative sensations may increase rapidly: Brightness of a light increases to obscure all vision or darkness advances to complete ictal amaurosis.

Unilateral visual phenomena as initial ictal events almost always reflect epileptic discharge in the contralateral occipital lobe (18–21). Ludwig and Ajmone Marsan (16), however, described in some patients an ipsilateral-to-contralateral (to seizure origin) movement of a simple image. Visual phenomena may arise in a hemianopic field (22): A patient described such an event to us as "nothing becoming black." Unilateral phenomena often are depicted by the patient as occurring in one eye.

Visual phenomena may just as commonly occupy all fields from onset (20–22; Wiebe et al., in preparation). Ictal origin in an occipital area with abundant interhemispheric connections, such as the peristriate cortex, may facilitate rapid propagation and bilaterality of symptoms (23,24). Moreover, a robust ictal discharge will more likely propagate throughout the occipital lobe, as shown by Collins and Gaston (25) by varying the units of the epileptogenic agent penicillin applied to rat occipital cortex. Such greater propagation would more likely engage areas with abundant callosal connections and therefore produce bilateral symptoms.

Unformed visual phenomena represent seizures arising from the occipital lobe, judging

TABLE 14.1. *Occipital seizure semiology*

Study (no. of patients)	Unformed visual aurae[a]	Formed visual aurae	Never visual	Non-visual aurae[a]	No aura	"Complex partial" seizures	Head, eye deviation	Unilateral clonic of limbs	Unilateral tonic of limbs	Total unilateral of limbs	Symmetrical motor
Ludwig and Ajmone Marsan, 1975 (55)	26 (47)	8 (15)	25 (45)[a]	~12 (22)[a]	18 (33)	16 (29)	16 (29)	18 (33)	8 (15)	26 (47)	≥29 (53)[b]
Blume et al., 1991 (19)	11 (58)	6 (32)	6 (32)	5 (26)	1 (5)	12 (63)	6 (32)	2 (11)	3 (16)	5 (26)	15 (79)
Salanova et al., 1992 (42)	29 (69)	9 (21)	8 (19)	16 (38)	6 (14)	25 (60)	29 (69)	16 (38)	6 (14)	22 (52)	3 (7)
Williamson et al., 1992 (25)	25 (100)	3 (12)	—	—	—	11 (44)	16 (64)	—	—	3 (12)	—
Totals	91 (65)	26 (18)	39 (34)	33 (28)	25 (22)	64 (45)	67 (48)	36 (31)	17 (15)	56 (40)	47 (41)

[a]Positive or negative (i.e., amaurosis).
[b]Estimated by current authors.
Parentheses in topic columns are percentages.

from the extensive experience of Penfield and Jasper (20). Palmini et al. (26) drew a similar conclusion from a depth electroencephalographic (EEG) study in which they found a consistent occipital lobe seizure onset among patients with only elementary visual aurae. Ictal blindness is also consistently associated with occipital lobe discharges (27,28). Finally, 19% to 45% of patients with verified occipital lobe seizures report no visual aura (16–18,26).

Motor Phenomena

Horizontal head and eye deviation have been commonly noted in most series of occipital lobe seizure patients (Table 14.1). Some investigators (16,18,29) found such deviation to occur only contralateral to seizure origin, whereas ipsiversion did occur in a minority of patients reported by Williamson et al. (19). These data reflect the representation of contralateral cortical pursuit movements in the anterior occipital lobe (30,31) and a lesser ipsiversive gaze function (30,32).

Krieger et al. (30) obtained contralateral oculoclonic movements by electrically stimulating the primate occipital lobe. Although most clinical reports cite oculoclonic movements as occurring contralateral to seizure origin (16,18), ipsiversive oculoclonic attacks have been described (33). Kanazawa et al. (34) and Gastaut and Roger (35) reported instances of status epilepticus manifested as contralateral oculoclonic events. Pulling or moving ocular sensations without detectable ocular movement are identified in a minority of patients of some series (19,36).

Ocular flutter and vigorous bilateral blinking accompany some occipital seizures (18,19, 37,38); this sign has been produced by occipital lobe stimulation in humans (20). Blinking also occurs in seizures arising elsewhere (39).

Ictal or postictal headache appears to occur more commonly with occipital seizures than with other partial seizures. Headache may be diffuse or confined to the ocular or periocular region, usually ipsilateral to seizure onset (20,40). Syndromes of headache with occipital seizures are described below.

SYMPTOMS CONSEQUENT TO ICTAL PROPAGATION

Many occipital lobe seizures may remain confined to the lobe of origin or spread only homotopically. Symptoms and signs correspond to those described in the previous section. Most occipital seizures of recent series, however, contain aspects that suggest propagation to other regions. From their video–EEG study of partial seizures induced by pentylenetetrazol, Ajmone Marsan and Ralston (41) postulated two principal routes of propagation: suprasylvian and infrasylvian.

Suprasylvian Spread

Anatomically, efferents from peristriate cortex project to premotor cortex (42). Therefore, suprasylvian spread to the ipsilateral premotor cortex (42) would produce asymmetric tonic seizures, as noted in 14% to 16% of several series (Table 14.1) (16–18). Spread to rolandic cortex would evoke clonic attacks as recorded in 11% to 38% of these reports. Symmetric motor attacks, compatible with spread bilaterally to the premotor cortex, primary motor cortex, thalamus, and brainstem, have been described in a variety of proportions of patients (16–18).

Infrasylvian Spread

Infrasylvian spread to the temporal lobe is associated with experiential and other limbic-like ictal events. Several studies documented such routes of propagation.

Spread to the temporal lobe has been the most commonly described ictal sequence as revealed by intracranial (18,19,26,43) and scalp recordings (16). Babb et al. (44) and Palmini et al. (26) described depth-recorded patients whose ictal clinical and electrographic manifestations evolved in synchrony from those of an occipital lobe discharge to those of a temporal ictus. Salanova et al. (18) and Williamson et al. (19) found a similar electrographic–clinical correlation with depth recordings. Olivier et al. (43) documented a seizure of occipital origin that became clinically evident only on reaching the temporal lobe. Figures 14.1 and 14.2 illustrate occipital-to-temporal propagation in two of our patients; the temporal lobe contralateral to occipital origin became principally involved in the second patient.

Comparative anatomic studies of mammals from the hedgehog to humans have shown that the temporal lobe has evolved in parallel with an increasing capability of vision (45). Anatomic connections between occipital and temporal lobes are expectedly abundant; however, Jones and Powell (46) and Turner et al. (47) found no direct connections between the rhesus monkey primary visual cortex and mesial temporal structures such as perirhinal

and prorhinal areas and the amygdala. Instead, these investigators demonstrated that efferents from visual cortex reach these structures via a multisynaptic pathway involving progressively more anterior regions of the temporal neocortex. Perhaps greater synaptic "efficiency" afforded by high-frequency action potentials in epileptic bursts (48) facilitates passage through such potential barriers. Collins and Gaston (25) demonstrated such occipital-to-hippocampal propagation in their ^{14}C-deoxyglucose study of penicillin-induced seizures in rats.

The foregoing experimental and clinical physiological data may underlie the common association of experiential phenomena and

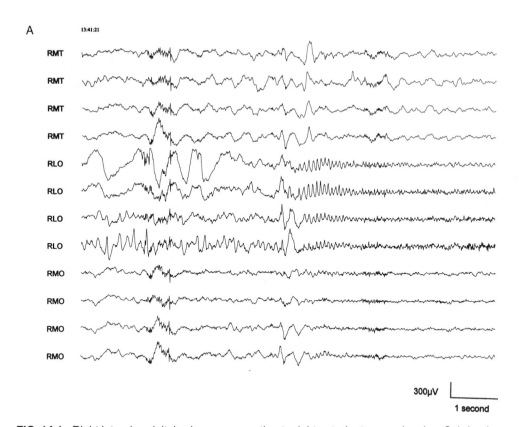

A   13:41:21

RMT

RMT

RMT

RMT

RLO

RLO

RLO

RLO

RMO

RMO

RMO

RMO

300μV

1 second

FIG. 14.1. Right lateral occipital seizure propagating to right anterior temporal region. Subdural recording. All segments of this and Fig. 14.2 are referentially recorded to an inactive subgaleal electrode. Segments are virtually contiguous. Only electrode positions with relevant data are shown. **A:** Following a background of mixed frequencies, principally as a 7-Hz irregular right lateral occipital *(RLO)* rhythm, a single RLO spike occurs, then a single wave followed by RLO and right mesial occipital *(RMO)* attenuation with a transient 10-Hz rhythm at RLO, followed by very high-frequency activity at RLO with slight spread to RMO. *(continued on next page)*

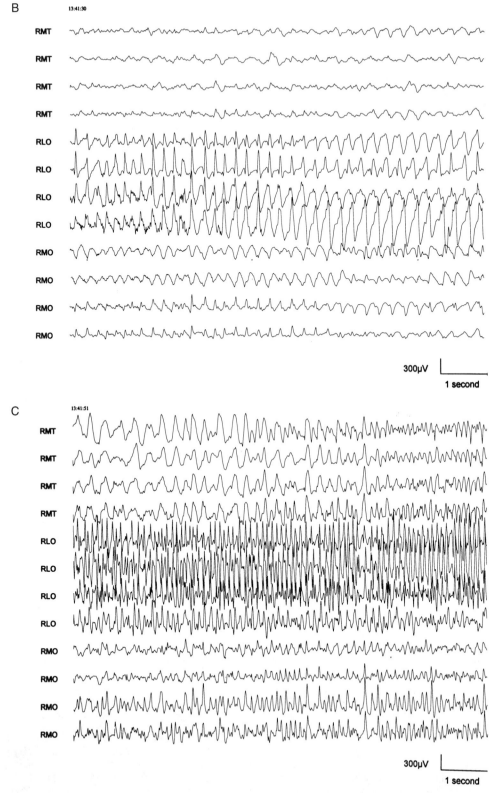

FIG. 14.1. *(Continued)* **B:** Features of Fig. 14.1A are followed immediately by sequential 4- to 5-Hz spikes at RLO with moderate spread to RMO. **C:** Ten seconds later, these spikes have increased markedly in frequency and have spread more widely throughout the occipital region; spread to the right mesial temporal *(RMT)* region occurs in the last two seconds as an 8- to 10-Hz rhythm with intermingled spikes.

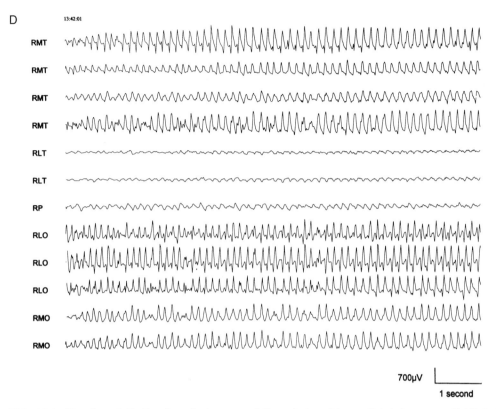

D 13:42:01

RMT
RMT
RMT
RMT
RLT
RLT
RP
RLO
RLO
RLO
RMO
RMO

700μV

1 second

FIG. 14.1. *(Continued)* **D:** Previous features are followed almost immediately by sequential 7- to 8-Hz spikes at RLO and RMT with minimal to no involvement in the right lateral temporal *(RLT)* and the right parietal *(RP)* regions. Note the decreased sensitivity of this last segment.

other manifestations of temporal lobe epileptogenesis in patients who also have occipital seizures. Formed visual hallucinations are reported in 12% to 31% of patients with occipital seizures (16,18,19,21,49) (Table 14.1). Wiebe et al. (in preparation) found a higher incidence of such phenomena among patients with lateral than with mesial occipital epileptogenesis. Animals, people, or scenes appearing unilaterally, centrally, or diffusely are examples of phenomena that have been described. Although such complex visual phenomena may be associated with memory recalls or an emotion to constitute a complete experience, the subject remains aware of its unreality (22,50). This latter feature distinguishes such hallucinatory experiences from those of psychiatric disorders. Head and eyes may deviate toward a unilateral image.

Visual illusions also may occur as distortions of shape, size, and stereoscopy and as alterations in movement, clarity, and illumination (22). Blurred vision may be the most common visual illusory experience.

Penfield and Perot (49) obtained visual experiential phenomena by electrically stimulating various points of the temporal neocortex at craniotomy. Gloor et al. (50) obtained such responses principally by stimulating the amygdala or hippocampus through depth electrodes. Relationships disclosed by each study appear to correlate somewhat with the structure(s) principally accessible to stimulation and recording with each approach. Each group maintained that involvement of "their" end of the temporal neocortex–allocortex axis in epileptic discharge (or dysfunction?) is essential for visual experiential phenomena.

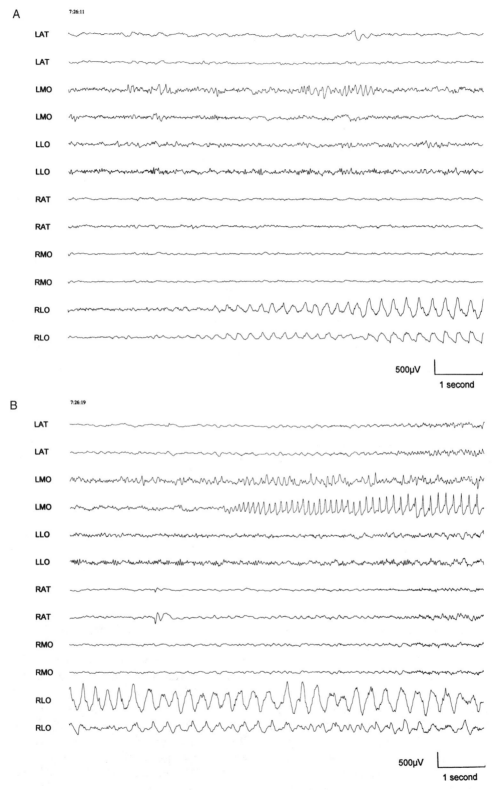

FIG. 14.2. Right occipital-originating seizure propagating bitemporally, principally left. Subdural recording. **A:** From a low-voltage background, 5-Hz rhythmic waves emerge at the right lateral occipital *(RLO)* region. **B:** This rhythm increases in voltage, and higher-frequency waves become superimposed on it. Spread to the left mesial occipital *(LMO)* region appears in the fourth second as a 9-Hz rhythm becoming sequential spikes.

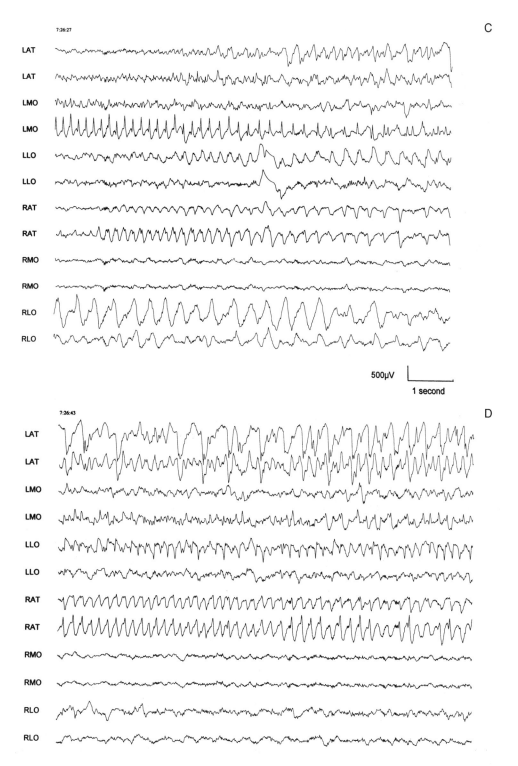

FIG. 14.2. *(Continued)* **C:** While the RLO seizure continues and spreads to the right anterior temporal *(RAT)* region, the LMO seizure becomes more prominent and spreads as a 10- to 11-Hz rhythm to the left anterior temporal *(LAT)* region. **D:** The seizure continues principally at the LAT region but also at the left lateral occipital *(LLO)* and RAT regions, with minimal involvement at its origin *(RLO)*.

(continued on next page)

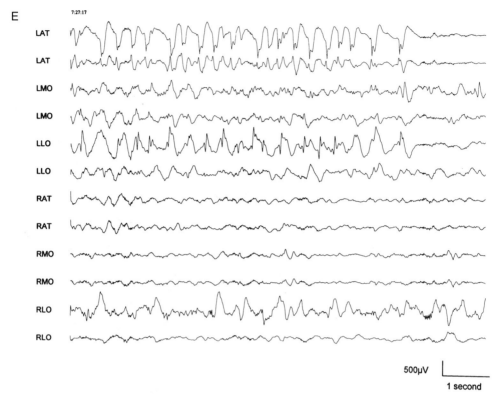

FIG. 14.2. *(Continued)* **E:** Near its termination, this seizure appears principally in the LLO and LAT leads as sequential spikes and semirhythmic delta and theta.

Our case report (51) supports a conclusion that paroxysmal epileptic dysfunction of this visual experiential *system*—neocortical *and* allocortical—produces such symptoms: temporal neocorticectomy converted ictal events of our patient from visual illusions to rising abdominal sensations. Later mesial temporal resection abolished all focal seizure phenomena. Requisite epileptic involvement—or at least dysfunction—of both components of this system would be more congruent with the anatomic relationships described by Gloor (45), Jones and Powell (46), and Turner et al. (47) and would be the interpretation most compatible with findings of both Penfield and Perot (49) and Gloor et al. (50). Note that temporal lobe stimulation by Penfield and Perot (49) and Gloor et al. (50) elicited visual experiential responses more commonly than auditory ones, a further illustration of the temporal lobe's principal role as an interpreter of visual experience.

Despite the abundant physiological and clinical evidence of visual function and dysfunction in the occipital lobe and its propagation targets, 19% to 45% of patients in the aforementioned series (16–18) reported no ictal visual component of any type.

Nonvisual aurae occurred in 22% to 38% of the preceding series (16–18); most of these, such as epigastric symptoms and fear, implicated limbic system involvement. Moreover, phenomena compatible with complex partial attacks appeared in 29% to 63% of patients in these series (16–19). Therefore, as suggested by experimental and clinical physiological data, there is abundant clinical evidence reflecting ictal spread from the occipital lobe to anterior mesial temporal regions.

VISUAL FIELD AND MOTOR ABNORMALITIES

Visual field abnormalities were detected in 20% to 60% of patients in several series (16–19; Wiebe et al., in preparation). When indicated, hemianopiae appeared more commonly than quadrantanopiae (17,18). A minority of patients in some series had unilateral motor deficits contralateral to seizure origin (17,18).

ELECTROENCEPHALOGRAPHY

Extracranial EEG

This may be normal in a minority of patients (e.g., 14% in Wiebe et al.'s series; in preparation). Several EEG abnormalities reflect focal occipital lobe dysfunction. The most obvious and time-honoured of these relates to alpha activity: its reduction, disruption, or slowing ipsilateral to a lesion. Unilateral reduction of "posterior slow waves of youth" in children or adolescents, paradoxically, may result in a more "regulated" alpha rhythm *ipsilateral* to a lesion.

Most studies focused on interictal spikes. Wiebe et al. (in preparation) found all such abnormalities to be regional, not focal at 01 or 02. As the generators of "occipital" (01,02) and most "posterior temporal" (T5,6) spikes appear to be within the occipital lobe and as the fields of posterior temporal spikes overlap principally with occipital ones (52), we have considered spikes from both positions together in reviewing previous series. Several series reported most active interictal spikes to appear over the epileptogenic occipital lobe in 79% to 97% of patients (17–19; Wiebe et al., in preparation). This close interictal–ictal spike topologic correlation also occurs with temporal lobe epilepsy (53) and in children (54).

As expected from the foregoing clinical and experimental data, temporal spikes have appeared in 24% to 64% of the subjects in several series (16–19). Wiebe et al. (in preparation) found a virtually equal proportion of patients harboring temporal spikes contralat-

eral to the epileptogenic occipital lobe (35%) as ipsilateral to the focus (41%).

Extracranial EEG regionalized seizures in 63% to 100% of seizures in the aforementioned series (17,18; Wiebe et al., in preparation). Origins of many scalp-recorded seizures were ambiguous (16–19), however. Mesial or inferior occipital origins and rapid contralateral or anterior propagation likely account for unclear EEG origins of some occipital seizures. Such circumstances require intracranial subdural EEG for clarification.

Intracranial EEG

The Montreal Neurological Institute series of six occipital patients studied with depth electrodes disclosed widespread areas of early seizure involvement involving mesial and lateral occipital cortices with virtually simultaneous engagement of supracalcarine and infracalcarine areas. Seizures began in a circumscribed manner in only one of their six patients. Mesial temporal structures were the principal targets of ictal spread. Williamson et al. (19) documented ictal occipital to mesial temporal spread in 12 of 17 patients and occipital-to-frontal spread in four patients. Subclinical seizures occurred in 59% of Wiebe et al.'s patients (in preparation). All remained confined to their region of origin.

ETIOLOGY

Occipital Epileptic Syndromes Unassociated with Surgically Treatable Structural Lesions

The often overlapping clinical entities described below contain two or more of the following features: occipital seizures, occipital spikes, and migraine-like headaches. Associated neurologic signs, course, and response to antiepileptic drugs help the clinician to distinguish among these entities.

Benign Epilepsy of Childhood with Occipital Spike and Wave Complexes

Gastaut (55,56) described an epileptic syndrome in children in which the attacks begin with visual symptoms and may be followed by sensory, motor, or complex partial ictal features. The seizures can be followed by headache and vomiting. Partial or complete visual loss is the most usual visual symptom occurring either alone or with other visual symptoms. Visual phenomena, such as phosphenes and colored or luminous disks, may appear; they may begin in the visual field either ipsilateral or contralateral to the focal occipital seizure onset and then spread to the entire field. Complex visual hallucinations appear less commonly. As with benign rolandic epilepsy, these children do not have other neurologic abnormalities, and neuroimaging is normal.

The interictal EEG contains abundant 3-Hz spike waves or slow spike waves at 2 to 3 Hz over the occipital area, either unilaterally or bilaterally. As with most occipital spike discharges, these appear principally with the eyes closed, with partial or complete suppression on eye opening (57). Ictally, a sustained discharge over one occipital lobe occurs.

Most patients apparently achieve complete seizure control by the end of adolescence (57). However, as features of this syndrome blend more with lesion-based occipital epilepsy than does benign rolandic epilepsy with its lesion-based counterpart, prognosis of an individual patient can be given less confidently. Some of the following syndromes illustrate this difficulty.

Occipital Seizures, Migraine, and Occipital Spikes

Several other clinical syndromes containing the components of occipital seizures, headache, and occipital EEG abnormalities have been described. Camfield et al. (58) reported four adolescents with basilar migraine, seizures, and active occipital epileptiform activity: spikes, spike waves, or slow spike waves resembling those described above. Attacks begin with unformed visual changes, such as white light or circular lights of many colors; they could be followed by total visual loss and then by a pounding headache. On some occasions, unilateral or generalised tonic–clonic

seizures would follow the migrainous aura. The seizures would less commonly occur independently of the migraine attack.

Andermann (59) described children and adults whose classic migrainous aura, usually visual, is followed by unilateral or generalized motor seizures. In most of these patients, the clinical course is benign. Although theoretically, prevention of the migraine also would control the seizures, the incomplete effectiveness of antimigraine agents usually means that an anticonvulsant is necessary. Andermann also found a group of patients with occipital epilepsy who have a history of common migraine and a family history of classic or common migraine. Two of his five patients with this constellation of abnormalities had hypodense occipital lesions on computed tomography (CT) scanning, raising the possibility that migraine produced occipital infarcts.

Occipital Seizures, Classical Migraine, and Stroke-like Episodes

Nine such patients (including eight male patients) were described by Dvorkin et al. (60). These patients had a history of migraine, usually classical, with visual symptoms. Some of these patients developed occipital seizures with elementary visual phenomena. A therapy-resistant partial and secondary generalized seizure disorder with episodes of status epilepticus gradually supervened. Seizures often were precipitated by prolonged migrainous symptoms, such as headache and vomiting. The course progressed unrelentingly with the appearance of multiple types of neurologic deficits, particularly blindness. Bilateral occipital lesions appeared on CT, occasionally extending to the parietal or temporal regions, always corresponding to the posterior cerebral artery territory.

Two such patients had serum lactic acidosis and ragged red fibers on muscle biopsy, suggesting a mitochondrial disorder, that is, a diagnosis of mitochondrial myopathy, encephalopathy, lactic acidosis, and stroke-like episodes (MELAS). In two others, ragged red fibers could not be found on muscle biopsy. Thus, patients with a clinical picture of

MELAS without ragged red fibers remain a diagnostic dilemma (61).

Epilepsy with Bilateral Occipital Calcifications

First reported by Gobbi et al. (62), this syndrome initially resembles benign occipital epilepsy, except that polyspike bursts may appear on sleep EEGs. In some cases, the seizure disorder subsequently may become refractory with atonic or tonic seizures accompanied by diffuse ictal and interictal EEG epileptiform abnormalities. Some, but not all, cases have celiac disease (63), which may result in folic acid malabsorption (63,64). Microscopic evidence of venous hemangiomas in deep cortical layers with calcium deposited in vessel walls and in parenchyma has been reported (65). Lack of leptomeningeal angiomatosis distinguishes this from Sturge–Weber syndrome.

Lafora's Disease

Of the progressive myoclonic epilepsies, focal occipital seizures with posterior spikes on the EEG suggest Lafora's disease (61,66). Seizures begin in adolescence, both occipital and generalized. Cognitive ability rapidly or gradually declines. The definitive diagnosis is made by demonstrating Lafora bodies—periodic acid-Schiff–positive inclusions—on skin or muscle biopsy. On skin biopsy, the storage material appears in the acinar and duct cells of the eccrine sweat glands and are confined by electron microscopy (67). These bodies are also present in brain, liver, and cardiac muscle.

Etiology of Focal Structural Lesions Causing Occipital Seizures

The occipital region is relatively unaffected by common insults such as trauma or febrile convulsions; therefore, no single type of structural lesion underlies the majority of occipital seizure disorders.

Cortical dysplasias and hamartomata constitute about 20% to 25% of some series (16,17,19). Glial tumours occur about equally as often (16–18). Vascular abnormalities, such as arteriovenous malformations and cav-

ernous angiomata, appeared in some series (16,17,19). Unilateral leptomeningeal angiomatosis (Sturge–Weber syndrome) occurs predominantly in the occipital and parietal areas (68), and occipital seizures may be present, along with partial motor and secondarily generalized attacks. Rarely, the characteristic facial nevus can be absent (69).

Birth trauma has been listed as an etiology in about 25% of some series (17,18). Remillard et al. (70) described occipital and complex partial seizures with hemianopia among eight patients with unilateral occipital–parietotemporal atrophy on air encephalography. All five patients undergoing vertebral angiography demonstrated occlusion of one or more branches of the posterior cerebral artery, presumably perinatally. Whether magnetic resonance imaging (MRI) of these cases would have reached a similar conclusion is unclear.

DIFFERENTIAL DIAGNOSIS

Three conditions contain symptoms which may mimic occipital epilepsy: migraine, syncope, and transient ischemic attacks (71,72).

Migraine

Migraine and occipital seizures share a common evolution: aura, ictus, and postictal phase. The most common initial symptoms of classical migraine are visual: unformed flashes of light or zigzag lines that traverse the visual field for several minutes, leaving an homonymous hemianopia. Migraine symptoms evolve over a few to several minutes, whereas those of epileptic seizures usually (although not always) do so in a few seconds. Sequential vomiting frequently occurs in migraine but is rare during an epileptic seizure.

The visual symptoms and impaired awareness of basilar artery migraine may overlap those of occipital seizures; however, the slower evolution and multiplicity of signs representing brainstem dysfunction favor migraine. Nonetheless, an entity combining features of occipital seizures and basilar artery migraine was described in an earlier section.

Syncope

Black and white dots with fading of vision may represent impending syncope. Consciousness is lost, and the patient may fall in a limp manner. Bilateral tonic or clonic events may supervene if loss of consciousness exceeds 20 seconds. All but the loss of muscle tone are also symptoms and signs of occipital seizures. Distinguishing features of syncope include (a) the setting or precipitating factors, such as upright posture, fright, pain, fasting state, hot and crowded area, fatigue, and cardiac dysrhythmia; (b) autonomic features, including facial pallor, sweating, and bradycardia; and (c) rapid recovery on recumbency without postictal confusion or other deficit.

Posterior Circulation Transient Ischaemia

Evolution and resolution of any occipital dysfunction would be slower than with seizures. Age and risk factors for vascular disease constitute additional distinguishing features.

ACKNOWLEDGMENTS

Mrs. Maria Raffa carefully typed this chapter.

REFERENCES

1. Maunsell JH, Newsome WT. Visual processing in monkey extrastriate cortex. *Annu Rev Neurosci* 1987;10:363–401.
2. Gennari F. *De Peculiari Structura Cerebri Nonnulisque Ejus Morbis.* Parma: Ex Regio Typographeo, 1782. Cited by Glickstein M, Whitteridge. *Trends in Neuroscience* 1987;20:350–353.
3. Munk H. *Über die Funktionen der Grosshirnrinde, A. Hirschwald.* [English translation in Von Bonin G, ed. (1960).] *The cerebral cortex.* Springfield, MA: Thomas, 1881:97–117.
4. Henschen SE. *Klinische und anatomische Beitrage zur Pathologie des Gehirns* (Pt 1). Almquist and Wiksell, 1890. Cited by Glickstein M, Whitteridge. *Trends in Neuroscience* 1987;20:350–353.
5. Inouye T. *Die Sehstörungen bei Schussverletzungen der kortikalen Sehsphäre nach Beobachtungen an Versundeten der letzten Japanische Kriege.* W Engelmann, 1909. Cited by Glickstein M, Whitteridge. *Trends in Neuroscience* 1987;20:350–353.
6. Holmes G, Lister WT. Disturbances of vision from cerebral lesions, with special reference to the cortical representation of the macula. *Brain* 1916;39:34–73.
7. Hubel DH, Wiesel TN. Receptive fields, binocular interaction, and functional architecture in the cat's visual cortex. *J Physiol (Lond)* 1962;160:106–154.
8. Hubel DH, Wiesel TN. Receptive fields and functional architecture of monkey striate cortex. *J Physiol (Lond)* 1968;195:215–243.
9. Mason C, Kandel ER. Central visual pathways. In: Kandel ER, Schwartz JH, Jessell TM, eds. *Principles of neural science.* New York: Elsevier, 1991:420–439.
10. Foerster O. Beitrage zur pathophysiologie der Sehbahn end der Sehsphare. *Psychol Neurol* 1929;39:463–485.
11. Penfield W, Rasmussen T. *The cerebral cortex of man.* New York: Macmillan, 1950.
12. Penfield W, Jasper H. *Epilepsy and the functional anatomy of the human brain.* Boston: Little, Brown, 1954:116.
13. Brodal A. *Neurological anatomy in relation to clinical medicine.* New York: Oxford University Press, 1981:474.
14. Ebersole JS, Chatt AB. Spread and arrest of seizures: the importance of layer 4 in laminar interactions during neocortical epileptogenesis. In: Delgado-Escueta AV, Ward AA Jr, Woodbury DM, Porter RJ, eds. *Basic mechanisms of the epilepsies: molecular and cellular approaches. Advances in Neurology,* vol 44. New York: Raven Press, 1986:515–558.
15. Cain DP. Kindling in sensory systems: neocortex. *Exp Neurol* 1982;76:276–283.
16. Ludwig B, Ajmone Marsan C. Clinical ictal patterns in epileptic patients with occipital electroencephalographic foci. *Neurology* 1975;25:463–471.
17. Blume WT, Whiting SE, Girvin JP. Epilepsy surgery in the posterior cortex. *Ann Neurol* 1991;29:638–645.
18. Salanova V, Andermann F, Olivier A, et al. Occipital lobe epilepsy: electroclinical manifestations, electrocorticography, cortical stimulation, and outcome in 42 patients treated between 1930 and 1991: surgery of occipital lobe epilepsy. *Brain* 1992;115:1655–1680.
19. Williamson PD, Thadani VM, Darcey TM, et al. Occipital lobe epilepsy: clinical characteristics, seizure spread patterns, and results of surgery. *Ann Neurol* 1992;31:3–13.
20. Penfield W, Jasper H. *Epilepsy and the functional anatomy of the human brain.* Boston: Little, Brown, 1954: 401–403.
21. Blume WT. Occipital lobe epilepsies. In: Lüders HO, ed. *Epilepsy surgery.* New York: Raven Press, 1991: 167–171.
22. Sveinbjornsdottir S, Duncan JS. Parietal and occipital lobe epilepsy: a review. *Epilepsia* 1993;34:493–521.
23. Brodal A. *Neurological anatomy in relation to clinical medicine.* New York: Oxford University Press, 1981:593.
24. Pandya DN, Rosene DL. Some observations on trajectories and topography of commissural fibers. In: Reeves AG, ed. *Epilepsy and the corpus callosum.* New York: Plenum Press, 1985:21–39.
25. Collins RC, Caston TV. Functional anatomy of occipital lobe seizures: an experimental study in rats. *Neurology* 1979;29:705–716.
26. Palmini A, Andermann F, Dubeau F, et al. Occipitotemporal epilepsies: evaluation of selected patients requiring depth electrodes studies and rationale for surgical approaches. *Epilepsia* 1993;34:84–96.
27. Huott AD, Madison DS, Niedermeyer E. Occipital lobe epilepsy: a clinical and electroencephalographic study. *Eur Neurol* 1974;11:325–339.
28. Bauer J, Schuler P, Feistel H, et al. Blindness as an ictal phenomenon: investigations with EEG and SPECT in two patients suffering from epilepsy. *J Neurol* 1991; 238:44–46.
29. Munari C, Bonis A, Kochens S, et al. Eye movements and occipital seizures in man. *Acta Neurochir Suppl (Wien)* 1984;33:47–52.

30. Krieger HP, Wagman IH, Bender MB. Eye movements obtained from the subcortex of the occipital lobe. *Trans Am Neurol Assoc* 1955;80:209–213.
31. Gay AJ, Newman NM, Keltner JL, et al. *Eye movement disorders*. St. Louis: CV Mosby, 1974:21.
32. Engel J Jr. *Seizures and epilepsy*. Philadelphia: FA Davis, 1989:138.
33. Trevisan C, Belasso M. Su di un case di nistagmo epilettico. *Riv Neurol* 1961;31:64–70.
34. Kanazawa O, Sengoku A, Kawai I. Oculoclonic status epilepticus. *Epilepsia* 1989;30:121–123.
35. Gastaut H, Roger J. Formes inhabituelles de l'épilepsie: le nystagmus épileptique. *Rev Neurol* 1954;90:130–132.
36. Holtzman RNN, Goldensohn ES. Sensations of ocular movement in seizures originating in the occipital lobe. *Neurology* 1977;27:554–556.
37. Gastaut H. Un aspect meconnu des decharges neuroniques occipitales: la crise oculo-clonique ou "nystagmus épileptique." In: Alajouanine P, ed. *Les grandes activites du lobe occipital*. Paris: Masson et Cie, 1960: 169–185.
38. Bancaud J. Les crises epileptiques d'origine occipitale (etude stereo-electroencephalographique). *Rev Otoneuroophthalmol* 1969;41:299–311.
39. Williamson PD. Seizures with origin in the occipital or parietal lobes. In: Wolf P, ed. *Epileptic seizures and syndromes*. England: John Libbey, 1994:383–390.
40. Young GB, Blume WT. Painful epileptic seizures. *Brain* 1983;106:537–554.
41. Ajmone Marsan C, Ralston BL. *The epileptic seizure: its functional morphology and diagnostic significance*. Springfield, IL: Charles C. Thomas, 1957:211–215.
42. Wiesendanger M. Organization of secondary motor areas of cerebral cortex. In: Brooks VB, ed. *Handbook of physiology: the nervous system. II. Motor control*. Bethesda, MD: American Physiology Society, 1981:1121–1147.
43. Olivier A, Gloor P, Andermann F, et al. Occipitotemporal epilepsy studied with stereotaxically implanted depth electrodes and successfully treated by temporal resection. *Ann Neurol* 1982;11:428–432.
44. Babb TL, Halgren E, Wilson C, et al. Neuronal firing patterns during the spread of an occipital lobe seizure to the temporal lobes in man. *Electroencephalogr Clin Neurophysiol* 1981;51:104–107.
45. Gloor P. *The temporal lobe and limbic system*. New York: Oxford University Press, 1997:80–85.
46. Jones EG, Powell TP. An anatomical study of converging sensory pathways within the cerebral cortex of the monkey. *Brain* 1970;93:793–820.
47. Turner BH, Mishkin M, Knapp M. Organization of the amygdalopetal projections from modality-specific cortical association areas in the monkey. *J Comp Neurol* 1980;191:515–543.
48. Lisman JE. Bursts as a unit of neural information: making unreliable synapses reliable. *Trends Neurosci* 1997; 20:38–43.
49. Penfield W, Perot P. The brain's record of auditory and visual experience: a final summary and discussion. *Brain* 1963;86:595–696.
50. Gloor P, Olivier A, Quesney LF, et al. The role of the limbic system in experiential phenomena of temporal lobe epilepsy. *Ann Neurol* 1982;12:129–144.
51. Blume WT, Girvin JP, Stenerson P. Temporal neocortical role in ictal experiential phenomena. *Ann Neurol* 1993;33:105–107.
52. Blume WT, Kaibara M. *Atlas of adult electroencephalography*. New York: Raven Press, 1995:242–245.
53. Blume WT, Borghesi JL, Lemieux JF. Interictal indices of temporal seizure origin. *Ann Neurol* 1993;34: 703–709.
54. Blume WT, Kaibara M. Localization of epileptic foci in children. *Can J Neurol Sci* 1991;18:570–572.
55. Gastaut H. L'epilepsie benigne de l'enfant a pointe-ondes occipitales. *Rev Electroencephalogr Neurophysiol Clin* 1982;12:179–201.
56. Gastaut H, Zifkin BG. Benign epilepsy of childhood with occipital spike and wave complexes. In: Andermann F, Lugaresi E, eds. *Migraine and epilepsy*. Boston: Butterworths, 1987:47–81.
57. Aicardi J. *Epilepsy in children*. New York: Raven Press, 1994:151–152.
58. Camfield PR, Metrakos K, Andermann F. Basilar migraine, seizures, and severe epileptiform EEG abnormalities. *Neurology* 1978;28:584–588.
59. Andermann F. Clinical features of migraine–epilepsy syndromes. In: Andermann F, Lugaresi E, eds. *Migraine and epilepsy*. Boston: Butterworths, 1987:3–30.
60. Dvorkin GS, Andermann F, Carpenter S, et al. Classical migraine, intractable epilepsy, and multiple strokes: a syndrome related to mitochondrial encephalopathy. In: Andermann F, Lugaresi E, eds. *Migraine and epilepsy*. Boston: Butterworths, 1987:203–232.
61. Berkovic SF, Andermann F, Carpenter S, et al. Progressive myoclonus epilepsies: specific causes and diagnosis. *N Engl J Med* 1986;315:296–305.
62. Gobbi G, Ambrosetto G, Parmeggiani A, et al. The malignant variant of partial epilepsy with occipital spikes in childhood. *Epilepsia* 1991;32(Suppl 1):16–17.
63. Ambrosetto G, Antonini L, Tassinari CA. Occipital lobe seizures related to clinically asymptomatic celiac disease in adulthood. *Epilepsia* 1992;33:476–481.
64. Lanzkowsky P, Erlandson ME, Bezan AI. Isolated defect of folic acid absorption associated with mental retardation and cerebral calcification. *Blood* 1969; 34:452–465.
65. Tiacci C, D'Alessandro P, Cantisani TA, et al. Epilepsy with bilateral occipital calcifications: Sturge–Weber variant or a different encephalopathy? *Epilepsia* 1993; 34:528–539.
66. Tinuper P, Aguglia U, Pellissier JF, et al. Visual ictal phenomena in a case of Lafora disease proven by skin biopsy. *Epilepsia* 1983;24:214–218.
67. Carpenter S, Karpati G. Sweat gland duct cells in Lafora disease: diagnosis by skin biopsy. *Neurology* 1981;31:1564–1568.
68. Wohlwill FJ, Yakovlev PI. Histopathology of meningofacial angiomatosis (Sturge–Weber disease). *J Neuropathol Exp Neurol* 1957;16:341.
69. Andriola M, Stolfi J. Sturge–Weber syndrome: report of an atypical case. *Am J Dis Child* 1972;123:507.
70. Remillard GM, Ethier R, Andermann F. Temporal lobe epilepsy and perinatal occlusion of the posterior cerebral artery. *Neurology* 1974;24:1001–1009.
71. Blume WT. Differential diagnosis of epileptic seizures. In: Wada JA, Ellingson RJ, eds. *Handbook of electroencephalography and clinical neurophysiology. Clinical neurophysiology of epilepsy* (revised series, Vol. 4). Amsterdam: Elsevier, 1990:407–431.
72. Pranzatelli MR, Pedley TA. Differential diagnosis in children. In: Dam M, Gram L, eds. *Comprehensive epileptology*. New York: Raven Press, 1991:423–447.

Neocortical Epilepsies.
Advances in Neurology, Vol. 84,
edited by P. D. Williamson, A. M. Siegel,
D. W. Roberts, V. M. Thadani, and M. S. Gazzaniga.
Lippincott Williams & Wilkins, Philadelphia © 2000.

15

Parietal Lobe Epilepsy

Adrian M. Siegel and *Peter D. Williamson

Department of Neurology, University Hospital of Zürich, 8091 Zürich, Switzerland;
*Section of Neurology, Dartmouth–Hitchcock Medical Center,
Lebanon, New Hampshire 03756

The enormous growth in centers that specialize in the management and surgical treatment of epilepsy emphasizes the importance of differentiating the varieties of localization-related epilepsies (1,2). Perhaps in agreement with the early writings of John Hughlings Jackson (3), traditional attempts to subclassify these epilepsies have focused on their lobe of origin. Although legitimately it could be argued that such a classification method is largely artificial because seizures do not respect anatomic boundaries, which themselves are partially artificial, this anatomic classification does serve a purpose: It allows investigators in the field to develop a system of communication and comparison. For example, it has long been recognized that most complex partial (psychomotor) seizures begin in the temporal lobes (4–7). The well-defined syndrome of mesial temporal lobe epilepsy (MTLE) has been identified as the most common type of localization-related epilepsy encountered in adult populations (8–11). Similarly, various seizures originating in the frontal lobes have clinical characteristics that differentiate them from the more common temporal lobe seizures (12–19). Recent reports also identified early signs and symptoms that help identify seizures originating in the occipital lobes, recognizing that multiple different potential spread patterns will define subsequent clinical events (20–22). Similarly, several reports and reviews described the clinical seizure characteristics and electroencephalographic (EEG) and neuroimaging findings of patients with carefully documented parietal lobe seizure origin (23–27); however, parietal lobe epilepsy has proven more difficult to define accurately (23,24).

EPIDEMIOLOGY

There is a paucity of epidemiologic data on patients with parietal lobe epilepsy. Moreover, studies that addressed epidemiologic issues suffered from methodologic deficits, in that they either included insufficiently confirmed cases (28) or studied exclusively surgical candidates (7,29).

Incidence

The first large epidemiologic study was performed by Gibbs and Gibbs (28), who reported an incidence of parietal lobe seizures of about 5% among patients with partial epilepsy. In recent comprehensive surgical series, parietal lobe seizures have been rare, constituting no more than 6% of all partial seizures (29,30).

Age at Onset

The early epidemiologic study by Gibbs and Gibbs (28) indicated a peak for parietal lobe epilepsy at an early age. The onset of parietal lobe seizures occurred in the first year of life in about 18% of the patients; however, the study by Gibbs and Gibbs must be interpreted cautiously because the diagnosis was based only on scalp EEG. In a large surgical series of 82 patients with nontumoral parietal lobe epilepsy, the age at seizure onset ranged from 1 to 50 years (mean, 14.1 years) (26).

Etiology

Among patients with parietal lobe epilepsy, brain tumors are the most common etiology. In large surgical series of tumoral epilepsy, about 10% of patients suffered from tumors of the parietal lobe (31,32). Compared with tumors localized elsewhere in the brain, tumors of the parietal lobe evidence a high epileptogenicity. In two large surgical series, parietal lobe tumors caused epilepsy in 46% and 68% of the patients (31,32).

Nontumoral lesions associated with parietal lobe seizures have been rare. In a surgical series of nontumoral epilepsy, parietal lobe lesions were found in only 3% of the patients (33). In 82 patients with nontumoral parietal lobe epilepsy, a history of head trauma and birth trauma as risk factors were found in 43% and in 16% of patients, respectively (26). The presumed etiology in 21% of these patients comprised a history of encephalitis, febrile convulsions, gunshot wounds to the head, forme fruste of tuberous sclerosis, hamartoma, vascular malformations, tuberculoma, arachnoid or porencephalic cysts, microgyria, and posttraumatic thrombosis of the middle cerebral artery. The etiology remained unknown in 20% of the patients.

CLINICAL FEATURES OF PARIETAL LOBE EPILEPSY

The epileptic significance of localized paresthesias has been recognized since antiquity (34). In the last century, several authors reported patients with tumors of the parietal lobe that caused seizures with paresthesias (35,36). The localizing and lateralizing significance of such "sensory fits" have been documented more vigorously in recent years (37–41).

Like all partial seizures, parietal lobe seizures consist of subjective and objective components. In parietal lobe seizures, the most common subjective sensations or auras are paresthesias, usually numbness and tingling, but also a sensation of "pins and needles" and, rarely, crawling or itching. In a series of 82 patients with parietal lobe seizures, 94% of the patients exhibited auras (26). Ictal paresthesias, however, occurred in fewer than half of the patients reported in recent parietal lobe epilepsy series (23,24). Furthermore, these somatosensory symptoms were not always lateralized. When lateralized, they were not always contralateral to the side of seizure origin, presumably reflecting activity in secondary sensory systems (23).

Objective manifestations of seizures confined to the parietal lobes consist mainly of positive or negative motor phenomena, such as focal motor clonic activity, head and eye deviation, and posturing of extremities. In contrast to frontal lobe epilepsy with predominantly nocturnal seizures, there is no clear part of the day during which parietal lobe seizures predominate (42).

Sveinbjornsdottir and Duncan (43) extensively reviewed the literature on parietal lobe seizures. They described paresthetic, dysesthetic, and painful seizures. They also described additional parietal lobe symptoms, including sexual sensations, apraxias, and disturbances of body image. Gustatory hallucinations have been associated not only with seizures or stimulation in the insula and the amygdala, but also with seizure activity in the parietal operculum (44). Other symptoms include asomatognosia, particularly if seizures are confined to the nondominant parietal lobe, and the feeling of body rotation (crise giratoires). Seizures confined to the dominant parietal lobe may produce disturbances in language function that are demonstrable with specific testing. One of our patients with a neurocytoma in the parietal lobe exhibited inhibitory motor seizures or ictal hemiplegia (patient 2).

The subjective ictal phenomenon of pain has been recognized for more than 100 years (45,46). Young and Blume (47) examined ictal pain in patients with this symptom as part of their seizures and identified three types of pain. The most common variety of pain was a burning dysesthesia, which involved part or all of the hemibody contralateral to the parietal lobe of seizure origin. Abdominal pain was the second most common type and was associated with temporal lobe seizure origin; however, abdominal pain also has been associated with parietal lobe seizure origin (24,43). Ictal head pain was the least common variety and lacked localizing value. We recently examined epileptic pain and reported contralateral peripheral dysesthesias and abdominal pain and unilateral head pain in seizures of parietal seizure origin (48).

Episodes that fulfill the diagnostic criteria for panic attacks have been described in patients with parietal lobe seizure origin (49). Rarely, parietal lobe seizures are precipitated by complex somatosensory afferent input (23) (see patient 1 in this chapter).

Much of the parietal lobe may be clinically silent in terms of seizure manifestations, however, or these may be demonstrable only under extraordinary circumstances. For example, while undergoing electrocorticography under local anesthesia, a patient of Penfield and Jasper suffered an electrically induced seizure that remained restricted to the parietal lobe (4). During the seizure, two-point discrimination was impaired in the contralateral hand, but it returned to normal when the seizure subsided. The patient was unaware of any specific symptoms.

All patients from two recent studies of parietal lobe epilepsy had probable epileptogenic lesions detected by magnetic resonance imaging (MRI) (23,24). The signs and symptoms of the patients' parietal lobe seizures were retrospectively analyzed. Although some findings suggested parietal lobe seizures, most patients displayed no clinical seizure manifestations until after the seizures had spread beyond the parietal lobe. These observations led to two conclusions. First, most of the parietal lobe is clinically silent in terms of seizures; second, most patients with parietal lobe seizure origin will not have a clinically localizable form of localization-related epilepsy. These observations, coupled with misleading scalp EEG findings,

almost certainly explain some of the surgical failures in patients with normal neuroimaging findings who were studied with invasive EEG that neglected coverage of the parietal lobe.

Clinical Characteristics of Seizures Originating from Different Parietal Regions

Certain clinical characteristics of seizures indicate the region of seizure origin within the parietal lobe. Seizures beginning in the anterior part are associated most often with contralateral sensorimotor phenomena, whereas seizures of posterior parietal origin are associated with automatisms, unresponsiveness, and other complex clinical manifestations (24,25). These seizures of posterior origin also have been described as *psychoparetic,* implying a psychic aura such as déjà vu or fear followed by an impairment of consciousness and motor arrest (25). Spatial disorientation is more common in seizures originating in the inferior parietal lobe. Vertiginous sensations are associated predominantly with seizures of temporoparietal origin (26). Seizures from the parietal operculum may be manifested in gustatory sensations. Some patients with parietal lobe seizure origin may experience elementary visual hallucinations or ictal amaurosis as the initial seizure symptoms, indicating a spread to the occipital lobe from "silent" posterior parietal foci (23,24). Seizures originating in the temporoparietooccipital region may be associated with complex visual symptoms.

Spread Pathways of Parietal Lobe Seizures

Most objective manifestations of parietal lobe seizures reflect seizure spread outside the parietal lobe (1) anteriorly into the frontal lobe (2), inferiorly into the temporal lobe, or (3) posteriorly into the occipital lobe, with seizure characteristics corresponding to the direction of spread. As such, tonic motor activity, automatisms, or both may occur in patients with parietal lobe seizure origin. Asymmetric tonic posturing was associated with a spread from the parietal lobe to the supplementary motor area (SMA) in a depth electrode study (23), but this finding was specifically not observed in another study of parietal lobe seizures using invasive monitoring (50).

Seizures that originate in the parietal lobes and spread to medial temporal structures have been well documented using intracranial recording (23,50). The clinical seizure characteristics of this event resemble temporal lobe seizures. Two patients with unsuspected parietal lobe seizure origin underwent unsuccessful temporal lobe surgeries in the Yale series (23), as did two patients from the series reported by Ho et al. (25). Parietal lobe seizure origin in the two patients from the Yale series was considered likely after parietal lobe lesions were detected using previously unavailable MRI. This was verified following successful surgery that removed the lesion and a limited area of surrounding brain. Ictal single-photon emission computed tomography (SPECT) was used to determine the parietal lobe seizure origin of the two unsuccessfully operated patients in the study by Ho et al. (25).

Electroencephalographic Findings

In a study of 11 patients with parietal lobe epilepsy documented by intracranial EEG, Williamson et al. (23) reported normal, nonspecific, or misleading scalp EEG findings. Scalp EEG clearly localized or lateralized the side of seizure origin in only one of 11 patients (23). In another scalp EEG study of 66 patients (26), interictal discharges were recorded frontocentroparietal in 33%, parietoposterior-temporal in 14%, parietal in 9%, parieto-occipital in 9%, fronto-centrotemporal in 4.5%, frontotemporoparietal in 4.5%, hemispheric with a posterior maximum in 9%, and bilateral in 4.5% of the patients. EEG was normal in 7.5%, and secondary bilateral synchrony was found in 32% of the patients. Salanova et al. (26) observed ictal discharges predominantly lateralized with a maximum over the centroparietal region or over the posterior head region.

Occasionally, the sleep EEG gives some nonspecific aid in the diagnosis of parietal lobe epilepsy. Whereas extrinsic stimuli dur-

ing non-rapid eye movement (REM) sleep (stage 2) usually induce vertex waves and K-complexes, the same stimuli may trigger seizures from parietal foci.

Neuropsychologic Examination

In a series of 11 patients with parietal lobe epilepsy (23), six had lateralized neuropsychological findings. Among these, the abnormality was congruent with the side of seizure origin in only three patients. Neuropsychological testing did not indicate the hemisphere of seizure origin in five patients. The most common neuropsychological deficits in patients with parietal lobe epilepsy were impairments in spatial ability, difficulties in the reproduction of complex pictorial material, left–right confusion, and hemispatial neglect.

ILLUSTRATIVE CASE REPORTS

Patient 1

This 41-year-old woman began having seizures when she was 13 years of age. The first episode consisted of left-sided numbness and left hemianopsia lasting several minutes, followed by a headache. She was diagnosed with migraine. These typical episodes ultimately evolved into generalized tonic–clonic seizures, and the diagnosis of epilepsy was established. After initiation of treatment with antiepileptic drugs, the seizures changed. She no longer had somatosensory symptoms. She experienced complete visual loss before some, but not all, seizures. She then had generalized tonic, but not clonic, motor activity. In most seizures, consciousness was lost, but when she was aware during seizures, she could hear but could not see or speak. Her seizures were brief, lasting about 15 seconds, but frequent, occurring many times daily. Several times a month, seizures occurred almost continuously for several hours. If in a standing position, she would fall and sustain injuries, some near fatal. Multiple antiepileptic drugs, alone and in combination, failed to control her seizures. She was evaluated for surgery. Interictal and ictal scalp EEG revealed an active right parietal spike focus (Fig. 15.1). This patient was the only one

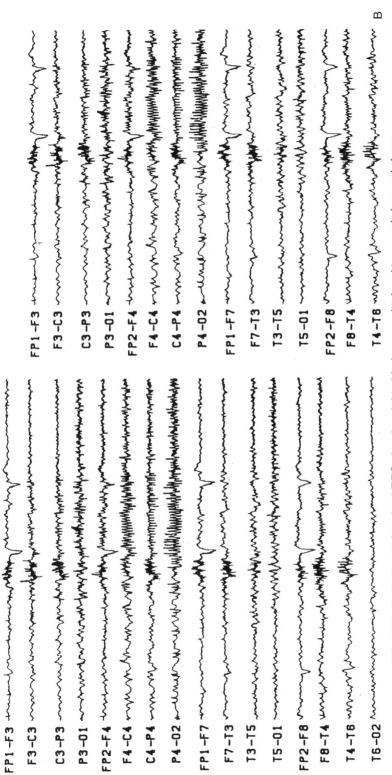

FIG. 15.1. A: Patient 1: Interictal EEG showing right-sided parasagittal and temporal slow and sharp waves. **B:** Patient 1: Ictal EEG showing right parietal discharge.

from the Yale series (23) who evidenced a relatively localized and lateralized EEG. There were less active, independent, sharp wave foci in the right temporal and left frontal regions. Ictal scalp recordings were obscured by muscle artifact. Videotaped seizures revealed tonic contraction of facial muscles, producing a grimace or pucker, tonic contraction of the hands and arms with clenched fists, and both arms held in flexion across her chest. Both legs were held in tonic extension. There was consistent right head deviation. During monitoring, seizures frequently occurred when she was trying to open a container or package. Only then was it learned that the patient was well aware that this type of kinesthetic input frequently precipitated seizures. Cranial CT was normal. Retrospectively, MRI from an early research 0.3-Tesla machine revealed a possible right parietal convexity lesion. Subdural and depth electrodes were placed to sample the left and right medial frontal regions, right medial and lateral occipital regions, right medial and lateral parietal regions, and right medial and anterior temporal lobe regions. Numerous subclinical and typical clinical seizures were recorded. Subclinical seizures were well localized to the right parietal convexity, but clinical seizures were associated with rapid spread to both supplementary motor areas. Early occipital lobe seizure spread occurred in some seizures, but ictal amaurosis was not described during intracranial recording.

At surgery, an intraaxial lesion was found in the middle of the right parietal convexity. Pathological diagnosis was hamartoma. During the first postoperative year, she had a few brief seizures, but then she became seizure free and has remained so for the past 14 years.

Comment

This patient, whose initial presentation was strongly suggestive of migraine, was ultimately found to have parietal lobe epilepsy. She had the unusual finding of kinesthetic precipitation of seizures. She also clearly described ictal amaurosis at the onset of some seizures, a symptom most often associated with occipital

lobe seizure origin (16). Presumably, this symptom was due to posterior seizure spread, but we were unable to document this during invasive monitoring. Finally, the consistent asymmetric tonic seizures, although more typical of frontal lobe seizure origin, have been described in well-documented, parietal lobe epilepsy, both with and without evidence of spread to the supplementary motor area (23,50).

Patient 2

This 37-year-old, right-handed man had a 3-month history of recurrent spells consisting of an unpleasant burning sensation in his right hand that would spread up his arm and into his face. His trunk and right leg were not involved. As soon as he experienced the painful dysesthesia, he developed right-sided weakness and could not speak. Occasionally, he also developed clonic twitching in his right face but no other tonic or clonic activity. The ictal aphasia and right hemiplegia would persist for as long as 10 minutes during the postictal period.

An MRI showed a lesion in the left parietal lobe that extended into the left posterior frontal lobe (Fig. 15.2). He was evaluated for surgery. Recorded seizures were described as showing ictal hemiplegia and aphasia associated with burning dysesthesias on the right, followed by prolonged right postictal hemiplegia and aphasia. There was no tonic or clonic motor activity. Interictal and ictal scalp EEGs provided no useful information. An 8 × 8 subdural grid was placed over the lesion for functional mapping and seizure recording. Resection of the entire lesion could not be done because of the risks to language and motor function. The region of brain and underlying lesion in the parietal lobe from which the intracranially recorded seizures appeared to originate consistently was partially resected. Pathological diagnosis was neurocytoma. Although postoperative seizures initially occurred infrequently, he was readmitted to the hospital 1 year after surgery, having seizures without pain but otherwise typical; these seizures were occurring every 30 minutes. He was ultimately

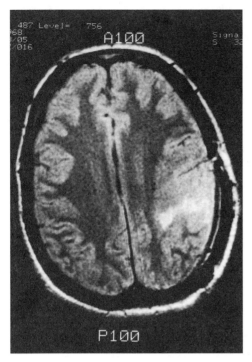

FIG. 15.2. Patient 2: MRI showing left parietal lesion. Pathological diagnosis was neurocytoma.

cent to the midline. The meningioma was resected. Four months later, he had two generalized convulsive seizures that were controlled by medications, but he then developed unusual seizures consisting of nausea, an "alien hand" on the left that he did not recognize as his own, loss of motor control on the left, and mild confusion. Four years ago, the character of the seizures changed dramatically. They began as described, but he would then develop severe cramping, left-sided abdominal pain, and intense "pins and needles" sensations in his left hand, arm, trunk, and leg, thus sparing the face. The seizures occurred weekly and would last for hours or until he was given intravenous benzodiazepines. Otherwise, seizures were not controlled with a variety of antiepileptic drugs, either alone and in combination. He was evaluated for surgery. An MRI revealed encephalomalacia in the right high parietal convexity extending to the midline (Fig. 15.3). Scalp

much better controlled by medications. Currently, 4 years after surgery, he continues to have one mild seizure per month.

Comment

This patient provides an example of lateralized ictal pain in seizures originating in the parietal lobe. The elimination of pain, but not the seizures, following a limited parietal cortical resection suggests that this symptom of pain was of parietal lobe origin. The ictal and postictal aphasia are not surprising findings, but ictal hemiplegia is an uncommon phenomenon.

Patient 3

Sixteen years previously, this 57-year-old man began having seizures consisting of 1-minute periods of confusion and disorientation. He was found to have a large right-sided meningioma overlying the parietal lobe adja-

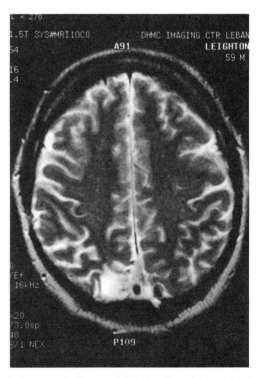

FIG. 15.3. Patient 3: MRI showing right parietal encephalomalacia at site of meningioma resection.

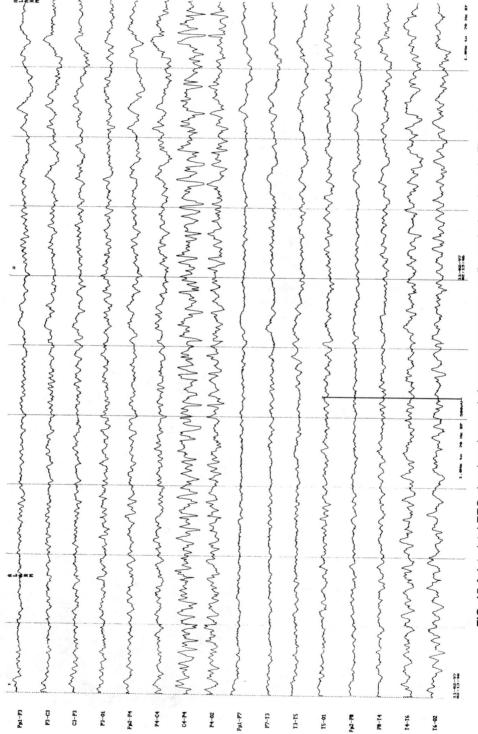

FIG. 15.4. Interictal EEG showing slow and sharp waves corresponding to lesion shown in Fig. 15.3.

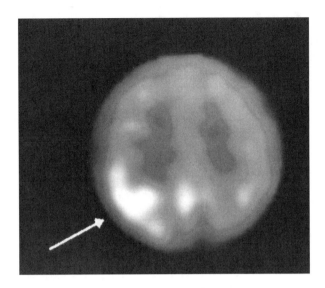

FIG. 15.5. Patient 3: Ictal SPECT scan showing increased radioactive tracer uptake in region of MRI and EEG abnormalities shown in Figs. 15.3 and 15.4.

EEG revealed continuous interictal sharp and slow activity over the right parietal lobe (Fig. 15.4). Ictal SPECT was strongly positive in the right parietal region (Fig. 15.5). During the evaluation, the alien hand sensation was described during the seizures, and the agonizing left abdominal pain was dramatically documented.

He underwent resection of the gliotic parietal tissue after intracranial subdural grid recording documented focal parietal lobe seizure origin. Immediately postsurgery, he developed touch-sensitive, left-sided choreoathetosis that resolved spontaneously in 1 week. Six weeks after surgery, he developed a progressive left hemiparesis over several days, culminating in an isolated left focal motor clonic seizure, followed by hemiparesis with a strong apractic component. MRI showed postoperative changes and right centroparietal edema. This complication, which was thought to be due to a cerebral venous occlusion, resolved completely over 3 weeks. There have been no habitual seizures during the year since surgery.

Comment

This patient provides a dramatic example of parietal lobe seizures with severe abdominal pain. This stoic former tractor–trailer driver was in such excruciating pain during seizures that reviewing his videotaped events was an unpleasant experience. The other ictal symptom of an alien hand is extremely uncommon. The unusual postoperative complications were not expected, but fortunately they resolved completely over time.

SUMMARY AND CONCLUSION

When symptoms such as lateralized paresthesias or pain occur prominently and early in partial seizures, parietal lobe seizure origin should be suspected. Most patients with parietal lobe seizures, however, have no symptoms or signs suggesting the parietal lobe. In the absence of detectable epileptogenic lesions, these patients without clinical seizure characteristics suggesting parietal lobe origin can present with misleading findings, resulting in erroneous localization, which can, in turn, lead to ineffective surgical intervention (23,25). Although ictal SPECT might provide vital evidence of parietal lobe seizure origin (25), as noted previously, this technology also can produce misleading data in some patients (52).

Even when parietal lobe seizure origin is suspected, in the absence of a structural lesion, documenting this with invasive monitoring can be difficult. The parietal lobes, like the frontal lobes, are large, diffuse structures, and the potential for sampling error is high (19). Spread patterns are unpredictable and can result in false localization (23). Even with extensive and repetitive invasive studies, localization can prove elusive (53). No well-documented series of patients with non-lesional parietal lobe epilepsy in the modern literature who have been cured by surgery have been reported as a result of a combination of the rarity of the condition, the lack of correct recognition, as well as the difficulty of localization.

Patients with medically intractable parietal lobe seizures, however, can experience excellent surgical results (23,24). Postoperative parietal lobe symptoms and signs, even when extreme, are usually not enduring (patient 3). One of our patients, however, did develop a chronic pain syndrome (48).

REFERENCES

1. Lüders HO. *Epilepsy surgery.* New York: Raven Press, 1992.
2. Engel J Jr, ed. *Surgical treatment of the epilepsies,* 2nd ed. New York: Raven Press, 1993:515–668.
3. Jackson JH. *Selected writings of John Hughlings Jackson.* London: Staples Press, 1874.
4. Penfield W, Jasper H. *Epilepsy and the functional anatomy of the human brain.* Boston: Little, Brown, 1954.
5. Ajmone-Marsan C, Ralston BL. *The epileptic seizure: its functional morphology and diagnostic significance.* Springfield, IL: Charles C. Thomas, 1957:211–215.
6. Bancaud J, Talairach J, Bonis A, et al. *La stereo-électro-encephalographie dans l'épilepsie.* Paris: Masson, 1965.
7. Rasmussen T. Surgical treatment of patients with complex partial seizures In: Penry JK, Daly DD, eds. *Complex partial seizures and their treatment.* New York: Raven Press, 1975:415–449.
8. Williamson PD, French JA, Thadani VM, et al. Characteristics of medial temporal lobe epilepsy. II. Interictal and ictal scalp electroencephalography, neuropsychological testing, neuroimaging, surgical results, and pathology. *Ann Neurol* 1993;34:781–787.
9. French JA, Williamson PD, Thadani VM, et al. Characteristics of medial temporal lobe epilepsy. I. Results of history and physical examination. *Ann Neurol* 1993;34:774–780.
10. Engel J Jr, Williamson PD, Wieser HG. Mesial temporal lobe epilepsy. In: Engel J Jr, Pedley TA, eds. *Epilepsy: a comprehensive textbook.* Philadelphia: Lippincott–Raven, 1997:2417–2426.
11. Williamson PD, Thadani VM, French JA, et al. Medial temporal lobe epilepsy: videotape analysis of objective clinical seizure characteristics. *Epilepsia* 1998;39:118.
12. Williamson PD, Spencer DD, Spencer SS, et al. Complex partial seizures of frontal lobe origin. *Ann Neurol* 1985;18:497–504.
13. Waterman K, Purves SJ, Kosaka B, et al. An epileptic syndrome caused by mesial frontal lobe foci. *Neurology* 1987;37:577–582.
14. Bancaud J, Talairach J. Clinical semiology of frontal lobe seizures. In: Chauvel P, Delgado-Escueta AV, Halgren E, Bancaud J, eds. *Frontal lobe seizures and epilepsies. Advances in Neurology,* vol 57. New York: Raven Press, 1992:3–58.
15. Wieser HG, Swartz BE, Delgado-Escueta AV, et al. Differentiating frontal lobe seizures from temporal lobe seizures. In: Chauvel P, Delgado-Escueta AV, Halgren E, Bancaud J, eds. *Frontal lobe seizures and epilepsies. Advances in Neurology,* vol 57. New York: Raven Press, 1992:267–285.
16. Williamson PD. Frontal lobe seizures: problems of diagnosis and classification. In: Chauvel P, Delgado-Escueta AV, Halgren E, Bancaud J, eds. *Frontal lobe seizures and epilepsies. Advances in Neurology,* vol 57. New York: Raven Press, 1992:289–309.
17. Williamson PD. Frontal lobe epilepsy: some clinical characteristics. In: Jasper HH, Riggio S, Goldman-Rakic PS, eds. *Epilepsy and the functional anatomy of the frontal lobe. Advances in Neurology,* vol 66. New York: Raven Press, 1995:127–152.
18. Williamson PD, Engel J Jr, Munari C. Anatomic classification of localization-related epilepsies. In: Engel J Jr, Pedley TA, eds. *Epilepsy: a comprehensive textbook.* Philadelphia: Lippincott–Raven, 1997:2405–2416.
19. Williamson PD, Engel J Jr. Complex partial seizures. In: Engel J Jr, Pedley TA, eds. *Epilepsy: a comprehensive textbook.* Philadelphia: Lippincott–Raven, 1997:557–566.
20. Williamson PD, Thadani VM, Darcey TM. Occipital lobe epilepsy: clinical characteristics, seizure spread patterns, and results of surgery. *Ann Neurol* 1992;31:3–13.
21. Salanova V, Andermann F, Olivier A, et al. Occipital lobe epilepsy: electroclinical manifestations, electrocorticography, cortical stimulation, and outcome in 42 patients treated between 1930 and 1991. *Brain* 1992;115:1655–1680.
22. Blume WT. Occipital lobe epilepsies. In: Lüders HO, ed. *Epilepsy surgery.* New York: Raven Press, 1991:167–171.
23. Williamson PD, Boon PA, Thadani VM, et al. Parietal lobe epilepsy: diagnostic considerations and results of surgery. *Ann Neurol* 1992;31:193–201.
24. Cascino GD, Hulihan JF, Sharbrough FW, et al. Parietal lobe lesional epilepsy: electroclinical correlation and operative outcome. *Epilepsia* 1993;34:522–527.
25. Ho SS, Berkovic SF, Newton MR, et al. Parietal lobe epilepsy: clinical features and seizure localization by ictal SPECT. *Neurology* 1994;44:2277–2284.
26. Salanova V, Andermann F, Rasmussen T, et al. Parietal lobe epilepsy: clinical manifestations and outcome in 82 patients treated surgically between 1929 and 1988. *Brain* 1995;118:607–628.
27. Salanova V, Andermann F, Rasmussen T, et al. Tumoural parietal lobe epilepsy: clinical manifestations and outcome in 34 patients treated between 1934 and 1988. *Brain* 1995;118:1289–1304.
28. Gibbs FA, Gibbs EL. *Atlas of electroencephalography,* vol 2. *Epilepsy.* Cambridge: Addison-Wesley, 1952:163–252.

29. Rasmussen T. Surgery for epilepsy arising in regions other than the temporal and frontal lobes. In: Purpura DP, Penry JK, Walter RD, eds. *Neurosurgical management of the epilepsies.* New York: Raven Press, 1975: 207–226.

30. Rasmussen T. Focal epilepsies of nontemporal and nonfrontal origin. In: Wieser HG, Elger CE, eds. *Presurgical evaluation of epilepsies: basics, techniques, implications.* Berlin: Springer-Verlag, 1987:301–305.

31. Penfield W, Erickson TC, Tarlov I. Relation of intracranial tumors and symptomatic epilepsy. *Arch Neurol Psychiatr* 1940;44:300–315.

32. White JC, Liu CT, Mixter WJ. Focal epilepsy: a statistical study of its causes and the results of surgical treatment. I. Epilepsy secondary to intracranial tumors. *N Engl J Med* 1948;238:891–899.

33. Bhatia R, Kollevold T. A follow-up study of 91 patients operated on for focal epilepsy. *Epilepsia* 1976;17:61–66.

34. Temkin O. *The falling sickness.* Baltimore: Johns Hopkins Press, 1945.

35. Bremer L, Carson NB. A case of brain tumor (angioma cavernosum), causing spastic paralysis and attacks of tonic spasms. Operation. *Amer J Med Sciences* 1890; 100:219–242.

36. McNaughton FL, Rasmussen T. Criteria for selection of patients for neurosurgical treatment. *Adv Neurol* 1975; 8:37–48.

37. Foerster O, Penfield W. The structural basis of traumatic epilepsy and results of radical operation. *Brain* 1930;53: 99–119.

38. Foerster O. The cerebral cortex in man. *Lancet* 1931;2: 309–312.

39. Cushing H. The parietal tumors: inaugural sensory fits. In: Cushing H, ed. *Meningiomas: their classification, regional behaviors, life history, and surgical end results.* Springfield, IL: Charles C. Thomas, 1938: 632–656.

40. Penfield W, Jasper H. *Epilepsy and the functional anatomy of the human brain.* London: J & A Churchill, 1954:773.

41. Mauguière F, Courjon J. Somatosensory epilepsy: a review of 127 cases. *Brain* 1978;101:307–332.

42. Janz D. The grand mal epilepsies and the sleeping-waking cycle. *Epilepsia* 1996;3:69–109.

43. Sveinbjornsdottir S, Duncan JS. Parietal and occipital lobe epilepsy: a review. *Epilepsia* 1993;34:493–521.

44. Hauser-Hauw C, Bancaud J. Gustatory hallucinations in epileptic seizures: electrophysiological, clinical, and anatomical correlates. *Brain* 1987;110:339–359.

45. Reynolds JR. *Epilepsy: its symptoms, treatment, and relation to other chronic convulsive diseases.* London: J & A Churchill, 1861.

46. Gowers W. *Epilepsy and other chronic convulsive disorders: their causes, symptoms, and treatment.* London: J & A Churchill, 1901:29–58.

47. Young GB, Blume WT. Painful epileptic seizures. *Brain* 1983;106:537–554.

48. Siegel AM, Williamson PD, Roberts DW, et al. Localized pain associated with seizure origin in the parietal lobe. *Epilepsia* 1999;40:845–855.

49. Alemayehu S, Bergey GK, Barry E, et al. Panic attacks as ictal manifestations of parietal lobe seizures. *Epilepsia* 1995;38:824–830.

50. Geier S, Bancaud J, Talairach J, et al. Ictal tonic postural changes and automatisms of the upper limb during epileptic parietal lobe discharges. *Epilepsia* 1977;18: 517–524.

51. Kolb B, Whishaw IQ. *Fundamentals of human neuropsychology.* San Francisco: WH Freeman, 1980.

52. Thadani VM, Darcey TM, Williamson PD, et al. Consistent and inconsistent findings with ictal SPECT. *Epilepsia* 1995;36 (Suppl 4):14.

53. Siegel AM, Roberts DW, Thadani VM, et al. The role of intracranial electrode re-evaluation in epilepsy patients failing initial invasive monitoring. *Epilepsia* 2000; 41:571–580.

Neocortical Epilepsies.
Advances in Neurology, Vol. 84,
edited by P.D. Williamson, A.M. Siegel,
D.W. Roberts, V.M. Thadani, and M.S. Gazzaniga.
Lippincott Williams & Wilkins, Philadelphia © 2000.

16

Semiology of Neocortical Temporal Lobe Epilepsy

Heinz Gregor Wieser

Neurologische Klinik, Universitätsspital Zürich, 8091 Zürich, Switzerland

The semiology of neocortical temporal lobe epilepsy (NTLE) is a controversial topic. Epileptic seizures and syndromes of the temporal lobe (TL) may be divided into the following types:

The syndrome of mesiotemporal epilepsy (MTLE)
So-called "cryptogenic" TL epilepsy
Lateral NTLE

The syndrome of MTLE is now widely recognized and accepted. It is common and often drug resistant but surgically remediable. Its clinical features are relatively homogeneous, as are the findings on investigational tests, including histology, magnetic resonance imagine (MRI), positron emission tomography (PET), and electroencephalography (EEG). It can be characterized in terms of genetic and environmental factors, natural history, pathogenesis, and prognosis. Most important, however, is its association with the histopathological finding of hippocampal sclerosis (1–3).

At present, it is difficult to estimate the incidence of so-called "cryptogenic" TLE (i.e., TLE without a pathological substrate). Available figures from surgical series are heavily biased, as are the figures of the recently identified familial TLE syndrome with a benign course (4). Whereas in Mathieson's surgical series no histopathological abnormality was found in 173 of 857 (20%) resected temporal lobes (5), more recent reviews give a lower

figure, about 10% (6–13). In our 1993 Zürich study, no histologic abnormality was found in only 2% of 224 available mesial TL tissue specimens (14).

Because the surgical outcome of patients in whom abnormalities are not found is usually poorer compared with those with histologic abnormalities, it cannot be ruled out that in patients without histopathologic abnormalities who did not become seizure free following TL resection, the origin of the seizure was not the TL. Therefore, in the near future, this category might disappear in surgical series with more sophisticated diagnoses.

TLE is etiologically most often a "lesional" epilepsy and NTLE an epilepsy with lesions in the temporal lobe other than hippocampal sclerosis. "Lesions," of course, differ with respect to their nature, size, and localization. Furthermore, they may be well circumscribed or more diffuse and without easy-to-define borders.

In the Montreal series of surgically excised epileptogenic temporal lobes (1928–1973), of 878 patients Mathieson (5) studied 857 and found in 202 patients the following "discrete focal lesions":

Gliomas and gangliogliomas (n = 105)
Meningocerebral cicatrix and remote contusion (n = 39)
Vascular malformations of the brain or pia (n = 19)

Hamartomas (n = 14)
Residuum of cerebral abscess (n = 10)
Tumors other than gliomas (n = 10)
Tuberous sclerosis and formes frustes (n = 4)
Residuum of old infarct (n = 1)

Even higher percentages of lesions were found in our neuropathological study of the amygdalohippocampectomy series. In 1993, Plate et al. (14) enrolled 247 patients with mesial temporal lobe resections and found neoplasms and microscopic clusters of oligodendroglia-like foci of 30 to 100 cells (interpreted as precursor lesions for neuroepithelial tumors) in 126 patients (51%). In the updated study (14a), in a total of 405 patients, we found 41% neoplasms, 11% vascular malformations, 3% hamartomas, and 2% other pathological abnormalities. The remaining subjects had hippocampal sclerosis alone (33%; patients with dual pathology were not listed under the category of hippocampal sclerosis), were without significant pathology, or the specimen could not be analyzed reliably because it was needed for other studies (10%).

Thus, neuroectodermal tumors, predominantly low-grade gliomas and gangliogliomas, are frequently encountered in TLE. In the "lesional" TLE group, *focal dysplasia* (15), *dysembryoplastic neuroepithelial tumors* (DNET) (16,17), and several other types of *cortical dysgenesis* (Table 16.1) have gained increased importance as a result of improved in vivo diagnosis owing to the advent of high-resolution MRI (18).

At present, however, *microdysgenesis* is still not visible on neuroimaging and remains a diagnosis based on pathology. It is thus likely that several subtle forms of migrational disorders are underdiagnosed in most series (19). Without histology this is self-evident, but even in surgical series, the pathologically abnormal tissue might be left in situ in some patients, in particular those with a poorer outcome. It would be worthwhile to restudy in particular all patients who did not become seizure free following a limited mesial temporal resection.

Although related to MTLE at a first glance, dysgenesis of the archicortex (duplication/dis-

TABLE 16.1. *Classification scheme for cortical dysgenesis presenting with epilepsy*

Abnormalities of gyration (agyria, macrogyria, polymicrogyria; focal, diffuse, or associated with a cleft; and minor gyral abnormalities)
Heterotopias (subependymal; subcortical gray-matter; nodular, diffuse, laminar; subarachnoid glioneuronal heterotopias)
Tuberous sclerosis
Focal cortical dysplasia/microdysgenesis
Cortical dysgenesis associated with neoplasia (DNET, ganglioglioma, low-grade astrocytoma)
Dysgenesis of the archicortex (duplication/dispersion of the dentate fascia, i.e., most probably some forms of hippocampal sclerosis)

DNET, dysembryoplastic neuroepithelial tumors.
From Raymond AA, Fish DR, Sisodiya SM, et al. The developmental basis of epilepsy. In: Shorvon S, Dreifuss F, Fish D, Thomas D, eds. *The treatment of epilepsy.* London: Blackwell Science, 1996:20–54, with permission.

persion of the dentate fascia) is a good example to illustrate that subtle changes most probably escaped description in many older studies. Duplication/dispersion of the dentate fascia is a particularly interesting and, at the same time, a controversial issue. Whereas experimental work suggests that this phenomenon occurs as a consequence of seizures, some authors have listed arguments in favor of a migrational defect. Arguments for both prenatal and postnatal mechanisms have been put forward as has evidence for being both the cause and the effect of epilepsy. The arguments in favor of a migrational defect are the following (20):

The occurrence of granule cells in the molecular layer suggests that they have migrated beyond their target position.
The presence of granule cells in the hilus of the dentate gyrus suggests that some cells have not completed their normal migration.
Their elongated form is reminiscent of developing forms.
Their alignment in vertically oriented rows is similar to the radial arrangement of migrating cells (21,22).

Although the older literature in fact did not pay much attention to this type of pathology, it might be a frequent finding. Mello et al. (23), for example, in 34 TL specimens from patients with TLE, found that the granule cells were normally arranged in 44%, generally dispersed in 38%, and displayed in a bilaminar arrangement in 18%; varying degrees of hippocampal sclerosis were observed in all cases.

In an attempt to study whether we had overlooked this phenomenon of disorganization of the dentate gyrus in TLE, we recently reviewed the histopathological specimens of 81 patients with a diagnosis of hippocampal gliosis from our series of patients with selective amygdalo hippocampectomy (AHE) (currently 405). The histopathological evaluation assessed the following hippocampal abnormalities, including a ranking of the degree of the pathology: gliosis, neuronal loss, alteration of the hippocampal Cornu Ammonis (CA) regions, and granule cell dispersion of the fascia dentata.

To correlate the histopathology with clinical data, an additional 32 AHE patients without hippocampal pathology were included in the statistical analyses. The types and the degrees of the histopathological findings are shown in Table 16.2.

As expected, patients with hippocampal pathology differed significantly from those with normal histologic findings. Some of the results of the correlation analysis between the clinical data of all the patients and the hippocampal pathology are given in Table 16.3. Apart from significant correlations between the various hippocampal pathology categories, highly significant correlations were seen between seizure outcome and gliosis, neuronal loss, and granule cell dispersion of the fascia dentata. Patients with hippocampal pathology had significantly better seizure outcome. Patients with febrile convulsions had a trend toward a severe granule cell dispersion and better seizure outcome. Seizure onset at an older age correlated with a destroyed architecture of the CA regions. Patients with hippocampal pathology had a longer duration of illness, but not significantly so, and were significantly older at the time of surgery.

Lateral neocortical temporal lobe seizures are much rarer than seizures originating in the mesial TL structures. NTLE usually is associated with a morphologic lesion invading the lateral TL cortex alone or in combination with the insula. In contrast to MTLE, NTLE has not been characterized thoroughly. Patients with NTLE without a preoperatively diagnosed gross lesion account for a small minority of surgical cases successfully treated by epilepsy surgery; however, seizures of lateral TL origin and without a gross morphologic lesion do exist and have been documented by stereotactic depth recording (stereo-EEG) (Tables 16.4 and 16.5) (24). Such seizures, as a rule, spread to the ipsilateral mesial TL structures, which may act as a kind of "amplifier," sustaining and prolonging the seizure discharges (Fig. 16.1). This spreading pattern of seizures with onset in the lateral neocortical TL represents a further complication in studying the semiology of NTLE, as is the fact that often a considerable sample problem prevents firm conclusions that only the lateral and not the mesial TL is discharging. It is therefore not surprising that several studies failed to find clinical features that differentiate between MTL and

TABLE 16.2. *Patients with hippocampal pathology (reevaluated) (n = 81)*

Degree of pathology	Gliosis	%	Neuronal loss	%	Cornu Ammonis (CA) regions	%	GC dispersion	%
Normal			7	13.5	31	38.3	15	21.1
Slight	2	2.8	7	13.5	11	13.6	19	26.8
Moderate	32	45.1	10	19.3	12	14.8	18	25.4
Severe	37	52.1	28	53.8	27	33.3	19 (4)[a]	26.8
Reevaluation not possible	10		29				10	

GC dispersion, granule cells dispersion of the fascia dentate.
[a]Bilaminar arrangement of the fascia dentate.

TABLE 16.3. *Correlation coefficients for clinical data and hippocampal pathology (reevaluated) (n = 81)*

Correlation coefficients	Gliosis	Neuronal loss	CA regions	GC dispersion	Age at seizure onset	Duration of illness	Age at surgery	Febrile convulsions
Gliosis								
Neuronal loss	0.78***							
CA regions	0.51***	0.25***						
GC dispersion	0.66***	0.88***	0.21**					
Age at seizure onset	0.14	−0.15	0.22**	−0.06				
Duration of illness	0.09	0.20**	−0.02	0.16*	−0.45***			
Age at surgery	0.21*	0.02	0.20**	0.10	0.46***	0.55***		
Febrile convulsions	0.10	0.20**	0.01	0.26***	−0.14	−0.06	−0.15	
Outcome	0.33***	0.43***	0.11	0.34***	−0.14	0.11	−0.02	0.18*

CA regions, alteration of CA-regions; GC-dispersion, granule cells dispersion of the fascia dentata.
*$p < 0.10$; **$p < 0.05$; ***$p < 0.01$.

TABLE 16.4. *Differentiation MTLE versus NTLE (clinical studies)*

Authors/Main conclusion	MTLE	NTLE	Sample size/characteristics
O'Brien et al., 1966			
A number of clinicoelectrical differences between patients with MTLE and patients with NTLE, but none is sufficient to allow a distinction to be made in an individual patient	History of febrile seizures 58%	26% [$p < 0.005$]	N_{MTLE} 31 N_{NTLE} 15 (discrete lesions)
	History of significant cerebral event at <4 yr of age 22%	0% [$p < 0.005$] (no significant difference)	
	Auras (Incidence and nature)		
	Seizure semiology: dystonic posturing 52%	26% [$p < 0.005$]	
	Facial grimacing/twitching later ($\bar{x} = 35$ s)	Earlier ($\bar{x} = 19$ s) [$p < 0.005$] (no significant difference)	
	Interictal EEG		
	Ictal-EEG		
	Increased frequency of fast rhythmic sharp waves (>4 Hz) 81%	60%, [$p = 0.005$]	
	Bilateral ictal EEG changes: Less often 26% Less rapidly ($\bar{x} = 74$ s) At onset: bilateral less often (4%)	55% [$p < 0.005$] rapidly ($\bar{x} = 23$ s) [$p < 0.005$] more often (20%) [$p < 0.005$]	
	Postsurgical outcome; seizure free 87%	60% [$p = 0.057$]	
Foldvary et al., 1997			
It may be possible to differentiate lesional NTLE from MTLE on the basis of historical features, seizure symptomatology, and ictal surface EEG recordings. This may assist in the identification of patients with medically refractory nonlesional NTLE who frequently require intracranial monitoring and more extensive or tailored resections	Historical features: younger at onset of habitual seizures, more likely to have a prior history of febrile seizures, CNS infection, perinatal complications, or head injury		N_{MTLE} 20; seizure-free after ant TL ectomy. N_{NTLE} 8; lesional, seizure-free after neocortical temporal resection with preservation of mesial structures. Seizure semiology of 107 seizures (28 NTLE, 79 MTLE), 101 ictal EEGs (19 NTLE, 82 MTLE)
	Seizure semiology	NTLE seizures lacked features commonly exhibited in MTLE, including automatisms, contralateral dystonia, searching head movements, body shifting, hyperventilation, and postictal cough or sigh.	
	Surface EEG at seizure onset [presence, distribution, and frequency of LRA] and distribution of postictal slowing: LRA in MTLE seizures was maximal over the ipsilateral temporal region	NTLE ictal EEG recordings demonstrated lower mean frequency of LRA that frequently had a hemispheric distribution	
Lee et al., 1997			
Surgical outcome is influenced by the type of epileptic syndromes rather than the etiology of seizures	Clinical characteristics: age of the time of CNS infection was significantly younger and the latent period of nonfebrile seizures after CNS infection was longer		N_{MTLE} 12; Engel I & II after ant TL ectomy. N_{NTLE} 8; patients with intractable epilepsy associated with previous CNS infections; localization of epileptic regions by means of standard presurgical evaluation (11 patients had intracranial EEG monitoring)
	Location of epileptogenic regions by MRI		
	MRI: 11/12 hippocampal atrophy and hippocampal signal changes	MRI: 5/6 patients had normal MRI and one showed cerebral hemiatrophy.	
	Surgical outcomes: success (class I & II) in all patients	Seizure-free results were not achieved in any patients after resective surgery and only 2 patients achieved class II outcomes after a second epilepsy surgery consisting of neocortical resection	

TABLE 16.4. *Continued*

Authors/Main conclusion	MTLE	NTLE	Sample size/characteristics
Pacia et al., 1996	In contrast to MTLE, with seizure free intervals between the initial cerebral insult or first seizure and habitual seizures	Mean age at the time of first seizure: 14 yr (range, 1–41 yr) Febrile seizures: in only 2 patients (9.5%) Seizure-free intervals: uncommon Possible or known risk factors for epilepsy: in 13 patients (62%) Seizure semiology: Auras: 15 patients (71%) Experiential phenomena: most common type Most common at ictal onset was a motionless stare (48%) MRI: normal or nonspecific in 15 patients; mild hippocampal atrophy in 2, tumors in 2, heterotopic gray matter and hippocampal atrophy in 1, and cortical dysgenesis in 1 patient Neuropsychological testing: deficits consistent with the seizure focus in 13 patients (62%); Wada test: ipsilateral memory deficits in 10 (48%) EEG: In contrast to prior studies of MTLE, only 1 NTLE patient had frequent independent, contralateral temporal lobe epileptiform spikes on scalp EEG	21 patients with NTLE, defined by intracranial EEG, who have been seizure free for 1 yr or more following temporal lobectomy

CNS, central nervous system; EEG, electroencephalography; LRA, lateralized rhythmic activity; MRI, magnetic resonance imaging; MTLE, mesial temporal lobe epilepsy; NTLE, neocortical temporal lobe epilepsy.

TABLE 16.5. *Paraclinical studies that might be useful in differentiating MTLE versus NTLE[a]*

Author(s)/Main conclusion	Technique/test	Patients/Type of study
Savic et al., 1997 Useful in distinguishing between NS and MTLS	Olfactory bedside test, using the University of Pennsylvania Smell Identification Test (quality discrimination and delayed recognition memory) MTLE patients were correctly identified with a sensitivity of 85% and a specificity of 90%, offering a correct lateralization in 74% of patients.	N_{MTLS}: 27 N_{NTLES}: 10 $N_{control}$: 10 All patients were referred for presurgical evaluation. The results were related to regional glucose metabolism measured with 18 FFDG PET
Ebersole & Pacia, 1996	Scalp EEG: Initial patterns of ictal discharges Categorization of seizure patterns; 5–9 Hz inferotemporal rhythms (type 1A) correlated with hippocampal seizure onset; Seizures without a clear lateralized EEG discharge (type 3) correlated with neocortical TL onset	Ictal recordings of scalp EEG of 93 epilepsy surgery candidates referred directly for TL-ectomy (n = 35) or who underwent intracranial EEG monitoring (n = 58)

TABLE 16.5. *Continued*

Author(s)/Main conclusion	Technique/test	Patients/Type of study
Assaf & Ebersole, 1997 Can provide information about the origin of TL seizures that is useful in presurgical planning. In particular, it can reliably distinguish seizures of mesial temporal origin from those of lateral temporal origin.	Advanced scalp EEG: Continuous source imaging of scalp ictal rhythms. Source analysis technique with multiple fixed dipoles.	Retrospective analysis of earliest scalp ictal rhythms in 40 patients with TLE; categorization of ictal activity according to its most prominent source components: Verification with intracranial EEG studies and successful surgery
King & Spencer, 1995	Invasive EEG of spontaneous seizures The presence of periodic spikes before seizure onset has a significant correlation with reduced CA1 cell counts. This phenomenon is followed, in spontaneous seizures, by 13–25 Hz discharge in medial temporal lobe structures. Temporal neocortical seizure onsets have significantly faster frequencies than hippocampal onsets	60% of MTLE ictal onsets initially propagate to the ipsilateral temporal neocortex. 30% propagate to the contralateral hippocampus, before involvement of the ipsilateral or contralateral temporal neocortex. Time to propagation to the contralateral hippocampus is lengthened in direct proportion to CA4 cell loss. Long interhemispheric propagation times are associated with good surgical outcomes and with the presence of MTS.
Knowlton et al., 1997 MEG can reliably localize sources of spike discharges in patients with temporal and extratemporal lobe epilepsy. MEG sometimes provides noninvasive localization data that are not otherwise available with MRI or conventional scalp ictal EEG	Magnetoencephalography: interictal epileptiform activity (observed in 16 of 22 patients) MEG localization yield was greater in patients with neocortical epilepsy (92%) than in those with mesial temporal lobe epilepsy (50%)	N_{MTLS}: 10 N_{NTLES}: 3 $N_{extratemporal}$: 9 A 37-channel biomagnetometer was used for simultaneously recording MEG with EEG (2–3-hour MEG recording session)
Vermathen et al., 1997 May help to distinguish between neocortical epilepsies and MTLE	Magnetic resonance spectroscopy: Hippocampal N-acetylaspartate (NAA) NAA is not reduced in the hippocampus of patients with neocortical epilepsies, neither ipsilateral nor contralateral to the seizure focus, but is reduced in MTLE	$N_{MTLE\ Unilateral)}$: 23 N_{NE}: 10 $N_{control}$: 16
Hamberger et al., 1996 Can help to distinguish between NTLE and MTLE	Intracarotid amobarbital procedure (IAP): IAP mean memory asymmetry scores were significantly lower in NTLE than in MTLE groups	$N_{MTLE\ Unilateral)}$: 23 N_{NE}: 10 (lateral TL lesion or lateral TL onset in intracranial recordings; absence of MTS). All patients had good (Engel I or II) postoperative seizure outcome $N_{control}$: 16
Hajek et al., 1993 Can help to distinguish between NTLE and MTLE as groups	18F-FDG PET, quantitative ROI analysis	$N_{MTLE\ unilateral,\ with\ MTS}$: 15 $N_{MTLE\ with\ tumors}$: 5 N_{NTLE}: 5

[a]Except magnetic resonance imaging.
   EEG, electroencephalographic, MTLE, mesial temporal epilepsy; MTS, medial temporal sclerosis; NTLE, neocortical temporal lobe epilepsy; TL, temporal lobe; TLE, temporal lobe epilepsy.

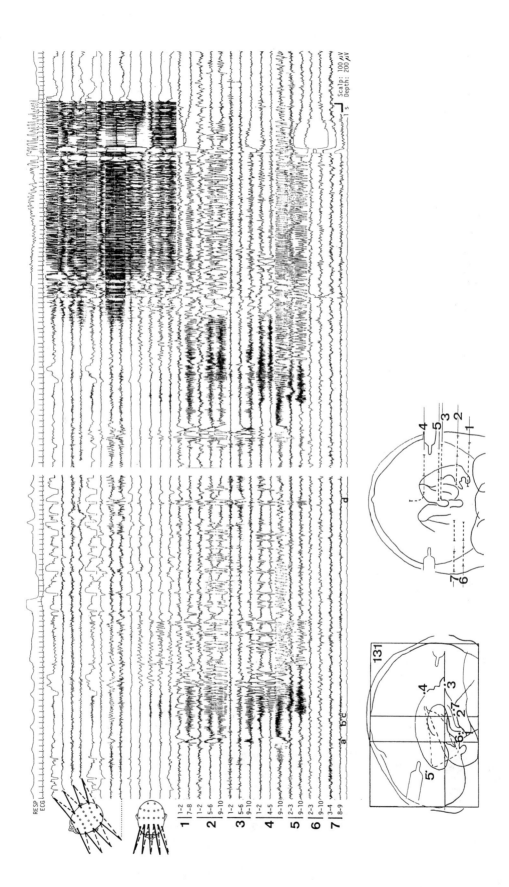

NTLE (25). Seizures with unilateral mesial TL origin usually spread to the ipsilateral neocortex (26), and clinical signs and symptoms supportive of seizures arising from the lateral TL neocortex commonly derive from epileptic discharges involving cortex of more than one lobe. It is therefore not uncommon that the diagnosis of a NTLE is based more on negative findings otherwise typical for MTLE. As already mentioned, MTLE has a characteristic set of findings in paraclinical tests, some of which are listed in Tables 16.4 and 16.5. Besides MRI, PET with [18]Fluoro-desoxyglucose (27) and 11C-Flumazenil PET (28) and proton magnetic resonance spectroscopy (^{1}H MRS). (29–31) can help in differentiating between MTLE and NTLE.

In a group of 31 patients who were seizure free 18 months after temporal lobectomy, only three patients (10%) had NTLE (32). Moreover, in those patients diagnosed as NTLE with subdural grids and without hippocampal sclerosis who underwent neocortical TL resections sparing the mesial TL structures, the postoperative seizure outcome was suboptimal: 50% of patients became seizure free, in contrast to MTLE, with 80% seizure-free after mesial TL resection. Most of these patients had cortical dysplasia (33). It is obvious that the diagnosis of NTLE must be questioned in patients who did not become seizure free after lateral temporal resection. Evidence for such a reasoning can be found in many studies, for example, that of Sisodiya et al. (34), who described 27 patients with proven hippocampal sclerosis who underwent quantitative postprocessing of preoperative MRIs. These authors found extrahippocampal structural abnormalities in 14 patients, 10 of whom did not become seizure free. In contrast, 11 of 13 patients without such changes did become seizure free following surgery. In other respects, the 27 patients were identical, and on visual inspection all patients had normal MRIs. Li et al. (35) recently specifically addressed the issue of periventricular nodular heterotopia in patients with intractable temporal lobe epilepsy. Ten patients with periventricular nodular heterotopia and electroclinical features of TLE underwent TL resection. None of the nine patients with a follow-up of more than 1 year was seizure free. Two patients were initially seizure free for 18 months, but then seizures reoccurred. Marsh et al. (36) studied specifically extrahippocampal areas in patients with TLE who were otherwise candidates for TL resection. In their MRI study, they compared 21 patients with 49 age range–matched controls. They found widespread volume abnormalities bilaterally in both temporal and extratemporal cortical areas compared with controls, indicating that structural abnormalities are more widespread than first thought.

SIGNS AND SYMPTOMS OF SEIZURES ORIGINATING IN THE NEOCORTICAL TL CORTEX

It is said that cephalic, auditory, vertiginous, and visual auras are more common in NTLE than in MTLE (Table 16.4 and Figs. 16.2 and 16.3). In MTLE visceral sensations, fear and olfactory–gustatory auras prevail.

FIG. 16.1. Combined scalp- and depth EEG-recorded seizures with similar left lateral temporal onset (4/9–10) close to Wernicke's area. **Left:** Note early involvement of the posterior cingulate cortex (4/1–2) and spread to the ipsilateral frontal cortex (5/9–10). Seizure semiology speech arrest and inability to speak **(a)**, flush **(b)**, and tonic contraction of the right corner of the mouth **(c)**, Language reappeared 30 seconds after seizure onset **(d)**, **Right:** Compared with the seizure illustrated at left, this seizure was accompanied by a longer aphasic state and more pronounced tonic–clonic motor phenomena of the right face and the right arm. This is indicated by the coinciding muscle activity in the scalp EEG. Aphasia persisted about 2 min into the postictal period. The position of the depth electrodes is indicated in the brain map. Large numerals indicate the electrode, small numerals the contacts. Each electrode has ten contacts, which are numbered from inside-out. (From Wieser HG, Müller RU. Neocortical temporal seizures. In: Wieser HG, Elger CE, eds. *Presurgical evaluation of epileptics.* Berlin, Heidelberg: Springer, 1987:252–266, with permission.)

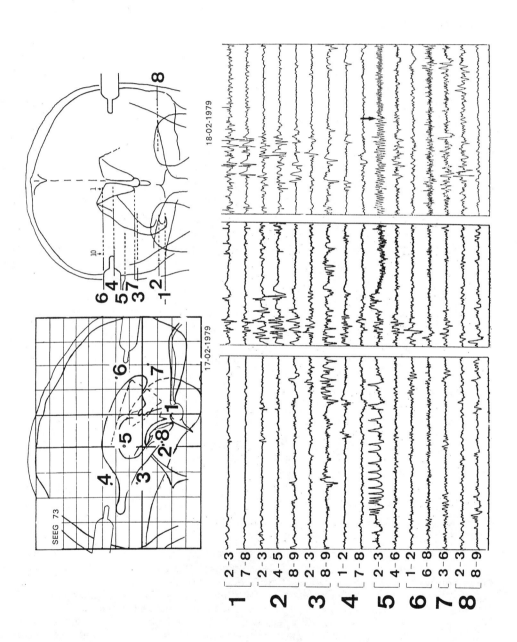

Extrahippocampal seizures are usually shorter than hippocampal seizures (lasting 46 seconds compared with 68 seconds) (37), and early somatomotor involvement is more fre-hemisphere). They are accompanied by *auditory hallucinations,* if the posterior insula (Heschl's gyrus) and the superior temporal gyrus are involved (Fig. 16.2) (38,39). *Vestibular hallucinations* are documented with posterior–temporal–parietal discharges (24). *Visual hallucinations* and *motor symptoms* are frequent.

Visual hallucinations often are encountered with discharges in the lateral temporal cortex and temporo–parieto–occipital junction but also inferotemporal cortex (24). They comprise often complex sceneries in the sense of a panoramic vision (déjà vu recollection), but they also may consist of macropsia and micropsia, *teleopsia* (distorted perception of distance), *plagiopsia* (object appears with an inclination), *dysplatopsia* (object appears flattened or elongated), *achromatopsia* (object is perceived as without color) or *erythropsia* (object is perceived with a red color), and *xanthopsia* (object is perceived with a yellow color). There might be loss *(astereognosia)* or enhancement of three-dimensional apperception. An object might be apperceived as doubled or even multiplied *(monocular diplopia, polyopia)* and can perseverate *(paliopsia).* The movement of an object can be judged as being accelerated *(quick motion)* or slowed *(slow motion).*

The question of whether dreamy states allow a differentiation between MTLE and NTLE must be answered in the negative. Jackson (40) observed that seizures arising in the medial temporal lobe may result in a "dreamy state," consisting of vivid memory-like hallucinations, or the sense of having previously lived through exactly the same situation (déjà vu). The dreamy state could occur alone but often was associated with epigastric phenomena and fear, followed by loss of contact and oroalimentary automatisms, and then by simple gestural automatisms, all characteristic of partial seizures beginning in the medial temporal lobe. Seldom is it associated with sensory illusions. Penfield et al. (41) demonstrated that the dreamy state sometimes can be evoked by electric stimulation of the lateral temporal neocortex, especially the superior temporal gyrus. Halgren et al. (42) showed that the dreamy state can be evoked by stimulation of the hippocampal formation and amygdala, and Gloor et al. (43) suggested that it is evoked by lateral stimulation only when the resulting afterdischarge spreads medially.

Bancaud et al. (44) studied 16 patients, all with seizures involving the temporal lobe, who experienced the dreamy state either as a result of spontaneous seizures (9 dreamy states in 6 patients), or due to electrical stimulation (43 in 14) or to chemical activation (5 in 3). Stimulation of either the neocortex (15 occurrences), anterior hippocampus (17), or amygdala (10) could evoke a dreamy state. The proportion of medial temporal electrodes in which dreamy states could be evoked was much higher than in the neocortex, fitting well with the results of our own study (45). Most responsive lateral temporal sites were located in the superior temporal gyrus rather than in the middle temporal gyrus, which was significantly less responsive. In 85% of dreamy states evoked by medial temporal lobe stimulation, the discharge spread to the temporal neocortex, and in 53% of dreamy states evoked by lateral temporal stimulation, the discharge spread medially. Considering all

FIG. 16.2. Spontaneous seizure discharge originating in the right Heschl's gyrus and accompanied by complex auditory, that is, musical hallucination. This discharge lasted 2 days [see the left and middle section (17-02-1979)], which are 19 seconds apart, and the right section (18-02-1979). The condition of the patient progressed into a psychomotor status epilepticus. The seizure discharge in the Heschl's gyrus could be modified by listening to a Portuguese song similar to that the patient was hallucinating. *Arrow* in the right section shows the sudden change of the discharge characteristics at the moment the patient was confronted with this Portuguese song. (Modified from Wieser HG. Temporal lobe or psychomotor status epilepticzus: a case report. *Electroencephalogr Clin Neurophysiol* 1980;48:558–572. 1980, with permission.)

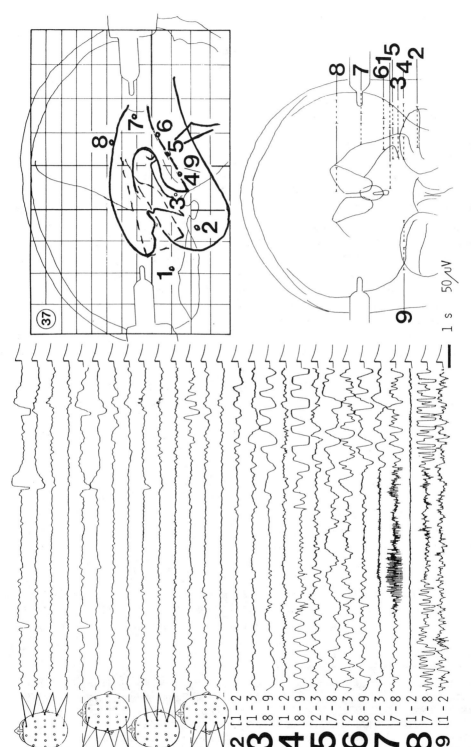

FIG. 16.3. Spontaneous short-lived seizure discharge in the left posterior temporal neocortex (7/7–8) accompanied by a vertiginous sensation pulling the patient to the right. (From Wieser HG, Müller RU. Neocortical temporal seizures. In: Wieser HG, Elger CE, eds. *Presurgical evaluation of epileptics.* Berlin, Heidelberg: Springer, 1987:252–266, with permission.)

dreamy states, the amygdala was involved (as the stimulated structure or as the site of ictal or after discharge) in 73% of cases, the anterior hippocampus in 83%, and the temporal neocortex in 88%. Motor symptoms with contralateral tonic–clonic manifestations and head–eye deviation are more frequent in neocortical lateral than in mesiobasal seizures, whereas dystonic posturing occurs more frequently (in about 40% of patients) with mesial TL onset seizures.

Besides MTLE, the differential diagnosis of NTLE comprises benign childhood epilepsy with centrotemporal spikes (BCEwCTS). Clinical signs and symptoms might be similar in BCEwCTS and MTLE. Both can begin in childhood with generalized seizures. In MTLE, however, there is usually an earlier age of seizure onset, a positive history of complicated febrile seizures, and an increased incidence of family members with seizures. Partial seizures of BCEwCTS usually manifest themselves with sensory or motor lateralized symptoms localized around the mouth or upper extremity.

Interictal EEG spikes are also different: In BCEwCTS the broad EEG spike is located more posteriorly-superiorly, and there is a characteristic transverse dipole direction. In MTLE the spike-wave discharges are located more anteriorly–basally, and there is a characteristic oblique dipole direction.

Today, the differential diagnosis of NTLE versus TLE attributable to other lesions in or close to the mesial TL usually is made by MRI. In the differential diagnosis NTLE versus complex partial seizures of extratemporal neocortical origin, the semiology is more important. Complex partial seizures of extratemporal neocortical origin often have an aura consisting of symptoms pointing more closely to the involved primary epileptogenic area (46–50). In addition, the scalp ictal EEG may differ (51).

CONCLUSION

Although the repertoire of the ictal signs and symptoms of NTLE and MTLE are similar as a result of the spread of ictal discharges within and outside the TL, careful analysis of the early symptoms, of the order of symptom appearance, and of the preferential spread

patterns may give hints for distinguishing seizures of mesial versus lateral–neocortical TL onset. In many instances, definitive proof, however, requires the intracranial recording from neocortical and mesial TL structures.

REFERENCES

1. Engel J Jr. Recent advances in surgical treatment of temporal lobe epilepsy. *Acta Neurol Scand* 1992 (Suppl);140:71–80.
2. Wieser HG, Williamson PG. Ictal semiology. In: Engel J Jr, ed. *Surgical treatment of the epilepsies,* 2nd ed. New York: Raven Press, 1993:161–171.
3. Engel J Jr, Williamson PD, Wieser HG. Mesial temporal lobe epilepsy. In: Engel J Jr, Pedley J, eds. *Epilepsy: a comprehensive textbook.* New York: Raven Press, 1997:2417–2426.
4. Berkovic SF, Howell RA, Hopper JL. Familial temporal epilepsy: a new symdrome with adolescent/adult onset and a benign course. In: Wolf P, ed. *Epileptic seizures and syndromes.* London: John Libbey, 1994:257–263.
5. Mathieson G. Pathology of temporal lobe foci. In: Penry JK, Daly DD, eds. *Complex partial seizures and their treatment. Advances in Neurology,* vol 11. New York: Raven Press, 1975:163–185.
6. Green JR, Scheetz DG. Surgery of epileptogenic lesions of the temporal lobe. *Arch Neurol* 1964;10:135–148.
7. Jensen I, Klinken L. Temporal lobe epilepsy and neuropathology: histological findings in resected temporal lobes correlated to surgical results and clinical aspects. *Acta Neurol Scand* 1976;54:391–414.
8. Duncan JS, Sagar HJ. Seizure characteristics, pathology, and outcome after temporal lobectomy. *Neurology* 1987;37:405–409.
9. Bruton C. *The neuropathology of temporal lobe epilepsy.* New York: Oxford University Press, 1988.
10. Berkovic SF, McIntosh AM, Kalnins RM, et al. Preoperative MRI predicts outcome of temporal lobectomy: an actuarial analysis. *Neurology* 1995;45:1358–1363.
11. Falconer MA, Serafetinides EA, Corsellis JAN. Etiology and pathogenesis of temporal lobe epilepsy. *Arch Neurol* 1964;10:233–248.
12. Babb TL, Brown WJ. Pathological findings in epilepsy. In: Engel J Jr, ED. *Surgical treatment of the epilepsies.* New York: Raven Press, 1987:511–540.
13. Zentner J, Hufnagel A, Wolf HK, et al. Surgical treatment of temporal lobe epilepsy: clinical, radiological, and histopathological findings in 178 patients. *J Neurol Neurosurg Psychiatry* 1995;58:666–673.
14. Plate KH, Wieser HG, Yasargil MG, et al. Neuropathological findings in 224 patients with temporal lobe epilepsy. *Acta Neuropathol (Berl)* 1993;86:433–438.
14a. Wieser HG. Epilepsiechirurgie in der Schweiz–unter besonderer Berücksichtigung der Zürcher selektiven Amygdala-Hippokampektomie-Serie. *Aktuelle Neurologie* 2000;27:77–85.
15. Taylor DC, Falconer MA, Bruton CJ, et al. Focal dysplasia of the cerebral cortex in epilepsy. *J Neurol Neurosurg Psychiatry* 1971;34:369–387.
16. Daumas-Duport C, Scheithauer BW, Chodkiewicz JP, et al. Dysembryoplastic neuroepithelial tumor: a surgically curable tumor of young patients with intractable partial seizures—report of thirty-nine cases. *Neurosurgery* 1988;23:545–556.

17. Daumas-Duport C. Dysembryoplastic neuroepithelial tumors. *Brain Pathol* 1993;3:283–295.
18. Lehericy S, Dormont D, Semah F, et al. Developmental abnormalities of the medial temporal lobe in patients with temporal lobe epilepsy. *Am J Neuroradiol* 1995; 16:617–626.
19. Palmini A, Andermann F, Olivier A, et al. Neuronal migration disorders: a contribution of modern neuroimaging to the etiologic diagnosis of epilepsy. *Can J Neurol Sci* 1991;18:580–587.
20. Raymond AA, Fish DR, Sisodiya SM, et al. The developmental basis of epilepsy. In: Shorvon S, Dreifuss F, Fish D, et al., eds. *The treatment of epilepsy.* London: Blackwell Science, 1996:20–54.
21. Houser CR. Granule cell dispersion in the dentate gyrus of humans with temporal lobe epilepsy. *Brain Res* 1990; 535:195–204.
22. Houser CR, Swartz BE, Walsh GO, et al. Granule cell disorganization in the dentate gyrus: possible alterations of neuronal migration in human temporal lobe epilepsy. In: Engel J Jr, Wasterlain C, Cavalheiro EA, et al., eds. *Molecular neurobiology of epilepsy.* Amsterdam: Elsevier, 1992:41–49.
23. Mello LEAM, Cavalheiro EA, Tan AM, et al. Granule cell dispersion in relation to mossy fiber sprouting, hippocampal cell loss, silent period, and seizure frequency in the pilocarpine model of epilepsy. In: Engel J Jr, Wasterlain C, Cavalheiro EA, et al., eds. *Molecular neurobiology of epilepsy.* Amsterdam: Elsevier, 1992:51–60.
24. Wieser HG, Müller RU. Neocortical temporal seizures. In: Wieser HG, Elger CE, eds. *Presurgical evaluation of epileptics.* Berlin, Heidelberg: Springer, 1987:252–266.
25. Burgerman RS, Sperling MR, French JA, et al. Comparison of mesial versus neocortical onset temporal lobe seizures: neurodiagnostic findings and surgical outcome. *Epilepsia* 1995;36:662–670.
26. King D, Spencer S. Invasive electroencephalography in mesial temporal lobe epilepsy. *J Clin Neurophysiol* 1995;12:32–45.
27. Hajek M, Antonini A, Leenders KL, et al. Mesiobasal versus lateral temporal lobe epilepsy: metabolic differences in the temporal lobe shown by interictal 18F-FDG positron emission tomography. *Neurology* 1993;43:79–86.
28. Henry TR, Frey KA, Sackellares JC, et al. In vivo cerebral metabolism and central benzodiazepine-receptor binding in temporal lobe epilepsy. *Neurology* 1993;43: 1998–2006.
29. Peeling J, Sutherling G. 1H magnetic resonance spectroscopy of extracts of human epileptic neocortex and hippocampus. *Neurology* 1993;43:589–594.
30. Wieser HG, Duc C, Meier D, et al. Clinical experience with magnetic resonance spectroscopy in epilepsy. In: Pawlik G, Stefan H, eds. *Focus localization.* Berlin: German Section of ILAE, 1994:63–74.
31. Wieser HG, Russ W, Bösiger P, et al. Examination of the profile and changes of brain metabolites in epilepsy patients suffering from complex partial seizures of mesial temporal lobe origin before and after treatment with vigabatrin by means of proton magnetic resonance spectroscopy. In: Stefan H, Krämer G, Mamoli B, eds. *Challenge epilepsy—new antiepileptic drugs.* Berlin: Blackwell Science, 1998:229–235.
32. Kotagal P. Neocortical temporal lobe epilepsy. *Ninth International Symposium Epilepsy Surgery:* Syllabi and Abstracts. Cleveland: The Cleveland Clinic Foundation, June 22–26, 1998;Syllabus 4:14–15.
33. Comair J, Najm I, Foldvary N, et al. The surgical management of neocortical temporal lobe epilepsy. *Ninth International Symposium Epilepsy Surgery:* Syllabi and Abstracts. Cleveland: The Cleveland Clinic Foundation, June 22–26, 1998;Syllabus 64:82.
34. Sisodiya SM, Moran N, Free SL, et al. Correlation of widespread preoperative magnetic resonance imaging changes with unsuccessful surgery for hippocampal sclerosis. *Ann Neurol* 1997;41:490–496.
35. Li LM, Dubeau F, Andermann F, et al. Periventricular nodular heterotopia and intractable temporal lobe epilepsy: poor outcome after temporal lobe resection. *Ann Neurol* 1997;41:662–668.
36. Marsh L, Morrell MJ, Shear PK, et al. Cortical and hippocampal volume deficits in temporal lobe epilepsy. *Epilepsia* 1997;38:576–587.
37. Foldvary N, Lee N, Thwaites G, et al. Clinical and electrographic manifestations of lesional neocortical temporal lobe epilepsy. *Neurology* 1997;49:757–763.
38. Wieser HG. Temporal lobe or psychomotor status epilepticus: a case report. *Electroencephalogr Clin Neurophysiol* 1980;48:558–572.
39. Wieser HG, Engel J Jr, Williamson PD, et al. Surgically remediable temporal lobe syndromes. In: Engel J Jr, ed. *Surgical treatment of the epilepsies,* 2nd ed. New York: Raven Press, 1993:49–63.
40. Jackson JH, Colman WS. Case of epilepsy with testing movements and "dreamy state": very small patch of softening in the left uncinate gyrus. [*Brain* 1898;21: 580–90]. In: Taylor J, ed. *Selected Writings of John Hughlings Jackson,* Vol 1. *On epilepsy and epileptiform convulsions.* New York: Basic Books, 1958.
41. Penfield W, Jasper H. *Epilepsy and the functional anatomy of the human brain.* Boston: Little, Brown, 1954.
42. Halgren E, Walter RD, Cherlow DG, et al. Mental phenomena evoked by electrical stimulation of the human hippocampal formation and amygdala. *Brain* 1978; 101:83–117.
43. Gloor P, Olivier A, Quesney LF, et al. The role of the limbic system in experiential phenomena of temporal lobe epilepsy. *Ann Neurol* 1982;12:129–144.
44. Bancaud J, Brunet-Bourgin F, Chauvel P, et al. Anatomical origin of déjà vu and vivid "memories" in human temporal lobe epilepsy. *Brain* 1994;117:71–90.
45. Wieser HG. Ictal manifestations of temporal lobe seizures. In: Smith DB, Treiman D, Trimble M, eds. *Neurobehavioral problems in epilepsy. Advances in Neurology,* vol 55. New York: Raven Press, 1991:301–315.
46. Wieser HG. *Electroclinical features of the psychomotor seizure.* Stuttgart, London: Gustav Fischer–Butterworths.
47. Williamson PD, Wieser HG, Delgado-Escueta AV. Clinical characteristics of partial seizures. In: Engel J Jr, ed. *Surgical treatment of the epilepsies.* New York: Raven Press, 1987:101–120.
48. Saygi S, Spencer SS, Scheyer R, et al. Differentiation of temporal lobe ictal behavior associated with hippocampal sclerosis and tumors of temporal lobe. *Epilepsia* 1994;35:737–742.
49. Blume WR, Girvin JP, Stenerson P. Temporal neocortical role in ictal experiential phenomena. *Ann Neurol* 1993;33:105–107.
50. Walczak R. Neocortical temporal lobe epilepsy: characterizing the syndrome. *Epilepsia* 1995;36:633–635.
51. Walczak R, Bazil C, Lee N, et al. Scalp ictal EEG differs in temporal neocortical and hippocampal seizures. *Epilepsia* 1994;35:134(abst).

Neocortical Epilepsies.
Advances in Neurology, Vol. 84,
edited by P.D. Williamson, A.M. Siegel,
D.W. Roberts, V.M. Thadani, and M.S. Gazzaniga.
Lippincott Williams & Wilkins, Philadelphia © 2000

17

Frontal Lobe Epilepsy

Peter D. Williamson and Barbara C. Jobst

Section of Neurology, Dartmouth–Hitchcock Medical Center, Lebanon, New Hampshire 03756

Descriptions of seizures of probable frontal lobe origin can be found in writings from ancient times (1), but the first detailed account of frontal lobe seizures in the form of focal clonic activity was reported by Bravais in 1827 (2). In the second half of the nineteenth century, Jackson described these focal motor seizures and added anatomic perspectives (3). The first successful epilepsy surgery was performed on a patient with a depressed frontal skull fracture (4). In 1951, Penfield first described supplementary motor area (SMA) epilepsy (5). In 1954, Penfield and Jasper published their classic monograph entitled *Epilepsy and the Functional Anatomy of the Human Brain* (6). This landmark work contains a number of descriptions of seizures beginning in the frontal lobes. It also states in passing that frontal lobe automatisms are different from temporal lobe automatisms (pages 516–520). In 1957, Ajmone-Marsan and Ralston, in their monograph, *The Epileptic Seizure,* provided detailed descriptions of asymmetric tonic seizures (7). In the 1970s, several articles from both the United States and Europe described frontal lobe epilepsy with some unusual behavioral characteristics (8–12). These unusual behaviors associated with frontal lobe seizure origin were examined in greater detail in several papers from the mid-1980s (13,14). Several years later, the clinical characteristics of seizures originating in the SMA were more precisely defined (15–17). Early in the last

decade of this century, two major symposia specifically examining frontal lobe epilepsy convened (18,19). Finally, an autosomal-dominant form of familial frontal lobe epilepsy was reported (20–26) with documentation of the specific genetic defect as it appeared in certain families (27–32). The recent heightened interest in frontal lobe seizures and epilepsy is reflected in a greater than sixfold (415:65) increase in citations in this decade compared with the previous 10 years (Medline bibliographic search).

GENERAL FEATURES OF FRONTAL LOBE SEIZURES

As our understanding of temporal lobe seizures has increased over the past 20 years, it has become apparent that most temporal lobe seizures, at least those originating in the medial structures, represent variations on a theme (33–36). That is, temporal lobe seizures, although they differ in detail among patients, are more similar than they are different. The same is not true for frontal lobe seizures (37,38). A wide variety of entirely different types of seizures can occur with frontal lobe origin.

Most seizures of frontal lobe origin have prominent motor manifestations that include focal clonic motor activity; asymmetric tonic posturing; and peculiar, fairly specific, agitated semipurposeful motor activity (13,14,

17,39). There are, however, notable exceptions, with some frontal lobe seizures manifesting little or no motor activity. For example, absence seizures with 3-Hz spike-wave electroencephalographic (EEG) patterns have been described in patients with frontal lobe epilepsy (39–41). Nonconvulsive status epilepticus with EEG patterns characteristic of spike-wave stupor may be a fairly common form of frontal lobe seizures, particularly in older patients (42,43). In fact, all varieties of convulsive and nonconvulsive status epilepticus are reported with frontal lobe seizure origin (38,44–46). These different seizure patterns are discussed in greater detail and examples provided in subsequent sections. Suffice it to say that frontal lobe seizures can present with a wide variety of different clinical patterns.

Frequent, rapid evolution into tonic–clonic seizures has been described as a common feature of frontal lobe seizures (6,7,47), but in well-documented series of patients with frontal lobe seizures, rapid, frequent generalization was not a prominent feature in most patients (48,49). Generic features of frontal lobe seizures include frequent brief seizures occurring in clusters with a nocturnal preponderance (50,51). Whereas this may be true for certain types of frontal lobe seizures, it does not apply to all types. Furthermore, significant deviations from these patterns may be found, even in frontal lobe seizures associated with such features.

SPECIFIC TYPES OF FRONTAL LOBE SEIZURES

Frontal lobe seizures with complex behaviors and seizures originating in the SMA are described in some detail because they are better defined than other frontal lobe seizure types. Focal clonic motor seizures, although common, are not location specific but can occur with small, circumscribed lesions in or near the primary motor area, or they can occur in diffuse hemispheric syndromes, and they can occur with seizure origin outside of the frontal lobes. They are only briefly described here. Finally, several variably specific seizure types have been associated with frontal lobe origin. These are described here and, when possible, examples are given.

Frontal lobe seizures with complex behaviors (frontal lobe complex partial seizures, frontal lobe seizures with hypermotor automatisms, frontal lobe seizures with frenetic automatisms, frontal lobe seizurea with agitated behavior, frontal lobe psychomotor seizures) have attracted considerable attention in the past 15 years, but they had been described earlier (9–12). These unusual seizures now have been well defined (9,13, 14,17,52). Clinically, they consist of a constellation of rather peculiar signs (13,14). Motor activity is prominent, and onset is often explosive with an agitated, frenetic appearance. Patients may vigorously rock to and fro, kick or cycle with their legs, pound the bed or other objects with their hand, and jump or scramble about. If standing, they might hop or run in circles. Sexual automatisms with pronounced pelvic thrusting or aggressive genital manipulation can be a prominent feature in these seizures (53). Vocalization is also common during these bizarre motor manifestations. The patient may yell, growl, shout expletives, bark, laugh, whistle, or hum. These seizures constitute one of the types of frontal lobe seizures that tend to be brief and frequent, occur in clusters, and often have a nocturnal preponderance. They begin explosively and end suddenly, often with no demonstrable postictal state. Indeed, there may be no alteration of awareness, even during complex episodes. When this happens, patients will say they can hear and understand but have no control over their motor activity and cannot respond. When the seizure is over, test phrases will be accurately recalled and repeated. Later, in a flurry of such seizures, or if they become more intense, consciousness becomes impaired. In their mildest form, these seizures may consist only of sudden awaking and briefly scrambling about the bed on all four extremities. In their most blatant form, they are among the most unusual and dramatic of epileptic events. Although these seizures are said to be easily confused with nonepileptic psychogenic seizures, particularly when EEG findings are not helpful, they are almost too bizarre to be psychogenic attacks. If the examiner is familiar with this type of seizure and is able to obtain an accurate description from a reliable observer, the correct diagnosis is usually obvious from the history alone. When videotaped examples are shown to those not familiar with this type of frontal lobe seizure, convincing them of the epileptic nature of these episodes is often quite difficult. The contention, however, that they cannot be clinically separated from the more common temporal lobe seizures is no longer acceptable (54).

There are two important observations concerning this type of frontal lobe seizure that are often not appreciated. First, whereas the clinical characteristics alone are usually reliable for identifying frontal lobe seizure origin, they do not localize or lateralize within the frontal lobes. Although these seizures often are associated with medial or orbital frontal lobe origin, there are well-documented examples with origin elsewhere in the frontal lobe (45,48). The second feature that is often overlooked is that these seizures in their typical form do not spread beyond the confines of the frontal lobe. When secondary spread to the temporal lobe occurs, clinical features will resemble temporal lobe seizures (38,55,56). That is, episodes start out clinically like frontal lobe seizures and end with features of temporal lobe seizures.

Supplementary Motor Area Seizures

In 1941, Penfield and Ericson (57) reported their results from stimulating the SMA of humans. They were able to reproduce some of the synergistic complex postures and speech arrest associated with seizures originating in that part of the brain

(5,6). In 1957, Ajmone-Marsan and Ralston, in their classic monograph, *The Epileptic Seizure,* described asymmetric tonic postures that are now associated with SMA seizure origin (7). They considered this posture one of the basic elements of epileptic seizures and, for unclear reasons, labeled it *M2e.* As an interesting aside, "larval M2e's" were described and well illustrated in patients with presumed temporal lobe epilepsy. This was the first description of the recently rediscovered contralateral dystonic posturing, which is commonly seen during typical mesial temporal lobe seizures (36,58–60).

Despite the fact that SMA seizures were described more than 50 years ago, they still are not often appreciated outside the world of epileptology, and this can lead to the erroneous impression of psychogenic, nonepileptic seizures (61,62). Any observer familiar with these seizures, however, should make the correct diagnosis without difficulty. Because they often have a somatosensory component, the Cleveland Clinic group prefers the term *supplementary sensory motor area* (63,64). To avoid confusion with the supplementary sensory area, the more common SMA is preferred.

Typically, SMA seizures consist of the sudden, often explosive, assumption of a tonic posture, usually asymmetric (15,16,38,63,65). The classic description of these seizures includes contralateral deviation of the head and eyes, abduction and external rotation of arm at the shoulder, and flexion of the elbow. The patient has the appearance of turning to look at his or her up-raised hand. The arm ipsilateral to seizure origin and both legs can be held in tonic extension, or they are not involved in the seizure. Often the patient is fully conscious and yet unable to speak.

Many variations of this typical presentation exist (38). For example, the seizure may consist of the arm contralateral to the side of seizure origin suddenly shooting straight out or up without other motor activity. Conversely, the contralateral arm may be flexed, held tight to the body, with the fist clenched. One or both legs may exhibit kicking, stepping, or cycling movements. When the tonic seizure involves predominantly one side of the body, the uninvolved hand may reach over and attempt to control or assist the seizing side. Speech may be unaffected, in which case patients will often cry out for help or complain bitterly. Some patients have seizures that are more symmetric in the beginning, but usually there is some asymmetry, even if it is subtle.

Warnings are common but not specific. The patient may note some mild twitching or muscle stiffening before the sudden onset of obvious tonic posturing. Somatosensory sensations, such as paresthesias or numbness, may be experienced at the beginning of seizures. When a warning occurs, the patient sometimes will cry out or shout an expletive in anticipation of what is about to occur.

As with frontal lobe seizures with complex behaviors, SMA seizures tend to be brief, frequent, and to have a nocturnal preponderance. They differ from frontal lobe complex partial seizures in that, when they occur in their typical form with predominantly unilateral tonic posturing, the clinical signs are both localizing and lateralizing. Caution, however, must be exercised because asymmetric tonic seizures and adversive seizures can occur with seizures originating in other regions of the frontal lobe or even outside the frontal lobe (37,49,66–69). Finally, frontal lobe seizures without prominent tonic components but with complex behaviors can begin near and probably in the SMA (61).

Focal Motor Clonic Seizures

Focal clonic motor seizures are a common, well-recognized variety of seizures that have been described since antiquity (1). Focal clonic seizures can be unifocal and nearly continuous, lasting weeks or months *(epilepsy partialis continua)* (70,71). They can march in a pattern that follows the motor homunculus *(Jacksonian March)* (6,72), or they can be multifocal with different body parts seizing at different rhythms and fre-

quencies *(Rasmussen's encephalitis)* (73,74). Although the typical clonic motor pattern in these seizures is usual, when the face is involved early or initially in the seizure, there is often a strong tonic contraction of the facial muscles.

Clonic motor seizures, insofar as they clearly involve the contralateral motor cortex, are localizing and lateralizing, but their occurrence does not necessarily imply that the seizure originated in the prerolandic gyrus. Even if focal clonic seizure activity is the only manifestation of the seizure, the origin could be at a distance, in any one of the numerous clinically "silent" areas in the frontal lobe, or in cortical areas outside of the frontal lobe (37).

Other Frontal Lobe Seizure Types

Several other seizure types have been described in patients with presumed frontal lobe epilepsy. Documentation of region of seizure origin and seizure descriptions have been uneven. A listing with descriptions and comments follows:

1. *Frontal lobe seizures resembling temporal lobe seizures:* As noted previously, when the seizures spread from the frontal lobe to the temporal lobe, a change in clinical pattern can occur. If the seizure is a frontal lobe type and then evolves into a temporal lobe type seizure, an astute observer should suspect the correct diagnosis. If, however, frontal lobe seizure origin was clinically silent and all clinical manifestations reflected spread to temporal lobe structures, the diagnostic impression would not correctly localize seizure origin. How often this occurs is simply not known, but there is no doubt it does (case 5).

2. *Frontal lobe "absence":* Not all frontal lobe seizures have dramatic motor components. Bland seizures resembling absence episodes have been described in patients with frontal lobe seizure origin (39). Some of these frontal lobe absence seizures are associated with 3-Hz spike-wave EEG patterns

(39,48,75), whereas others have a more disorganized, diffuse ictal EEG pattern (case 6). In addition to isolated absence seizures, prolonged episodes of absence status or spike-wave stupor have been well documented in patients with frontal lobe seizure origin (case 7). Some older patients who present with absence status have evidence of frontal lobe seizure origin (42,43). Therefore, both isolated and prolonged nonconvulsive seizures with little or no motor activity also can be included in the diverse variety of frontal lobe seizures.

3. *Frontal opercular seizures:* Seizures involving the frontal operculum have been described in detail but only rarely documented with careful investigations and surgical cure. Nevertheless, frontal opercular seizures characterized by mastication, salivation, laryngeal sensations, swallowing, and (when involving the language-dominant hemisphere) speech arrest and aphasia have been described (39,76,77). Case 8 is an example of left-sided frontal opercular seizures, even though the results of subpial resection were equivocal. In a recent report of six patients with lateral frontal lobe seizure origin, two patients with opercular lesions did not exhibit any of the preceding characteristics (78). Finally, because the clinical characteristics described for opercular seizures resemble those of benign rolandic epilepsy (79), caution is necessary when evaluating children for possible surgery with these seizure characteristics.

4. *Anterior cingulate gyrus seizures:* Earlier reports of cingulate gyrus seizures described episodes resembling those seen in idiopathic generalized epilepsy with tonic–clonic seizures and absences (80–82). Although these reports are often cited when discussing cingulate gyrus seizures, the examples provided were not well described or documented. More recently, cingulate gyrus seizures consisting of fear, prominent vocalization with screaming and shouted expletives, complex agitated motor activity, autonomic findings, and partial retention of consciousness have been described (39,76).

This description is also contained in the current International Classification of the Epilepsies and Epileptic Syndromes (51). Bancaud and Talairach provided a fairly convincing description of a patient with seizures of this type who was studied with intracranial electrodes and cured with surgery (39). These descriptions, however, are clearly identical to those of frontal lobe seizures with complex behaviors that can originate in many regions of the frontal lobes in addition to the anterior cingulate gyrus (cases 3 and 4) (13,14). Therefore, the concept of specific or diagnostic anterior cingulate gyrus seizures cannot be supported.

DIAGNOSIS OF FRONTAL LOBE EPILEPSY

Clinical Seizure Characteristics

The single most important factor in the diagnosis of frontal lobe epilepsy is awareness of the wide variety of entirely different seizure types that can occur (45). Not only is this true for unusual seizures with minimal EEG findings (SMA seizures, frontal lobe seizures with complex behaviors), but it is also true for seizures that might mimic other types of seizures (frontal lobe absence seizures, frontal lobe seizures that closely resemble temporal lobe seizures). Although seizure descriptions by patients or reliable witnesses can suggest the correct diagnosis, examination of videotaped events provides the most accurate means of assessing clinical seizure characteristics. Features such as frequent brief seizures, nocturnal preponderance, and a history of nonconvulsive status should suggest the possibility of frontal lobe seizure origin (14,38,45,83,84).

Scalp Electroencephalography

Ictal and interictal scalp EEG findings in patients with medial temporal lobe epilepsy are often helpful in terms of lateralizing and localizing the region of seizure origin (35,85–87). The same is not true for many patients with frontal lobe seizure origin. Although scalp EEGs in patients with frontal lobe epilepsy can be correctly localizing and lateralizing, often they are not (87–90). Secondary bisynchronous epileptiform activity occurs in patients with medial frontal lobe seizure origin (91). Some patients will have consistently normal or nonspecific scalp EEG recordings (14,52,89). This is often the case in patients with SMA seizure origin and in patients who have the peculiar seizures with complex behaviors. Ictal EEGs in these same patients are often normal or nonspecific, thus further promoting the erroneous diagnosis of psychogenic, nonepileptic seizures (14,62,90). Other patients with frontal lobe seizures, particularly those with orbital frontal cortex origin, can have ictal and interictal EEG findings suggestive of temporal lobe epilepsy (14,89).

In conclusion, whereas scalp EEG results may help to localize frontal lobe seizure origin, often they are uninformative or misleading. In fact, the absence of clear ictal or interictal scalp EEG findings in patients with stereotyped asymmetrical tonic seizures or with bizarre behavior events might even be used to suggest the diagnosis of frontal lobe seizures rather than psychogenic events (13, 14,16,37,38,52,89).

Imaging Studies

The use of magnetic resonance imaging (MRI) in the detection of potentially epileptogenic lesions is enormously important in patients with localization-related epilepsy and hardly needs elaboration (92–94). When such lesions are found in the frontal lobe of patients with seizures suggestive of frontal lobe origin, they are usually the cause of the seizures unless other data are markedly discordant (95). More subtle findings, such as blurring of the cortical gray–white matter junction or abnormal gyral anatomy, can suggest disorders of neural migration or early injury (96,97). High-resolution MRI should be performed as an early screening test in all patients with localization-related epilepsy.

Baseline or routine single-photon emission computed tomography (SPECT) is not sensitive and is of limited value in patients with epilepsy, but ictal SPECT can provide potentially important localizing data that are otherwise not available (98). The test is logistically difficult to perform, and the best timing for injection of the radioligand has not been established. With relatively brief frontal lobe seizures, injection early in the seizure is essential (99). When the interictal SPECT is subtracted from the ictal study and the result is coregistered with the MRI, the sensitivity of the study is improved (100). Ictal SPECT has specifically been shown to be of value in frontal lobe epilepsy (99).

Although positron emission tomography (PET) has proven value in detecting temporal lobe epilepsy (101–104), it has been disappointing in locating extratemporal seizure foci in the absence of MRI-detectible lesions (105,106). Possibly, new radiopharmaceuticals will improve results, but so far this has not been the case. MRI spectroscopy is still in its infancy but might prove valuable in localizing regions of potential seizure origin in patients with frontal lobe epilepsy (107–111). This is likely to improve as magnet strength increases.

Intracranial Electrode Investigations

Patients with medically intractable frontal lobe epilepsy being considered for surgery will often require invasive EEG investigations. This is usually mandatory for those patients who do not have obvious potentially epileptogenic lesions on MRI. Although the specifics of invasive evaluations and electrode-placement strategies are beyond the scope of this communication, suffice it to say, that data from all the preceding evaluation are used when making decisions (112). In the absence of MRI findings in the large, anatomically diffuse frontal lobes, however, the potential for sampling error is high (37). The results of ictal SPECT are playing an increasingly important role in directing electrode placement in patients with frontal lobe epilepsy who are being considered for surgery (98,113,114). In some patients, more than one invasive study may be required to localize adequately the region of seizure origin (77,115). This type of aggressive approach will allow patients to have potentially curative epilepsy surgery who otherwise would not have been offered surgery (116,117).

ILLUSTRATIVE CASE REPORTS

These case reports were selected to demonstrate both the different types of frontal lobe seizures and the types of presurgical evaluations undertaken that lead to successful surgery. Ictal SPECT scans are now routinely done in patients with normal or nonlocalizing MRI findings, but these were not available when some of the described cases were evaluated.

Patient 1

This 21-year-old man developed seizures at age 6 consisting of right-sided stiffening. Other than mild head trauma without loss of consciousness, there were no risk factors for epilepsy. These episodes would cause him to fall if he was standing. He was started on carbamazepine, which he took for only 1 month. No additional seizures were observed until he was 12 years old, but he had frequent, unexplained enuresis. When seizures returned at 12, they were similar to previous episodes with right-sided stiffening, but the seizures were longer and more severe. Some secondarily generalized into tonic–clonic seizures. There was a strong nocturnal preponderance for all seizures. They would occur in flurries of many episodes every 2 to 3 nights, lasting all night. Seizures were medically refractory, and he was referred for surgery.

Neurologic examination was normal, but neuropsychological testing suggested some right-sided motor deficits. MRI was normal. During scalp video/EEG monitoring, he had

35 seizures. Seizures were brief, lasting about 30 seconds, and consisted of rigid tonic posturing of the right upper extremity with adduction at the shoulder, flexion of the elbow, and tight fisting of the hand. In some seizures, his head and eyes would deviate strongly to the right, but in others he looked straight ahead. In some seizures, he exhibited bicycling activity of both legs, whereas in others his right leg was held in tonic extension while his left foot and leg kicked. Frequently during seizures, his left hand and arm would reach across purposefully and grab the tonic right arm. The patient stated that he was fully awake throughout most of his seizures, but he could not speak. All recorded seizures occurred out of sleep. Interictal scalp EEGs were normal, and ictal records revealed only artifact. There was no postictal slowing.

A subdural electrode study was designed to sample posterior medial frontal regions bilaterally and both frontal convexities. Interictal recording revealed rare but definite spiking in the left SMA. Habitual seizures demonstrated SMA seizure origin with an emphasis on the left side. Electric stimulation through the subdural electrodes elicited complex motor responses. Stimulation of a restricted area in the left SMA consistently produced motor responses identical to the right arm posture seen in spontaneous seizures.

A limited resection of the left SMA was done (Fig. 17.1). Pathological examination of the resected tissue was unremarkable. The patient has had no seizures during the 7 years since surgery. He has taken no antiepileptic drugs for the past 3 years.

Comment: This patient presented with fairly typical SMA seizures. The 6-year hiatus between seizure onset and seizure recurrence off all antiepileptic drugs is unusual with this type of seizure. The enuresis during that period may have reflected unrecognized nocturnal seizures. The surgical success following a limited cortical resection in a patient with a normal MRI reflects utilization of all the pertinent localizing data gathered during the entire presurgical evaluation.

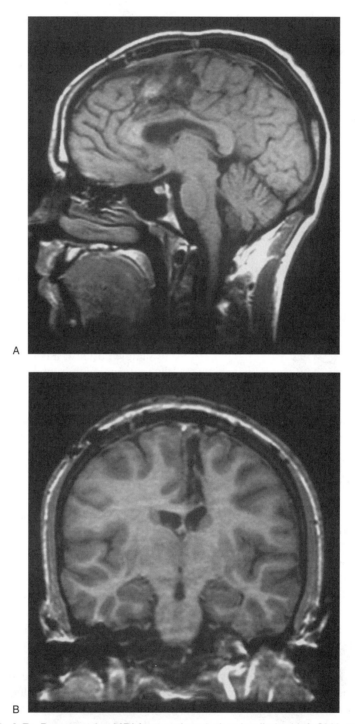

FIG. 17.1. A,B: Postoperative MRI from patient 1 showing limited left SMA resection.

Patient 2

This 33-year-old man had an unprovoked partial seizure that secondarily generalized when he was 31 years of age. Subsequent evaluation revealed an arteriovenous malformation in the left medial inferior frontal polar region. The lesion was resected without incident, but he continued to have seizures, which occurred without warning every 1 to 2 months and were described as generalized tonic–clonic convulsions. The patient also described a different type of episode occurring only once that consisted of confusion, difficulty understanding or speaking, recurrent right head deviation, and uncontrollable posturing of his right arm. The episode lasted over 1 hour, during which the patient felt as if he were fading in and out of contact. A variety of antiepileptic drugs, alone and in combination, failed to provide enduring seizure control, and he was evaluated for surgery.

The neurologic examination was normal. MRI revealed a well-circumscribed region of postoperative encephalomalacia in the left medial frontopolar region (Fig. 17.2). EEG during monitoring showed mild left frontal slowing but was otherwise normal. He had two seizures while undergoing video/EEG monitoring. Both were similar, occurring without warning while the patient was awake. They began with strong head and eye adversion to the right with the right arm flexed and elevated and then evolved into generalized tonic–clonic convulsions. The ictal EEG revealed a gradual left frontal slow wave buildup that began as long as 17 minutes prior to any clinical seizure activity (Fig. 17.3). The patient underwent resection of the left frontal gliotic scar. He has had no seizures in the year following surgery while being maintained on carbamazepine monotherapy.

Comment: This patient had fairly typical adversive (contraversive) asymmetric tonic seizures that secondarily generalized. Because invasive EEG studies were not done, it cannot be determined whether the clinical seizure manifestations represented spread to the left SMA. The unexpected finding was the prolonged subclinical EEG buildup that preceded seizures by many minutes. Frontal lobe seizures usually are associated with rapid spread patterns (37). Also, the history of the prolonged confusional episode strongly suggests that he had an episode of nonconvulsive status epilepticus that was not documented during inpatient monitoring.

Patient 3

This 29-year-old man developed seizures at age 17. There were no risk factors. Seizures initially were exclusively nocturnal and consisted of his awaking, shouting, and jumping in bed. The seizures increased in frequency until he was having them all night long. The diagnosis of epilepsy was made, and antiepileptic drugs initially dramatically reduced seizure frequency to one or two per month. Seizures then increased in frequency and also began occurring when he was awake. When seizures occurred while he was awake, he had an aura of fear. The patient stated that he was conscious during some, but not all, seizures. When medications failed to control seizures, he was evaluated for surgery.

The neurologic examination was normal, and neuropsychological testing did not provide localizing or lateralizing information. Numerous habitual seizures were recorded. These dramatic events usually came out of sleep and consisted of his awaking suddenly and shouting meaningless phrases similar to those associated with the cartoon character Fred Flintstone. At the same time, he would violently rock back and forth in bed. The seizures would begin explosively and end as suddenly as they began. During scalp monitoring, the interictal EEG, awake and asleep, was normal. Seizures were associated with bilateral, frontally preponderant delta activity, but they were largely obscured by artifact. Based on clinical seizure characteristics, an intracranial electrode study was planned using bilateral subdural electrodes to cover medial and orbital frontal cortex and

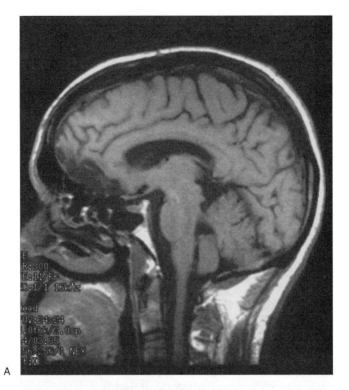

A

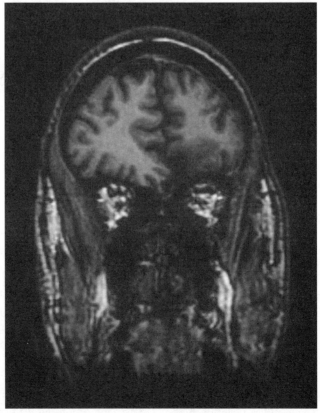

B

FIG. 17.2. A,B: MRI from patient 2 showing medial frontopolar encephalomalacia from prior surgery.

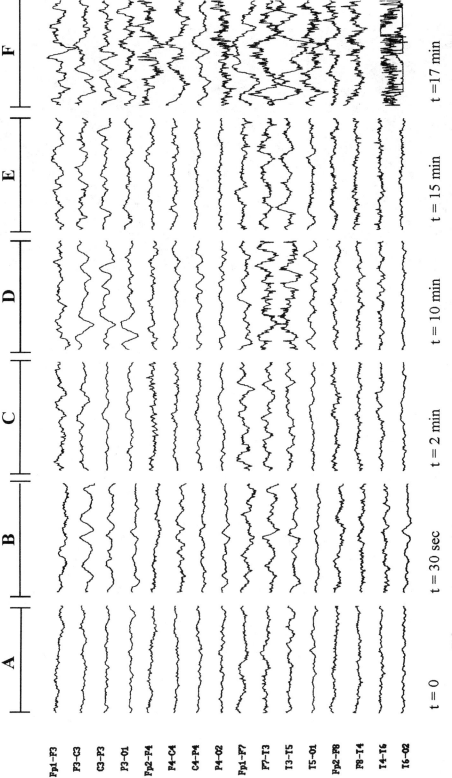

FIG. 17.3. Scalp EEG from patient #2 showing gradual buildup of left frontotemporal slowing during 17 minutes prior to clinical seizure onset.

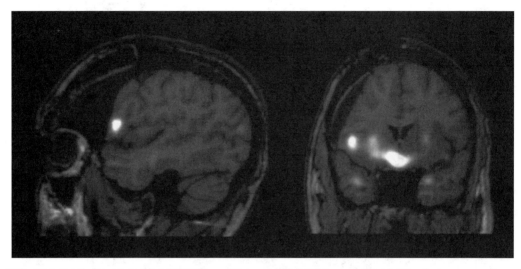

FIG. 17.4. Ictal minus interictal SPECT coregistered with MRI from patient 3 after first surgery showing region of increased perfusion in margin of previous resection.

frontal convexity. Seizure origin localized imprecisely but consistently to the right orbital frontal region. He underwent a limited right orbital frontal resection at age 24. Three months after surgery, seizures recurred. Even though postoperative seizures were much less severe and less frequent, they were still disruptive. Two years after surgery, he underwent a second presurgical evaluation. An ictal SPECT scan demonstrated an area of increased activity in the inferior lateral margin of the previous resection (Fig. 17.4). A subdural electrode study confirmed seizure origin in this location, and he underwent a limited extension of his previous resection. Three months after his second surgery, the patient had an episode of focal motor status epilepticus and several isolated staring spells. He then became and has remained seizure free during the next 3 years. He remains on antiepileptic drugs.

Comment: This patient with a normal MRI and unlocalized scalp EEG had the typical bizarre hypermotor, nocturnally preponderant seizures associated with seizure origin in various regions in the frontal lobes. This case also underlines the difficulties of accurately identifying the region of seizure origin in patients with normal MRIs even with invasive monitoring. It also demonstrates the utility of re-evaluation when initial surgery is unsuccessful.

Patient 4

This 23-year-old woman began having seizures at the age of 3 years. There were no risk factors. Initial seizures consisted of her appearing frightened, screaming, and shaking both hands. Sometimes seizures were associated with urinary incontinence. Despite frequent nocturnal seizures, she was not correctly diagnosed until she had a generalized tonic–clonic seizure several months after the seizures began. This was the only generalized tonic–clonic seizure she ever had. She was started on phenytoin. Seizures persisted at a much reduced frequency. An attempt to switch her rapidly to carbamazepine resulted in a several-hours episode of nonconvulsive status epilepticus. Despite trials of multiple antiepileptic drugs, alone and in combination, seizures persisted with nocturnal clusters occurring two to six times per month. Rare seizures while she was awake had an aura of fear.

She was evaluated for surgery at age 16. Her neurologic examination was normal. Her

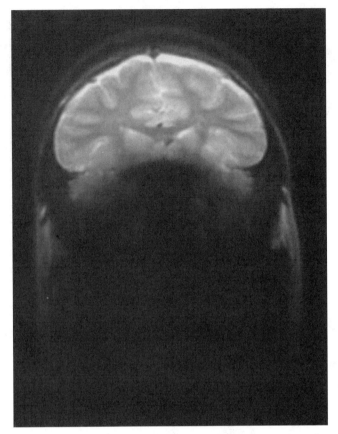

FIG. 17.5. MRI from patient 4 showing obscuration of orbital frontal anatomy by artifact.

MRI was interpreted as normal, but the orbital frontal regions were distorted and partially obscured by artifact from orthodontic devices (Fig. 17.5). Interictal scalp EEG was normal while she was awake and showed left anterior temporal epileptiform sharp waves during sleep. Ictal scalp EEG recordings of numerous seizures were associated with no apparent changes or left temporal buildup of rhythmic theta activity. All but one seizure occurred out of sleep. They consisted of sudden awaking with growling and yelling followed by pronounced pelvic thrusting movements accompanied by grunting noises. After some seizures, she seemed bewildered and dysphasic. These latter seizures were those with a delayed left temporal electrographic seizure buildup.

Because the clinical seizure characteristics strongly suggested frontal lobe origin, an MRI was repeated after her orthodontic devices had been removed and revealed a circumscribed lesion in the left lateral posterior orbital frontal region that previously had been obscured by artifact (Fig. 17.6). A limited intracranial study verified seizure origin from the region of the lesion and also documented inconsistent spread to the left temporal lobe. The subdural intracranial electrodes also were used to map Broca's area.

The lesion was resected. Pathological diagnosis was ganglioglioma. The patient has had no seizures during the 7 years since surgery. She has taken no antiepileptic drugs for 3 years.

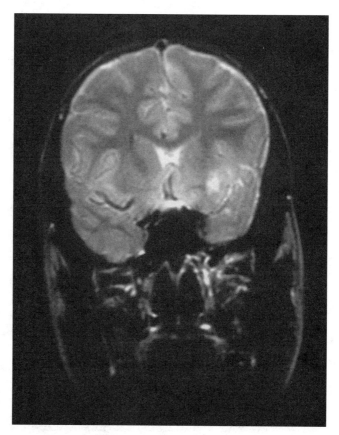

FIG. 17.6. MRI from patient 4 after removal of orthodontic devices and showing lesion in the left posterior orbital frontal cortex.

Comment: This is another example of a patient with typical nocturnally preponderant frontal lobe seizures with complex behaviors that included prominent sexual automatisms. Some of her seizures evolved into a temporal lobe pattern with confusion and aphasia resulting from seizure spread from orbital frontal cortex to the adjacent temporal lobe. Interictal and ictal scalp EEG suggested temporal lobe epilepsy, but the clinical seizure characteristics were strongly suggestive of frontal lobe seizure origin.

Patient 5

This 36-year-old man began having seizures at the age of 10 years. There were no risk factors. Initially, the seizures consisted of a dreamy feeling as if he were being "closed in." These episodes, which were not associated with altered consciousness, occurred several times a week throughout his teenage years. They gradually increased in frequency. When he was 31 years of age, seizures were occurring 10 to 15 times per day. They also began to be associated with altered consciousness and semipurposeful motor activity, such as walking in circles or stamping his feet. He had inappropriate speech and posturing of his right hand and arm. The diagnosis of epilepsy was made. An MRI revealed a cystic lesion in the left posterior medial orbital frontal cortex adjacent to the lamina terminalis (Fig. 17.7). The pathological diagnosis from a biopsy done at another institution was dysembryoplastic neuroepithelial tumor. He was told that sur-

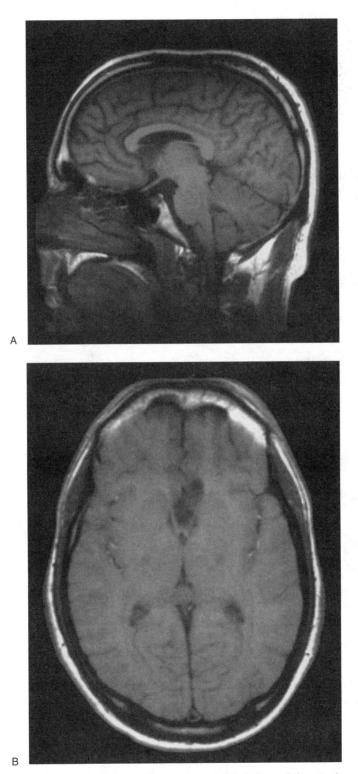

A

B

FIG. 17.7. A,B: MRI from patient 5 showing cystic lesion in left medial posterior orbital cortex.

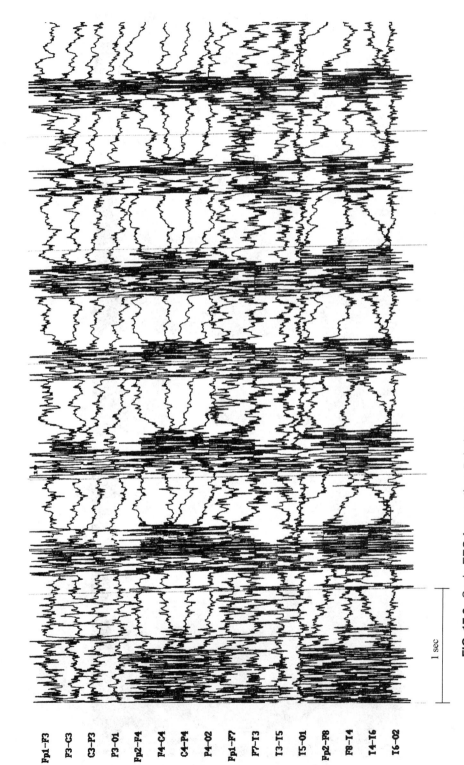

Fp1-F3
F3-C3
C3-P3
P3-O1
Fp2-F4
F4-C4
C4-P4
P4-O2
Fp1-F7
F7-T3
T3-T5
T5-O1
Fp2-F8
F8-T4
T4-T6
T6-O2

1 sec

FIG. 17.8. Scalp EEG from patient 5 during seizure showing maximal buildup of rhythmic theta over left temporal area. Artifact is from lip smacking and chewing automatisms.

gical resection was not advisable because of the location of the lesion. Seizures persisted despite trials with a wide variety of antiepileptic drugs, alone and in combination, and were seriously interfering with his life.

He was evaluated for surgery. Neurologic examination was normal. Interictal scalp EEG showed epileptiform sharp complexes in the left anterior temporal region and in the left frontopolar region. Ictal scalp recording revealed maximal seizure buildup over the left temporal region (Fig. 17.8). An ictal SPECT scan demonstrated increased blood flow in the left medial temporal lobe and the left basal ganglia but not in the region of the lesion (Fig. 17.9). Clinically, seizures consisted of his habitual aura followed by loss of contact, lip smacking and chewing, right hand and arm dystonia, and left hand fumbling automatisms. Because of the EEG and clinical seizure patterns, he underwent a limited intracranial study using subdural electrodes to sample the orbital frontal cortex and lateral and medial temporal lobe regions.

This verified seizure origin in the region of the lesion with rapid spread to the left temporal lobe. Clinical seizure manifestation occurred only after spread to the left temporal lobe, and the lesion was resected. The portion of the lesion invading the frontal lobe was completely removed, but it was probable that tumor remained in the region of the hypothalamus. Pathological examination of the resected tissue confirmed the findings from biopsy. The patient made an uneventful recovery from surgery. He has been seizure free during the year since surgery and continues to take antiepileptic drugs, but in reduced amounts.

Comment: This is an example of a patient with frontal lobe seizure origin who presented with temporal lobe type seizures, both clinically and electrographically. Temporal lobe seizure activity was further documented with an ictal SPECT scan that did not demonstrate orbital frontal enhancement. Although it might be argued that the invasive study was not warranted, it was considered that the seizure characteristics,

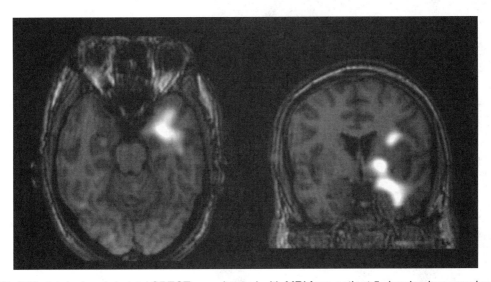

FIG. 17.9. Ictal minus interictal SPECT coregistered with MRI from patient 5 showing increased perfusion in left medial temporal region. There was no signal change in the region of the orbital frontal lesion.

the scalp EEG findings, and the location of the lesion justified the limited invasive study.

Patient 6

This 43-year-old man began having seizures at the age of 14 years. There were no risk factors. Initial seizures were described as simple staring spells without motor activity. Later seizures consisted of unresponsiveness and staring followed by some restless motor activity. Bland seizures lasted 1 to 2 minutes and were associated with postictal agitated confusion and combativeness. Seizures occurred without warning with a nocturnal preponderance. Occasionally, they would secondarily generalize into tonic–clonic seizures. They occurred as frequently as four times per night, but he could go a month without seizures. Medications failed to control seizures, and he was evaluated for surgery at age 38.

Other than borderline intelligence, his neurologic examination was normal. MRI revealed a questionably significant small left frontal lobe, but there were no definite structural abnormalities (Fig. 17.10). Interictal scalp EEG showed right anterior temporal sharp waves. Ictal recording consisted of diffuse bifrontal sharp–slow complexes with a delayed buildup over the right temporal area (Fig. 17.11). Clinically, seizures began with a blank stare and unresponsiveness. Other than some mild restless fidgeting, there was no motor activity for 2 to 3 minutes. He then would develop variable bilateral tonic posturing and left facial clonic activity. Seizures could end there or progress to bilateral symmetric clonic activity. Postictally, he was confused, agitated, and exhibited escape behavior. Because of the atypical appearance of both the clinical seizures and the scalp

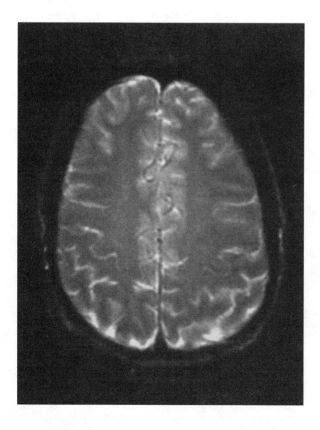

FIG. 17.10. MRI from patient 6 showing smallness of the left frontal lobe.

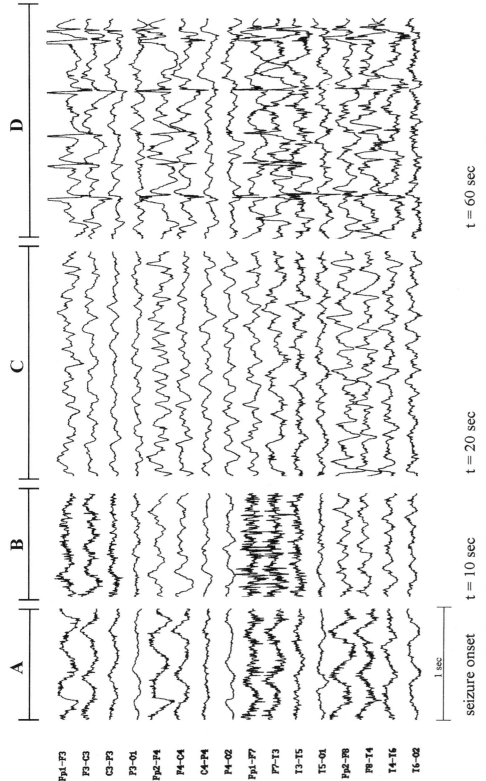

FIG. 17.11. Scalp EEG from patient 6; successive panels from same seizure. **A:** Seizure onset with diffuse 2- to 3-Hz activity. **B:** Continued diffuse rhythmic slow with a slight preponderance in right anterior temporal region. **C:** Continued diffuse slow with some sharp activity clear maximal in right anterior temporal region. **D:** Frontally maximal bilateral 3-Hz spike-and-slow activity 1 minute from seizure onset.

seizure onset   t = 10 sec   t = 20 sec   t = 60 sec

1 sec

Fp1–F3
F3–C3
C3–P3
P3–O1
Fp2–F4
F4–C4
C4–P4
P4–O2
Fp1–F7
F7–T3
T3–T5
T5–O1
Fp2–F8
F8–T4
T4–T6
T6–O2

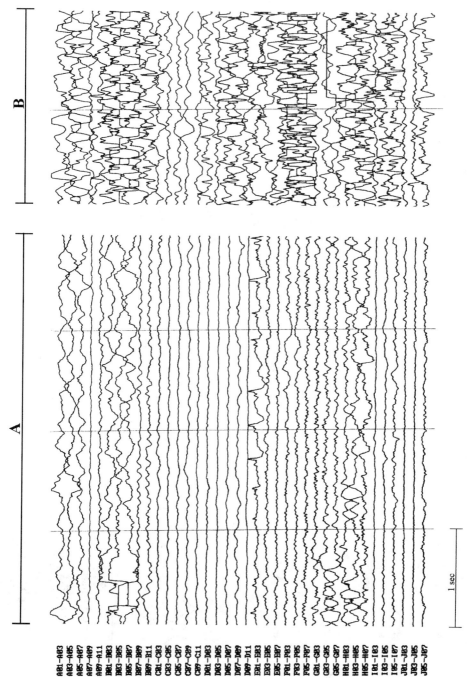

FIG. 17.12. Intracranial recording using a combination of bilateral 12-contact depth electrodes *(A–D)* and bilateral 8-contact subdural strip electrodes *(E–J)*. **A:** All seizures began with 3-Hz periodic sharp discharges from most distant contact of left frontal subdural strip electrode (E1). **B:** Maximal seizure buildup occurred in the right hippocampus (B1–B7), right frontal convexity (F1–F8) and right lateral temporal cortex (H1–7).

EEG, he underwent an extensive invasive evaluation using a combination of bilateral depth and subdural electrodes. Six seizures were recorded. Although the initial impression was that of poorly localized right hippocampal seizure onset, further evaluation with all 96 intracranial contacts displayed, showed consistent initial seizure activity in the left frontal polar region (Fig. 17.12). Because this left frontopolar seizure activity was confined to the most distant contact of an eight-contact subdural strip, a second invasive evaluation was undertaken to document better the left frontal seizure origin, which did confirm left frontal lobe origin. The patient underwent a left anterior frontal resection. Pathological examination of the resected tissue revealed nodular thickening of the molecular layer, abnormal neuronal orientation, and previously unrecognized regional microgyria.

Six months after surgery, the patient was admitted urgently in convulsive status epilepticus. There was no obvious explanation for this event. These were the first and last seizures since surgery. He has now been seizure free for 4.5 years but remains on antiepileptic medications.

Comment: This patient had "absence-like" frontal lobe seizures, both clinically and electrographically. He had misleading scalp EEGs and potentially misleading intracranial EEGs. In retrospect, the small left frontal lobe on MRI was probably significant and is an example of a carefully planned and well executed "fishing expedition."

Patient 7

This 49-year-old woman developed bifrontal headaches at the age of 35 years old. These headaches progressively increased in intensity over the next 2 years. She was found to have a large left medial superior frontopolar arteriovenous malformation, which was resected without incident. Two years after surgery, she had her first generalized tonic–clonic seizure. Convulsive seizures were controlled with antiepileptic drugs but she continued to have rare, brief seizures consisting of a giddy, "spacey" feeling without alteration of consciousness. When she was 46 years old, seizures increased in frequency and were followed by generalized tonic–clonic seizures. She then developed prolonged confusional episodes with variable loss of contact, often accompanied by uncontrollable laughter. These episodes would last hours to days and were medically refractory. She was evaluated for surgery.

Her neurologic examination and neuropsychological testing were normal. MRI revealed a well-circumscribed region of postoperative encephalomalacia in the left frontopolar region (Fig. 17.13). Scalp EEG demonstrated a left frontal spike focus. During video/EEG monitoring, several habitual seizures were recorded. Typically, they began with bifrontal continuous 3- to 4-Hz spike or sharp–slow activity that persisted unchanged throughout the seizure (Fig. 17.14). Initially, the patient was fully responsive, conversing with the staff. Later in the same seizure, she would stop speaking and appear bewildered. She would follow some, but not all commands. Finally, she would develop uncontrolled, infectious laughter. The documented episodes lasted up to 3 hours and were terminated rapidly with lorazepam. Some seizures evolved into right adversive seizures that rapidly generalized into tonic–clonic seizures. Despite the disabling nature of these seizures and the high likelihood of surgical success, the patient refused surgery.

Comment: This patient with an unequivocal left frontal lobe seizure focus developed frequent episodes of nonconvulsive status epilepticus that electrically resembled spike-wave stupor. These unusual clinical manifestations included a striking gelastic component. During episodes of nonconvulsive status, there was electroclinical dissociation in that clinical features varied, whereas the EEG seizure pattern did not.

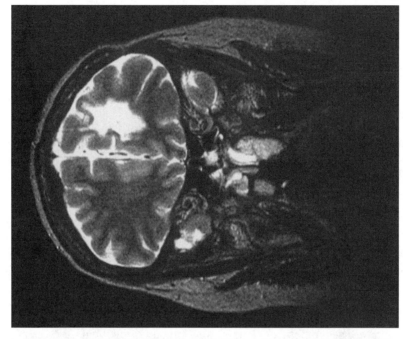

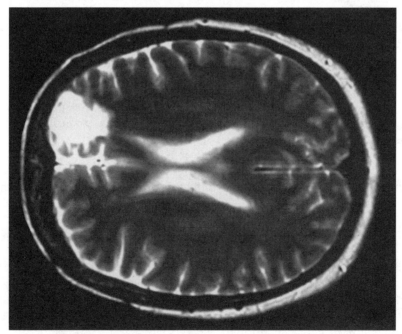

FIG. 17.13. MRI from patient 7 showing postoperative encephalomalacia in the left frontal polar region.

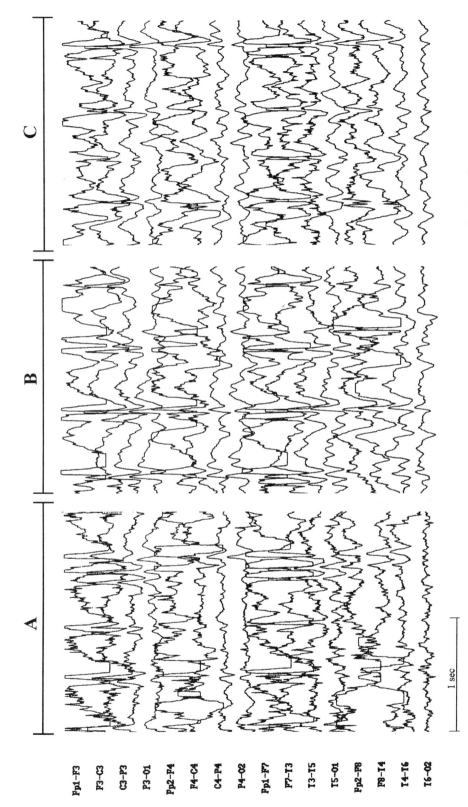

FIG. 17.14. Scalp EEG from patient 7 during an episode of nonconvulsive status epilepticus showing electroclinical obscuration. Panels A through C with similar 2- to 3-Hz bifrontal spike-wave patterns. **A:** Clinically, the patient is fully conversant and appears normal. **B:** She appears bewildered and would not respond. **C:** She appears unresponsive and had uncontrolled laughter.

Fp1–F3
F3–C3
C3–P3
P3–O1
Fp2–F4
F4–C4
C4–P4
P4–O2
Fp1–F7
F7–T3
T3–T5
T5–O1
Fp2–F8
F8–T4
T4–T6
T6–O2

1 sec

A   B   C

Patient 8

This 22-year-old man began having seizures at age 2. Initially, they were characterized by falling to the ground unresponsive. He had a number of these events in clusters, and the diagnosis of epilepsy was made. Multiple antiepileptic drugs, alone and in combination, failed to control the seizures. The seizures changed in character. They became predominantly nocturnal, occurring in clusters of up to 30 a night. They were characterized by profuse salivation, gulping, and swallowing, facial automatisms with grimacing, and the inability to speak. Consciousness and understanding were not impaired. He was evaluated for surgery at the age of 16 years. His neurologic examination was normal. The MRI and examination were normal. Scalp EEG during seizures revealed subtle slowing in the left frontal temporal region. An ictal SPECT scan showed increased uptake in the left inferior posterior lateral frontal lobe. He underwent an invasive study with two 4 × 8 subdural grids placed over the frontal convexity. Seizures began in the frontal operculum between Broca's area and the lower end of the primary motor strip. Because resection almost certainly would produce a language impairment, he had a subpial transection of the region of seizure origin. Initially, seizures were unaffected by surgery. Within a year from surgery, and possibly related to antiepileptic drug adjustments, he was having rare brief nocturnal seizures.

Comment: This patient had opercular onset seizures from the language-dominant side. This was well documented during presurgical evaluation and with invasive monitoring. Because he had been refractory to all antiepileptic medications before surgery, the subpial transection probably had some delayed beneficial effect.

CONCLUSION

Although frontal lobe epilepsy is common, the clinical presentation is diverse. No single seizure type stands out as specifically diag-

nostic or frontal lobe seizure origin, but some are suggestive. The following conclusions are based on current understanding of frontal lobe seizures and epilepsies:

1. Frontal lobe seizures with agitated, aggressive, complex motor behavior often accompanied by vocalization are identifiable from the clinical presentation alone. These seizures occur in their "pure" form when the seizure discharge remains confined to the frontal lobes, resulting in the typically brief, often nocturnally preponderant seizures, which tend to occur in clusters or as episodes of nonconvulsive status epilepticus. This constellation of clinical findings is almost diagnostic of frontal lobe seizure origin but not of side or site of origin. Scalp EEG findings are often normal, nonspecific, or misleading.

2. Brief, explosive seizures consisting of various patterns of asymmetric tonic posturing, often with preservation of consciousness, are highly suggestive of seizure origin in the supplementary motor area. These seizures tend to occur in clusters with a nocturnal preponderance. The tonic posturing is usually predominantly unilateral and contralateral to the side of seizure origin. Interictal and ictal scalp EEG recording is often not informative. Caution is required, however, because asymmetric tonic seizures can be associated with seizure origin from other frontal lobe regions and as well as seizures beginning outside of the frontal lobes.

3. Seizures beginning in the frontal lobes, particularly the orbital frontal region, can spread to the temporal lobes. When this happens, a frontal lobe seizure can evolve into a temporal lobe seizure with characteristic automatisms and postictal confusion. Conversely, the frontal lobe seizure discharges can be clinically silent with seizure manifestations appearing only after seizure spread to temporal lobe structures has occurred. This can occur with orbital frontal seizure onset, and the episodes will closely resemble temporal lobe seizures.

4. Focal clonic motor seizures always imply involvement of the primary motor (pre-

rolandic) gyrus. Seizure origin, however, can be from elsewhere in the brain, adjacent to the motor strip or from more remote areas. Therefore, whereas these common seizures are usually specific for lateralization, they are not specific for localization of the region of seizure origin.

5. Seizures resembling absence seizures and absence status can be seen in patients with frontal lobe seizure origin.

6. Frontal opercular seizures consisting of prominent face and jaw motor activity, deglutition, profuse salivation, and when from the language dominant side, Broca's aphasia (although infrequently described) are probably a recognizable variety of frontal lobe seizures.

7. Anterior cingulate gyrus seizures cannot be distinguished from the more generic frontal lobe seizures with complex behaviors that can originate in several frontal lobe regions.

Finally, surgical intervention in patients with frontal lobe seizures is said to be less successful than for temporal lobe epilepsy (78,118). Although this is still true, there has been improvement during the past 20 years. Advances in neuroimaging and improved understanding of frontal lobe seizures have allowed many more patients with refractory frontal lobe seizures to be considered for surgery. Surgical success in carefully studied patients with frontal lobe epilepsy now resembles that reported for temporal lobe epilepsy 20 years ago (49,78,119). Additional advances are sure to follow.

REFERENCES

1. Temkin O. *The falling sickness.* Baltimore: Johns Hopkins Press, 1945.
2. Bravais LF. *Recherche sur les symptômes et le traitement de l'épilepsie hemiplegique.* Paris: Thèse Fac Med, 1827.
3. Jackson JH, ed. *Selected writings of John Hughlings Jackson.* Reprinted in 1931 and edited by Taylor J. London: Staples Press, 1874.
4. Horsley SV. Brain-surgery. *BMJ* 1886;2:670–675.
5. Penfield W, Welch K. The supplementary motor area of the cerebral cortex. *Arch Neurol Psychiatry* 1951;66:289–317.
6. Penfield W, Jasper H. *Epilepsy and the functional anatomy of the human brain.* Boston: Little, Brown, 1954.
7. Ajmone-Marsan C, Ralston BL. *The epileptic seizure: its functional morphology and diagnostic significance.* Springfield, IL: Charles C. Thomas, 1957:211–215.
8. Geier S, Bancaud J, Talairach J, et al. Clinical note: clinical and tele-stereo–EEG findings in a patient with psychomotor seizures. *Epilepsia* 1975;16:119–125.
9. Geier S, Bancaud J, Talairach J, et al. Automatisms during frontal lobe epileptic seizures. *Brain* 1976;99:447–458.
10. Geier S, Bancaud J, Talairach J, et al. The seizures of frontal lobe epilepsy: a study of clinical manifestations. *Neurology* 1977;27:951–958.
11. Ludwig B, Ajmone-Marsan C, Van Buren J. Cerebral seizures of probable orbitofrontal origin. *Epilepsia* 1975;16:141–158.
12. Tharp BR. Orbital frontal seizures: a unique electroencephalographic and clinical syndrome. *Epilepsia* 1972;13:627–642.
13. Waterman K, Purves SJ, Kosaka B, et al. An epileptic syndrome caused by mesial frontal lobe foci. *Neurology* 1987;37:577–582.
14. Williamson PD, Spencer DD, Spencer SS, et al. Complex partial seizures of frontal lobe origin. *Ann Neurol* 1985;18:497–504.
15. Baumgartner C, Flint R, Tuxhorn I, et al. Supplementary motor area seizures: propagation pathways as studied with invasive recordings. *Neurology* 1996;l46:508–514.
16. Morris HH, Dinner DS, Lüders HO, et al. Supplementary motor seizures: clinical and electroencephalographic findings. *Neurology* 1988;38:1075–1082.
17. Salanova V, Morris H, Van Ness P, et al. Frontal lobe seizures: electroclinical syndromes. *Epilepsia* 1995;36:16–24.
18. Chauvel P, Delgado-Escueta A, Halgren E, Bancaud J, eds. *Frontal lobe seizures and epilepsies. Advances in Neurology,* vol 57. New York: Raven Press, 1992.
19. Jasper HH, Riggio S, Goldman-Rakic PS, eds. *Epilepsy and the functional anatomy of the frontal lobe. Advances in Neurology,* vol 66. New York: Raven Press, 1995.
20. Hayman M, Scheffer IE, Chinvarun Y, et al. Autosomal dominant nocturnal frontal lobe epilepsy: demonstration of focal frontal onset and intrafamilial variation. *Neurology* 1997;49:969–975.
21. Meierkord H, Fish DR, Smith SJM, et al. Is nocturnal paroxysmal dystonia a form of frontal lobe epilepsy? *Mov Disord* 1992;7:38–42.
22. Oldani A, Zucconi M, et al. Autosomal dominant nocturnal frontal lobe epilepsy: electroclinical picture. *Epilepsia* 1996;37:964–976.
23. Oldani A, Zucconi M, Asselta R, et al. Autosomal dominant nocturnal frontal lobe epilepsy: a video-polysomnographic and genetic appraisal of 40 patients and delineation of the epileptic syndrome. *Brain* 1998;121(Pt 2):205–23.
24. Provini F, Plazzi G, Tinuper P, et al. Nocturnal frontal lobe epilepsy: a clinical and polygraphic overview of 100 consecutive cases. *Brain* 1999;122(Pt 6):1017–1031.
25. Scheffer IE, Bhatia KP, Lopes-Cendes I, et al. Autosomal dominant frontal epilepsy misdiagnosed as sleep disorder. *Lancet* 1994;343:515–517.
26. Tinuper P, Cerullo A, Cirignotta F, et al. Nocturnal paroxysmal dystonia with short-lasting attacks: three

cases with evidence for an epileptic frontal lobe origin of seizures. *Epilepsia* 1990;31:549–556.

27. Figl A, Viseshakul N, Shafaee N, et al. Two mutations linked to nocturnal frontal lobe epilepsy cause use-dependent potentiation of the nicotinic ACh response. *J Physiol* 1998;513(Pt 3):55–70.

28. Nakken KO, Magnusson A, Steinlein OK. Autosomal dominant nocturnal frontal lobe epilepsy: an electroclinical study of a Norwegian family with ten affected members. *Epilepsia* 1999;40:88–92.

29. Phillips HA, Scheffer IE, et al. Localization of a gene for autosomal dominant nocturnal frontal lobe epilepsy to chromosome 20q13.2. *Nat Genet* 1995;10: 117–118.

30. Phillips HA, Scheffer IE, Crossland KM, et al. Autosomal dominant nocturnal frontal-lobe epilepsy: genetic heterogeneity and evidence for a second locus at 15q24. *Am J Hum Genet* 1998;63:1108–1116.

31. Steinlein OK, Magnusson A, Stoodt J, et al. An insertion mutation of the *CHRNA4* gene in a family with autosomal dominant nocturnal frontal lobe epilepsy. *Hum Mol Genet* 1997;6:943–947.

32. Steinlein OK, Mulley JC, et al. A missense mutation in the neuronal nicotinic acetylcholine receptor alpha 4 subunit is associated with autosomal dominant nocturnal frontal lobe epilepsy. *Nat Genet* 1995;11:201–203.

33. Engel J Jr, Williamson PD, Wieser HG. Mesial temporal lobe epilepsy. In: Engel J Jr, Pedley TA, eds. *Epilepsy: a comprehensive textbook.* Philadelphia: Lippincott–Raven, 1997:2417–2426.

34. French JA, Williamson PD, Thadani VM, et al. Characteristics of medial temporal lobe epilepsy. I. Results of history and physical examination. *Ann Neurol* 1993; 34:774–780.

35. Williamson PD, French JA, Thadani VM, et al. Characteristics of medial temporal lobe epilepsy. II. Interictal and ictal scalp electroencephalography, neuropsychological testing, neuroimaging, surgical results, and pathology. *Ann Neurol* 1993;34:781–787.

36. Williamson PD, Thadani VM, French JA, et al. Medial temporal lobe epilepsy. III. Videotape analysis of objective seizure characteristics. *Epilepsia* 1998;39 (Suppl 1):1182–1188.

37. Williamson PD. Frontal lobe seizures: problems of diagnosis and classification. In: Chauvel P, Delgado-Escueta AV, Halgren E, Bancaud J, eds. *Frontal lobe seizures and epilepsies. Advances in Neurology,* vol 57. New York: Raven Press, 1992:289–309.

38. Williamson PD. Frontal lobe epilepsy: some clinical characteristics. In: Jasper HH, Riggio S, Goldman-Rakic PS, eds. *Epilepsy and the functional anatomy of the frontal lobe. Advances in Neurology,* vol 66. New York: Raven Press, 1995:127–152.

39. Bancaud J, Talairach J. Clinical semiology of frontal lobe seizures. In: Chauvel P, Delgado-Escueta AV, Halgren E, Bancaud J, eds. *Frontal lobe seizures and epilepsies. Advances in Neurology,* vol 57. New York: Raven Press, 1992:53–58.

40. Quesney LF, Constain M, Fish DR, et al. The clinical differentiation of seizures arising in the parasagittal and anterolaterodorsal frontal convexities. *Arch Neurol* 1990;47:677–679.

41. So NK. Mesial frontal epilepsy. *Epilepsia* 1998;39 (Suppl 4):S49–S61.

42. Thomas P, Andermann F. Late-onset absence status

epilepticus is most often situation-related. In: Malafosse A, Genton P, Hirsch E, eds. *Idiopathic generalized epilepsies.* London: John Libbey, 1994.

43. Tomson T, Lindom U, Nilsson BY. Nonconvulsive status epilepticus in adults: thirty-two consecutive patients from a general hospital population. *Epilepsia* 1992;33:829–835.

44. Janz D. Status epilepticus and frontal lobe lesions. *J Neurol Sci* 1964;11:446–457.

45. Williamson PD, Engel J Jr, Munari C. Anatomic classification of localization-related epilepsies. In: Engel J Jr, Pedley TA, eds. *Epilepsy: a comprehensive textbook.* Philadelphia: Lippincott–Raven, 1997:2405–2416.

46. Williamson PD, Mattson RH, Spencer DD, et al. Complex partial status epilepticus: a depth electrode evaluation. *Ann Neurol* 1983;18:647–654.

47. Bancaud J, Talairach J, Bonis A, et al. *La stereo electroencephalographie dans l'épilepsie.* Paris: Masson, 1965.

48. Chauvel P, Kliemann F, Vignal JP, et al. The clinical signs and symptoms of frontal lobe seizures: phenomenology and classification. In: Jasper HH, Riggio S, Goldman-Rakic PS, eds. *Epilepsy and the functional anatomy of the frontal lobe. Advances in Neurology,* vol 66. New York: Raven Press, 1995:115–126.

49. Jobst BC, Siegel AM, Thadani VM, et al. Intractable seizures of frontal lobe origin. *Epilepsia* 2000. (In press.)

50. Commission on Classification and Terminology of the International League Against Epilepsy. Proposal for classification of epilepsies and epileptic syndromes. *Epilepsia* 1985;26:268–278.

51. Commission on Classification and Terminology of the International League Against Epilepsy. Proposal for revised classification of epilepsies and epileptic syndromes. *Epilepsia* 1989;30:389–399.

52. Laskowitz DT, Sperling MR, French JA, et al. The syndrome of frontal lobe epilepsy: characteristics and surgical management. *Neurology* 1995;45:780–787.

53. Spencer SS, Spencer DD, Williamson PD, et al. Sexual automatisms in complex partial seizures. *Neurology* 1983;33:527–533.

54 Wieser HG, Swartz BE, Delgado-Escueta AV, et al. Differentiating frontal lobe seizures from temporal lobe seizures. In: Chauvel P, Delgado-Escueta AV, Halgren E, Bancaud J, eds. *Frontal lobe seizures and epilepsies. Advances in Neurology,* vol 57. New York: Raven Press, 1992:267–285.

55. Munari C, Tassi L, Di Leo M, et al. Video-stereo–electroencephalographic investigation of the orbitofrontal cortex. In: Jasper HH, Riggio S, Goldman-Rakic PS, eds. *Epilepsy and the functional anatomy of the frontal lobe. Advances in Neurology,* vol 66. New York: Raven Press, 1995:115–126.

56. Quesney LF, Constain M, Rasmussen T. Seizures from the dorsolateral frontal lobe. In: Chauvel P, Delgado-Escueta AV, Halgren E, Bancaud J, eds. *Frontal lobe seizures and epilepsies. Advances in Neurology,* vol 57. New York: Raven Press, 1992:233–244.

57. Penfield W, Erickson TC. *Epilepsy and cerebral localization.* Baltimore: Charles C. Thomas, 1941:101–103.

58. Fakhoury T, Abou-Khalil B. Association of ipsilateral head turning and dystonia in temporal lobe seizures. *Epilepsia* 1995;36:1065–1070.

59. Kotagal P, Lüders HO, Morris HH, et al. Dystonic posturing in complex partial seizures of temporal lobe onset: a new lateralizing sign. *Neurology* 1989;39: 196–201.

60. Wieser HG. Ictal manifestations of temporal lobe seizures. *Adv Neurol* 1991;55:301–315.

61 Fusco L, Iani C, Faedda MT, et al. Mesial frontal lobe epilepsy: a clinical entity not sufficiently described. *J Epilepsy* 1990;3:123–135.

62. Kanner AM, Morris HH, Lüders HO, et al. Supplementary motor seizures mimicking pseudoseizures: some clinical differences. *Neurology* 1990;40: 1404–1407.

63. Connolly MB, Langill L, Wong PKH, et al. Seizures involving the supplementary sensorimotor area in children: a video-EEG analysis. *Epilepsia* 1995;36:1025–1032.

64. Lim SH, Dinner DS, Pillay PK, et al. Functional anatomy of the human supplementary sensorimotor area: results of extraoperative electrical stimulation. *Electroencephalogr Clin Neurophysiol* 1994;91:179–193.

65. Morris HH, Dinner DS, Lüders HO, et al. Supplentary motor seizures. *Neurology* 1998;38:1075–1082.

66. Delgado-Escueta AV, Swartz B, Chauvel P, et al. Clinical and CCTV-EEG evaluation in presurgical work-up of temporal and frontal lobe epilepsies. *Epilepsy Res Suppl* 1992;5:37–54.

67. Geier S, Bancaud J, Talairach J, et al. Ictal tonic postural changes and automatisms of the upper limb during epileptic parietal lobe discharges. *Epilepsia* 1977; 18:517–524.

68. Manford M, Fish DR, Shorvon SD. An analysis of clinical seizure patterns and their localizing value in frontal and temporal lobe epilepsies. *Brain* 1996; 119:17–40.

69. Williamson PD, Boon PA, Thadani VM, et al. Parietal lobe epilepsy: diagnostic considerations and results of surgery. *Ann Neurol* 1992;31:193–201.

70. Biraben A, Chauvel P. Epilepsia partialis continua. In: Engel J Jr, Pedley TA, eds. *Epilepsy: a comprehensive textbook.* Philadelphia: Lippincott–Raven, 1997: 2224–2453.

71. Thomas JE, Reggan TJ, Klass DW. Epilepsia partialis continua: a review of 32 cases. *Arch Neurol* 1977;34: 266–275.

72. Loiseau P. The Jacksonian model of partial motor seizures. In: Chauvel P, Delgado-Escueta AV, Halgren E, Bancaud J, eds. *Frontal lobe seizures and epilepsies. Advances in Neurology,* vol 57. New York: Raven Press, 1992:181–184.

73. Andermann F, Rasmussen TB. Chronic encephalitis and epilepsy: an overview. In: Andermann F, ed. *Chronic encephalitis and epilepsy: Rasmussen's syndrome.* Boston: Butterworth–Heinemann, 1991: 283–288.

74. Vining EPG, Freeman JM, Brandt J, et al. Progressive unilateral encephalopathy of childhood (Rasmussen's syndrome): a reappraisal. *Epilepsia* 1993;34:639–650.

75. Loiseau P, Cohadon F, Cohadon S. Recording of absences of petit mal type in a man of 40, with epileptic attacks since the age of 3, who had a frontal glioma. *Electroencephalogr Clin Neurophysiol* 1971;30:251.

76. Goldensohn E. Structural lesions of the frontal lobe: manifestations, classification, and prognosis. In: Chau-

vel P, Delgado-Escueta AV, Halgren E, Bancaud J, eds. *Frontal lobe seizures and epilepsies. Advances in Neurology,* vol 57. New York: Raven Press, 1992:435–447.

77. Williamson PD, Wieser HG, Delgado-Escueta AV. Clinical characteristics of partial seizures. In: Engel J Jr, ed. *Surgical treatment of the epilepsies.* New York: Raven Press, 1987:101–120.

78. Sutherling WW, Risinger MW, Crandall PH, et al. Focal functional anatomy of dorsolateral frontocentral seizures. *Neurology* 1990;40:87–98.

79. Lerman P. Benign childhood epilepsy with centrotemporal spikes (BECT). In: Engel J Jr, Engel TA, eds. *Epilepsy: a comprehensive textbook.* Philadelphia: Lippincott–Raven, 1997:2307–2314.

80. Mazars G. Cingulate gyrus epileptogenic foci as an origin for generalized seizures. In: Gastaut H, Jasper H, Bancaud J, Waltregny A, eds. *The physiolopathogenesis of the epilepsies.* Springfield, IL: Charles C. Thomas, 1969:186–189.

81. Mazars G. Criteria for identifying cingulate epilepsies. *Epilepsia* 1970;11:41–47.

82. Mazars G, Gotusso C, Merienne L. Criteria for identifying cingulate epilepsies. *Rev Neurol* 1966;114: 225–242.

83. Crespel A, Baldy-Moulinier M, Coubes P. The relationship between sleep and epilepsy in frontal and temporal lobe epilepsies: practical and physiopathic considerations. *Epilepsia* 1998;39:150–157.

84. Williamson PD, Spencer DD, Spencer SS, et al. Complex partial status epilepticus: a depth-electrode study. *Ann Neurol* 1985;18:647–654.

85. Pataraia E, Lurger S, Serles W, et al. Ictal scalp EEG in unilateral mesial temporal lobe epilepsy. *Epilepsia* 1998;39:608–614.

86. Sperling MR, O'Connor MJ, Saykin AJ, et al. A noninvasive protocol for anterior temporal lobectomy. *Neurology* 1992;42:416–422.

87. Walczak TS, Jayakzar P. Interictal EEG. In: Engel J Jr, Pedley TA, eds. *Epilepsy: a comprehensive textbook.* Philadelphia: Lippincott–Raven, 1997:831–848.

88. Quesney LF. Extratemporal epilepsy: clinical presentation, pre-operative EEG localization, and surgical outcome. *Acta Neurol Scand Suppl* 1992;140:81–94.

89. Quesney LF, Risinger MW, Shewmon DA. Extracranial EET evaluation. In: Engel J Jr, ed. *Surgical treatment of the epilepsies,* 2nd ed. New York: Raven Press, 1993:173–196.

90. Sperling MR, Clancy RR. Ictal EEG. In: Engel J Jr, Pedley TA, eds. *Epilepsy: a comprehensive textbook.* Philadelphia: Lippincott–Raven, 1997:849–885.

91. Tukel K, Jasper H. The electroencephalogram in parasagittal lesions. *Electroencephalogr Clin Neurophysiol* 1952;4:481–494.

92. Bergen D, Bleck T, Ramsey R, et al. Magnetic resonance imaging as a sensitive and specific predictor of neoplasms removed for intractable epilepsy. *Epilepsia* 1989;30:310–321.

93. Boon PA, Williamson PD, Fried I, et al. Intracranial, intraaxial, space-occupying lesions in patients with intractable partial seizures: an anatomoclinical, neuropsychological, and surgical correlation. *Epilepsia* 1991; 32:467–476.

94. Cascino GD. Structural brain imaging. In: Engel J Jr, Pedley TA, eds. *Epilepsy: a comprehensive textbook.* Philadelphia: Lippincott–Raven, 1997:937–946.

95. Cascino GD, Clifford RJ, Parisi JE, et al. MRI in presurgical evaluation of patients with frontal lobe epilespy and children with temporal lobe epilepsy: pathologic correlation and prognostic importance. *Epilepsy Res* 1992;11:51–59.

96. Barkovich AJ, Kuzniecky RI. Neuroimaging of focal malformations of cortical development. *J Clin Neurophysiol* 1996;13:481–494.

97. Palmini A, Andermann F, Olivier A, et al. Focal neuronal migration disorders and intractable partial epilepsy: a study of 30 patients. *Ann Neurol* 1991;30:741–749.

98. Berkovic SF, Newton MR. Single photon emission computed tomography. In: Engel J Jr, Pedley TA, eds. *Epilepsy: a comprehensive textbook.* Philadelphia: Lippincott–Raven, 1997:969–975.

99. Stefan H, Quesney LF, Feistel HK, et al. Presurgical evaluation in frontal lobe epilepsy: a multimethodological approach. *Adv Neurol* 1995;66:213–221.

100. O' Brien TJ, So EL, Mullan BP, et al. Subtraction ictal SPECT co-registered to MRI improves clinical usefulness of SPECT in localizing the surgical seizure focus. *Neurology* 1998;50:445–454.

101. Engel J Jr, Brown WJ, Kuhl DE, et al. Pathological findings underlying focal temporal lobe hypometabolism in partial epilepsy. *Ann Neurol* 1982;12:518–528.

102. Foldvary N, Lee N, Hanson MW, et al. Correlation of hippocampal neuronal density and FDG-PET in mesial temporal lobe epilepsy. *Epilepsia* 1999;40: 26–29.

103. Henry TR, Chugani HT. Positron emission tomography. In: Engel J Jr, Pedley TA, eds. *Epilepsy: a comprehensive textbook.* Philadelphia: Lippincott–Raven, 1997:947–968.

104. Radtke RA, Hanson MW, Hoffman JM, et al. Temporal lobe hypometabolism on PET: predictor of seizure control after temporal lobectomy. *Neurology* 1993;43 1088–1092.

105. Henry TR, Sutherling WW, Engel J Jr. Interictal cerebral metabolism in partial epilepsies of neocortical origin. *Epilepsy Res* 1991;10:174–182.

106. Radtke RA, Hanson MW, Hoffman JM, et al. Positron emission tomography: comparison of clinical utility in temporal lobe and extratemporal epilepsy. *J Epilepsy* 1994;7:27–33.

107. Connelly A, Van Paesschen W, Porter DA, et al. Proton magnetic resonance spectroscopy in MRI-negative temporal lobe epilepsy. *Neurology* 1998;51:61–66.

108. Garcia PA, Laxer KD, van der Grond J, et al. Phospho-

rus magnetic resonance spectroscopic imaging in patients with frontal lobe epilepsy. *Ann Neurol* 1994;35: 217–221.

109. Hugg JW, Laxer KD, Matson GB, et al. Lateralization of human focal epilepsy by ^{31}P magnetic resonance spectroscopic imaging. *Neurology* 1992;42:2011–2008.

110. Hugg JW, Laxer KD, Matson GB, et al. Neuron loss localizes human temporal lobe epilepsy by in vivo proton magnetic resonance spectroscopic imaging. *Ann Neurol* 1993;34:788–794.

111. Laxer KD, Garcia PA. Imaging criteria to identify the epileptic focus: magnetic resonance imaging, magnetic resonance spectroscopy, positron emission tomography scanning, and single photon emission computed tomography. *Neurosurg Clin North Am* 1993;4: 199–209.

112. Williamson PD. Evaluation of patients for epilepsy surgery at the West Haven VA/Yale–New Haven Epilepsy Unit. In: Spencer SS, Spencer DD, eds. *Surgery for epilepsy.* Boston: Blackwell, 1991:36–52.

113. Harvey AS, Hopkins IJ, Bowe JM, et al. Frontal lobe epilepsy: clinical seizure characteristics and localization with ictal 99m Tc-HMPAO SPECT. *Neurology* 1993;43:1966–1980.

114. Marks DA, Katz A, Hoffer P, et al. Localization of extratemporal epileptic foci during ictal single photon emission computed tomography. *Ann Neurol* 1992; 32:250–255.

115. Spencer SS. Intracranial recording. In: Spencer SS, Spencer DD, eds. *Surgery for epilepsy.* Boston: Blackwell, 1991:54–68.

116. Jobst BC, Siegel AM, Thadani VM, et al. Clinical characteristics and localizing signs in seizures of frontal lobe origin. Presented at the 23rd International Epilepsy Congress. Prague, Czech Republic, 1999. *Epilepsia* 1999;40(Suppl 2):266–267.

117. Williamson PD, Thadani VM, Siegel AM, et al. Nonlesional, medically intractable, localization-related epilepsy: a diagnostic challenge. *Epilepsia* 1997;38 (Suppl 8):65.

118. Rasmussen T. Surgery of frontal lobe epilepsy. In: Purpura DP, Penry JK, Walter RD, eds. *Neurosurgical management of the epilepsies.* New York: Raven Press, 1975:197–205.

119. Roberts DW, Williamson PD, Thadani VM, et al. Nonlesional supplementary motor area epilepsy: results of evaluation and surgery in four patients. *Epilepsia* 1995;36(Suppl 4):15.

Neocortical Epilepsies.
Advances in Neurology, Vol. 84,
edited by P.D. Williamson, A.M. Siegel,
D.W. Roberts, V.M. Thadani, and M.S. Gazzaniga.
Lippincott Williams & Wilkins, Philadelphia © 2000.

18

Neocortical Status Epilepticus

David M. Treiman

Department of Neurology, University of Medicine and Dentistry of New Jersey,
Robert Wood Johnson Medical School, New Brunswick, New Jersey 08901

The first reference to status epilepticus in the medical literature (1) was almost certainly an account of neocortical status epilepticus. Although it has been suggested that there are as many types of status epilepticus as there are types of epileptic seizures (2), most episodes of status epilepticus are neocortical in localization because they arise from a neocortical seizure focus, result from a diffuse neocortical insult such as hypoxia or infection, or engage the neocortex before evolving into status epilepticus. This chapter deals mainly with the three types of status epilepticus that are primarily neocortical: secondarily generalized convulsive status epilepticus (GCSE), complex partial status of neocortical origin, and simple partial status epilepticus. It considers other types of status epilepticus only as necessary to clarify issues related to these three types of status epilepticus.

DEFINITION OF STATUS EPILEPTICUS

Status epilepticus is defined in the International Classification of Epileptic Seizures (ICES) (3) as a "seizure which persists for a sufficient length of time or is repeated frequently enough that recovery between attacks does not occur." This definition has been criticized as lacking operational precision. Many investigators add a requirement that the seizures persist at least 30 minutes, but a recent editorial argued for a requirement of only 5 minutes' duration (4). Although it does lack operational criteria, the current ICES definition captures the essence of the pathophysiologic nature of status epilepticus that was suggested by the initial ICES definition of status epilepticus as "a term used whenever a seizure persists for a sufficient length of time, or is repeated frequently enough to produce a fixed or enduring epileptic condition" (5). The idea is that mechanisms exist that cause isolated seizures to be brief paroxysmal events that exhibit a characteristic evolution over a period of a few seconds to a few minutes and then stop abruptly. Then there is complete recovery from seizure-induced neurochemical and physiological changes during a refractory period, during which further seizures do not occur. When there is a loss of the mechanisms that limit the duration of seizures and that are responsible for the refractory state, so that subsequent seizures occur before complete normalization of brain chemistry and physiology, then the patient can be viewed as being in an enduring epileptic condition, that is, status epilepticus. Sometimes, however, seizures do not stop at all but continue for longer than the usual brief duration of most seizures. When this occurs, and there is a loss of the typical evolution for that type of seizure (e.g., from tonic to clonic activity, to abrupt cessation as seen in generalized tonic–clonic seizures), the patient also can be regarded as being in status epilepticus, regardless of the duration of the seizure activity. Operationally, continuous seizure activity for more than 10 minutes was used to diagnose the continuous presentation of GCSE in a recently published treatment study (6). The essential element for diagnosis is not the exact duration, which is necessarily arbitrary, but rather the loss of the characteristic evolution of the seizure, which is what tells us there has been a loss of seizure stopping mechanisms and that the patient is in status epilepticus.

PATHOPHYSIOLOGY

Mechanisms that start and stop seizures are as yet incompletely understood. More than 100 years ago, Gowers (7) suggested that epileptic seizures are the result of either too much excitation or too little inhibition acting on cortical neurons. We now know that under normal circumstances, depolarizing inward currents, such as Na^+ and Ca^{2+} ionic currents are balanced by repolarizing outward currents, such as voltage and Ca^{2+}-dependent K^+ currents. Ca^{2+}-dependent Cl^- and cation currents also influence neuronal excitability, as do a variety of intracellular events as a result of the activation of protein kinases and phosphatases. At the synaptic level, the effect of excitatory neurotransmitters, such as glutamate and acetylcholine, is balanced by the inhibitory effect of γ-aminobutyric acid (GABA), perhaps modulated by adenosine and other inhibitory agents. Focal seizures, the initial event in all seizures of neocortical origin, are the result of regional alterations of ionic or neurotransmitter balance. Interictal spikes or spike-wave complexes correspond to intracellular paroxysmal depolarization shifts (PDSs) (8) triggered by intrinsic bursting cells (9). Normally, few cortical neurons are bursting cells; however, alterations of the ionic milleau, such as downregulation of K^+ currents, may turn nonbursting neurons into bursting neurons, which may recruit other neurons into interictal discharges if excitatory forces are increased or inhibition is compromised (10,11). If a sufficient number of cells are recruited so that prolonged membrane depolarization occurs simultaneously in many neurons, high-frequency action potentials are generated, pro-

ducing the tonic phase of a seizure. As the excitatory force diminishes, membrane potentials repolarize and single PDSs can once again be recorded, which correspond to the clonic discharges recorded on the encephalogram (EEG). Similar mechanisms are probably responsible for seizure spread.

Under most circumstances, partial-onset seizures are limited to a single brief "tonic" phase followed by a brief "clonic" phase. A number of mechanisms are responsible for the termination of a seizure, including activation of Na^+-K^+ adenosine triphosphatase (12–14), acidification of the extracellular environment, which stabilizes neuronal membranes (15), blockade of N-methyl-D-aspartate channels by Mg^{2+}, and activation of K^+ conductances and thus repolarization of neurons (16,17). Endogenous opioids also may contribute to the termination of seizures and to the refractory period before another seizure can occur. Rocha et al. (18), in a model of temporal lobe epilepsy, showed that the postictal refractory period is markedly shortened by naloxone, an opioid antagonist. Failure of these seizure-stopping mechanisms, or the occurrence of a strong excitatory stimulus, may result in repeated or prolonged seizures, that is, in status epilepticus. Once status does occur, alteration of γ-aminobutyric acid (GABA) mechanisms may contribute to its continuation, especially during prolonged episodes of status epilepticus. Kapur and Macdonald (19), using perforated-patch recordings, found a marked reduction of GABA currents in CA1 pyramidal neurons during status epilepticus. Kapur et al. (20), using a paired-pulse technique in an electrogenic model of status epilepticus, showed a deterioration of GABA-mediated inhibition during continuous hippocampal stimulation. NMDA receptors become activated during hippocampal stimulation (21), and NMDA antagonists block the deterioration of GABA-mediated inhibition (22).

EPIDEMIOLOGY

Status epilepticus is surprisingly common, although this is a recent concept. In the nineteenth and early twentieth centuries, status epilepticus was considered rare (23,24), although Turner (25) thought it "more frequent than is generally supposed." These early references considered only generalized convulsive status, which is largely still the case in more recent population studies. In a prospective community-based study in Richmond, Virginia, DeLorenzo and colleagues (26) calculated an annual incidence of 41 per 100,000. The incidence in the white population, however, was 20 per 100,000. This figure is quite similar to that reported by Hesdorffer et al. (27), who found an incidence of 18.3 per 100,000 in Rochester, Minnesota, based on a retrospective study of medical records from 1965 through 1984. These data suggest a minimum of about 50,000 cases of neocortical status epilepticus in the United States each year, and likely many more when poor urban populations are included in the estimate.

GENERALIZED CONVULSIVE STATUS EPILEPTICUS

Generalized convulsive status epilepticus is by far the most common and the most threatening form of status epilepticus, although certain other forms of status epilepticus, especially in children, are extremely challenging. GCSE is characterized by paroxysmal or continuous tonic or clonic convulsive movements (which may be overt or subtle and symmetric or asymmetric) associated with coma (especially during ictal discharges) and with bilateral (but frequently asymmetric) ictal discharges on the EEG (28,29).

Treiman (28–31) emphasized that GCSE is a dynamic rather than static condition in which clinical presentation, associated EEG pattern, and response to treatment evolve over time and may even vary in their initial appearance, depending on the underlying cause of the episode. Most patients present with overt GCSE, in which the clinical appearance is one of repeated discrete generalized tonic seizures that evolve from tonic stiffening to clonic jerking and generally last less than 2 minutes (32). The convulsive activity is followed by postictal coma or

confusion, which may gradually resolve; however, if another seizure ensues before the patient has completely recovered normal mental and neurologic function, then by definition the patient is in GCSE. This is an important point because there is a tendency on the part of some clinicians to reject the diagnosis of status epilepticus if recovery of consciousness proceeds to the point of capacity for interaction with the examiner, even though there are still residual effects of the previous seizure. If status epilepticus is defined physiologically as continuous effects of seizure activity, either ictal or interictal, then any effects of the previous seizure—even a slight impairment of mental function or mild slowing on the EEG—still present when another seizure occurs requires the diagnosis of status epilepticus.

If overt GCSE is allowed to continue untreated or is treated inadequately, there is a gradual evolution from overt to subtle convulsive activity until eventually all convulsive activity may disappear. When convulsive activity is sufficiently attenuated so that only subtle twitching movements of fingers, facial muscles, or abdominal muscles or nystagmoid jerks of the eyes are seen but ictal discharges persist on the EEG, Treiman (28,33,34) suggested this presentation should be called *subtle generalized convulsive status epilepticus* (SGCSE); this term has begun to enter the literature (6,35,36). Because these patients are extremely ill, some investigators have questioned the use of the term *subtle*. A more accurate and less ambiguous modification of the term *SGCSE* that might have merit would be *GCSE with subtle motor manifestations*. If such a term were to be adopted, when convulsive movements disappear entirely during GCSE, an analogous term would be *GCSE with electrographic seizures only*.

Regardless of the terminology used, several points need to be emphasized. First is that a cardinal feature of GCSE is profound coma. Patients who have ictal discharges on the EEG but only a partial alteration of consciousness [what Treiman and Delgado-Escueta (37) referred to as an *epileptic twilight state*] by definition cannot be in GCSE;

TABLE 18.1. *Characteristics of overt and subtle generalized convulsive status epilepticus (GCSE)*

Characteristic	Overt GCSE	Subtle GCSE
Number of patients	384	134
Age (yr), mean ± SD	58.6 ± 15.6	62.0 ± 15.1
Veterans (%)	70.1	80.6
Male (%)	82.3	85.1
Not pretreated acutely (%)	51.3	51.5
Previous history of acute seizures (%)	54.2	25.4
Previous history of epilepsy (%)	42.4	12.7
Previous history of status epilepticus (%)	12.8	4.5
Median duration of status prior to enrollment (h)	2.8	5.8
Etiologic factors present:[a]		
Remote neurology (%)	69.5	34.3
Acute neurologic (%)	27.3	37.3
Life-threatening medical condition (%)	32	56.7
Cardiopulmonary arrest (%)	6.3	38.1
Therapeutic or recreational drug toxicity (%)	6.3	5.2
Alcohol withdrawal (%)	6.5	0.7

[a]Some patients had more than one etiologic factor present.
From Treiman DM, Meyers PD, Walton NY, et al. A comparison of four treatments for generalized convulsive status epilepticus. *N Engl J Med* 1998;339:792–798, with permission.

rather, these patients are in nonconvulsive status epilepticus (discussed further later). Second, it is not necessary that a patient start in overt GCSE to exhibit clinical characteristics of subtle GCSE. Such an evolution has been well documented in experimental models of GCSE in the rat (38,39) and has been observed in humans when pharmacologic treatment has failed to stop GCSE completely. The essential determinant of the clinical expression in GCSE is the degree of encephalopathy that is present. Thus, if an episode of GCSE develops as the result of a severe metabolic or infectious insult to the brain, such as hypoxia, it is likely that the clinical convulsions will be subtle from the beginning, even though there are ictal discharges on the EEG. Subtle GCSE evolves from overt GCSE when seizure activity is not completely controlled and the continuing seizure activity is itself encephalopathogenic.

Although part of a continuum, overt and subtle GCSE are quite different in their etiology and prognosis. Table 18.1 presents the demographic characteristics of 384 patients with overt GCSE and 134 patients with subtle GCSE who participated in a Veterans Administration comparison of four pharmacologic treatments of GCSE (6). Table 18.2 presents

the outcome at 30 days in these two groups. Treatment results from this study are discussed subsequently.

Just as there is an evolution of behavioral changes from overt to subtle convulsions in untreated or inadequately treated GCSE, there is also a predictable sequence of progressive changes of the EEG (40). Initially, discrete electrographic seizures are seen, which generally coincide with typical generalized convulsions. If GCSE is allowed to progress, however, the discrete seizures merge together to produce a pattern of waxing and waning amplitudes, frequencies, or extent of cortical engagement.

TABLE 18.2. *Outcome at discharge or 30 days after an episode of overt or subtle generalized convulsive status epilepticus (GCSE)*

	Overt GCSE (n = 377)	Subtle GCSE (n = 134)
Improved and discharged	50.0%	8.3%
Still in hospital	22.7%	27.1%
Died	27.3%	64.7

Data from Treiman DM, Meyers PD, Walton NY, et al. A comparison of four treatments for generalized convulsive status epilepticus. *N Engl J Med* 1998;339: 792–798, with permission.

Eventually, the ictal activity becomes relatively monomorphic and continuous and then begins to be punctuated by periods of relative flattening. These flat periods become longer as the ictal discharges become shorter, until finally periodic epileptiform discharges are seen on a relatively flat background. This sequence of progressive EEG changes was first suggested by Treiman and colleagues (40,41) after a study of 109 EEGs recorded during human GCSE and subsequently confirmed by observation of the same sequence in at least eight experimental models of status epilepticus in the rat (39,40,42–45).

Some controversy continues as to whether periodic epileptiform discharges (PEDs) are ictal or rather postictal evidence of brain injury. Four lines of evidence suggest that PEDs that develop during GCSE or a coma-producing encephalopathic insult are ictal discharges: (a) a transition to PEDs from the continuous ictal patterns has been seen in some human patients and in all the experimental models of status epilepticus in which the evolution of EEG patterns has been studied; (b) hypermetabolism on positron emission tomography has been seen in the same area in which periodic epileptiform discharges have been recorded on EEG and disappeared as the PEDs disappeared (46); (c) some areas of hypermetabolism observed in experimental status epilepticus in the rat during the EEG phase of continuous ictal discharges persist after the transition to PEDs (47); (d) and periodic epileptiform discharges in some patients and some experimental models of status epilepticus respond to pharmacologic treatment. For these reasons, Treiman argued that patients in SGCSE who exhibit PEDs on the EEG be treated as aggressively as patients with overt GCSE (28,48).

NEOCORTICAL COMPLEX PARTIAL STATUS EPILEPTICUS

Complex partial status epilepticus (CPSE) is defined as a state of recurrent or continuous epileptic seizures during which there is at least some alteration of contact with the environment and impairment of memory for the event, producing an epileptic twilight state but not coma. Automatisms may or may not be seen. CPSE is frequently assumed to be of mesial temporal origin, but recent data make it clear that CPSE may also arise from neocortical epileptic foci as well. Treiman and Delgado-Escueta (37,49) emphasized the cyclic nature of complex partial status epilepticus during which the patient exhibits an "epileptic twilight state" punctuated by periods of unresponsiveness and motor automatisms with associated rhythmic EEG discharges. Most of their cases were of mesial temporal origin; however, they also recognized that continuous behavioral alterations may occur in CPSE and suggested that cases with continuous behavioral and EEG symptomatology probably represent cases of prolonged CPSE and frequently may be of frontal origin (49).

Complex partial status epilepticus of frontal origin is now well recognized and has been reviewed by several authors (50,51), most recently by Thomas and colleagues (52). These investigators prospectively studied 10 patients with frontal origin nonconvulsive status epilepticus (NCSE). They identified two types of frontal origin NCSE. *Type 1* was characterized by mood disturbances associated with subtle impairment of cognitive function without overt confusion. The EEG showed normal background rhythms and unilateral frontal ictal discharges. Thomas and colleagues considered type 1 NCSE to be simple partial status epilepticus. In *type 2* NCSE, on the other hand, impaired consciousness was associated with bilateral, asymmetric, frontal EEG discharges occurring on an abnormal background. Such patients are similar to what others have considered CPSE of frontal origin, and Thomas and colleagues also considered these patients to be in CPSE. Many authors (53–58) consider type 2 patients to be examples of spike-wave stupor with focal features or to occupy a borderland between spike-wave stupor and CPSE. Although it is sometimes extremely difficult to differentiate spike-wave stupor and frontal origin CPSE when the EEG consists of bilaterally symmetric spike-wave discharges, the diagnosis is aided by consideration of other clinical parameters. When NCSE occurs in patients with established epilepsy, the type of epilepsy allows differentiation of the type of NCSE. Furthermore, even if NCSE occurs de novo, the presence of a frontal lesion on static or functional imaging studies suggests the diagnosis of CPSE.

SIMPLE PARTIAL STATUS EPILEPTICUS

Simple partial status epilepticus (SPSE) is operationally defined as a state of recurrent or continuous seizures without any impairment of consciousness. The behavioral manifestations of the seizures are determined by the cortical localization of the seizure activity (49). Thus, cases of focal motor status, pure sensory status, and epileptic aphasia as well as of other behavioral phenomena have been described. Simple partial status is relatively uncommon, but it is much more common than CPSE for reasons suggested later. SPSE accounted for 23% of the cases of status epilepticus in Richmond, Virginia, collected by DeLorenzo and colleagues (26), whereas CPSE accounted for only 3% of their cases.

NEOCORTICAL STATUS EPILEPTICUS: A UNIFYING CONCEPT

How then should we think about neocortical status epilepticus? SPSE and CPSE (including mesial temporal as well as neocortical CPSE) are both far less common than GCSE, although SPSE is observed much more frequently than CPSE. This is somewhat of a paradox because simple and complex partial seizures tend to be much more common than secondarily generalized convulsions, especially in the presence of vigorous pharmacolgic management. An explanation for this paradox may lie in the balance between mechanisms that allow seizures to spread (which, as noted, are probably the same mechanisms

that allow neuronal recruitment and focal seizure development initially) and mechanisms that cause seizures to terminate. In most cases, seizures spread before termination mechanisms fail. Thus, even seizures that start from a localized neocortical focus are likely to become generalized before they become repetitive. This would account for the relatively rare occurrence of CPSE commented on by many authors. Under some circumstances, there may be a local failure of seizure termination mechanisms and thus SPSE may occur. This would account for the much greater frequency of SPSE than CPSE. Once seizure spread has been sufficient to engage at least portions of both cortical hemispheres, however, as must happen to produce a complex partial seizure, further spread to produce generalized convulsive activity is likely to occur before the widespread failure of seizure termination mechanisms that would be necessary to produce complex partial status epilepticus.

TREATMENT

Only one study has directly compared the efficacy of standard antistatus drugs administered intravenously in the initial treatment of status epilepticus. Treiman et al. (6) compared the efficacy of intravenous lorazepam 0.1 mg/kg, phenobarbital 15 mg/kg, diazepam 0.15 mg/kg, followed by phenytoin 18 mg/kg in the initial treatment of overt and subtle generalized convulsive status epilepticus. The primary outcome of the study is shown in Fig. 18.1. Overall, 55.5% of the overt patients responded to the first treatment, and the frequency of success of lorazepam (64.9%) was statistically significantly greater than the frequency of success of phenytoin alone (43.6%). In the subtle group, all four of the treatments were much less effective than in the overt group. Overall, only 14.9% of the patients responded to the first treatment, and no statistically significant differences among treatment groups were found. Based on these results and the ease of use, lorazepam appears to be the treatment of choice for the management of secondary GCSE. Al-

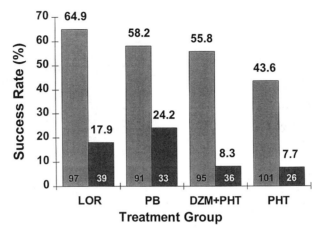

FIG. 18.1. Outcome from a comparison of the efficacy of four drug treatments in the initial management of generalized convulsive status epilepticus. Percent success of each of the four first-drug regimens is shown for overt and subtle GCSE (*gray bars,* overt patients; *black bars,* = subtle patients): in the overt patients, differences in frequency of success among treatments were statistically significant ($p = 0.02$). In pairwise comparisons, lorazepam was effective more often than phenytoin ($p = 0.002$). The percent success rate for each treatment is indicated above the bars. There was a total of 384 overt patients and 134 subtle patients, with the number in each treatment group shown within the bars. Treatment group abbreviations: *LOR,* lorazepam; *PB,* phenobarbital; *DZM + PHT,* diazepam followed by phenytoin; *PHT,* phenytoin. (Modified from Treiman DM, Meyers PD, Walton NY, et al. A comparison of four treatments for generalized convulsive status epilepticus. *N Engl J Med* 1998;339:792–798, with permission.)

though no comparative data exist, most physicians also view lorazepam as the drug of choice for primarily generalized status epilepticus and for CPSE; however, treatment for simple partial status should be initiated with a nonsedating drug such as phenytoin. Use of sedating drugs, such as benzodiazepines and barbiturates, in SPSE must be balanced between the clinical urgency to stop the ongoing seizure activity and the potential risk of producing coma in a conscious patient. The recent availability of valproic acid in an intravenous preparation may provide an alternative nonsedating therapeutic agent for this type of status epilepticus. The management of status epilepticus has been reviewed more fully elsewhere (35,48,59).

FUTURE RESEARCH

Our understanding of neocortical status epilepticus is far from complete, and many questions remain that require investigation. Certainly, there are fundamental differences in the underlying mechanisms of seizures that are focal in onset and those that are generalized from onset. Is this also true for mechanisms that allow single discrete partial onset seizures and primarily generalized seizures to present as status epilepticus? Are there fundamental differences in pathophysiology between neocortical status epilepticus and other types of status epilepticus? What are the mechanisms that underlie the evolution from overt to subtle clinical manifestations of GCSE and from discrete electrographic seizures to periodic epileptiform discharges? Why does GCSE become progressively refractory to treatment the longer it persists, especially the later the EEG stage? Why do only two thirds of the cases of overt GCSE respond to initial treatment? Can we find better drugs? Do neuroprotective agents have a role in the management of status epilepticus? Although much progress in understanding neocortical status epilepticus and developing more effective treatments has been made during the last century, the new century brings new challenges and leaves much work to be done.

REFERENCES

1. Wilson JVK, Reynolds EH. Translation and analysis of a Cuneiform text forming part of a Babylonian treatise on epilepsy. *Med Hist* 1990;34:185–198.
2. Gastaut H. Classification of status epilepticus. In: Delgado-Escueta AV, Wasterlain CG, Treiman DM, Porter RJ, eds. *Status epilepticus: mechanisms of brain damage and treatment. Advances in Neurology,* vol 34. New York: Raven Press, 1983:15–35.
3. Commission on Classification and Terminology of the International League Against Epilepsy. Proposal for revised clinical and electroencephalographic classification of epileptic seizures. *Epilepsia* 1981;22:489–501.
4. Lowenstein DH, Bleck T, Macdonald RL. It's time to revise the definition of status epilepticus. *Epilepsia* 1999; 40:120–122.
5. Gastaut H. Clinical and electroencephalographical classification of epileptic seizures. *Epilepsia* 1970;11: 102–113.
6. Treiman DM, Meyers PD, Walton NY, et al. A comparison of four treatments for generalized convulsive status epilepticus. *N Engl J Med* 1998;339:792–798.
7. Gowers W. *Epilepsy and other chronic convulsive disorders.* London: Churchill, 1881.
8. Matsumoto H, Ajmone-Marsan C. Cortical cellular phenomena in experimental epilepsy: interictal manifestations. *Exp Neurol* 1964;9:286–304.
9. Gutnick MJ, Connors BW, Prince DA. Mechanisms of neocortical epileptogenesis in vitro. *J Neurophysiol* 1982;48:1321–1335.
10. Mody I, Lambert JD, Heinemann U. Low extracellular magnesium induces epileptiform activity and spreading depression in rat hippocampal slices. *J Neurophysiol* 1987;57:869–888.
11. Traub RD, Knowles WD, Miles R, et al. Models of the cellular mechanism underlying propagation of epileptiform activity in the CA2-CA3 region of the hippocampal slice. *Neuroscience* 1987;21:457–470.
12. Heinemann U, Lux HD. Undershoots following stimulus-induced rises of extracellular potassium concentration in cerebral cortex of cat. *Brain Res* 1975;93:63–76.
13. Lewis DV, Schuette WH. NADH fluorescence, $[K^+]0$, and oxygen consumption in cat cerebral cortex during direct cortical stimulation. *Brain Res* 1976;110: 523–535.
14. Fukuda A, Prince DA. Excessive intracellular Ca^{2+} inhibits glutamate-induced $Na^{(+)}$-K^+ pump activation in rat hippocampal neurons. *J Neurophysiol* 1992;68: 28–35.
15. Caspers H, Speckmann EJ, Lehmenkuhler A. DC potentials of the cerebral cortex: seizure activity and changes in gas pressures. *Rev Physiol Biochem Pharmacol* 1987;106:127–178.
16. Spuler A, Grafe P. Adenosine, 'pertussis-sensitive' G-proteins, and K^+ conductance in central mammalian neurones under energy deprivation. *Neurosc Lett* 1989; 98:280–284.
17. Bennett MR, Kerr R, Nichol K. Adenosine modulation

18. Rocha L, Engel J Jr, Ackermann RF. Effects of chronic naloxone pretreatment on amygdaloid kindling in rats. *Epilepsy Res* 1991;10:103–110.
19. Kapur J, Macdonald RL. Status epilepticus: a proposed pathophysiology. In: Shorvon S, Dreifuss F, Fish D, Thomas D, eds. *The treatment of epilepsy.* Oxford: Blackwell Scientific Publications, 1996:258–268.
20. Kapur J, Stringer JL, Lothman EW. Evidence that repetitive seizures in the hippocampus cause a lasting reduction of GABAergic inhibition. *J Neurophysiol* 1989; 61:417–426.
21. Bertram EH, Lothman EW. NMDA receptor antagonists and limbic status epilepticus: a comparison with standard anticonvulsants. *Epilepsy Res* 1990;5:177–184.
22. Kapur J, Lothman EW. NMDA receptor activation mediates the loss of GABAergic inhibition induced by recurrent seizures. *Epilepsy Res* 1990;5:103–111.
23. Clark LP, Prout TP. Status epilepticus: a clinical and pathological study in epilepsy. *American Journal of Insanity* 1904;60:645–699.
24. Clark LP, Prout TP. Status epilepticus: a clinical and pathological study in epilepsy. *American Journal of Insanity* 1904;61:81–108.
25. Turner WA. *Epilepsy—a study of the idiopathic disease.* London: Macmillan, 1907.
26. DeLorenzo RJ, Hauser WA, Towne AR, et al. A prospective, population-based epidemiologic study of status epilepticus in Richmond, Virginia. *Neurology* 1996;46: 1029–1035.
27. Hesdorffer DC, Logroscino G, Cascino G, et al. Incidence of status epilepticus in Rochester, Minnesota, 1965–1984. *Neurology* 1998;50:735–741.
28. Treiman DM. Generalized convulsive status epilepticus in the adult. *Epilepsia* 1993;34(Suppl 1):S2–S11.
29. Treiman DM. Generalized convulsive status epilepticus. In: Engel J Jr, Pedley TA, eds. *Epilepsy: a comprehensive textbook.* Philadelphia: Lippincott–Raven, 1997: 669–680.
30. Treiman DM. Status epilepticus. In: Laidlaw J, Richens A, Chadwick D, eds. *A textbook of epilepsy.* Edinburgh: Churchill Livingstone, 1993:205–220.
31. Treiman DM. Generalized convulsive, nonconvulsive, and focal status epilepticus. In: Feldman E, ed. *Current diagnosis in neurology.* St. Louis: Mosby-Yearbook, 1994:11–18.
32. Theodore WH, Porter RJ, Albert P, et al. The secondarily generalized tonic–clonic seizure: a videotape analysis. *Neurology* 1994;44:1403–1407.
33. Treiman DM, DeGiorgio CM, Salisbury S, et al. Subtle generalized convulsive status epilepticus. *Epilepsia* 1984;25:653.
34. Treiman DM. Status epilepticus. In: Johnson RT, ed. *Current therapy in neurologic disease.* Philadelphia: BC Decker, 1987:38–42.
35. Shorvon S. *Status epilepticus: its clinical features and treatment in children and adults.* Cambridge: Cambridge University Press, 1994.
36. Privitera M, Hoffman M, Moore JL, et al. EEG detection of nontonic–clonic status epilepticus in patients with altered consciousness. *Epilepsy Res* 1994;18: 155–166.
37. Treiman DM, Delgado-Escueta AV. Complex partial sta-

tus epilepticus. In: Delgado-Escueta AV, Wasterlain CG, Treiman DM, Porter RJ, eds. *Status epilepticus: mechanisms of brain damage and treatment. Advances in Neurology,* vol 34. New York: Raven Press, 1983:69–81.

38. Walton NY, Treiman DM. Experimental secondarily generalized convulsive status epilepticus induced by D,L-homocysteine thiolactone. *Epilepsy Res* 1988;2:79–86.

39. Handforth A, Treiman DM. A new, non-pharmacologic model of convulsive status epilepticus induced by electrical stimulation: behavioral/electroencephalographic observations and response to phenytoin and phenobarbital. *Epilepsy Res* 1994;19:15–25.

40. Treiman DM, Walton NY, Kendrick C. A progressive sequence of electroencephalographic changes during generalized convulsive status epilepticus. *Epilepsy Res* 1990;5:49–60.

41. Treiman DM, Walton NY, Wickboldt C, et al. Predictable sequence of EEG changes during generalized convulsive status epilepticus in man and three experimental models of status epilepticus in the rat. *Neurology* 1987;7(Suppl 1):244.

42. Lothman EW, Bertram EH, Bekenstein JW, et al. Self-sustaining limbic status epilepticus induced by 'continuous' hippocampal stimulation: electrographic and behavioral characteristics. *Epilepsy Res* 1989;3:107–119.

43. Mikati MA, Chronopoulos A, Holmes GL. Stages of kainic acid (KA)-induced status epilepticus (SE) in the prepubescent brain and response to phenobarbital (Pb). *Neurology* 1992;42:364.

44. Kim J-M, Walton NY, Treiman DM. EEG patterns of high dose pilocarpine-induced status epilepticus in rats. *Epilepsia* 1997;38(Suppl 8):225.

45. Koplovitz I, Skvorak JP. Electrocorticographic changes during generalized convulsive status epilepticus in soman intoxicated rats. *Epilepsy Res* 1998;30:159–164.

46. Handforth A, Cheng JT, Mandelkern MA, et al. Markedly increased mesiotemporal lobe metabolism in a case with PLEDs: further evidence that PLEDs are a manifestation of partial status epilepticus. *Epilepsia* 1994;35:876–881.

47. Handforth A, Treiman DM. Functional mapping of the late stages of status epilepticus in the lithium-pilocarpine model in rat: a 14C-2-deoxyglucose study. *Neuroscience* 1995;64:1075–1089.

48. Treiman DM. Treatment of status epilepticus. In: Engel J Jr, Pedley TA, eds. *Epilepsy: a comprehensive textbook.* Philadelphia: Lippincott–Raven, 1997:1317–1323.

49. Delgado-Escueta AV, Treiman DM. Focal status epilepticus: modern concepts. In: Lüders HO, Lesser RP, eds. *Epilepsy: electroclinical syndromes.* Berlin: Springer-Verlag, 1987:347–391.

50. Williamson PD, Spencer DD, Spencer SS, et al. Complex partial status epilepticus: a depth-electrode study. *Ann Neurol* 1985;18:647–654.

51. Takeda A. Complex partial status epilepticus of frontal lobe origin. *Jpn J Psychiatry Neurol* 1988;42:525–530.

52. Thomas P, Zifkin B, Migneco O, et al. Nonconvulsive status epilepticus of frontal origin. *Neurology* 1999; 52:1174–1183.

53. Hess R, Scollo-Lavizzari G, Wyss FE. Borderline cases of petit mal status. *Eur Neurol* 1971;5:137–154.

54. Geier S. Prolonged psychic epileptic seizures: a study of the absence status. *Epilepsia* 1978;19:431–445.

55. Niedermeyer E, Fineyre F, Riley T, et al. Absence status (petit mal status) with focal characteristics. *Arch Neurol* 1979;36:417–421.

56. Aguglia U, Tinuper P, Farnarier G. État confusionnel critique à point de départ frontal chez le sujet âgé. *Rev Electroencephalogr Neurophysiol Clin* 1983;13:174–179.

57. Guberman A, Cantu-Reyna G, Stuss D, et al. Nonconvulsive generalized status epilepticus: clinical features, neuropsychological testing, and long-term follow-up. *Neurology* 1986;36:1284–1291.

58. Rey M, Papy JJ. État d'obnubilation critique d'origine frontale chez le sujet âgé: un diagnostic difficile. *Rev Electroencephalogr Neurophysiol Clin* 1987;17:377–385.

59. Dodson WE, DeLorenzo RJ, Pedley TA, et al. Treatment of convulsive status epilepticus: recommendations of the Epilepsy Foundation of America's Working Group on Status Epilepticus. *JAMA* 1993;270:854–859.

60. Treiman DM, Meyers PD, Walton NY. DVA Status Epilepticus Cooperative Study Group. Factors that predict prognosis in generalized convulsive status epilepticus. *Epilepsia* 1993;34(Suppl 6):30.

Neocortical Epilepsies.
Advances in Neurology, Vol. 84,
edited by P.D. Williamson, A.M. Siegel,
D.W. Roberts, V.M. Thadani, and M.S. Gazzaniga.
Lippincott Williams & Wilkins, Philadelphia © 2000.

19

Intracranial EEG Investigation in Neocortical Epilepsy

L.F. Quesney

Division of EEG and Clinical Neurophysiology, Montreal Neurological Institute, McGill University,
Montreal, Quebec, Canada H3A 2B4

EEG LOCALIZATION IN NEOCORTICAL EPILEPSY: PROBLEMS AND PITFALLS

Neocortical epilepsy comprises seizures arising in the cortical mantle that are usually short lived and display a rapid seizure propagation. The nature of their clinical behavioral manifestations is largely dependent on the anatomic regions involved at seizure onset and during early spread.

Much of the nosologic ground of neocortical seizures derives from the pioneer work of Penfield and Jasper (1), particularly their experiences with intraoperative cortical electric stimulation and elicitation of clinical responses, often associated with afterdischarges involving the neocortex. Clinical behavioral manifestations elicited by cortical electric stimulation not only identified the functional anatomy of different brain regions, but also highlighted the constellation of symptoms and signs usually seen at seizure onset or during the early stages of seizure evolution.

Electroencephalographic (EEG) localization of seizure generators originating in the neocortical mantle is a difficult endeavour because of the inherent anatomic and biophysical limitations, which equally affect EEG recordings obtained with scalp, cortical, or intracranial electrodes (2–23).

The success of surgical therapy in neocortical epilepsy is critically dependent on an accurate localization and excision of the cortical substrate responsible for the generation of the patients' habitual seizures. Understandably, this is not an easy task. The limitations commonly encountered during the preoperative investigation in patients with neocortical epilepsy are listed in Table 19.1 and are reviewed thoroughly in the first section of this chapter.

Undersampling and Nearsightedness of Recording Electrodes

This common problem potentially affects any EEG recording obtained from the neocortex and is essentially dependent on the folding of the cortical mantle into hidden sulci and convolutions. As elegantly illustrated by means of magnetic resonance imaging (MRI), brain-surface reconstruction, and generation

TABLE 19.1. Localization of seizure onset in neocortical epilepsy: Problems and pitfalls

Undersampling and near-sightedness of recording electrodes: missing the seizure generator
Rapid seizure propagation: reduced localization of the seizure generator (regional, lobar, hemispheric seizure onset)
Seizure generator located in a clinically silent area: risk of a "double miss" phenomenon
Large as opposed to restricted epileptogenic zones
Low incidence of specific neuroimaging abnormalities: difficulty in interpretation of results
Lack of consensus regarding what neocortical seizures should be like

of cortical flat maps. Van Essen and Drury (24) clearly documented that approximately 70% of the cortical surface is convoluted and therefore not directly accessible to extracranial, epidural, or subdural electrodes.

If we assume that the generator of a synchronized EEG activity, such as an interictal or ictal epileptic discharge, is located horizontally along the cortical surface of a gyrus (thus constituting a vertical dipole), scalp, cortical, epidural, or subdural electrodes will record an electronegative potential proportional to the solid angle subtended by the electrode and inversely proportional to the square factor of the distance between the recording electrode and the generator (25). Convoluted generators are so called because they are located in one or both sulcal walls without involvement of the cortical surface or crown (25). A dipole layer involving both walls of a sulcus with a concave distribution produces conflicting electric fields (Fig. 19.1). The solid angle subtended by electrode P1 is extremely small, and therefore the amplitude of the EEG potential recorded will be minimal.

This explains why EEG electrodes located immediately above a restricted cortical generator may record a small-amplitude EEG signal. In the same figure, electrode P2 is looking at the electropositive layer of the proximal sulcal wall and simultaneously recording from the electronegative layer of the distal sulcal wall. If the potential value of these two layers is similar, the resultant potential difference will be close to zero; therefore, electrode P2 would not record any significant electrocerebral potential (25). These considerations illustrate how the electrical activity generated by convoluted generators, even if synchronized, could be easily missed by extracranial, epidural, subdural, or cortical electrodes.

Small ictal generators located in an area of convoluted cortical gray matter at a depth of 1.5 to 2 cm may produce restricted electric fields that could be missed by epidural or subdural electrodes recording from the cortical surface. This situation is illustrated in Fig. 19.2, which depicts a patient with seizure onset in the left superior frontal gyrus, as suggested by rhythmic polyspike activity in the

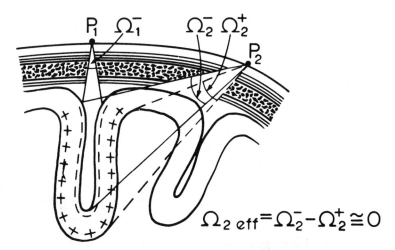

FIG. 19.1. The difficulty of obtaining a surface recording from a dipole layer occupying both walls of a sulcus is shown. At P1, the solid angle subtended is extremely small, and at P2 the effective solid angle $\Omega_{2\ eff}$ is nearly zero because the solid angles subtended by the positive and negative portion of the dipole layer seen by the electrode at P2 are nearly equal and their difference cancels out. (From Gloor P. Contribution of electroencephalography and electrocorticography to the neurosurgical treatment of the epilepsies. In: Purpura DP, Penry JK, Walter RD, eds. *Advances in Neurology,* vol 8. New York: Raven Press, 1975:59–63, with permission.)

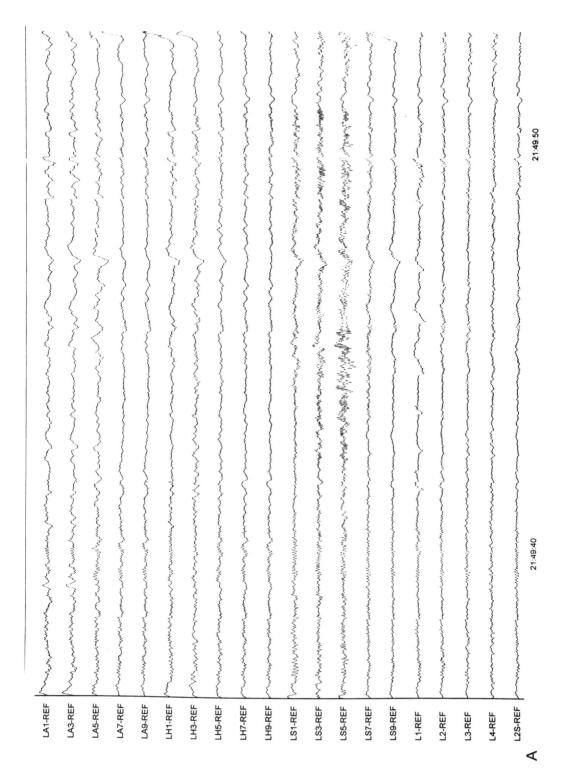

FIG. 19.2. Referential EEG recording **(A)** showing an electrographic seizure discharge in the gamma frequency band (48–50 Hz) recorded mostly from contact 5 of depth electrode LS. *Continued on next page.*

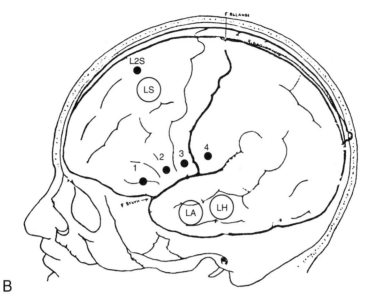

B

FIG. 19.2. *Continued.* **(B)** located at a depth of 2 cm. Note that the cortical surface electrode contact (LS9) shows no epileptic activity. See time display at the bottom. Note: In this and subsequent brain diagrams illustrating intracranial electrode placement, depth electrodes are represented by *empty circles* and epidural electrodes as smaller *black circles*.

gamma frequency band recorded from electrode contacts LS5 and LS3. Note that the more superficial contact of this electrode (LS9) would be comparable to an epidural or subdural electrode and does not record any seizure activity. This is also the case for an epidural electrode placed approximately 1.5 cm above the insertion point of depth electrode LS.

Conversely, intracerebral electrodes provide mostly tunnel vision with good resolution in the depth but with a low yield at the cortical surface (2). This is illustrated in Fig. 19.3, which portrays a continuous electrographic seizure activity recorded from the more superficial contacts of an electrode inserted through the third frontal gyrus on the right side, with the deepest contacts aimed at the orbitofrontal cortex. Bursts of polyspike activity in the gamma frequency band are recorded from electrode contacts RF06-9, but the anatomic extension of the epileptogenic

zone around the depth electrode remains unknown.

Coregistration with intracerebral and epidural or subdural electrodes (13,26–32) can improve some of these limitations. This situation is illustrated by M.F., a 37-year-old patient with recurrent complex partial seizures despite a left anterior temporal lobectomy including amygdalectomy and hippocampectomy performed 17 years earlier. The patient underwent implantation of four depth electrodes along the remnant of the second temporal gyrus and extending into the left occipital lobe (LC, LD, LP, and LO). In addition, nine epidural electrodes were implanted in the postcentral, posterior temporal, and parietal regions of the left hemisphere (Fig. 19.4). The EEG tracing shows rhythmic periodic spikes with a widespread distribution involving the second temporal gyrus behind the excision (see phase reversals at depth electrode contacts LC5) simultaneously reflecting

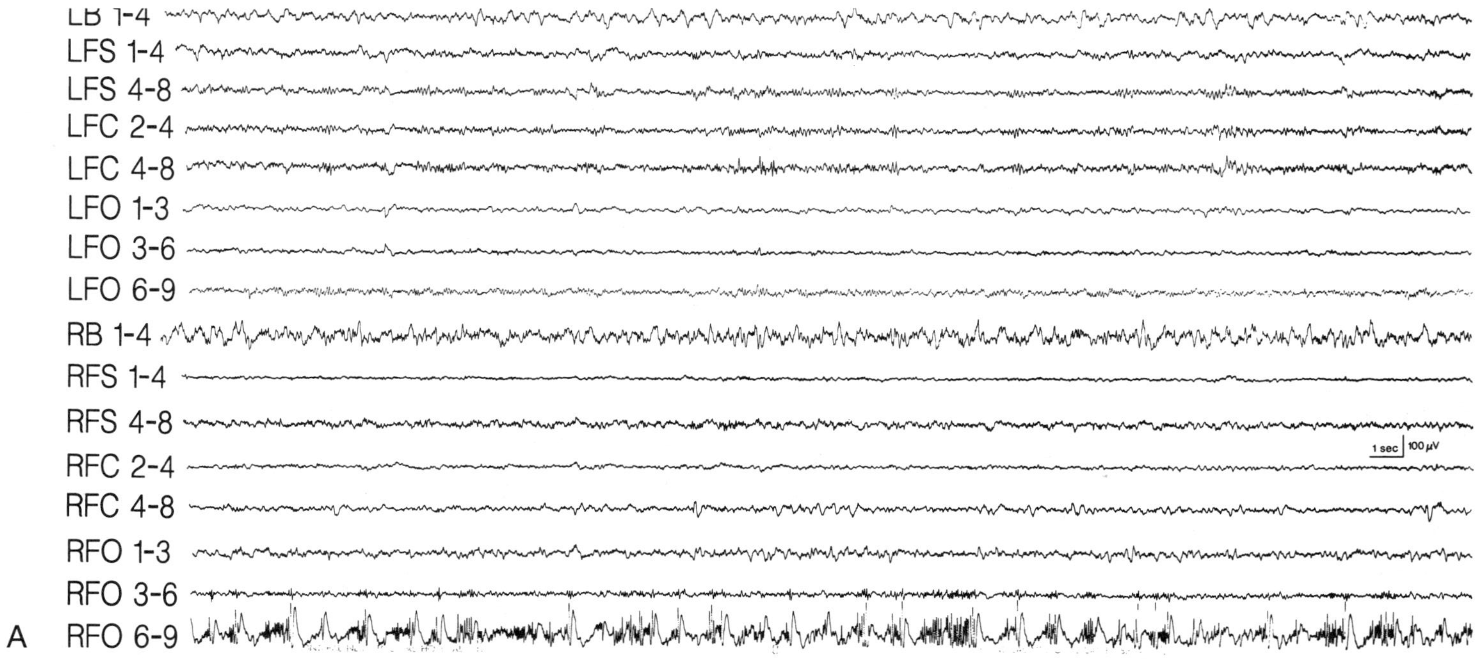

FIG. 19.3. Bipolar EEG recording **(A)** illustrating rhythmic periodic spiking intermingled with trains of polyspike activity in the beta frequency band recorded from the more superficial contacts (RFO6-9) of a depth electrode inserted through the third frontal gyrus **(B)**.

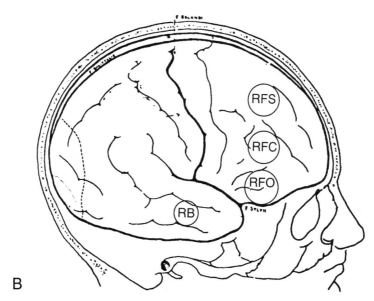

FIG. 19.3. *Continued.*

along the midsuperficial contacts of the left occipital depth electrode (LO5) and epidural electrode T3 located in the posterior aspect of the first temporal gyrus.

It is evident from this illustration that the most superficial contacts of the left posterior temporal (LC7-9) and left occipital depth electrodes (LO7-9) failed to record the electrographic seizure activity produced by a generator that is most likely located in a folded convolution at a depth of approximately 2 cm. Epidural or subdural electrodes undoubtedly would have recorded ictal EEG changes in the vicinity of epidural electrode T3 (one could say the "tip of the iceberg"), thereby inadvertently contributing to the false localization of a large epileptogenic zone. The last 12 channels of this figure represent a vertical bipolar montage linking the epidural electrodes to the more superficial contacts of the depth electrodes, thus providing adequate EEG recording resolution at a neocortical level (similar to an epidural grid) and in addition providing EEG coverage from specific sites in the brain's depth.

Large Epileptogenic Zones

Several reports in the literature documented that the ictal generators in extratemporal epilepsy may range along a continuum from a restricted to a large epileptogenic zone (4,6–8,10–21). Our last review of 18 patients with frontal lobe epilepsy investigated using depth electrodes (13) found that a focal or regional EEG onset confined to the frontal lobe was recorded in only seven patients (39%). A bifrontal seizure onset was documented in another seven patients (39%), and a bilobar distribution of ictal EEG onset involving frontal and temporal lobe structures was recorded in four patients (22%). A similar trend was reported elsewhere in parietal and occipital lobe epilepsy (12,14,16,18,21–23).

Excluding cortical dysplasia as well as tumoral and vascular lesions, large epileptogenic zones may be due to posttraumatic and postencephalitic meningocerebral cicatrix, porencephalic cysts (33,34), and extensive gliosis. Secondary epileptogenesis also may play a role (35). Similar pathological substrates have been reported in parietal and occipital lobe epilepsy (12,14).

Large epileptogenic zones may have independent multifocal generators responsible for the generation of the patient's habitual seizures (8,10). Somewhat arbitrarily, large epileptogenic zones can be anatomically classified as follows.

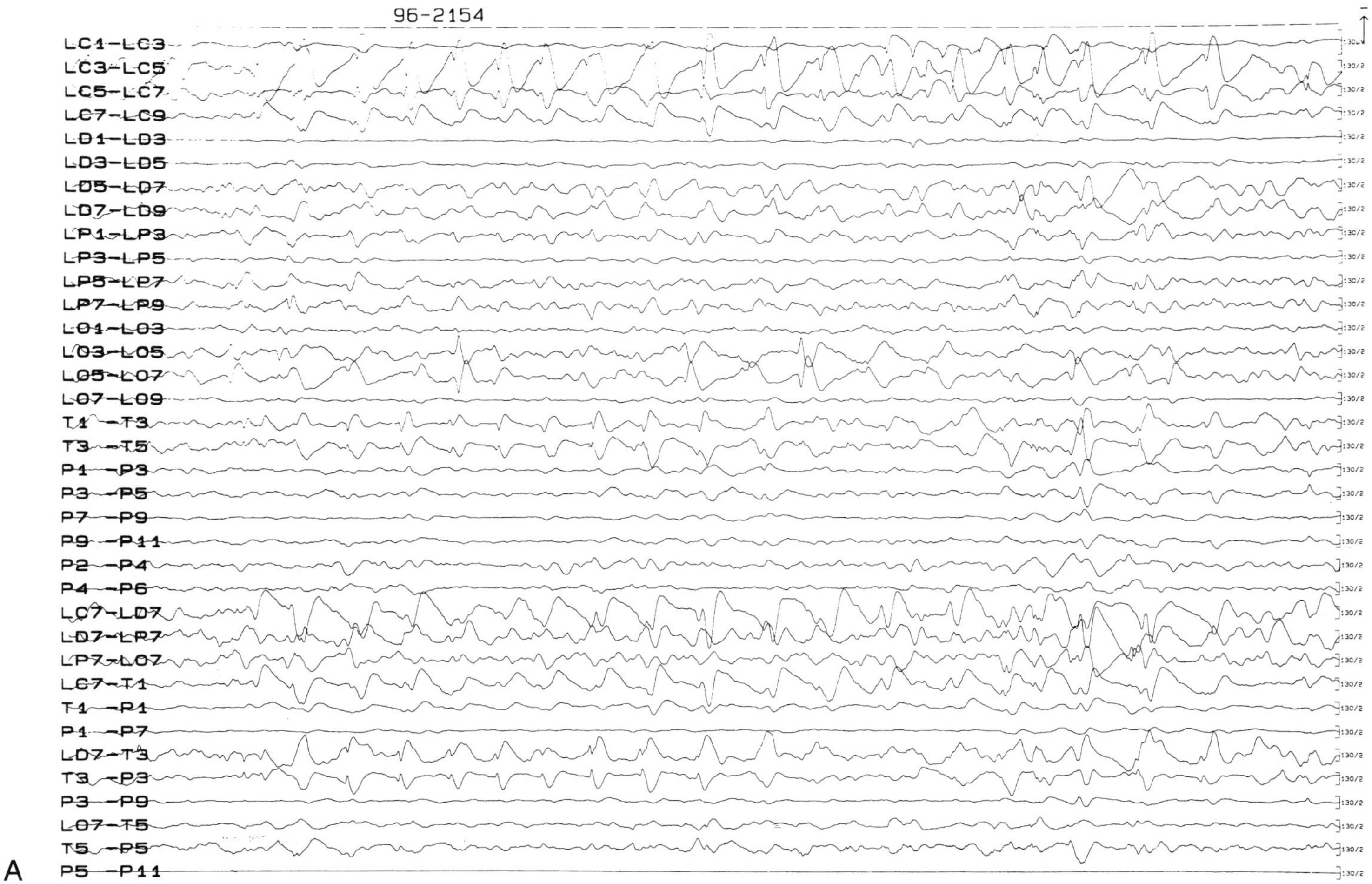

FIG. 19.4. Rhythmic continuous sharp and slow-wave activity (**A**) recorded from the superficial contacts of depth electrodes inserted through the left posterior–temporal and occipital regions. *Continued on next page.*

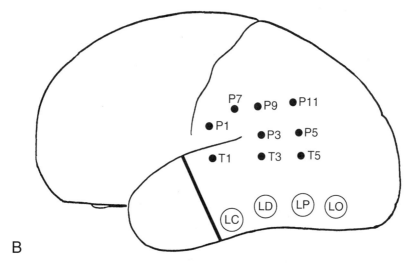

FIG. 19.4. Rhythmic continuous sharp and slow-wave activity **(A)** recorded from the superficial contacts of depth electrodes inserted through the left posterior–temporal and occipital regions **(B)**. Phase reversals of the abnormal potentials are seen at LC5, LO5, and at epidural electrode T3. Note the absence of spiking activity at LC7-9 and at LO7-9.

Restricted to Neocortical Structures

Usually in these cases, the anatomic extent of the epileptogenic zone is regional and involves different gyral compartments of the same lobe. Ictal generators independently involving the anterior, mid, or posterior neocortical boundaries of a lobe are not uncommon, creating uncertainty as to the extent of surgical excision to be performed, particularly in the absence of a neuroimaging lesion. Patient S.M. illustrates this situation. His habitual seizures could show either a regional EEG onset involving the left mid and anterior temporal neocortical regions (Fig. 19.5A,B) or could start in the left posterior and midtemporal neocortical structures (Fig. 19.6). Of 14 of this patient's recorded habitual seizures, ten originated in the left anterior or midtemporal neocortex, and the remaining four involved the left mid and posterior temporal neocortical structures.

Involving Neocortical as Well as Deep Sulcal or Mesial Structures

With the advent of three-dimensional MRI-based image guiding, a technique that allows

neurosurgeons to perform "frameless stereotactic" implantation of intracerebral electrodes, it is possible to know the exact anatomic location of a given depth electrode contact in the patient's MRI and its correlation with deep sulcal, cortical gray or white matter (36). In a large series comprising 464 clinical seizures of temporal lobe origin recorded with depth electrodes in 61 patients (37), 165 clinical seizures (35%) showed a focal EEG onset and 299 events (65%) displayed a regional EEG onset. Most of the latter seizures (212/299; 71%), showed involvement of more than one mesial temporal lobe structure, occasionally with simultaneous recruitment (4%) of the temporal neocortex. Although the incidence of simultaneous mesial–neocortical seizure onset is acknowledged low, it should be considered that patients in this series had a limited epidural electrode coverage restricted to the first temporal gyrus, which may underestimate the true extent of the neocortical epileptogenicity.

Bilobar or Multilobar Distribution

Despite utilization of state of the art EEG–video monitoring techniques, exact lo-

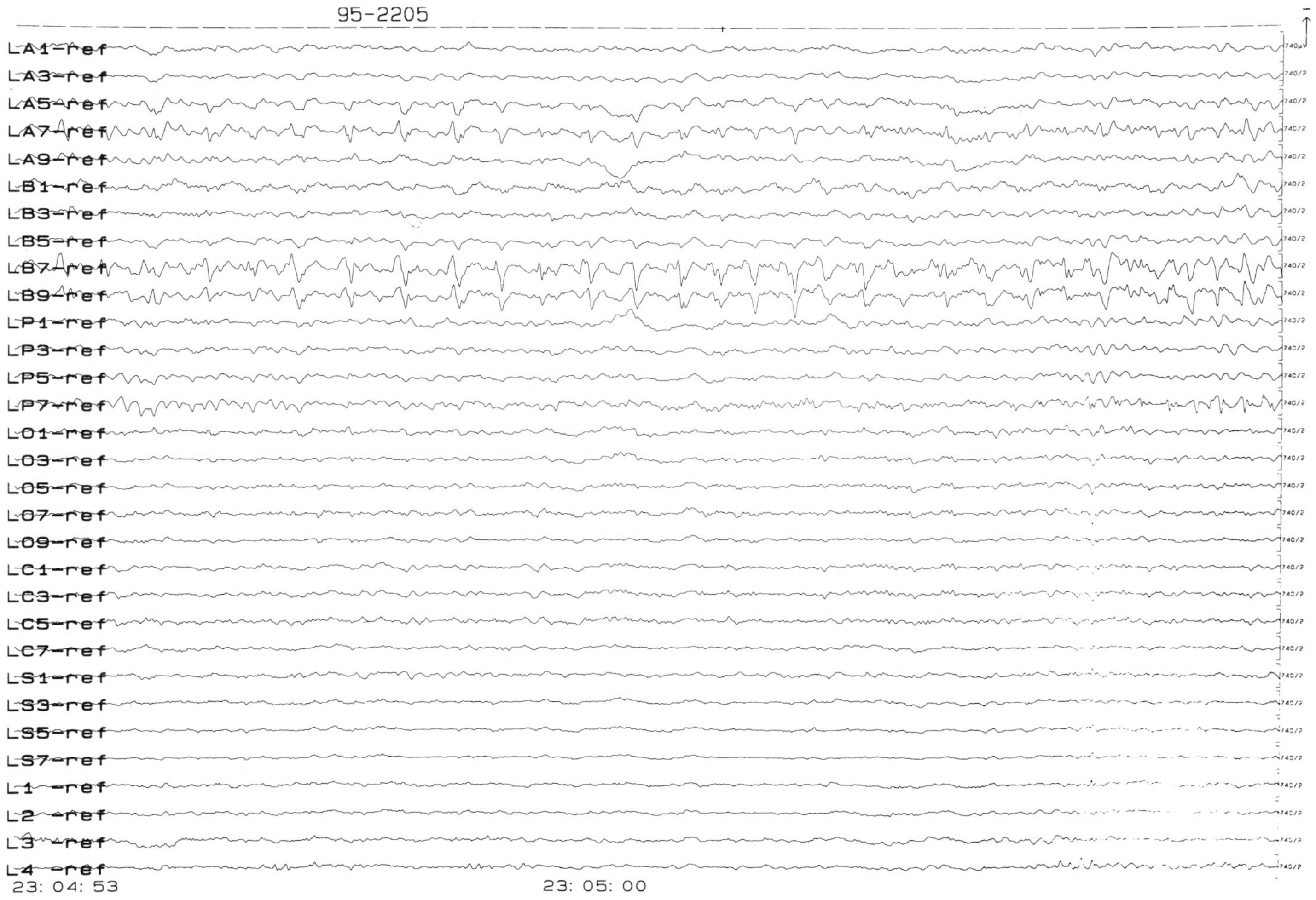

FIG. 19.5. A: Referential EEG recording showing rhythmic continuous sharp and slow-wave activity resembling triphasic waves recorded from the more superficial contacts of depth electrodes inserted through the anterior (LA7) and mid portion (LB7 and LB9) of the second temporal gyrus. *Continued on next page.*

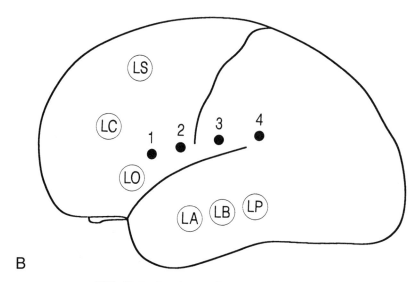

FIG. 19.5. *Continued.* **B:** Electrode placement.

calization of epileptogenic zones involving the frontotemporal or temporoparieto-occipital convexities is a difficult task (2,4,7, 10–13,15,38).

This difficulty is illustrated by S.B., a 14-year-old patient with intractable complex partial seizures. Extensive preoperative EEG investigation using extracranial electrodes showed a persistent focal interictal epileptic disturbance recorded from the left frontotemporal region (see phase reversals at F7), occasionally leading to secondary bilateral synchrony (Fig. 19.7). Several of the patient's habitual seizures were recorded without reliable localization or lateralization of the epileptogenic zone. This led to an EEG investigation with chronically implanted depth electrodes in the frontal and temporal lobes bilaterally. Interictally, rhythmic periodic spiking was recorded from the more superficial contacts of a depth electrode inserted through the third frontal gyrus (LAF5-8, Fig. 19.8). Seizures recorded were either bifrontal

in onset, or they showed a widespread EEG onset involving the neocortical structures of the left frontal and temporal lobes (Fig. 19.8).

Rapid Seizure Propagation

Rapid seizure spread from a focal generator located in the frontal lobe has been discussed elsewhere (3,4,38,39). In a review of 279 frontal lobe seizures recorded in ten patients who were being investigated by stereotactically implanted depth electrodes, Quesney (39) reported a mean time for seizure propagation of 6 seconds. A fast seizure spread is also common in parietal and occipital epilepsy (22).

Although the exact pathophysiological mechanisms of seizure propagation are not well known, one could postulate that seizure spread from a focal generator will depend on a network of pathways, permitting seizure spread within and outside the lobe where the seizure originates. The frontotemporal propagation, which is bidirectional, could be medi-

FIG. 19.6. Referential EEG recording in the same patient as Fig. 19.5A showing continuous electrographic seizure activity recorded from the left mid (LB7 and LB9) and posterior (LP7) temporal neocortical structures (see Fig. 19.5B for electrode placement).

95-2205

23:05:09   23:05:10   23:05:20

LA1-ref
LA3-ref
LA5-ref
LA7-ref
LA9-ref
LB1-ref
LB3-ref
LB5-ref
LB7-ref
LB9-ref
LP1-ref
LP3-ref
LP5-ref
LP7-ref
LO1-ref
LO3-ref
LO5-ref
LO7-ref
LO9-ref
LC1-ref
LC3-ref
LC5-ref
LC7-ref
LS1-ref
LS3-ref
LS5-ref
LS7-ref
L1-ref
L2-ref
L3-ref
L4-ref

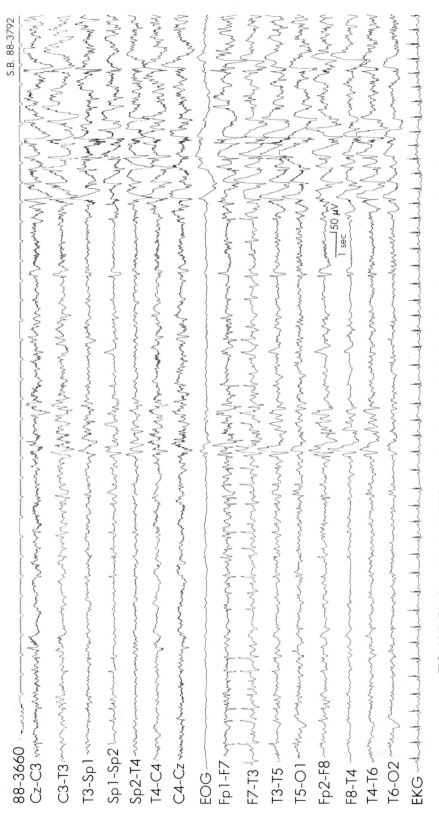

FIG. 19.7. Bipolar extracranial EEG recording showing rhythmic spiking with phase reversals at electrode F7, leading to secondarily generalized spike and slow wave complexes. (Reproduced from Quesney LF, Fish DR, Rasmussen T. Extracranial EEG and electrocorticography in children with medically refractory partial seizures. *J Epilepsy* 1990;3(Suppl):55–67, with permission.)

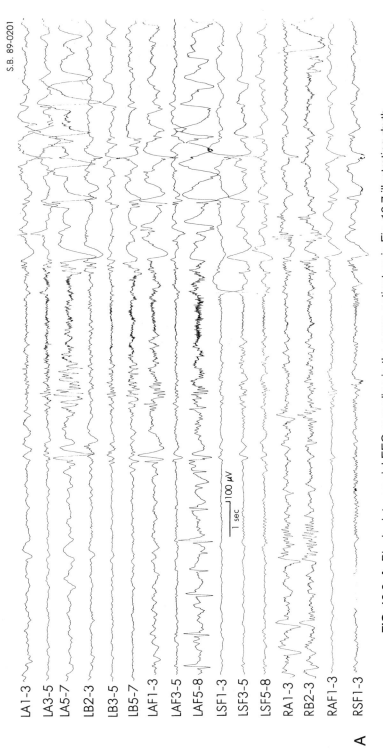

LA1-3
LA3-5
LA5-7
LB2-3
LB3-5
LB5-7
LAF1-3
LAF3-5
LAF5-8
LSF1-3
LSF3-5
LSF5-8
RA1-3
RB2-3
RAF1-3
A   RSF1-3

S.B. 89-0201

1 sec ⌐100 µV

FIG. 19.8. A: Bipolar intracranial EEG recording in the same patient as in Fig. 19.7 illustrating rhythmic periodic spikes recorded from the more superficial contacts (LAF5-8) of a depth electrode inserted through the third frontal gyrus (see **B**) leading subsequently to a widespread seizure discharge recorded from the intermediate and superficial contacts of the depth electrodes inserted through the left second temporal gyrus (LA3-5, LA5-7, LB3-5, and LB5-7). Note: depth electrode implantation was bilateral and symmetrical. Only intracranial electrodes implanted in the left hemisphere are shown in B. (Reproduced from Quesney LF, Fish DR, Rasmussen T. Extracranial EEG and electrocorticography in children with medically refractory partial seizures. *J Epilepsy* 1990;3 (Suppl):55–67, with permission.)

265

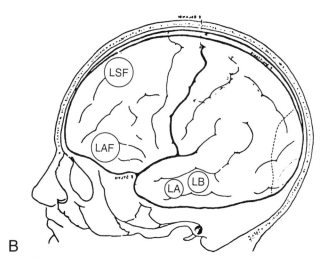

FIG. 19.8. *Continued.*

ated by the uncinate fasciculus, the cingulum, or the arcuate fasciculus (2,3,40). The occipito-temporal seizure spread (15,18,21) is dependent on the inferior longitudinal fasciculus (40).

A recent study supported the view that seizure propagation is proportional to the size of the ictal generator (37) because a large generator is likely to recruit more pathways. Neuromodulatory factors affecting seizure spread, such as the predominant inhibitory role of the hippocampus in modifying seizure propagation in mesial temporal lobe epilepsy (37), are essentially unknown in neocortical epilepsy. Seizure propagation from a common ictal generator through different pathways may be responsible for different clinical seizure patterns, which in turn may suggest a bilobar or multilobar seizure onset (12,14,18,21).

Rapid seizure propagation from a restricted ictal generator located at a distance from the recording electrodes may result in a regional, lobar, or hemispheric EEG seizure onset, thus mimicking a large epileptogenic zone. This limitation is thoroughly explained elsewhere (2–4,8,10–14,38).

Seizure Generator Located in a Clinically Silent Area

Intracerebral and cortical electric stimulation studies demonstrate that a handful of brain regions may elicit clinical manifestations in response to electric stimulation (41). Nevertheless, a large proportion of brain regions appear to be silent or less eloquent.

Theoretically, one could conceive of seizure onset in a silent region of the brain, such as the third frontal gyrus of the nondominant frontal lobe. Rapid seizure spread to the temporal lobe through the uncinate or arcuate fasciculus could be responsible for temporal lobelike ictal behavioral manifestations. If the electrographic seizure onset is missed, but the first or second stages of seizure propagation are recorded instead from the temporal lobe, the temptation to localize seizure onset in this region mistakenly is strong. This situation is illustrated by patient D.F., a 10-year-old boy with intractable complex partial seizures characterized by vocalization and early loss of consciousness followed by prominent automatisms. A right anterior temporal lobectomy performed at a different center produced no significant changes in his seizure trend. An electrocorticogram (ECoG) performed during reoperation documented rhythmic electrographic seizure activity in the third frontal gyrus of the right hemisphere (Fig. 19.9).

Low Incidence of Specific Neuroimaging Abnormalities

Compared with temporal lobe epilepsy, particularly if neuronal migration disorders and tumoral or vascular lesions are excluded as etiopathological factors of neocortical epilepsy, the incidence of MRI, positron emission tomography (PET), and single-photon emission computed tomography (SPECT) abnormalities, although encouraging, is not impressive (42–48). In a recent review of 42 patients with frontal lobe epilepsy (49), MRI studies found no lesions in 28 patients (67%).

COREGISTRATION WITH INTRACEREBRAL AND EPIDURAL ELECTRODES IN NEOCORTICAL EPILEPSY: THE MONTREAL NEUROLOGICAL INSTITUTE (MNI) APPROACH

Two main types of intracranially recorded ictal electrographic patterns have been reported in seizures involving mesial temporal lobe structures. From a historical perspective, the first pattern described consisted of a hypersynchronous seizure onset characterized by rhythmical polyspike activity usually at a high frequency, which correlated with increased extracellular unitary firing, presumably as a result of increased excitation (50). More recently, an electrographic pattern consisting of rhythmic periodic spikes has been found by different authors to be highly specific to mesial temporal lobe seizure onset (51–53). Both patterns may coexist and correlate with significant hippocampal neuronal loss (51,54–56).

The electrographic features that provide a "neocortical" imprinting to an intracranially recorded ictal EEG discharge are largely unknown. We undertook a review of 515 neocortical seizures to study their electrographic pattern at seizure onset, with particular emphasis on their localizing effectiveness and possible lobar morphological differences.

Materials and Methods

This series included 23 patients with neocortical epilepsy investigated with intracranial electrodes following an unsuccessful attempt to localize the ictal generator by serial 24-hour extracranial EEG–video monitoring sessions. The intracranial EEG investigation was interpreted by a single electroencephalographer. The series currently presented corresponds to approximately half the patients with neocortical epilepsy investigated with intracranial electrodes at the MNH from 1974 through 1997.

All patients underwent computed tomography (CT) or MRI examination and neuropsychological testing. Complementary neuroimaging investigation with PET, interictal or ictal SPECT, and MR spectroscopy was available in the patients investigated during the 1990s. Except for one patient with an oligodendroglioma, intracranial EEG investigation was performed in an attempt to localize the epileptogenic zone in the absence of CT or MRI abnormalities, suggesting a specific pathological substrate. Our series, in contrast to others (see Chapter 20), included no patients with neuronal migration disorder.

We studied 515 seizures of neocortical onset recorded with chronically implanted epidural and/or intracerebral electrodes in 23 patients. The anatomic compartmentalization was as follows: frontal lobe, ten patients (339 seizures); temporal lobe, six patients (71 seizures); centroparietal, five patients (98 seizures); and occipital, two patients (7 seizures).

The strategy for intracranial electrode implantation was tailored to the patients' needs. Intracerebral and epidural electrodes were chronically implanted initially using a CT or MRI-guided stereotactic technique (26) and more recently using a frameless stereotactic approach based on three-dimensional image guidance (36). The sites of depth electrode implantation were selected for each patient to

Pre-Excision ECoG

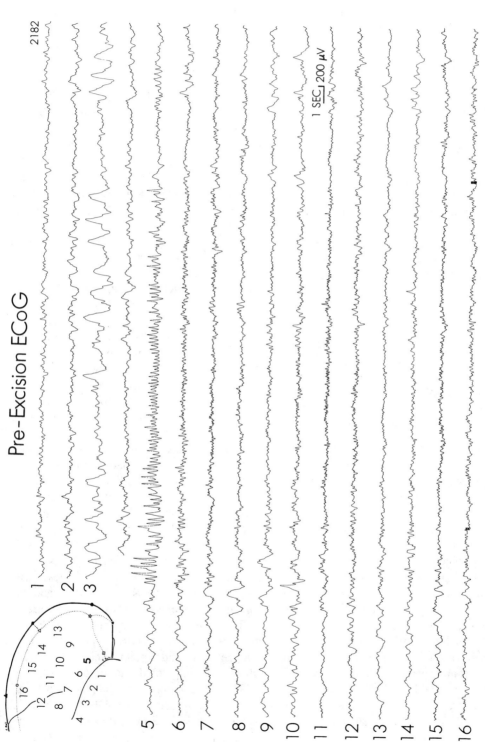

FIG. 19.9. Referential ECoG recording showing rhythmic sharp wave activity mainly at electrode 5 located in the third frontal gyrus. Cortical electrode placement as indicated in the diagram. (Reproduced from Quesney LF, Fish DR, Rasmussen T. Extracranial EEG and electrocorticography in children with medically refractory partial seizures. *J Epilepsy* 1990;3(Suppl):55–67, with permission.)

confirm a localization of the seizure generator hypothesized from a comprehensive review of clinical data, surface EEG, neuropsychological testing, and neuroimaging findings. Each depth electrode comprised nine contacts 5 mm apart, thus providing EEG recording from deep, intermediate, and neocortical structures (2,13).

A few patients in this series were studied during the 1970s and early 1980s before we started using simultaneous implantation of intracerebral and epidural electrodes. We used 24-hour computer-assisted EEG video monitoring with either 16 or 32 channels in the 1980s and 64 channels in the 1990s, according to previously described techniques (57,58).

The following exclusion criteria were applied: seizure onset missed or poorly recorded; patients with orbitofrontal, cingular, or mesial interhemispheric seizure onset; and seizures that originated simultaneously in the mesial and neocortical structures of the temporal lobe. Arbitrarily, a seizure was considered *focal* (small epileptogenic zone) when the initial ictal EEG changes involved one to three neighboring depth electrode contacts or one epidural electrode in a referential montage. The minimal electrographic expression of a regional seizure onset included initial EEG involvement of at least four depth electrode contacts or two epidural electrodes in referential montage.

Results

Our findings indicated that the success of localizing neocortical seizures depends on the anatomic location of their onset. The ratio between small and large epileptogenic zones (SEZ:LEZ) varies according to the anatomic localization of seizure onset (Table 19.2). The highest ratio of SEZ:LEZ is seen in seizures arising in the centroparietal convexity (86/4) and the lowest in the frontal lobe as a result of a high proportion of seizures showing a bifrontal synchronous onset (155/18). A similar phenomenon was reported elsewhere (13). Temporal lobe seizures occupy an intermedi-

TABLE 19.2. Localization and anatomic extent of neocortical seizure onset (498 seizures)

	SEZ	LEZ	Bilobar
Frontal	155	18	166[a]
Temporal	49	12	
Centroparietal	86	4	8[b]
Total	290	34	174

[a]Synchronously.
[b]Independently.
LEZ, large epileptogenic; SEZ, small epileptogenic.

ate position (49/12). Occipital lobe seizures were too few to be considered.

The topographic distribution of focal seizure onsets (SEZ) in the beta and gamma frequency band is illustrated in Fig. 19.10. Restricted focal seizure onset in the beta and gamma frequency band occurred mostly in the frontal lobe (123/155 seizures). Only a small fraction of temporal (9/51) or centroparietal (3/86) seizures presented with initial ictal electrographic changes in the beta or gamma frequency band. The topographic distribution of focal seizure onsets at a frequency of 5 to 14 Hz is shown in Fig. 19.11. Focal seizures in this frequency band were distributed mostly in

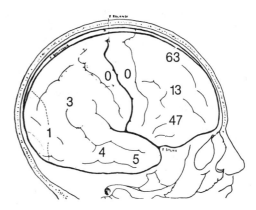

Frontal lobe: 155 sz
Centro-parietal: 86 sz
Temporal lobe: 51 sz
Occipital lobe: 1 sz

FIG. 19.10. Topographic distribution of focal seizure onsets in the beta and gamma frequency band.

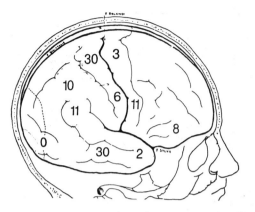

Frontal lobe: 155 sz
Centro-parietal: 86 sz
Temporal lobe: 51 sz
Occiptal lobe: 0 sz

Frontal lobe: 155 sz
Centro-parietal: 86 sz
Temporal lobe: 51 sz
Occipital lobe: 1 sz

FIG. 19.11. Topographic distribution of focal seizure onsets at a frequency of 5 to 14 Hz.

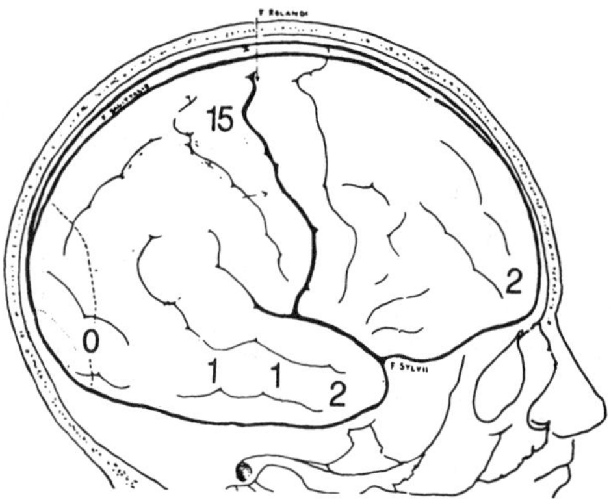

FIG. 19.12. Topographic distribution of focal seizure onsets at a frequency of 2 to 4 Hz.

the central parietal convexity (60/86) and in the temporal neocortex (43/51) with scarce representation (8/155) in the frontal lobe.

Seizures with an initial frequency at 2–4 Hz were less numerous. Their topographic distribution (Fig. 19.12) shows a comparatively higher incidence in the central region.

Some patients in this series were studied in the 1970s and early 1980s, before MRI availability. The latter technique was available in six frontal lobe patients with positive findings (oligodendroglioma) in only one of them. Four patients in the centroparietal series underwent MRI examination; abnormalities (atrophy) were found in only one of these patients. The MRI results were slightly better in the temporal lobe group, which comprised five patients (asymmetry of the temporal horn in one patient and hippocampal gliosis with diffuse temporal atrophy in another patient).

Discussion

The current study deals with the biophysical and electrophysiological properties of seizure onset and evolution in patients with neocortical epilepsy who underwent intracra-

nial EEG investigation. Most patients included in this series presented with conflicting EEG lateralization or localization of the epileptogenic zone in the absence of diagnostic MRI abnormalities. Only one of these patients had a specific structural lesion on neuroimaging. From this perspective, our population of patients is different from that presented by Spencer and Lee in this volume.

Our results clearly showed that electrographic seizure onset in the beta or gamma frequency band strongly correlates with an ictal generator located in the neocortical mantle of the frontal lobe (Figs. 19.2, 19.3, and 19.9). Similar findings have been reported in smaller series (59–61). We admit, however, that this is not an exclusive finding because a high-frequency discharge at seizure onset can be seen in other lobes as well.

Focal electrographic seizure onset in the beta or gamma frequency band does not provide "fool-proof" localization of the ictal generator because an ictal discharge at a similar frequency can be observed during seizure spread. The physiopathological mechanism responsible for the genesis of high frequency seizure discharge in the frontal lobes remains largely unknown.

We believe that high-frequency seizure onset in the frontal lobe is related to an intrinsic network that operates under physiologic and physiopathological conditions. The genesis of electrographic seizure discharge in the beta and gamma frequency band would be a pathophysiologic expression of this network, whereas the genesis of beta and sleep spindle activity would constitute a physiologic expression. The main ictal EEG frequency of seizures arising in the centroparietal and temporal neocortical structures was 5 to 14 Hz.

With regard to neuropathological correlation, extratemporal neocortical seizure onset at high frequency can be associated with cortical dysplasia (62,63) or with extensive cortical gliosis (64,65). For correlation of electrographic findings with neuroradiologic abnormalities, pathological substrates, and surgical outcome, the reader is referred to Chapter 20.

The success of localizing neocortical seizures seems to correlate with their anatomic location at onset. The SEZ:LEZ ratio was highest in the centroparietal convexity and lowest in the frontal lobe. This is probably related to a "hard wiring" network arrangement in the centroparietal convexity, in contrast to the frontal lobe, which allows small epileptogenic zones to express themselves electrographically and clinically as part of an integrated somatomotor cortical system subserving specific topographic functions. It is also possible that local inhibitory networks may reduce the main frequency of seizure discharge, thereby acting as neuromodulators of the electrophysiologic properties of seizure initiation and evolution (37). A lower inhibitory "tone" could explain the predominance of beta and gamma electrographic activity at seizure onset as well as a highest incidence of bilateral synchrony observed in frontal lobe epilepsy.

Rhythmic periodic spiking at seizure onset. which is a distinctive electrographic pattern in mesial temporal lobe epilepsy (51–54), was seen only occasionally in seizures of neocortical origin (approximately 1%; Fig. 19.8). Background activity flattening at seizure onset was documented in approximately 10% of focal neocortical seizures and almost always evolved into beta and gamma rhythmical polyspike activity.

In the first section of this chapter, we reviewed the electrophysiologic limitations commonly encountered during the preoperative investigation of patients with neocortical epilepsy. We provided electrographic evidence that small ictal generators located in an area of convoluted cortical gray matter could be easily missed by epidural, subdural, or cortical electrodes. Conversely, it is also evident that intracerebral electrodes provide "tunnel vision" with reliable EEG resolution in the depth and low yield at the level of the cortical mantle.

In our experience, which is also shared by others (26–32,66), coregistration with intracerebral and epidural or subdural electrodes is the most practical approach to recording neocortical seizures accurately. A significant limiting factor in the EEG localization of neocortical ictal generators resides in their fast propagation following seizure onset (2–4,12, 14,18,21,22,36,38,39). This is even more of a complication if the electrographic seizure onset is missed or not properly recorded, such that EEG abnormalities actually recorded do not represent the anatomic site of ictal onset, but rather they are the first or even second stages of seizure propagation.

Traditionally, electroencephalographers with experience in the interpretation of EEG tracings obtained with intracranial electrodes have assumed that a focal seizure discharge in the beta or gamma frequency probably originates in the immediate vicinity of the ictal generator, thus providing reliable localization. The correlation between focal EEG changes of an ictal nature recorded with intracranial electrodes and the anatomical extent of the epileptogenic zone remains controversial, particularly in the absence of a pathological lesion (67). Similar questions have been posed regarding the feasibility of differentiation between electrographic seizure onset and EEG changes secondary to seizure spread. In this regard, a recent publication provided evidence that focal seizure onset in the gamma frequency band in extratemporal epilepsy is preferentially seen at sites of seizure onset, in contrast to anatomic sites of seizure spread (68).

A promising approach to differentiating between initial versus propagated ictal EEG changes is offered by a recently developed technique that searches as an "EEG microscope" for focal electric discharges in the brain's depth prior to the appearance of ictal EEG changes in the scalp (see Chapter 22).

REFERENCES

1. Penfield W, Jasper HH. *Epilepsy and the functional anatomy of the human brain.* Boston: Little, Brown, 1954.
2. Quesney LF, Gloor P. Localization of epileptic foci. Long-term monitoring in epilepsy. *Electroencephalogr Clin Neurophysiol* 1985;(Suppl 37):327–340.
3. Quesney LF. Seizures of frontal lobe origin. In: Meldrum B, Pedley T, eds. *Recent advances in epilepsy,* vol 3. London: Churchill Livingstone, 1986:81–110.
4. Quesney LF. Extracranial EEG evaluation. In: Engel J Jr, ed. *Surgical treatment of the epilepsies.* New York: Raven Press, 1987:129–166.
5. Quesney LF, Abou-Khalil B, Cole A, et al. Pre-operative and intracerebral EEG investigation in patients with temporal lobe epilepsy: trends, results, and review of pathophysiologic mechanisms. *Acta Neurol Scand Suppl* 1988;78:52–61.
6. Quesney LF, Olivier A. Pre-operative EEG evaluation in frontal lobe epilepsy. *Acta Neurologica Scand Suppl* 1988;78:61–72.
7. Quesney LF, Fish DR, Rasmussen T. Extracranial EEG and electrocorticography in children with medically refractory partial seizures. *J Epilepsy* 1990;3(Suppl): 55–67.
8. Quesney LF, Constain M, Rasmussen T, et al. How large are frontal lobe epileptogenic zones? EEG, ECoG, and SEEG evidence. In: Chauvel P, Delgado-Escueta AV, Halgren E, Bancaud J, eds. *Frontal lobe seizures and epilepsies. Advances in neurology,* vol 57. New York: Raven Press, 1992:311–323.
9. Quesney LF. Pre-operative electroencephalographic investigation in frontal lobe epilepsy: electroencephalographic and electrocorticographic recordings. *Can J Neurol Sci* 1991;18:559–563.
10. Quesney LF. Extratemporal epilepsy: clinical presentation, pre-operative EEG localization, and surgical outcome. *Acta Neurol Scand Suppl* 1992;86:81–94.
11. Quesney LF, Constain M, Rasmussen T, et al. Presurgical EEG investigation in frontal lobe epilepsy. In: Theodore WH, ed. *Surgical treatment of the epilepsy.* New York: Elsevier, 1992:55–69.
12. Salanova V, Andermann F, Olivier A, et al. Occipital lobe epilepsy: electroclinical manifestations, electrocorticography, cortical stimulation, and outcome in 42 patients treated between 1930 and 1991. *Brain* 1992; 115:1655–1680.
13. Quesney LF, Cendes F, Olivier A, et al. Intracranial electroencephalographic investigation in frontal lobe epilepsy. In: Jasper HH, Riggio S, Goldman-Rakic PS, eds. *Epilepsy and the functional anatomy of the frontal lobe. Advances in neurology,* vol 66, 1995:243–260.
14. Salanova V, Andermann F, Rasmussen T, et al. Parietal lobe epilepsy: clinical manifestations and outcome in 82 patients treated surgically between 1929 and 1988. *Brain* 1995;118:607–627.
15. Palmini A, Andermann F, Dubeau F, et al. Occipitotemporal epilepsies: evaluation of selected patients requiring depth electrodes studies and rationale for surgical approaches. *Epilepsia* 1993;34:84–96.
16. Williamson PD, Van Ness PC, Wieser H-G, et al. Surgically remediable extratemporal syndromes. In: Engel J Jr, ed. *Surgical treatment of the epilepsies,* 2nd ed. New York: Raven Press, 1993:65–76.
17. Williamson PD. Frontal lobe seizures: problems of diagnosis and classification. In: Chauvel P, Delgado-Escueta AV, Halgren E, Bancaud J, eds. *Frontal lobe seizures and epilepsies. Advances in neurology,* vol 57. New York: Raven Press, 1992:289–309.
18. Williamson PD, Boon PA, Thadani VM, et al. Parietal lobe epilepsy: diagnostic considerations and results of surgery. *Ann Neurol* 1992;31:193–201.
19. Williamson PD, Spencer DD, Spencer SS, et al. Complex partial seizures of extratemporal origin. *Ann Neurol* 1985;18:497–504.
20. Williamson PD, Spencer SS. Clinical and EEG features of complex partial seizures of extratemporal origin. *Epilepsia* 1986;27(Suppl 2):46–93.
21. Williamson PD, Thadani VM, Darcey TM, et al. Occipital lobe epilepsy: clinical characteristics, seizure spread patterns, and results of surgery. *Ann Neurol* 1992; 31:3–13.
22. Sveinbjornsdottir S, Duncan JS. Parietal and occipital lobe epilepsy: a review. *Epilepsia* 1993;34:493–521.
23. Cascino GD, Hulihan JF, Sharbrough FW, et al. Parietal lobe lesional epilepsy: electroclinical correlation and operative outcome. *Epilepsia* 1993;34:522–527.
24. Van Essen DC, Drury HA. Structural and functional analyses of human cerebral cortex using a surface-based atlas. *J Neurosci* 1997;17:7079–7102.
25. Gloor P. Contribution of electroencephalography and electrocorticography to the neurosurgical treatment of the epilepsies. In: Purpura DP, Penry JK, Walter RD, eds. *Neurosurgical management of the epilepsies. Advances in neurology,* vol 8. New York: Raven Press, 1975:59–63.
26. Olivier A. Surgery of frontal lobe epilepsy. In: Jasper HH, Riggio S, Goldman-Rakic P, eds. *Epilepsy and the functional anatomy of the frontal lobe. Advances in neurology,* vol 66. New York: Raven Press, 1995: 321–348.
27. Spencer SS, SO NK, Engel J Jr, et al. Depth electrodes. In: Engel J Jr, ed. *Surgical treatment of the epilepsies,* 2nd ed. New York: Raven Press, 1993:359–376.
28. Arroyo S, Lesser RP, Awad IA, et al. Subdural and epidural grids and strips. In: Engel J Jr, ed. *Surgical treatment of the epilepsies,* 2nd ed. New York: Raven Press, 1993:377–386.
29. Wyler AR, Wilkus RJ, Blume T. Strip electrodes. In: Engel J Jr, ed. *Surgical treatment of the epilepsies,* 2nd ed. New York: Raven Press, 1993:387.
30. Spencer SS, Williamson PD, Spencer DD, et al. Human hippocampal seizure spread studied by depth and sub-

dural recording: the hippocampus commissure. *Epilepsia* 1987;28:479–489.

31. Awad IA, Assirati JA, Burgess R, et al. A new case of electrodes of "intermediate invasiveness": preliminary experience with epidural pegs and foramen ovale electrodes in the mapping of seizure foci. *Neurol Res* 1991; 13:177–183.
32. Lüders HO, Lesser RP, Dinner DS, et al. Commentary: chronic intracranial recording and stimulation with subdural electrodes. In: Engel J Jr, ed. *Surgical treatment of the epilepsies.* New York: Raven Press, 1987:197–321.
33. Rasmussen T. Surgical treatment of complex partial seizures: results, lessons, and problems. *Epilepsia* 1983; 24(Suppl):S65–S76.
34. Robitaille Y, Rasmussen T, Dubeau F, et al. Histopathology of nonneoplastic lesions in frontal lobe epilepsy: review of 180 cases with recent MRI and PET correlations. In: Chauvel P, Delgado-Escueta AV, Halgren E, Bancaud J, eds. *Frontal lobe seizures and epilepsies. Advances in neurology,* vol 57. New York: Raven Press, 1992:499–513.
35. Morrell F. Varieties of human secondary epileptogenesis. *J Clin Neurophysiol* 1989;6:227–275.
36. Alonso-Vanegas MA, Olivier A, Quesney LF. Applications of image-guided and surgery to intraoperative electrophysiology. In: Quesney LF, Binnie CD, Chatrian G-E, eds. *Electrocorticography: current trends and future perspectives. Electroencephalogr Clin Neurophysiol Suppl* 1998;48:140–156.
37. Quesney LF, Arruda F, Olivier A, et al. Seizure evolution analyzed by depth electrodes. In: *Epileptic seizures: pathophysiology and semiology.* Philadelphia: Lippincott Williams & Wilkins, 2000 (in press).
38. Quesney LF, Risinger M, Shewmon A. Extracranial EEG evaluation. In: Engel J Jr, ed. *Surgical treatment of the epilepsies,* 2nd ed. New York: Raven Press, 1993: 173–196.
39. Quesney LF. Electroencephalographic and clinical manifestations of frontal and temporal lobe epilepsy. *Clin Neurol Neurosurg* 1987;89(Suppl):41–42.
40. Schneider RC, Crosby EC, Farhat SM. Extratemporal lesions triggering the temporal lobe syndrome. *J Neurosurg* 1965;22:246–263.
41. Fish DR, Gloor P, Quesney LF, et al. Clinical responses to electrical brain stimulation of the temporal and frontal lobes in patients with epilepsy. *Brain* 116;1993: 397–414.
42. Franck G, Maquet P, Sadzot B, et al. Contribution of positron emission tomography to the investigation of epilepsies of frontal lobe origin. In: Chauvel P, Delgado-Escueta AV, Halgren E, Bancaud J, eds. *Frontal lobe seizures and epilepsies. Advances in neurology,* vol 57. New York: Raven Press, 1992:471–485.
43. Swartz B, Theodore WH, Sanabria E, et al. Positron emission and single proton emission computed tomographic studies in the frontal lobe with emphasis on the relationship to seizure foci. In: Chauvel P, Delgado-Escueta AV, Halgren E, Bancaud J, eds. *Frontal lobe seizures and epilepsies. Advances in neurology,* vol 57. New York: Raven Press, 1992:487–497.
44. Cascino GD, Jack CR Jr, Parisi JE, et al. MRI in the presurgical evaluation of patients with frontal lobe epilepsy and children with temporal lobe epilepsy: pathologic correlation and prognostic importance. *Epilepsy Res* 1992;11:51–59.
45. Kuzniecky RI, Cascino GD, Palmini A, et al. Structural neuroimaging. In: Engel J Jr, ed. *Surgical treatment of the epilepsies,* 2nd ed. New York: Raven Press, 1993: 197–209.
46. Swartz BE, Halgren E, Delgado-Escueta AV, et al. Neuroimaging in patients with seizures of probable frontal lobe origin. *Epilepsia* 1898;30 547–558.
47. Stefan H, Quesney LF, Feistel HK, et al. Pre-surgical evaluation in frontal lobe epilepsy: a multimethodological approach. In: Jasper HH, Riggio S, Goldman-Rakic PS, eds. Epilepsy and the functional anatomy of the frontal lobe. *Adv Neurol* 1995;66:213–221.
48. Stanley JA, Cendes F, Dubeau F, et al. Proton magnetic resonance spectroscopic imaging in patients with extratemporal epilepsy. *Epilepsia* 1998;39:267–273.
49. Gross DW, Dubeau F, Gotman J, et al. Surface EEG recording in patients with lesional and nonlesional frontal lobe epilepsy. *Epilepsia* 1998;39(Suppl 8):75.
50. Babb TL, Wilson CL, Isokawa-Akesson M. Firing patterns of human limbic neurons during stereoencephalography (SEEG) and clinical temporal lobe seizures. *Electroencephalogr Clin Neurophysiol* 1987; 66:467–482.
51. Spencer SS, Guimaraes P, Katz A, et al. Morphological patterns of seizures recorded intracranially. *Epilepsia* 1992;33:537–545.
52. Reiher J, Quesney LF. Classification of intracranial spikes in 48 operated patients with bitemporal extracranial epileptiform abnormalities. *Electroencephalogr Clin Neurophysiol* 1993;86:57P–78P.
53. Quesney LF, Reiher J, Olivier A. Rhythmic limbic spiking: a reliable predictor of impending mesial temporal seizures in man. *Epilepsia* 1994;35(Suppl 8):28.
54. Arruda F, Quesney LF, Wennberg R, et al. Initial spread in focal and regional onset mesial temporal seizures. *Epilepsia* 1997;38(Suppl 8):116.
55. Babb TL, Lieb JP, Brown WJ, et al. Distribution of pyramidal cell density and hyperexcitability in the epileptic human hippocampal formation. *Epilepsia* 1984;25: 721–728.
56. Babb TL, Lieb JP, Brown WJ, et al. Distribution of pyramidal cell density and hyperexcitability in the epileptic human hippocampal formation. *Epilepsia* 1984;25:721–728.
57. Gotman J. Automatic recognition of epileptic seizures in the EEG. *Electroencephalogr Clin Neurophysiol* 1982;54:530–540.
58. Gotman J, Ives JR, Gloor P, et al. Monitoring at the Montreal Neurological Institute. In: Gotman J, Ives JR, Gloor P, eds. *Long-term monitoring in epilepsies.* New York: Elsevier, 1985:327–340.
59. Quesney LF, Krieger C, Leitner C, et al. Frontal lobe epilepsy: clinical and electrographic presentation. In: Porter RJ, Mattson RH, Ward AA, Dam M, eds. *Advances in epileptology:* XVth Epilepsy International Symposium. New York: Raven Press, 1984:503–508.
60. Fisher RS, Webber WRS, Lesser RP, et al. High frequency EEG activity at the start of seizures. *J Clin Neurophysiol* 1992;9:441–448.
61. Allen PJ, Fish DR, Smith SJM. Very high frequency rhythmic activity during SEEG suppression in frontal lobe epilepsy. *Electroencephalogr Clin Neurophysiol* 1992;82:155–159.
62. Palmini A, Gambardella A, Andermann F, et al. Intrinsic epileptogenecity of human dysplastic cortex as sug-

gested by corticography and surgical results. *Ann Neurol* 1995;37:476–487.

63. Gambardella A, Palmini A, Andermann F, et al. Usefulness of focal rhythmic discharges on scalp EEG of patients with focal cortical dysplasia and instractable epilepsy. *Electroencephalogr Clin Neurophysiol* 1996;98:243–249.

64. Jasper H. Electrocorticogram in man. *Electroencephalogr Clin Neurophysiol* 1949;2(Suppl):216–229.

65. Guerreiro M, Quesney LF, Salanova V, et al. Continous ECoG epileptiform discharges due to brain gliosis. *Epilepsia* 1998;39(Suppl 6):209.

66. Brekelman GJF, van Emde Boas W, Velis DN, et al. Comparison of combined versus subdural or intracerebral electrodes alone in presurgical focus localization. *Epilepsia* 1998;39:1290–1301.

67. Schiller Y, Cascino GD, Sharbrough FW. Chronic intracranial EEG monitoring for localizing the epileptogenic zone: an electroclinical correlation. *Epilepsia* 1998;39:1302–1308.

68. Schiller Y, Cascino GD, Busacker NE, et al. Characterization and comparison of local onset and remote propagated electrographic seizures recorded with intracranial electrodes. *Epilepsia* 1998;39:380–388.

Neocortical Epilepsies.
Advances in Neurology, Vol. 84,
edited by P.D. Williamson, A.M. Siegel,
D.W. Roberts, V.M. Thadani, and M.S. Gazzaniga.
Lippincott Williams & Wilkins, Philadelphia © 2000.

20

Invasive EEG in Neocortical Epilepsy: Seizure Onset

Susan S. Spencer and Sang-Ahm Lee

Department of Neurology, Yale University School of Medicine, New Haven, Connecticut 06520-8018

Although intracranial EEG is widely held to be necessary in the localization of the epileptogenic zone for purposes of resective surgical treatment in refractory epilepsy of neocortical onset, remarkably little information is available to define the characteristics of seizure onset in the epileptogenic neocortex. Our experience at Yale was used to describe neocortical seizures with respect to intracranial EEG features of onset patterns, frequency, and distribution in relation to substrate and surgical outcome.

Of 53 neocortical epileptic patients evaluated and operated at Yale from 1989 to 1996 (23 temporal, 30 extratemporal), the substrate was developmental in 28 (neuronal migrational disorder, focal cortical dysplasia, mesial temporal sclerosis), mature in 14 (neoplastic, trauma, vascular), and negative (gliosis only) in 11. Only 16 of the total group were completely seizure free after resective surgery. Surgical outcome was significantly related to pathology, better in mature substrates than normal or developmental ones ($p = 0.037$), and significantly related to morphology of seizure onset, worse in patients with semirhythmic slow activity, or slow- or fast-spike activity at seizure onset than in patients with low voltage fast or sinusoidal wave activity at seizure onset ($p = 0.02$). Surgical outcome was *not* significantly related to frequency or distribution of seizure onset.

Neocortical seizure onsets recorded from intracranial electrodes had frequencies that were significantly related to the lobe of onset (extratemporal seizures had significantly higher onset frequency, in the gamma range, than temporal seizures, which were usually in the beta range, $p = 0.017$). Seizure onset distribution was significantly related to frequency (beta onset was commonly focal whereas gamma was regional, $p < 0.005$). These seizure features were *independent* of the substrate. Morphology of seizure onset was significantly related to the pathologic *substrate,* with low voltage, fast and rhythmic slow spike onset most commonly observed in developmental substrates, and rhythmic sinusoidal wave onset *only* in mature ones ($p = 0.02$).

The electric signal of neocortical seizure onset is thus a complicated product of the specific substrate (which is significantly related to waveform and outcome) and anatomic localization (which is significantly related to frequency and distribution of seizure onset). These observations have implications for pathophysiology, diagnosis, and prognosis in neocortical epilepsy.

Understanding differences in the pathophysiology and expression of different types of epilepsy, particularly neocortical compared with mesiotemporal, is of theoretical as well as practical value. It makes sense that neocortical epilepsies, being generated in anatomically distinct brain structures with different networks and connections, should manifest unique patterns on various tests of cortical function (and dysfunction) compared with epilepsies arising in limbic structures. In a practical sense, this is of most interest in the localization of the epileptogenic region for surgical treatment of refractory patients. Considerable experience has accumulated in the study of mesiotemporal lobe epilepsy (MTLE), and rules have evolved to help in interpretating the depth and subdural electroencephalographic (EEG) signals in that entity (1–4). Similarly, the positron emission tomography (PET), single-photon emission computed tomography (SPECT), and magnetic resonance imaging (MRI) signatures as well as the common historical features of MTLE have been defined to a considerable extent (5). In neocortical epilepsies, however, the anatomic representation, the metabolism and perfusion characteristics on functional imaging, and the historical features that point to specific etiology and location of onset are largely unknown. This difficulty extends to the interpretation of the intracranial EEG signals as they relate to definition and localization of seizure onset (6). Because cortical structure, layering, and connections of these locations are different, one might expect the EEG expression of seizures arising in the neocortex to differ from those in mesiotemporal structures, but analysis of neocortical seizure onset patterns recorded with intracranial electrodes is more problematic than in MTLE because we are so often unsuccessful in defining the epileptogenic region fully. Furthermore, some of the findings in MTLE have been amenable to quantitative analyses, specifically the imaging and pathological data, but such quantitation of the substrate has not yet been done in the neocortex. It remains true, despite these vagaries, that localization of seizure onset by implanted electrodes is taken as the most important piece of localizing information for the purposes of resective surgery in the neocortex as well as mesiotemporal structures.

To help define the intracranial EEG in this situation, we investigated 53 refractory neocortical epilepsy patients at the Yale Epilepsy Center who were studied with implanted intracranial electrodes, had seizure onset recorded and stored for review, and subsequently had resective surgical treatment with pathological analysis and at least 1 year of follow-up. Using outcome and pathology to judge the success or failure of localization by the detected signals, we analyzed the characteristics of seizure onset in the neocortex. In this study, we underline several aspects:

1. It *is* possible to do a systematic study of neocortical epileptogenic signals recorded from implanted electrodes.
2. Those signals enable prediction of substrate and of surgical outcome.
3. Those signals are dependent on the neocortical location of seizure onset (and implicitly on its anatomical connections).
4. Further systematic analysis in greater numbers of patients may allow more understanding of the pathophysiology of medically refractory neocortical epilepsies.

METHODS

Patient Selection

Patients studied at the Yale Epilepsy Center with implanted intracranial electrodes (including any combination of depth, subdural, and grid electrodes) between the years of 1989 and 1996 were included in this analysis. Our database was reviewed, and *all* patients within those years of study were included if they additionally fulfilled the following criteria:

1. Multiple spontaneous seizures were recorded by any array of implanted intracranial electrodes.
2. Recorded seizures were stored for reanalysis.
3. Subsequent resective surgery was performed.
4. Follow-up of at least 12 months was available.
5. Pathological analysis of resective tissue was done.

All patients underwent initial evaluation as previously described (7–9), including structural imaging with epilepsy protocol MRI study: functional imaging, including interictal PET and SPECT; ictal SPECT when available;

neuropsychological evaluation; detailed historical and neurological examinations; and intensive video–EEG monitoring using scalp electrodes and recording of multiple spontaneous seizures as well as interictal spike activity and background analysis. Medication withdrawal in a controlled fashion was used for the video–EEG monitoring. Except for space-occupying lesions with concordant EEG data, all candidates for resective surgery in neocortical areas underwent repeat video–EEG with some combination of intracranial electrodes. Specific electrodes used and their placement were selected based on the prior noninvasive data.

Whether any abnormalities were identified by structural neuroimaging was not a factor in the selection of patients for this study; however, the group is biased in that certain anatomic lesions identified by MRI may demand surgical treatment *independent* of electrographic evidence of seizure onset in the region, and those patients are necessarily excluded from this analysis because they did not undergo implanted electrode study. Precise medications, actual age, and concomitant neurologic or psychological conditions were not exclusionary criteria. Certain patients had multiple intracranial EEG studies, and in those situations the last study was used for our analysis because it was in that study that localization was determined for the purposes of resective surgery.

Surgery and Follow-up

Patients underwent resective surgery within 3 months of intracranial electrode study. Resection location was determined by localization from seizure recording from implanted electrodes. Tissue was resected to at least 1 cm (or maximal) margins around the identified epileptogenic region of onset, defined by normal cytoarchitecture, or limited by regions of cortical function. Mapping was performed when necessary. Interictal spikes did not affect the determination of extent of resection.

Patients had follow-up at 6-month intervals postoperatively by outpatient visits or telephone consultation. Postoperative seizure frequency and occurrence were verified by discussion with family members or other persons in a position to observe the patients. Outcome for the purpose of this analysis was characterized by the Engel criteria 1 through 4 as well as by the designation of *seizure free* or *not seizure-free*. Seizures occurring during hospitalization were *not* included in the assessment of outcome.

Electroencephalographic Analysis

All seizures recorded for these 53 patients were reformatted and printed for visual analysis in referential and bipolar montages, with displays employing all contacts recorded. The seizures were analyzed independently by the two authors. *Seizure onset* was defined as a sustained rhythmic change in the EEG accompanied by subsequent clinically typical seizure activity, at a frequency of greater than 2 Hz, not explained by level of arousal and clearly distinguished from background EEG and interictal activity. The seizure onset characteristics of the *first two seconds* were analyzed visually. Seizure frequency, waveform, and spatial distribution of the signal were tabulated.

Frequency was assessed visually and characterized in traditional EEG frequency bands of delta, theta, alpha, beta, and gamma. In addition, these frequencies were grouped for further analysis into *fast* (beta and gamma) and *slow* (all others). Morphology of seizure onset was defined in five groups, including low-voltage fast activity, generally over 13 Hz; rhythmic slow spike or spike wave at 4–13 Hz of moderate amplitude; rhythmic sinusoidal waves of alpha frequency; semirhythmic slow waves under 5 Hz; and high amplitude fast-spike activity in the beta frequency band. Distribution of seizure onset was classified as *focal* or *regional,* where focal was defined as seizure onset involving one to four contacts of one electrode or two adjacent electrodes, and regional included seizure onset involving five contacts or more on a single or adjacent electrodes within a single lobe. Preictal spikes lasting longer than 5 seconds at a frequency of 2 Hz or lower were not considered part of seizure onset for this analysis, nor were subclinical seizures, seizures without clear localization, onset characterized by diffuse electric changes in all recorded contacts, and atypical seizures. Anatomic location of seizure onset was defined by lobe and by medial or lateral region of the lobe. When multiple seizure-onset locations or patterns were recorded in a patient, the *predominant* pattern was used for the analysis.

Pathological Analysis

Resected tissue was subjected to routine staining and analysis. The pathological diagnoses were divided into those of *mature* or *developmental* origin. Developmental etiologies included focal cortical dysplasia, neuronal migrational disorder, heterotopia, hamartoma, microdysgenesis, and other cortical dysgenesis, mesial temporal sclerosis. Mature pathological entities included neoplasm, trauma, and vascular events, including ischemia and prior hemorrhage. Patients with mild or nonspecific glial proliferation were characterized as normal, as were patients with no detected pathological abnormalities.

Electrodes

A combination of electrodes was used for recording in all patients and consisted of a variable representation of subdural grid electrodes, subdural strip electrodes, and intracerebral depth electrodes. The subdural strip and grid electrodes consisted of multiple contacts with 1-cm intercontact placement. Grids varied in size from 4×4 to 8×8. Multicontact intracerebral depth electrodes had intercontact spacing of 5 to 10 mm along their length and were inserted stereotactically. Specific electrode type and distribution were individualized depending on the results of the noninvasive evaluation. The electrodes used in each individual patient were tabulated, and note was made of the specific electrode in which seizure onset was first detected in each patient.

Analysis

Features of seizure onset recorded from implanted electrodes, including waveform, frequency, distribution, location, and electrode type, were analyzed with respect to surgical outcome, pathological findings, and anatomic location. Chi-square statistics were applied. Age of onset and duration of epilepsy also were analyzed by analysis of variance with respect to the different EEG characteristics.

RESULTS

General

Of the 53 patients with neocortical seizure onset, 23 were in the temporal lobe, and the others were extratemporal (16 frontal, 10 occipital, 4 parietal). Eleven patients had lesions identified by structural neuroimaging prior to the electrode implantation study.

We recorded 333 seizures, of which 103 were recorded from temporal lobe. The age of onset for these patients was a mean of 11 years and ranged from 0.5 to 42 years. Temporal and extratemporal age at onset did not differ statistically: 13.6 years in the temporal and 9.0 years in the extratemporal group. A trend toward earlier onset in the extratemporal group was noted, however. Epilepsy duration had an overall mean of 16.9 years, ranging from 1 to 50 years, and did not differ significantly in temporal and extratemporal patients, although again a trend toward longer duration in the extratemporal group was identified. The mean duration of epilepsy in temporal neocortical patients was 14 years, in extratemporal patients, 18.5 years. The 53 patients comprised 29 with a negative medical history; 8 gave a history of febrile seizures, 6 of significant trauma, 5 of central nervous system infection, and 2 of significant prenatal injuries.

Pathological Substrates

The 53 patients included 28 with developmental etiologies, 14 with mature etiologies, and 11 who were diagnosed as normal. The developmental lesions included 7 focal cortical dysplasia, 4 heterotopia, 1 hamartoma, 1 tuberous sclerosis, and 15 microdysgenesis. Mature substrates, representing 26% of the total group, included 5 neoplasms, 5 ischemic lesions, 2 prior hemorrhages, and 2 AVMs.

Onset Electrodes

Of the total group of patients, 7 were studied only with subdural strip electrodes, 2 with only intracerebral depth electrodes, and 1 with only a subdural grid. The other patients had combinations of electrodes including grid and strip electrodes in 27, depth and strip electrodes in 10, and a grid, strip and depth electrodes in 6. In the subgroup of patients who had *at least* strip and grid electrodes, 18 were localized by the grid and 24 by the strips (not significantly different).

The type of electrode in which seizure onset was diagnosed was examined with respect to pathology, the presence or absence of an identified lesion prior to implantation, the medial and lateral lobar location, the regional or focal distribution, and the specific lobe of seizure onset (Table 20.1). Of the 28 patients with developmental pathology, 54% were localized by strip electrodes and 43% by grid electrodes (Fig. 20.1). Strip electrodes accounted for the majority of localization in most comparisons, with three notable exceptions. Fifty-five percent of lesions were localized by grids compared with only 27% by strips and 18% by depth electrodes. Fifty-eight percent of diagnoses of seizure onset in a lateral lobar location were made by grids

compared with 39% by strips and 4% by depth electrodes. On the other hand, 87% of medial locations of seizure onset were detected first by strips. Finally, frontal lobe localization was slightly more common in grids than in strips: 53% versus 47%. A distinct minority, never more than 20%, of any group was localized by implanted depth electrodes. The single *significant* difference was the ability of specific electrodes to diagnose seizure onset in medial (strips) versus lateral (grids) locations. This difference may be related to the selection of electrode type for the study of those regions. Nevertheless, all frequencies, morphologies, distributions, and lobar locations *sometimes* were detected by *any* electrode type; and detection of seizure onset in any lobe with any specific pathology, frequency, distribution, and outcome was *not* significantly related to the type of electrode.

Frequency of Seizure Onset

Most patients had seizures with onset frequency greater than 13 Hz (62%). Overall, seizures included 17 with gamma onset (32%), 16 with beta onset (30%), 8 with alpha onset (15%), 9 with theta onset (17%), and three with delta onset (6%). The onset frequency was significantly related to anatomic location ($p = 0.017$); extratemporal seizures were faster, mostly gamma onset, than temporal seizures, which were mostly within the

TABLE 20.1. *Electrode sensitivity in neocortical epilepsy*

Diagnosis	Grid (%)	Strip (%)	Depth (%)
Developmental	12/28 (43)	15/28 (54)	1/28 (4)
Mature	4/14 (29)	8/14 (57)	2/14 (14)
Gliosis	3/11 (27)	8/11 (73)	0
Lesional	6/11 (55)	3/11 (27)	2/11 (18)
Nonlesional	13/42 (31)	28/42 (67)	1/42 (2)
Medial location	1/23 (4)	20/23 (87)	2/23 (9)
Lateral location	15/26 (58)	10/26 (39)	1/26 (4)
Regional	10/21 (48)	10/21 (48)	1/21 (5)
Focal	9/32 (28)	21/32 (66)	2/32 (6)
Temporal	8/23 (35)	14/23 (61)	1/23 (4)
Extratemporal	11/30 (37)	17/30 (57)	2/30 (7)
Parietal	0	3/3 (100)	0
Frontal	9/17 (53)	8/17 (47)	0
Occipital	2/10 (20)	6/10 (60)	2/10 (20)

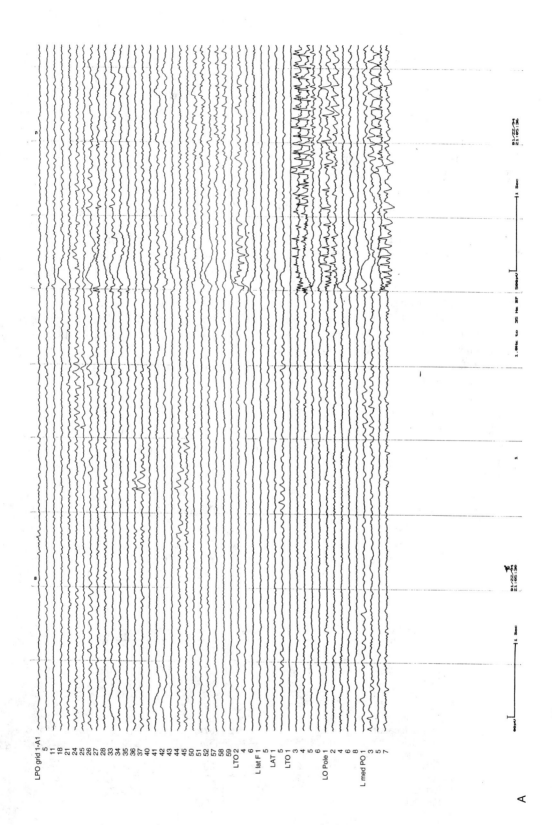

280

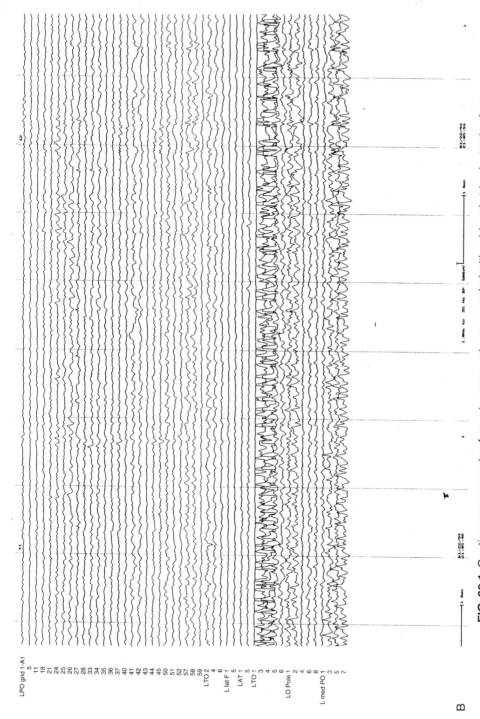

FIG. 20.1. Continuous segments of spontaneous seizure recorded with grid and strip electrodes from the left occipital cortex in a patient with final pathology of laminar heterotopia. Seizure has alpha frequency regional onset in five selected contacts of three adjacent strip electrodes (LTO 3,4; LO pole 1,2; Lmed PO 7). Each division = 1 second; calib = 500 μV. LPO grid, 64 contact left parieto-occipital grid; *LTO*, left temporo-occipital strip; *L latF*, left lateral frontal strip; *LAT*, left anterior temporal strip; *LO pole*, left occipital polar strip; *Lmed PO*, left medial parieto-occipital strip. Strips named for point of insertion—point of termination. Contacts numbered deep (1) to superficial.

281

beta frequency range (Table 20.2). Onset frequency was not significantly related to pathological substrate or surgical outcome (by Engel criteria or by classification of seizure free or not).

Distribution of Seizure Onset

Focal onset was more common than regional onset: 60% versus 40%. Distribution of onset was significantly related to the frequency of seizure onset ($p = 0.03$); regional onsets usually were expressed in the gamma frequency band, and focal onsets in the beta, alpha, or theta frequency bands (Table 20.3). Distribution of onset was not significantly related to pathology, surgical outcome, lobe, or location (Table 20.4).

Morphology of Seizure Onset

Morphology of seizure onset was divided into five groups as described. The low-voltage fast waveform at onset was the most common (30 patients, 57%) whereas rhythmic sinusoidal wave onset was seen in seven patients (13%), slow spike onset in seven (13%), slow onset in six (11%), and fast spike onset in three (6%). Onset morphology was significantly related to pathologic substrate ($p = 0.02$); low voltage fast and slow spike onset morphologies were seen significantly more often in patients with developmental etiologies, whereas rhythmic sinusoidal wave onset was observed *only* in mature substrates (Table 20.5). The onset morphology was *not* significantly related to the lobe, frequency, or distribution of seizure onset.

Predictors of Surgical Outcome

Of all the EEG characteristics, only morphology was significantly related to surgical outcome ($p = 0.02$); low voltage fast and rhythmic sinusoidal wave onset predicted good outcome (15 of 16 seizure-free patients) (Table 20.6). Outcome also was related to pathology, being significantly worse in the developmental and normal groups than in ma-

TABLE 20.2. *Onset frequency and anatomic location*

	Gamma	Beta	Alpha	Theta	Delta
Frontal	11	3	1	2	1
Temporal	2	10	3	6	2
Parietal	3	1	0	0	0
Occipital	3	2	4	1	0
Total	17	16	8	9	3

TABLE 20.3. *Distribution and frequency of seizure onset*

	Focal	Regional	Total
Gamma	5	12	17
Beta	13	3	16
Alpha	6	2	8
Theta	6	3	9
Delta	2	1	3
Total	32	21	53

TABLE 20.4. *Onset distribution and anatomic location*

Area	Focal	Regional
Frontal	8	8
Temporal	17	6
Parietal	2	2
Occipital	5	5
Total	32	21

TABLE 20.5. *Seizure onset morphology and pathology*

	Developmental	Mature	Normal
Low-voltage fast	17	6	7
Rhythmic sinusoidal	0	5	2
Slow spike/wave	6	1	0
Slow	4	0	2
Fast spike	1	2	0
Total	28	14	11

TABLE 20.6. *Seizure onset morphology and outcome*

	Seizure free	Not seizure free
Low-voltage fast	11	19
Rhythmic sinusoidal	4	3
Slow spike/wave	0	7
Slow	1	5
Fast spike	0	3
Total	16	37

TABLE 20.7. *Pathology and outcome*

	Seizure free	Not seizure free
Developmental	6	22
Mature	8	6
Normal	2	9

ture substrates ($p = 0.037$) (Table 20.7). Outcome was not significantly related to seizure onset, frequency, or distribution.

Certain combinations of factors predicted outcome. Thus, patients with slow frequency onset *plus* developmental substrates, regional onset, or extratemporal location almost always failed to achieve seizure control by undergoing surgery. Patients with slow morphology at onset associated with mature substrate, focal distribution, and temporal location were usually seizure free.

Periodic Spike Preictal Pattern

The preictal pattern described as a periodic spike discharge less than 2 Hz in frequency, which has been found in MTLE to be significantly related to certain pathologic findings, also was seen in neocortical patients. Thirteen patients (7 temporal, 4 frontal, 2 occipital) demonstrated this preictal pattern; 62% of the group had developmental etiology, only 53% were temporal, and 77% had fast frequency at seizure onset. Half of the patients with this preictal pattern were seizure free.

DISCUSSION

Invasive EEG characteristics in neocortical epilepsy, particularly with respect to seizure onset, have not been systematically studied. Prior studies examined specific issues in small homogeneous groups of patients (10–12). Gamma frequency seizure onset is described frequently, sometimes preceded by a direct current (DC) shift or electrodecremental pattern (13–15). The highest reported onset frequencies, up to 200 Hz, were found in neocortical seizures of frontal lobe onset (13,16,17). Despite the common teaching that ictal discharges of higher frequency are

more accurately localizing than those of slower frequencies, Quesney et al. found that seizure onset frequency in neocortical epilepsy of occipital, parietal, or temporal origin was slower than that of frontal origin (18). Studies have reported low-voltage fast activity at seizure onset to be associated with good surgical outcome; and conversely, that slow activity at seizure onset carries a poor prognosis (16,19–22). Similarly, prior reports suggest that regional seizure onset is predictive of poor surgical outcome, whereas focal onset is more clearly localizing to the actual epileptogenic zone (23–25). Some authors suggested a relationship between "focal" seizure onset and underlying pathology, at least in medial temporal lobe epilepsy. Lieb and colleagues reported that focal seizure onset in the medial temporal lobe recorded with depth electrodes was associated with mesial temporal sclerosis of the classic variety (26). Babb and associates demonstrated that focal seizure onset in the hippocampal region recorded with depth electrodes predicted selective loss of pyramidal cells in anterior hippocampus (27). Recent literature does not, however, support the association between focal or regional distribution of initial seizure change on intracranial EEG in neocortical epilepsy and surgical outcome or pathological substrate (28,29).

In our study, slow onset itself was not predictive of poor outcome, nor was regional seizure onset. In fact, we found no significant association of distribution *or* frequency of onset with outcome *or* pathology. We found, on the other hand, that frequency and distribution of seizure onset in neocortex recorded with implanted electrodes are characteristic of the anatomic region itself. This association of frequency and distribution of seizure onset with anatomic location has not been reported previously.

Many investigators recognize variability in the morphologic expression of seizure onset (30). Only rare attempts have been made to understand the meaning of different waveforms at seizure onset. Those attempts were restricted predominantly to medial temporal lobe epilepsy, in which a beta frequency seizure onset was associated with abnormal substrate, particularly mesial temporal sclerosis (1–4,12). In this neocortical analysis, we found two particular morphologies of seizure onset, low-voltage fast-activity and rhythmic sinusoidal waves, that predicted good surgical outcome. They were not, however, associated with specific substrates.

The preictal periodic spike discharge, previously characterized as typical of mesial temporal sclerosis, was observed in 14 neocortical seizure patients (31). This observation establishes that the pattern is not associated strictly with limbic epilepsy or its anatomic connections. The pattern was found in all lobes and many substrates, although predominantly in developmental ones. Because morphology of seizure onset seems to be related to substrate, and the periodic spiking is characteristic of mesial temporal sclerosis, we would predict that the neocortical substrates with which it is associated might bear some resemblance to mesial temporal sclerosis. In fact, this preictal spike pattern was more common among the developmental substrates, of which we consider mesial temporal sclerosis one. In MTLE, a preictal spike pattern has been linked to neuronal loss and to glial proliferation (31,32). The neocortical developmental substrates also may have a prominent glial component that contributes to epileptogenesis.

The practical issues of successfully recording neocortical seizure onset raise the issue of type of electrode best suited for these studies. It is difficult to analyze these data because the electrodes varied across the patient groups and are selected based on preconceived notions about which electrodes will provide better localization in any given scenario. Thus, the significant relationships of strip electrodes to medial seizure onset determination, and of grid electrodes to lateral neocortical seizure onset detection, are probably purely artifacts of patient selection for those types of electrodes. Nevertheless, this analysis does demonstrate that in neocortical epilepsy, any type of intracranial electrode is capable of

demonstrating any type of morphology, frequency, or distribution of seizure onset.

Our results prompt a hypothesis. The frequency, lobe, and distribution of seizure onset recorded by implanted electrodes in medically uncontrolled neocortical epilepsy are significantly correlated with one another but *not* with outcome or pathology, suggesting that these features are determined by the anatomic location and its networks or connections, independent of the etiology of the epilepsy, cellular alterations, or mechanism of epileptogenesis. On the other hand, the morphology or waveform of seizure onset, the underlying pathology, and surgical outcome are significantly correlated with one another (but not with the lobe, frequency, or distribution of onset). This observation suggests that waveform is a characteristic of specific pathophysiology and might be used to predict the underlying substrate. By this reasoning, because the morphology of seizure onset is the seizure characteristic that derives from the type of abnormal tissue and reflects the process of seizure generation in that substrate, both the waveform and the substrate should predict surgical outcome, and they do.

Our observations are only a first step in understanding and analyzing the signature of neocortical epilepsy on intracranial EEG. They suggest, however, that such analyses can be fruitful and can facilitate interpretation, direct future patient management, and identify features that provide clues to pathogenesis and epileptogenesis.

REFERENCES

1. King D, Spencer SS. Invasive electroencephalography in mesial temporal lobe epilepsy. *J Clin Neurophysiol* 1995;12:32–45.
2. Spencer SS. Temporal lobectomy: selection of candidates. In: Wyllie E, ed. *The treatment of epilepsy: principles and practices.* Philadelphia: Lea & Febiger, 1993:1062.
3. Spencer SS, So NK, Engel J, et al. Depth electrodes. In: Engel J Jr, ed. *Surgical treatment of the epilepsies,* 2nd ed. New York: Raven Press, 1993:359–376.
4. Spencer SS, Sperling MR, Shewmon DA. Intracranial electrodes. In: Engel J Jr, Pedley TA, eds. *Epilepsy: a comprehensive textbook.* Philadelphia: Lippincott–Raven, 1997:1719–1747.

5. Spencer SS. Substrates of localization-related spilepsies: biologic implications of localizing findings in humans. *Epilepsia* 1998;39:114–123.
6. Sperling MR. Clinical challenges in invasive monitoring in epilepsy surgery. *Epilepsia* 1997;38(Suppl 4): S6–S12.
7. Spencer DD, Spencer SS. Surgery for epilepsy. In: Krantzler L, ed. *Advances in neurosurgery. Neurologic clinics,* vol 3. Philadelphia: WB Saunders, 1985: 313–330.
8. Spencer SS. Surgical options for uncontrolled epilepsy. In: Theodore WH, Porter RJ, eds. *Epilepsy. Neurologic clinics,* vol 4. Philadelphia: WB Saunders, 1986: 669–695.
9. Spencer DD, Spencer SS, Fried I. Presurgical localization: neurophysiological and neuroimaging studies. In: Apuzzo M, ed. *Neurosurgical aspects of epilepsy.* Park Ridge, IL: American Association of Neurological Surgeons, 1991:73–86.
10. Arroyo S, Lesser RP, Awad IA, et al. Subdural and epidural grids and strips. In: Engel J Jr, ed. *Surgical treatment of the epilepsies,* 2nd ed. New York: Raven Press, 1993:377–386.
11. Wyler AR, Wilkus RJ, Blume WT. Strip electrodes. In: Engel J Jr, ed. *Surgical treatment of the epilepsies,* 2nd ed. New York: Raven Press, 1993:387–397.
12. Spencer SS, Guimaraes P, Katz A, et al. Morphological patterns of seizures recorded intracranially. *Epilepsia* 1992;33:537–545.
13. Fisher RS, Webber WRS, Lesser RP, et al. High frequency EEG activity at the start of seizures. *J Clin Neurophysiol* 1992;9:441–448.
14. Ikeda A, Terada K, Mikuni N, et al. Subdural recording of ictal DC shifts in neocortical seizures in humans. *Epilepsia* 1996;37:662–674.
15. Olivier A, Gloor P, Andermann F, et al. Occipitotemporal epilepsy studied with stereotactically implanted depth electrodes and successfully treated by surgical resection. *Ann Neurol* 1982;11:428–432.
16. Allen PJ, Fish DR, Smith SJM. Very high-frequency rhythmic activity during SEEG suppression in frontal lobe epilepsy. *Electroencephalogr Clin Neurophysiol* 1992;82:155–159.
17. Quesney LF, Krieger C, Leitner C, et al. Frontal lobe epilepsy: clinical and electrographic presentation. In: Porter RJ, Mattson RH, Ward AA, Dam M, eds. *Advances in epileptology:* XVth Epilepsy International Symposium. New York: Raven Press, 1984:503–508.
18. Quesney LF, Wennberg R, Olivier A. Morphologic patterns of electrographic seizure onset in neocortical epilepsy. *Epilepsia* 1997;38(suppl 8):213(abst).
19. Faught E, Kuzniecky RI, Hurst DC. Ictal EEG waveforms from epidural electrodes predictive of seizure control after temporal lobectomy. *Electroencephalogr Clin Neurophysiol* 1992;9:441–448.
20. Weinand ME, Wyler A, Richey ET, et al. Long-term ictal monitoring with subdural strip electrodes: prognostic factors for selecting temporal lobectomy candidates. *J Neurosurg* 1992;77:20–28.
21. Schiller Y, Cascino GD, Busacker NE, et al. Characterization and comparison of local onset and remote propagated electrographic seizures recorded with intracranial electrodes. *Epilepsia* 1998;39:380–388.
22. Alarcon G, Binnie CD, Elwes RDC, et al. Power spectrum and intracranial EEG patterns at seizure onset in partial epilepsy. *Electroencephalogr Clin Neurophysiol* 1995;94:326–337.
23. Engel J, Crandall PH. Intensive neurodiagnostic monitoring with intracranial electrodes. In: Gumnit RJ, ed. *Intensive neurodiagnostic monitoring. Advances in neurology,* vol 46. New York: Raven Press, 1986: 85–106.
24. Wieser H. Data analysis. In: Engel J Jr, ed. *Surgical treatment of the epilepsies.* New York: Raven Press, 1987:335–360.
25. So NK. Depth electrode studies in mesial temporal epilepsy. In: Lüders HO, ed. *Epilepsy surgery.* New York: Raven Press, 1992:371–384.
26. Lieb JP, Engel J, Brown WJ, et al. Neuropathological findings following temporal lobectomy related to surface and deep EEG patterns. *Epilepsia* 1981;22: 539–549.
27. Babb TL, Lieb JP, Brown WJ, et al. Distribution of pyramidal cell density and hyperexcitability in the epileptic human hippocampal formation. *Epilepsia* 1984;25: 721–728.
28. Kuzniecky R, Faught E, Morawetz R, et al. Epidural ictal patterns: correlations in temporal lobe epilepsy. *Epilepsia* 1989;30:703(abst).
29. Mathern GW, Babb TL, Pretorius JK, et al. The pathophysiologic relations between lesion pathology, intracranial ictal EEG onsets, and hippocampal neuron losses in temporal lobe epilepsy. *Epilepsy Res* 1995;21: 133–147.
30. Sperling MR, O'Connor MJ. Electrographic correlates of spontaneous seizures. *Clin Neurosci* 1994;2:17–46.
31. Spencer SS, Kim J, Spencer DD. Ictal spikes: a marker of specific hippocampal cell loss. *Electroencephalogr Clin Neurophysiol* 1992;83:104–111.
32. Spencer SS, Kim J, deLanerolle N, et al. Intracranial EEG seizure patterns and pathology in temporal lobe epilepsy. *Epilepsia* 1997;38(Suppl 8):212(abst).

Neocortical Epilepsies.
Advances in Neurology, Vol. 84,
edited by P.D. Williamson, A.M. Siegel,
D.W. Roberts, V.M. Thadani, and M.S. Gazzaniga.
Lippincott Williams & Wilkins, Philadelphia © 2000.

21

Propagation of Neocortical Extratemporal Seizures

Dennis J. Dlugos and *Michael R. Sperling

Division of Neurology, The Children's Hospital of Philadelphia, Philadelphia, Pennsylvania 19104;
*Jefferson Comprehensive Epilepsy Center, Department of Neurology,
Jefferson Medical College of Thomas Jefferson University, Philadelphia, Pennsylvania 19107

One of the primary aims of the electrophysiologic evaluation in an epilepsy surgery candidate is to identify the region in which seizures begin. This region, known as the *ictal onset zone,* is the area of cortex that is usually resected in the attempt to abolish seizures, although cortical areas containing prominent interictal spikes also may be removed. In contrast, how and where seizures spread beyond the zone of ictal onset generally are not factored into the surgical decision-making process; emphasis has always been given to extirpating the primary epileptogenic region. Limited attention has been paid to seizure propagation; consequently, little is known about how seizure propagation characteristics should influence surgical decisions, particularly in the extratemporal neocortical epilepsies. In part, this lack of knowledge relates to the difficulty of studying seizure spread. Accurate studies of seizure propagation require intracranial electroencephalographic (EEG) recording because scalp EEG is relatively insensitive. Moreover, analyses of invasive EEG recordings may be misleading as a result of limited spatial sampling. Even with extensive subdural and depth electrode placement, large cortical regions of necessity remain unsurveyed. Subcortical nuclei, which may play

an essential role in seizure propagation, generally cannot be studied at all for ethical reasons. Thus, it is difficult to know whether the propagation patterns identified in the cortical EEG accurately reflect what really occurs.

Despite these challenges and limitations, the study of seizure propagation is important. Understanding seizure propagation can provide insight into behavior observed during seizures and may offer clues that aid in localizing the region to be removed. If predictable propagation patterns occur in certain types of seizures, one may be able to infer correct localization, even in the absence of electrodes that sample from the ictal onset zone. For example, the ictal onset zone may be clinically silent and not evident from scalp EEG recordings. If invasive coverage is planned solely on the basis of clinical semiology and scalp EEG, the area of "onset" identified may, in fact, be an area of propagation, with the true area of ictal onset lying outside the region surveyed by invasive electrodes. Knowledge of common seizure propagation patterns allows thorough and logical placement of invasive electrodes and, one hopes, accurate identification of the ictal onset zone. Furthermore, studying seizure propagation allows more accurate electroclinical correlation of ictal behavior. Finally, seizure propagation patterns provide insight into synaptic pathways and may improve understanding of clinical neuroanatomy.

The earliest analyses of seizure propagation were based on ictal semiology, and such studies remain critical. This work has been supplemented in recent years by a few reports on ictal propagation patterns from invasive EEG recording. This chapter reviews the propagation of neocortical seizures arising in the frontal, parietal, and occipital lobes.

BACKGROUND AND LITERATURE REVIEW

Occipital Lobe Seizures

Occipital seizures have been studied with analyses of ictal behavior, scalp EEG, and intracranial EEG. Studies in animals, however, indicate that the complexities of seizure propagation cannot be fully appreciated, even from intracranial recordings with extensive cortical sampling. Studies of occipital lobe seizures in rats using the carbon 14-labeled 2-deoxyglucose autoradiography technique (1) suggest the existence of complex interactions between cortical and subcortical structures. Mild seizures induced by local occipital injection of 25 to 30 U of penicillin are associated with increased me-

tabolism in primary visual cortex, extrastriate cortex, ipsilateral thalamus, pretectal nuclei, and superior colliculus. Seizures with more severe behavioral manifestations induced by 60 to 100 U of penicillin cause increased metabolism in the bilateral occipital cortex, posterior cingulum, subiculum, and bilateral hippocampus. Greater spread to limbic regions was seen with seizures originating in the occipital pole compared with seizures beginning in visual cortex. Such studies trace the metabolic anatomy of focal seizures but do not specifically identify the route of propagation. It is unclear whether the occipital–temporal spread seen with severe seizures occurs as a result of direct cortex to cortex seizure propagation, by subcortical relays, or both.

Descriptions of seizure semiology have suggested likely seizure propagation patterns in patients with occipital lobe epilepsy. Ajmone-Marsan and Ralston (2) postulated that occipital lobe seizures had three primary propagation routes (Fig. 21.1).

Infrasylvian spread to the temporal lobes resulted in seizures with impairment of consciousness and automatisms, lateral suprasylvian propagation resulted in focal motor or sensory seizures, and medial suprasylvian propagation produced asymmetric tonic seizures (2,3). Takeda et al. (4) reported similar spread patterns and advanced the notion that temporal spread was preferred if the site

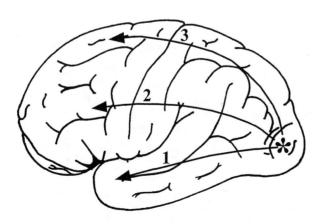

FIG. 21.1. The pathways by which occipital seizures spread are shown in this diagram. Seizures most often preferentially spread to the ipsilateral temporal lobe, although suprasylvian spread also may be seen. The preferred route may depend on the origin of the discharge within the occipital lobe.

of seizure origin was inferior to the calcarine fissure, parietal spread being more likely if origin was superior to the calcarine fissure. Salanova et al. (5) reported 42 patients with medically refractory occipital epilepsy. Seventy-three percent of patients reported visual auras. During the course of complex partial seizures, 50% developed typical temporal lobe automatisms, and 38% had focal motor activity. These clinical symptoms suggest that temporal lobe spread is more common than frontal lobe spread. Moreover, these data indicate that the location to which seizures spread may be responsible for much of the ictal semiology observed during occipital seizures.

More recent work using intracranial EEG added to this understanding. Williamson et al. (6) reported that 12 of 17 patients with occipital-onset seizures had preferential occipital-to-medial temporal propagation. In four patients, occipital–frontal propagation was documented by intracranial EEG; such spread was inferred on clinical grounds in three other patients. In some patients, both infrasylvian and suprasylvian spread were observed during different seizures. An example of occipital–temporal propagation recorded with intracranial EEG is shown in Fig. 21.2.

Parietal Lobe Seizures

The variety of ictal behaviors reported in patients with parietal lobe epilepsy also suggests multiple propagation routes. Salanova et al. (7) reported 82 patients with parietal lobe epilepsy, and using clinical seizure characteristics, suggested ictal spread to the frontal, supplementary motor, or temporal–limbic areas. Specifically, 28% of patients exhibited tonic posturing, 57% had unilateral clonic activity, 17% had oral or gestural automatisms, and 4% had complex automatisms. Two preferential propagation patterns were postulated. There was strong evidence for superior parietal lobe origin and frontal spread of the ictal discharge in

patients with tonic posturing, whereas 79% of patients with automatisms had ictal activity involving the inferior parietal lobe, suggesting temporal lobe spread in these patients.

One study that analyzed parietal lobe seizure propagation in 12 patients using subdural EEG recording (8) noted two seizure spread patterns (Fig. 21.3). Nine patients had seizure onset in the superior parietal region with spread to the frontal and central cortex. Clinical symptoms included tingling, followed by extremity posturing and variable secondary generalization. Three patients had seizure onset in the low parietal region with spread to the temporal lobe. Clinical symptoms included behavioral arrest, automatisms, and occasional facial twitching and drooling.

Often, patients with parietal lobe epilepsy exhibit no symptoms at the start of seizures or the symptoms are too vague to suggest definite parietal localization; the initial ictal symptoms often reflect seizure propagation rather than seizure onset (7–9). Hence, when examining ictal behavior, it is crucial to recall that clinical signs can be misleading.

Frontal Lobe Seizures

Because of the large size of the frontal lobe and its extensive connections with other cortical and subcortical regions, both clinical and electrophysiologic studies of frontal lobe epilepsy are particularly complex. Animal studies using carbon 14-labeled 2-deoxyglucose autoradiography suggest the presence of important interactions between cortical and subcortical structures (10). Behaviorally mild seizures induced by intracortical injection of 25 U of penicillin caused increased metabolic activity locally in injected cortex, ipsilateral basal ganglia and thalamus, and contralateral cerebellum (Fig. 21.4). More severe seizures induced by local injection of 350 U of penicillin caused increased metabolic activity in bilaterally in medial frontal cortex, basal ganglia, thalamus, cerebellum, and limbic struc-

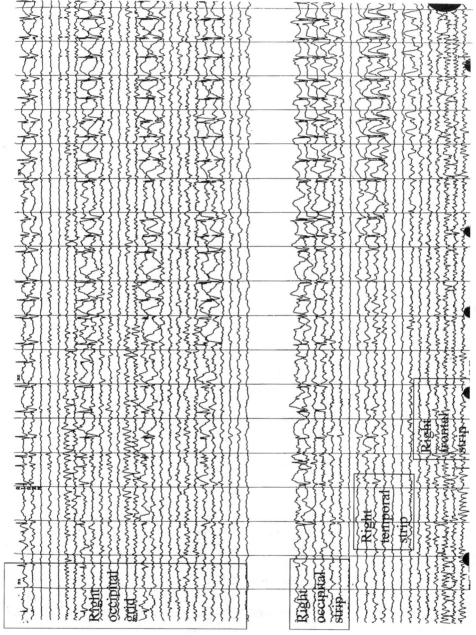

FIG. 21.2. EEG recorded with intracranial electrodes demonstrating a seizure starting in the right occipital lobe, which then spread to the temporal lobe 10 seconds later.

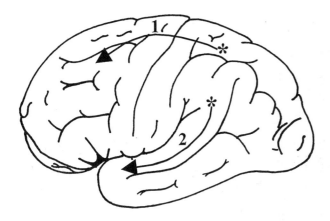

FIG. 21.3. Patterns of parietal seizure spread are illustrated here. At present, there are no identifiable preferred routes of propagation to either suprasylvian or infrasylvian areas.

tures (Fig. 21.5). A unilateral frontal seizure can spread to the contralateral hemisphere directly across the corpus callosum, via the callosum after spread to ipsilateral parietal, temporal, or occipital lobes, or via polysynaptic subcortical pathways. Similarly, frontal–temporal spread could be direct via cortical–cortical association fibers or indirect via subcortical relays. Animal studies suggest that subcortical nuclei, including the thalamus (11), caudate (12), and substantia nigra (13), can play a role in the regulation of cortical excitability and can influence seizure propagation.

In humans, a distinction is often made between medial frontal seizures (including the supplementary motor area, or SMA), dorsolateral frontal seizures, and orbitofrontal seizures

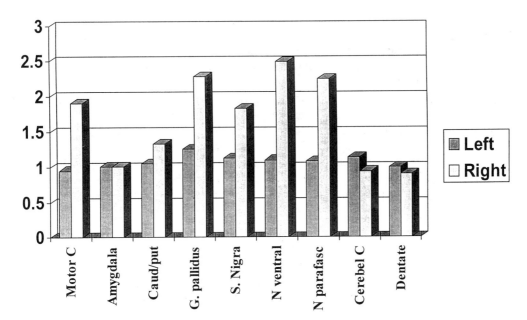

FIG. 21.4. Graph showing 2-deoxyglucose uptake in cortical and subcortical regions after inducing behaviorally mild seizures with intracortical injection of 25 U of penicillin. Note the increased metabolic activity in injected cortex, ipsilateral basal ganglia and thalamus, and contralateral cerebellum.

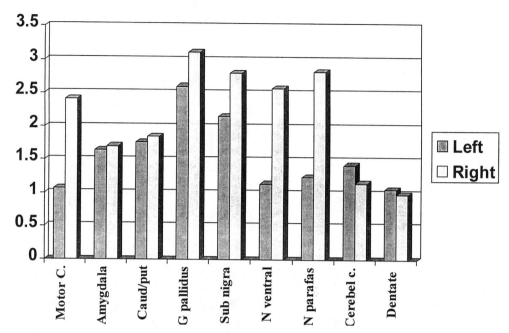

FIG. 21.5. Graph showing 2-deoxyglucose uptake in cortical and subcortical regions after inducing behaviorally severe seizures with intracortical injection of 350 U of penicillin. Note the increased metabolic activity in bilaterally in medial frontal cortex, basal ganglia, thalamus, cerebellum, and limbic structures.

(14) (Table 21.1). Medial frontal seizures are often characterized by tonic posturing of the extremities or by complex, bilateral, large-amplitude movements. Less frequently, absence seizures may occur. These clinical features, along with scalp EEG recordings, support the belief that rapid, interhemispheric seizure propagation via the corpus callosum is common with medial frontal seizures. Dorsolateral frontal seizures are characterized by simple partial seizures and versive head and eye movements, suggesting less rapid propagation outside the frontal lobe to the contralateral hemisphere. Lastly, orbitofrontal seizures are characterized by complex automatisms and autonomic features, suggesting spread to the cingulate gyrus or temporal lobe (14,15) or activation of the same subcortical structures as in temporal lobe seizures.

Studies of frontal lobe seizures using intracranial EEG provide a view of the complexity of their propagation patterns. Williamson et al. (16) described ten patients whose seizures began in medial frontal or orbitofrontal cortex.

TABLE 21.1. *Frontal lobe seizures*

Site of onset	Clinical manifestations
Medial frontal lobe	Complex bilateral motor movements, tonic posturing of extremities, rarely absence seizures
Dorsolateral frontal lobe	Contralateral clonic movements, forced head and eye deviation
Orbitofrontal lobe	Complex auto matisms, autonomic symptoms

Eight patients had brief clinical seizures confined to the frontal lobe. Rapid spread to the contralateral frontal lobe also occurred commonly, precluding consistent lateralization in four patients. Finally, spread to the temporal lobe occurred in two patients. Sperling and O'Connor (17) noted the rapidity of spread of medial frontal seizures and observed that anterior corpus callosotomy was needed before correct lateralization could take place in one of their patients.

In a series limited to medial frontal lobe seizures, Toczek et al. (18) were able to define clearly the ictal onset zone in seven of nine patients. Of 73 clinical seizures recorded from the seven patients, ictal onset was "well-localized" in 53 (73%). The term *well-localized* onset implied that the ictal discharge was confined to the area of ictal onset or that ictal propagation was limited to adjacent regions. The initial ictal pattern displayed low-amplitude beta or gamma frequency activity in six of seven patients and high amplitude spike and polyspike and wave discharges in one patient. Baumgartner et al. (19) emphasized a different aspect of medial frontal lobe seizures by analyzing the connections between the supplementary motor cortex and ipsilateral primary motor cortex in five patients. Ictal discharges in the SMA either preceded primary motor cortex discharges by 85 to 125 ms, or they occurred simultaneously. The initial ictal pattern was either paroxysmal fast activity or repetitive spiking. Despite the rapid spread or simultaneous onset in both the SMA and primary motor areas, outcome was favorable with resections sparing the primary motor cortex. Interhemispheric propagation of ictal discharges was not reported in this study.

Scant data are available regarding the propagation of dorsolateral frontal seizures using intracranial EEG; however, there is a suggestion that dorsolateral seizures spread more slowly than medial frontal seizures. Ociepa and Blume (20) noted that six seizures beginning in the frontal convexity propagated to the contralateral frontal lobe after a median of 13.5 seconds, whereas four medial frontal seizures propagated within 2.75 seconds.

Cortical–subcortical interactions, which are undoubtedly important in the regulation and propagation of seizures in humans, have been the subject of a few case reports. Ispilateral thalamic hypermetabolism was seen on positron emission tomography scan in a patient with epilepsia partialis continua (21). Corticothalamic coupling of metabolism was observed on a functional magnetic resonance imaging scan between a left frontal cortical seizure focus and the left ventrolateral thalamus (22). These data provide metabolic evidence for the subcortical spread of ictal activity in humans and offer a link to animal studies.

ORIGINAL DATA

We analyzed 25 seizures in 10 patients with extratemporal neocortical epilepsy recorded using combinations of intracranial electrodes, including subdural strips, subdural grids, and depth electrodes as clinically indicated. All patients had medically intractable epilepsy and were being evaluated for epilepsy surgery at Graduate Hospital, Children's Hospital of Philadelphia, or Thomas Jefferson University Hospital. The sample included 14 seizures from 5 patients with frontal lobe epilepsy, 4 seizures from 3 patients with parietal lobe epilepsy, and 7 seizures from 2 patients with occipital lobe epilepsy. Frontal lobe cases were further divided into medial frontal (1 seizure, 1 patient), dorsolateral frontal (5 seizures, 2 patients), and orbitofrontal (8 seizures, 2 patients). The following variables were examined:

1. *Ipsilateral propagation time* (IPT): the time from electrographic seizure onset to first spread to an adjacent ipsilateral lobe
2. *Contralateral propagation time* (CPT): the time from electrographic seizure onset to first spread to the contralateral hemisphere
3. *Propagation route*
4. Ictal frequency and waveform at seizure onset

5. Ictal frequency and waveform at time of the earliest spread to another cortical region, either ipsilateral or contralateral

The CPT could be analyzed only in patients with bilateral intracranial EEG implants. This was possible in 13 of 14 frontal lobe seizures, and 1 of 4 parietal lobe seizures. No occipital seizures were recorded using bilateral implants. The results are summarized in Table 21.2.

In one medial frontal seizure, IPT to the ipsilateral temporal lobe was 8.0 seconds, whereas CPT to the contralateral frontal lobe was zero; the ictal onset appeared simulataneously in both medial frontal cortices in a homotopic distribution. After an anterior corpus callosotomy, seizures could be lateralized to one medial frontal lobe because CPT to the contralateral frontal lobe slowed to 8.0 seconds following the disconnection. (A medial frontal focal resection then was performed, and abolition of seizures resulted.) The delay in CPT following anterior callosal section indicated that direct callosal spread was the route of propagation of ictal discharges to the contralateral hemisphere and that cortical–subcortical pathways were not crucial for contralateral seizure propagation.

In five dorsolateral frontal seizures, the mean IPT to the ipsilateral temporal lobe was 6.8 seconds (range, 0–22 seconds) and mean CPT to the contralateral frontal lobe was 8.3 seconds (range, 0.4–26.6 seconds). Excluding from the analysis one seizure that was an out-

lier because of excessively slow propagation, mean IPT was 1.7 seconds (range, 0–2.8 seconds) and mean CPT was 3.7 seconds (range, 0.4–6.2 seconds).

In eight orbitofrontal seizures, mean IPT to the ipsilateral temporal lobe was 47.4 seconds (range, 12.5–85 seconds). Mean CPT to the contralateral frontal lobe was 41.5 seconds (range, 9.8–92 seconds).

Parietal lobe seizures showed variable propagation patterns. Initial spread was noted in the ipsilateral frontal lobe in two cases, in ipsilateral occipital lobe in one case, and in ipsilateral temporal lobe in one case. Mean IPT was 2.0 seconds (range, 0.4–4.0 seconds). In one patient with bilateral intracranial electrode placement, IPT to the ipsilateral temporal lobe was 3.2 seconds and CPT to the contralateral parietal lobe was 5.0 seconds.

All seven occipital lobe seizures showed a consistent propagation pattern, and each demonstrated initial spread to the temporal lobe. Mean IPT was 7.4 seconds (range, 0–19 seconds).

At the time of seizure onset, EEG patterns varied. Repetitive sharp waves in the delta frequency range (9 seizures), theta frequency sharp waves (1 seizure), alpha frequency sharp waves (2 patients), and low amplitude beta activity (13 seizures) were noted. At the time that spread first was noted in the EEG, low-amplitude beta activity was present in 20 seizures, and repetitive sharp waves in the delta range were seen in 4 seizures.

TABLE 21.2. *Seizure propagation data*

Region of onset	Number of seizures	Ipsilateral propagation time (mean in seconds, range)	Contralateral propagation time (mean, range)	Route(s) of propagation
Medial frontal	1	8.0	0	Contralateral frontal lobe
Dorsolateral frontal	5	6.8 (0–22)	8.3 (0.4–26.6)	Ipsilateral temporal; contralateral frontal lobe
Orbitofrontal	8	47.4 (12.5–85)	41.5 (9.8–92)	Ipsilateral temporal; contralateral frontal lobe
Parietal	4 (1 bilateral coverage)	2.0 (0.4–4.0)	5.0	Ipsilateral frontal, occipital, temporal lobes; contralateral parietal lobe
Occipital	7 (no bilateral coverage)	7.4 (0–19)	NA	Ipsilateral temporal lobe

CONCLUSION

Despite the challenges and limitations of studying seizure propagation in humans, some preliminary observations can be made from this review of the literature and the original data presented in this chapter. It appears that different anatomic regions have distinct seizure propagation characteristics. Knowledge of these features may be useful in confirming a hypothesis regarding seizure localization in individual patients.

The propagation of seizures probably relates mostly to two factors. First, it may rely on the richness of efferent and afferent connections of different cortical areas, which may be further modulated by subcortical and cortical inputs that can either dampen or enhance the tendency of seizure discharges to spread. The strength of callosal connections differs strikingly, depending on cortical area, and these connections are quite important for spread of some seizures to the opposite hemisphere. The medial frontal lobe appears to be most tightly bound to the contralateral homotopic regions, whereas other regions, particularly orbitofrontal cortex, have weaker connections to the opposite hemisphere. The tendency for consistent propagation routes also varies with the location. The occipital lobe has the most predictable routes for disseminating seizures, whereas parietal seizures, in contrast, exhibit marked variability. Second, the strength of the ictal discharge, perhaps related to the amount of neurons recruited locally, and the firing frequency may play a crucial role in influencing the extent to which the seizures propagate beyond the ictal onset zone. The latter hypothesis is suggested by the finding that high-frequency activity usually accompanied spread of seizures beyond the region of their origin.

The site of seizure origin correlates with where seizures spread and how rapidly they get there. Occipital lobe seizures tend to spread first to the ipsilateral temporal lobe, undoubtedly because of the presence of robust occipitotemporal connections (23). That some occipital seizures preferentially propagate to the frontal lobe confirms the relevance of occipitofrontal connections as well. These findings aid in understanding the variability of clinical symptoms in occipital seizures. The variability in occipitotemporal propagation time, ranging from 0 to 19 seconds in our small series, forces one to be flexible in interpreting ictal behavior. Temporal or frontal lobe signs appearing early in the course of a seizure are not necessarily inconsistent with posterior seizure origin; because visual auras are present in only three quarters of patients with occipital seizures, knowledge of propagation characteristics may aid in designing appropriate investigations to identify the epileptogenic zone.

Parietal lobe seizures propagate quite variably, to frontal, temporal, or occipital lobes. Some parietal seizures are clinically silent when they begin; therefore, the first behavioral symptoms often reflect seizure propagation. Hence, parietal seizures are particularly challenging to localize, especially in patients without lesions on neuroimaging studies. Therefore, surveying parietal cortex should be considered in nonlesional patients undergoing intracranial EEG evaluation.

The frontal lobe has a number of cytoarchitecturally distinct regions and a wealth of ipsilateral, contralateral, and subcortical connections. Subdividing frontal lobe seizures may be somewhat artificial, but it conforms to distinct behavioral and electrographic patterns observed in many patients. Medial frontal seizures can propagate quickly to the contralateral homotopic cortex, but how reliably this happens and whether they consistently spread faster than dorsolateral frontal, parietal, or occipital seizures remains to be determined. Contralateral frontal lobe seizure propagation probably occurs mainly via direct callosal connections, but spread via subcortical nuclei must still be considered a possibility. Spread of frontal lobe seizures to other lobes in the same hemisphere varies by location and seizure, and ipsilateral connections sometimes appear to be preferentially activated sooner than contralateral connections. For example, SMA seizures rapidly propagate first to ipsilateral primary motor cortex, and distinguishing between primary motor and supplementary onset may not be possible with EEG recording. Other frontal lobe seizures in our series showed a fairly stately progression of ictal discharges, and ipsilateral temporal lobe propagation preceded contralateral frontal spread in some circumstances. This was most pronounced in orbitofrontal seizures, which tended to propagate slowly. As in occipital and parietal seizures, the first symptoms of orbitofrontal seizures may be produced by cortex to which the seizures have spread rather than the cortex in which they begin. In the original data presented here, seizures from every location except the orbitofrontal region displayed the potential to propagate extremely rapidly, with an IPT or CPT of 0 to 0.4 seconds in some seizures. In contrast, the fastest propagation time of an orbitofrontal seizure was 9.8 seconds. This finding suggests less efficient or poorer connections in orbitofrontal cortex, although a larger sample will be needed for a more definitive statement.

The frequency of the seizure discharge at ictal onset is variable, but propagation is usually accompanied by low-amplitude beta activity. Often, the EEG evolves from repetitive sharp waves to low-amplitude beta activity immediately before seizures spread to other cortical areas. Ictal beta could reflect a strengthening of the discharge, with greater propensity to spread, which could be due to intracortical mechanisms, to a failure of subcortical modulation of excitability, or both. Animal models suggest complex interactions between cortical and subcortical structures during seizure propagation. Because the thalamus, caudate, and substantia nigra regulate cortical excitability in experimental models, perhaps they also regulate seizure propagation.

Further study of seizure propagation might improve our understanding of basic mechanisms involved in the regulation of ictal activity, could lead to improvements in localizing an epileptogenic zone in patients considered for surgery, and possibly will

lead to new avenues of treatment for patients with intractable epilepsy. For example, augmenting or interrupting pathways that regulate seizure propagation might improve seizure control in patients who are not helped by current therapeutic techniques. Corpus callosotomy (24) is the prototypical procedure that works solely by altering pathways of seizure spread and seizure modulation. More refined procedures targeting specific pathways between cortical regions also may enjoy success at lower cost. Further attention to the fundamental role of the connections between subcortical nuclei and cortex in regulating seizure propagation might enhance our understanding of epilepsy and also provide new means of treating people with epilepsy.

REFERENCES

1. Collins RC, Caston TV. Functional anatomy of occipital lobe seizures: an experimental study in rats. *Neurology* 1979;29:705–716.
2. Ajmone-Marsan C, Ralston BL. *The epileptic seizure: its functional morphology and diagnostic significance.* Springfield, IL: Charles C. Thomas, 1957:211–215.
3. Ludwig BI, Ajmone-Marsan C. Clinical ictal patterns in epileptic patients with occipital electroencephalographic foci. *Neurology* 1975;25:463–471.
4. Takeda A, Bancaud J, Talairach J, et al. Concerning epileptic attacks of occipital origin. *Electroencephalogr Clin Neurophysiol* 1970;28:644–649.
5. Salanova V, Andermann F, Olivier A, et al. Occipital lobe epilepsy: electroclinical manifestations, electrocorticography, cortical stimulation, and outcome in 42 patients treated between 1930 and 1991. *Brain* 1992;115:1655–1680.
6. Williamson PD, Thadani VM, Darcey TM, et al. Occipital lobe epilepsy: clinical characteristics, seizure spread patterns, and results of surgery. *Ann Neurol* 1992;31: 3–13.
7. Salanova V, Andermann F, Rasmussen T, et al. Parietal lobe epilepsy: clinical manifestations and outcome in 82 patients treated surgically between 1929 and 1988. *Brain* 1995;118:607–627.
8. Resnick TJ, Duchowny M, Jayakar P, et al. Clinical semiology of parietal lobe epilepsy. *Epilepsia* 1993;34 (Suppl 6):29.
9. Cascino G, Hulihan JF, Sharbrough FW, et al. Parietal lobe lesional epilepsy: electroclinical correlation and operative outcome. *Epilepsia* 1993;34:522–527.
10. Collins RC, Kennedy C, Sokoloff L, et al. Metabolic anatomy of focal motor seizures. *Arch Neurol* 1976;33:536–542.
11. Gale K. Subcortical structures and pathways involved in convulsive seizure generation. *J Clin Neurophysiol* 1992;9:264–277.

12. La Grutta V, Amato G, Zagami MT. The importance of the caudate nucleus in the control of convulsive activity in the amygdaloid complex and the temporal cortex of the cat. *Electroencephalogr Clin Neurophysiol* 1971;31: 57–69.

13. Depaulis A, Vergnes M, Marescaux C. Endogenous control of epilepsy: the nigral inhibitory system. *Prog Neurobiol* 1994;42:33–52.

14. Bautista RE, Spencer DD, Spencer SS. EEG findings in frontal lobe epilepsies. *Neurology* 1998;50:1765–1771.

15. Laskowitz DT, Sperling MR, French JA, et al. The syndrome of frontal lobe epilepsy: characteristics and surgical management. *Neurology* 1995;45:780–787.

16. Williamson PD, Spencer DD, Spencer SS, et al. Complex partial seizures of frontal lobe origin. *Ann Neurol* 1985;18:497–504.

17. Sperling MR, O'Connor MJ. Electrographic correlates of spontaneous seizures. In: Spencer SS, ed. *Clinical neuroscience, 2.* New York: Wiley-Liss,1994:17–46.

18. Toczek MT, Morrell MJ, Risinger MW, et al. Intracra-nial ictal recordings in mesial frontal lobe epilepsy. *J Clin Neurophysiol* 1997;14:499–506.

19. Baumgartner C, Flint R, Tuxhorn I, et al. Supplementary motor area seizures: propagation pathways as studied with invasive recordings. *Neurology* 1996;46: 506–514.

20. Ociepa D, Blume WT. Propagation pathways of subdurally recorded frontal lobe seizures. *Epilepsia* 1998; 39(Suppl 6):120.

21. Hajek M, Antonini A, Leenders KL, et al. Epilepsia partialis continua studied by PET. *Epilepsy Res* 1991;9:44–48.

22. Detre JA, Alsop DC, Aguirre GK, Sperling MR. Coupling of cortical and thalamic ictal activity in human partial epilepsy: demonstration by functional magnetic resonance imaging. *Epilepsia* 1996;37:657–661.

23. Gloor P. *The temporal lobe and limbic system.* New York: Oxford University Press, 1997:163–201.

24. Spencer S, Gates JR, Reeves AR, et al. Corpus callosum section. In: Engel J Jr, ed. *Surgical treatment of the epilepsies.* New York: Raven Press, 1987:425–444.

Neocortical Epilepsies.
Advances in Neurology, Vol. 84,
edited by P.D. Williamson, A.M. Siegel,
D.W. Roberts, V.M. Thadani, and M.S. Gazzaniga.
Lippincott Williams & Wilkins, Philadelphia © 2000.

22

Can Seizure Analysis Tell Us Where the Focus Is?

Jean Gotman

Montreal Neurological Institute, McGill University, Montreal, Quebec, Canada H3A 2B4

THE ELUSIVE FOCUS

When a seizure discharge is present in the scalp electroencephalogram (EEG), even if it appears focal, a relatively large region of cortex must be involved, estimated to be about 6 to 8 cm^2 (1). We confirmed the order of magnitude in a recent study comparing scalp and intracerebral EEG in the same subject (2). It is likely that in many cases, the discharge started in a much smaller area, spread to involve a larger region, and thus became visible on the scalp. In addition, even if a large brain region is involved but is far from the skull, its activity may not be seen. We sometimes can gain more precise information about seizure onset with intracranial recordings. We must remain acutely aware, however, that when a discharge appears focally in the intracerebral EEG, we really do not know its extent: It can indeed be very focal, or it may be extensive, including vast regions in which there are no electrodes. It may have started before the visible onset, even in regions close to the recording electrodes. If clinical signs follow the seizure onset, and the seizure onset is focal, one tends to assume that the region of onset *is the focus*. In fact, there is no formal way to exclude the possibility that the seizure has started in another region but remained clinically silent.

It has been said (3) that a regional seizure onset is more likely the result of propagation from a focus, in contrast to a focal onset, which is more likely to represent *the focus*. We accept, however, the concept of generalized seizures, seizures starting at once over a large fraction of the brain probably as a result of tight coupling between distant regions (most often subthalamic nuclei, the thalamus, and the cortex). Similarly, we can have a *regional* onset, where a seizure starts in a whole lobe, for instance. Why would a regional onset reflect propagation then? One also can question whether a focal onset is likely to represent *the* focus: When a seizure starts at a limited set of intracerebral contacts, there is no *a priori* reason to think it has not propagated from somewhere else, as illustrated by Fig. 22.1.

We can therefore argue that we can never know whether we have recorded the real onset because we cannot record everywhere. It is also possible to ask the question, Can careful analysis of seizure discharges help us in determining that a discharge is likely to be at the focus as opposed to having propagated to the recording site?

SEIZURE MORPHOLOGY IN RELATION TO PATHOLOGY

One possible avenue of investigation is to compare the morphology of EEG discharges

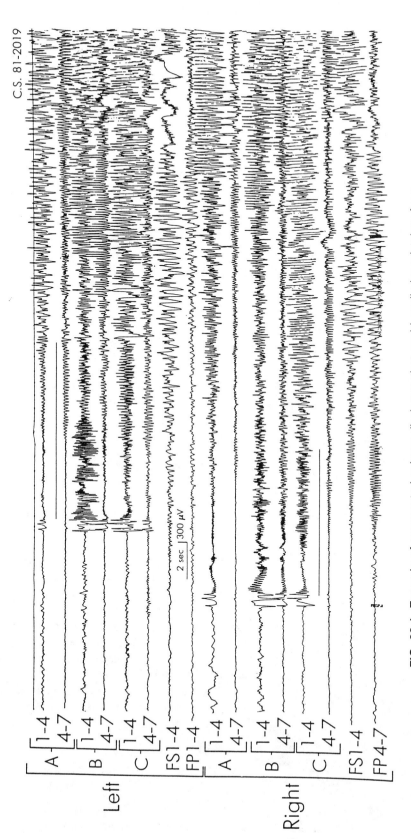

FIG. 22.1. Example of propagated seizure discharge that could easily be mistaken for a seizure onset: The discharge in the left hemisphere **(top)** is focal, limited to the hippocampus, and has the morphologic characteristics often associated with seizure onset. It is clear, however, that there is an earlier discharge, with remarkably similar morphology, in the right hippocampus. Of course, we cannot be absolutely sure where the seizure really started. Depth electrodes are implanted laterally and aimed at the amygdala **(A)**, anterior hippocampus **(B)**, and middle hippocampus **(C)**; contacts are 5 mm apart, and contact 1 is deepest.

taking place near regions of known pathology to discharges taking place in regions with no apparent pathology. One can assume that discharges taking place in a pathological region are more likely to represent the focus than are discharges taking place in normal regions. If discharges associated with pathological regions have a specific EEG morphology, the presence of this morphology, even in the absence of pathology, might increase the probability that the discharge is at the focus.

In one such study (4), we compared several aspects of intracerebral EEG discharges, their morphology, rapidity, and likelihood of spread with the degree of presumed sclerosis measured by volumetry of the hippocampus and amygdala. We divided the EEG morphologies at onset into seven categories, largely representing the frequency of the EEG discharge. There was little difference between discharges starting in atrophic mesiotemporal structures and discharges starting in mesial structures with a normal volume, with the exception that high frequencies at onset tended to be found more often in apparently normal tissue. We also examined whether seizures starting in atrophic regions had a higher tendency to spread than seizures starting in apparently normal regions; this was not the case. We also found that seizures did not have a higher tendency to spread *to* atrophic regions than *to* normal regions, independently of where they started. When they spread, propagation time was independent of the presence of pathology in the target region.

This last finding is in apparent contradiction with the results of Lieb et al. (5), who had found that surgical outcome was worse in patients in whom seizures spread quickly to the side contralateral to the focus, implying that seizures spread faster to a potentially epileptogenic region than to a normal region.

The study of Spanedda et al. (4) can be criticized because all the regions examined (mesial temporal regions on both sides in patients with bitemporal epilepsy) were potentially epileptogenic, even if some had normal volume measurements. It might be of interest to compare the morphologies of discharges starting in the presumed focus with that of discharges starting in regions that are "presumed" normal and far from the focus (one can argue that any region where a seizure starts is, by definition, abnormal). It may be noted, however, that in the experimental model of focal epilepsy, where penicillin is applied topically to the cortex, the discharge at the focus has the same morphology as the discharge that spread to the contralateral homotopic point, which is obviously normal. It may be that, in the end, it is impossible to distinguish a discharge taking place at the focus from one that has spread from the focus to the recording site.

SEIZURE MORPHOLOGY IN RELATION TO SIZE OF EPILEPTOGENIC ZONE

In another study (6), we investigated whether seizures starting in a small region had frequency characteristics different from those of seizures starting over a widespread region. Although, as stated, one cannot be sure that we have a better knowledge of the location of the focus in one case than in the other, it is *statistically* more likely that seizures starting in a small zone reflect a small focus, and the seizures starting in a large zone reflect a wide epileptogenic area. We found that the frequency of the EEG at onset, as well as the maximum frequency of the EEG discharge, which did not necessarily occur at onset, were significantly higher when discharges started in a spatially restricted region than when they started over a widespread area (Fig. 22.2). This finding indicates that the EEG discharge tends to be faster when the epileptogenic zone is small. The high-speed discharge may occur at seizure onset or later in the seizure (Fig. 22.3). The results do not support the commonly held view that the discharge is faster early in the seizure, when the discharge is spatially limited, and becomes slower as the discharge occupies a larger brain

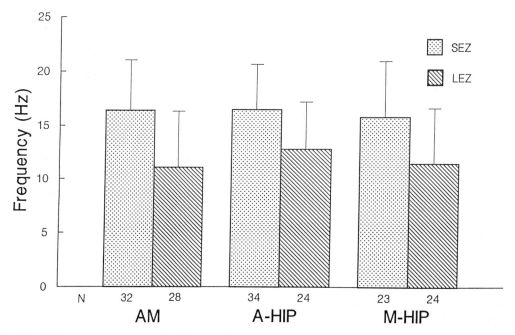

FIG. 22.2. Average and standard deviation of peak frequencies in the first 8 seconds of rhythmic activity in amygdala *(AM),* anterior hippocampus *(A-HIP),* and middle hippocampus *(M-HIP)* for the seizures with onset in a small epileptogenic zone *(SEZ)* and seizures with onset in a large epileptogenic zone *(LEZ).* Frequencies are higher for seizures from a SEZ. (From Gotman J, Levtova V, Olivier A. Frequency of the electroencephalographic discharge in seizures of focal and widespread onset in intracerebral recordings. *Epilepsia* 1995;36:697–703, with permission.)

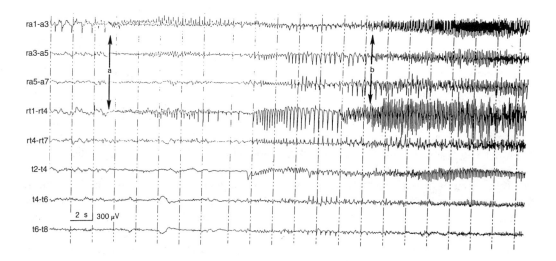

volume. They indicate that the EEG discharge, even when the seizure has spread, may remain influenced by the size of the region in which it started because it tends to include faster frequencies when it has started in a small region.

This result was obtained, of course, by statistical analysis of a group of subjects and does not hold for every patient. It is noteworthy, however, that frequencies above 20 Hz were almost never seen in seizures starting in a wide epileptogenic zone. This study was performed in the temporal lobe, and it is not clear whether its findings are applicable to extratemporal regions. It has been shown (7) that seizures of temporal neocortical origin tend to have a faster discharge than seizures of mesial temporal origin; it also has been shown that there is some regional specificity in frequency characteristics of seizure onset (see Chapter 19). These studies indicate that there is no simple way to separate an activity that is really at the focus from one that has propagated, although there are a few group differences.

RELATIONSHIPS BETWEEN BRAIN REGIONS DURING SEIZURES

A different avenue of investigation is to analyze seizure discharges occurring simultaneously in different regions to determine whether one of the regions appears to *drive* the discharge. This can be done by measuring the coherence and phase between the two discharges or by using other measures of similar type. Sometimes it can be determined that the discharge in one region leads that in another region by a few milliseconds or that one region appears causal to the others, without any time measurement.

To assess the relationships between two or more channels, one first must determine whether the two channels have information in common. It is possible that two regions both are involved in a seizure but are discharging independently of each other. In such a case, there is no discussion of causality. If a relationship between two discharges does exist, one can ask whether one appears causal to the other. Relationships between two channels have been measured most often with the coherence function. This measures only relationships that are *linear*, in the mathematical sense. Other measures, such as the average amount of mutual information (AAMI) (8), can measure linear and nonlinear relationships and therefore are theoretically more general. Using the coherence, we were able to show that interhemispheric coherence was high only during the few seconds when a unilateral temporal seizure becomes bilateral and also often at the end of seizures (9). A parallel finding was obtained by Duckrow and Spencer (10), who found that "the process of neuronal entrainment during seizure onset involves a transient interaction between brain regions but the maintenance of this interaction is not required for sustained seizure activity." Lieb et al. (11) found few instances of high interhemispheric coherence in seizures of mesial temporal onset and concluded that propagation was unlikely to take place through the main commissures and was more likely to take place through brainstem structures. Bertashius (12) found similar results but also documented interhemispheric propaga-

FIG. 22.3. High discharge frequencies are more frequent in seizures starting in a small epileptogenic zone. This maximum frequency is often not at seizure onset, as illustrated here. Eight bipolar channels are from the right temporal lobe; depth electrodes are implanted laterally and aimed at the amygdala **(a)** and anterior hippocampus **(b)**; contacts are 5 mm apart, and contact 1 is deepest; the last three channels are epidural contacts over the first temporal convolution. The onset of rhythmic activity is at *a*, but activity in amygdala and hippocampus electrodes (RA1-3 and RB1-4, where the seizure started) is fastest at about time *b*, approximately 25 seconds after onset. Maximum frequency is 16 Hz in amygdala and 10 Hz in the hippocampus.

tion through the thalamic nuclei; he used the correlation function rather than coherence, but the basic principle is the same.

If it is established that the coherence or the AAMI is sufficiently large, it is possible to measure the time difference between the discharges in two channels (9,11,13,14). Establishing that channel A leads channel B by a few milliseconds gives valuable information as to the direction of spread (A leads B), although we must be careful about the interpretation: it does not prove that the seizure starts in A unless one is sure that it must start either in A or in B. It does prove, however, that the seizure does not start in B.

In a phase and coherence study of amygdala–hippocampus relationships in temporal seizures, we found that seizures that were limited to mesiotemporal lobe structures tended to show a lead from the hippocampus to the amygdala, whereas the amygdala led the hippocampus in seizures that tended to be more diffuse, involving the temporal lobe in a widespread fashion (15).

Another method of studying interactions between brain regions during seizures was proposed more recently: the Directed Transfer Function (16,17). This method analyzes all the channels at once. It was shown that, in some seizures, the region in which the seizure started remained the driving region throughout the seizures, even after it became widespread. In other seizures, a region different from that of onset was driving the late part of the seizure.

THE ELECTROENCEPHALOGRAHIC MICROSCOPE

In an attempt to resolve the uncertainty that always plagues intracerebral recordings because of the necessarily limited spatial sampling (the "tunnel vision"), a new method was developed that can scan the whole intracerebral volume in an unbiased way (i.e., not using any a priori knowledge of where the generator might be). The method assumes that the discharge at seizure onset is spatially restricted to a small

region and therefore contributes only minimally to the scalp EEG; because this contribution is spread among several channels, it may not be visible by traditional examination of the scalp EEG. It therefore can be likened to viewing the scalp EEG through an "EEG microscope" (18,19). We have been able to find focal activity in the depth of the temporal neocortex at a time when visual examination of the scalp EEG does not show any clear ictal discharge. The localization and frequency content of this activity was confirmed by subsequent SEEG recordings.

The domain of applicability of this method remains to be established: How deep under the skull can it "see" seizure discharges? How focal do the discharges have to be for them to be visible by this "microscope"?

DISCUSSION

We reviewed some of the attempts made at identifying a seizure focus given the fundamental limitation that a seizure can always start in a region that is not accessible to our recording methodology. It appears impossible to overcome fully this limitation, and one therefore must always remain skeptical when thinking that the seizure focus has been found. From a theoretical point of view, successful surgical excision does not localize the seizure onset with certainty because a clinically silent discharge still could be present. Even if such a discharge is not present, the surgical excision is likely to be much larger than the seizure focus. We have seen that it is possible to analyze the seizure discharge and gain some statistical knowledge with respect to the likelihood that it is indeed of focal origin. We also have seen that there is little relationship between the pathological substrate generating a seizure and the morphology of the EEG discharge. One must be careful not to think that some patterns (for instance, focal flattening or repetitive spikes) are more indicative than others (e.g., slow discharge) of proximity to the epileptic focus. Even though to do so is tempting from an empirical point of view and from the knowledge of how some patterns resemble those seen in experimental epilepsy, there is really no objective evidence linking particular patterns to the focus.

We also have discussed various methods to measure interactions during seizures. It is sometimes possible to measure the strength of the functional connection between two discharging regions and to measure a time delay that might be interpreted as corresponding to neuronal conduction. When finding that one region discharges a few milliseconds before another, one major question remains: Does this reflect propagation from a focus to a passively responding normal region, or does it reflect a widespread epileptogenic area where one region simply predominates? Even when we know that one region is more epileptogenic than a second one, we do not know whether this second region is able to generate a seizure on its own.

ACKNOWLEDGMENTS

This work was supported in part by grant MT-10189 of the Medical Research Council of Canada.

REFERENCES

1. Cooper R, Winter AL, Crow HJ, et al. Comparison of subcortical, cortical, and scalp activity using chronically indwelling electrodes in man. *Electroencephalogr Clin Neurophysiol* 1965;18:217–228.
2. Merlet I, Gotman J. Reliability of dipole models of epileptic spikes. *Clin Neurophysiol* 1999;110:1013–1028.
3. Ojemann GA, Engel J Jr. Acute and chronic intracranial recordings and stimulation. In: Engel J Jr, eds. *Surgical treatment of the epilepsies.* New York: Raven Press, 1986:263–288.
4. Spanedda F, Cendes F, Gotman J. Relations between EEG seizure morphology, interhemispheric spread, and mesial temporal atrophy in bitemporal epilepsy. *Epilepsia* 1997;38:1300–1314.
5. Lieb JP, Engel J Jr, Babb TL. Interhemispheric propaga-tion time of human hippocampal seizures. I. Relationship to surgical outcome. *Epilepsia* 1986;27:286–293.
6. Gotman J, Levtova V, Olivier A. Frequency of the electroencephalographic discharge in seizures of focal and widespread onset in intracerebral recordings. *Epilepsia* 1995;36:697–703.
7. Javidan M, Katz A, Tran T, et al. Frequency characteristics of neocortical and hippocampal onset seizures. *Epilepsia* 1992;33:58(abst).
8. Lopes da Silva FH, Mars NJI. Parametric methods in EEG analysis. In: Gevins AS, Rémond A, eds. *Methods of analysis of brain electrical and magnetic signals. Handbook of electroencephalography and clinical neurophysiology,* vol 1. Amsterdam: Elsevier, 1987:243–260.
9. Gotman J. Interhemispheric interactions in seizures of focal onset: data from human intracranial recordings. *Electroencephalogr Clin Neurophysiol* 1987;67:120–133.
10. Duckrow RB, Spencer SS. Regional coherence and the transfer of ictal activity during seizure onset in the medial temporal lobe. *Electroencephalogr Clin Neurophysiol* 1992;82:415–422.
11. Lieb JP, Hoque K, Skomer CE, et al. Inter-hemispheric propagation of human mesial temporal lobe seizures: a coherence/phase analysis. *Electroencephalogr Clin Neurophysiol* 1987;67:101–119.
12. Bertashius KM. Propagation of human complex-partial seizures: a correlation analysis. *Electroencephalog Clin Neurophysiol* 1991;78:333–340.
13. Brazier MAB. Spread of seizure discharges in epilepsy: anatomical and electrophysiological considerations. *Exp Neurol* 1972;36:263–272.
14. Gotman J. Measurement of small time differences between EEG channels: method and application to epileptic seizure propagation *Electroencephalogr Clin Neurophysiol* 1983;56:501–514.
15. Gotman J, Levtova V. Amygdala–hippocampus relationships in temporal lobe seizures: a phase–coherence study. *Epilpesy Res* 1996;25:51–57.
16. Franaszczuk PJ, Bergey GK, Kaminski MJ. Analysis of mesial temporal seizure onset and propagation using the directed transfer function method. *Electroencephalogr Clin Neurophysiol* 1994;91:413–427.
17. Franaszczuk PJ, Bergey GK, Durka PJ, et al. Time–frequency analysis using the matching pursuit algorithm applied to seizures originating from the mesial temporal lobe. *Electroencephalogr Clin Neurophysiol* 1998;106:513–521.
18. Kobayashi K, Nakahori T, Ohmori I, et al. Estimation of obscure ictal epileptic activity in scalp EEG. *Brain Topogr* 1996;9:125–134.
19. Kobayashi K, James CJ, Yoshinaga H, et al. The electroencephalogram through a software microscope: noninvasive and visualization of epileptic seizure activity from inside the brain. *Clin Neurophysiol* 2000;111:134–149.

Neocortical Epilepsies.
Advances in Neurology, Vol. 84,
edited by P.D. Williamson, A.M. Siegel,
D.W. Roberts, V.M. Thadani, and M.S. Gazzaniga.
Lippincott Williams & Wilkins, Philadelphia © 2000.

23

Detection of Epileptiform Activity Using Artificial Neural Networks

Ronald P. Lesser and *W.R.S. Webber

*Departments of Neurology and Neurosurgery, The Johns Hopkins University, Baltimore, Maryland 21287-7247; *Department of Neurology, The Johns Hopkins University, Baltimore, Maryland 21287*

When one designs a computer program to detect epileptiform discharges, one either implicitly or explicitly assumes that this detector will perform similarly to an expert human. More specifically, the electroencephalographer (EEGer) or epileptologist would expect a computer-based detector to find, event by event, all existing interictal seizure discharges as well as, event by event, all existing seizures. That individual might look through a record, page by page, to determine whether the detector "found" every instance of a spike, sharp wave, or spike and wave complex; had found every instance of a seizure; and had not incorrectly marked normal variants as being artifacts and other patterns as being epileptiform in character.

Electroencephalographers, however, do not agree among themselves regarding individual events, even though often there can be agreement about the overall composition of a record (1–17). We might agree that most of the sharp waves in a particular record are located in the left temporal region but might not agree about whether the particular event that occurred at 3:00 p.m. was a sharp wave. Moreover, many factors can affect how an individual reader assesses a record, including how that person was trained, how alert, how distracted, and how motivated he or she was at the time of assessment. Some features in the record itself might affect how the EEGer assessed it, including the frequency of occurrence of events in a record, the similarity of epileptiform discharges (EDs) to normal variants and artifacts, the overall frequency of artifacts in the record, the state of awakeness or sleep, and others.

The problem is that to develop a computer-based detector, we must tell the computer what to find. If we do not agree among ourselves about what the detector should detect, it becomes much more difficult to develop a detector that will be 100% accurate. Moreover, because we do not agree with one another, we may be expecting of the detector something that we do not even expect of ourselves. In a more formal sense, one could ask several EEGers to mark a particular EEG file or group of files. One could then take two approaches in developing a detector. A more *inclusive* approach would require the detector to find every event that had been marked by even one EEGer. The problem with this apparoach is that such a detector might mark up a large number of events that would be taken to be false-positives by a single EEGer who might have marked some, but not all, of the events in the set. A *less inclusive* approach might be to require the detector to find the events, and only the events, marked by all the EEGers. In this case, an individual

EEGer who had marked events not marked by others might see the computer program as producing a large number of false-negatives (Fig. 23.1).

To assess this problem in a more formal sense, we (17) studied what might be called the *EEG marking behavior* of eight EEGers. Twelve records were obtained from ten patients, each of which comprised continuous recordings 3 to 5 minutes long and consisting of 10 to 16 channels with electrodes placed according to the international 10 to 20 system. The montages primarily consisted of "bipolar chains," but there were some "referentially recorded" channels as well. The records included some with many EDs, some with few, and some with artifacts

that resembled EDs. The EEGers were asked to read the records as they normally would and to mark each found epileptiform discharge.

In this study, 1,739 events were marked by at least one or more readers, but only 1,071 events were marked by at least two readers, and 668 events were marked by only one reader. Only 316 events were marked by all eight readers. In this case, what would constitute a "gold standard" spike? Would it be the 1,739, the 1,071, the 668, or the 316 events? For the eight readers, there were 28 possible pairs of readers, and for these 28 possible pairs, the mean overlap in marked events was 52%. On the other hand, there was relatively good agree-

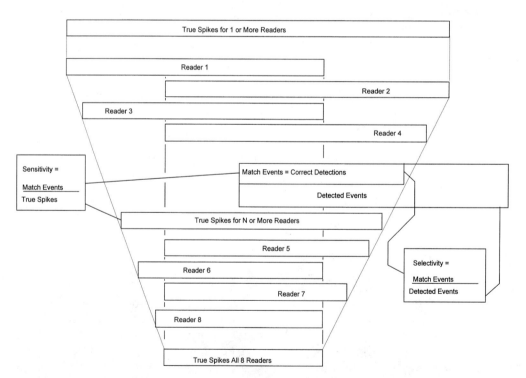

FIG. 23.1. How many readers are needed to define "true spikes"? As shown, different people identify different events as being epileptiform. We can define true spikes as being those so identified by one person, by everyone who reads the record, or by a subset of people reading the record. Each definition will leave us with a different set of events that have been identified and thus will change what we ask a computer detector to find.

ment among the readers with respect to the overall interpretation of the record. Gottman et al. (4) arrived at a similar conclusion, finding that the overall agreement as to the findings in EEG was much higher (72%–84%) than was the agreement regarding the count of individual events. Moreover, there appeared to be consistent characteristic styles of reading for individual EEGers: Some marked more events and some fewer. These findings are similar to those reported by others (3,18). Gevins et al. (3) reported that 401 events were considered EDs by at least one reader, of which 184 were marked by only one reader and only 69 were marked by all. Ehrenberg and Penry (18) studied the markings of three EEGers and found that 1,447 events were marked by at least one reader and 609 by all three. Hostetler et al. (5) found that from 7% to 68% of EDs were marked by at least one reader of five. We therefore assessed the average sensitivity and selectivity of each reader in finding events. Let us say that a gold standard ED is one detected by a reader or group of readers. We then can define sensitivity and selectivity as follows:

Sensitivity = The number of gold standard EDs detected by reader(s) or by the computer/The total number of gold standard EDs

Selectivity = The number of gold standard EDs marked/The total number of EDs marked by reader(s) or by the computer

If a gold standard ED is one found by all readers, the curve should look different from that if a gold standard is defined as an event found by only one reader or by one particular reader. We assessed the markings of each reader compared with the gold standard of EDs marked by a given number of other readers with that particular reader eliminated from the defining set (17). As one might expect, as more readers are required to define a gold standard ED, sensitivity increases, but selectivity decreases. In this study, we found

that the sensitivity and selectivity curves intersected at three readers. In other words, when we took as the gold standard events that were marked by three of the eight readers, this crossover point was optimal with respect to the combination and sensitivity and selectivity. We thought, therefore, that this crossover point might be a reasonable gold standard.

If one wants to improve both sensitivity and selectivity, however, one would have to decide how this is defined (Fig. 23.2). If one wants to define this with respect to all EEGers, both sensitivity and selectivity cannot be improved simultaneously. A broader definition of EDs would increase sensitivity but decrease selectivity. A more restricted definition would increase selectivity but not sensitivity. On the other hand, microprocessor-based techniques ultimately have the possibility of allowing the algorithm to define mathematically a set of events, which humans then could evaluate. Over time, an interactive process of this sort might result in a greater consensus regarding what events are to be considered EDs; if such a consensus is reached, the sensitivity and selectivity conundrum might be solved, at least partially.

These considerations in essence simply imply that questions remain about how one can best devise an algorithm for detecting seizure discharges. Notwithstanding these considerations, an algorithm eventually should be able to answer certain fundamental questions. From the clinical perspective, one wants to know whether epileptiform discharges are present. One wants to know where they are and whether one or more than one region of epileptogenesis exist. One wants to know what the relative frequencies of discharges are in various regions and whether epileptiform discharges spread in a regular fashion from one to another. Seen from this perspective, a detection algorithm is simply a tool to answer these and similar questions.

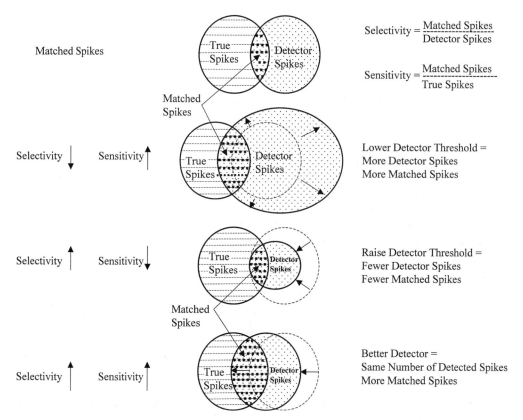

$$\text{Selectivity} = \frac{\text{Matched Spikes}}{\text{Detector Spikes}}$$

$$\text{Sensitivity} = \frac{\text{Matched Spikes}}{\text{True Spikes}}$$

Lower Detector Threshold =
More Detector Spikes
More Matched Spikes

Raise Detector Threshold =
Fewer Detector Spikes
Fewer Matched Spikes

Better Detector =
Same Number of Detected Spikes
More Matched Spikes

FIG. 23.2. The detection problem. Assume that a certain number of spikes are truly epileptiform discharges—"true spikes." There also are a certain number of events that are found by a given computer detector or, for that matter, by a person reading the EEG. One then can determine how many "spikes" there really are, how many events are detected, and how many are matched because they are both "true spikes" and detected events. The selectivity and sensitivity are then as shown. If the detector is made to find more events, that is if we lower the detector threshold, there may be more matched events, but there also may be more false-positives—events found by the computer detector that really are not spikes. The opposite would occur if we have more stringent criteria for the detector. Ideally, we want a detector that imitates "truth" as closely as possible. Current detectors, at least those used for scalp EEG recordings, do not do this, in part because epileptiform activity, normal variant patterns, and scalp recorded artifacts closely resemble one another.

ARTIFICIAL NEURAL NETWORKS

Artificial neural networks (ANNs) (19–23) are potentially a way to solve this problem because they do not rely on a fixed set of rules, rules that might insist that the algorithm behave like reader one, like three of eight readers, or like all readers. They can be trained to do any one of these; because they learn by example, however, they also can adapt to new situations, for example, learn to accept anything marked by three of eight readers but then learn to use more stringent, or less stringent, rules. They would do this to accept anything marked by a different, larger, or smaller, set of readers. The disadvantage of these ANNs is that they can be computationally intensive (23). With improvements in the speed of microprocessors over the last several years, these are no longer major limitations to the successful use of neural networks in electrophysiology. Because neural networks can "learn," they have been used in a number of medical applications, including dementia, drug monitoring, anesthesia, and epilepsy (24–30).

A number of groups have applied ANNs to the analysis of EEG activity (31–36). The methods used all have included the use of feed-forward neural networks that employ the back-propagation learning algorithm. These programs operate either on line or off line, depending on the specifics of the application. Similarly, various approaches to the detection of epileptiform discharges have been attempted, including the number of subjects studied, the relationship between the training and test sets, the size of the individual data set (including number of channels and time), and the speed with which the ANN would operate. The most important difference is the nature of the data presented to the neural network: Is it raw EEG data or data that has been processed in one way or another? Another significant distinguishing feature of spike and seizure detectors is whether and how data from several channels are combined to produce the final result. For example, Ozdamar et al. (33) and Yaylali et al. (36), when detecting epileptiform discharges, used raw data and a three-layer artificial neural network for each of 16 channels of EEG, the outputs of which were fed to another three-layer artificial neural network. Jando et al. (27) compared raw data input with input from a fast Fourier transform of the raw data for detecting spike and wave patterns. In their study, the ANN performed better when trained on the transformed data. The methodology we used (37,38) first parameterizes the data and then presents the parameters obtained to the ANN. The parameters measure a variety of aspects of the raw data, such as amplitude, duration, and sharpness of the individual events in the case of spikes. For seizures, for example, 31 parameters from both the time and frequency domains are presented, but we believe fewer parameters are

probably necessary, and we are currently studying ways to optimize our method.

The ANN itself is therefore the second stage of our detector, implemented as a generic three-layer feed-forward neural network trained by the back-propagation method with input, hidden, and output layers. The weights of our network were adjusted by training beginning with relatively high values for the learning coefficient, 0.02 for spikes and 0.015 for seizures. The momentum was set to 0.9 for both the spikes and seizure ANNs. There is a third stage that consists of a few simple rules used to assess the output of the neural network. We are similarly assessing this stage in an effort to optimize our method. The training set was presented a thousand times, and the network then was tested individually against each patient set.

One EEGer (R.P.L.) directly marked the training files on a computer screen. This allowed us to log the choices of selected events automatically and precisely. Ten EEG files were between 3 and 5 minutes long, chosen by W.R.S.W. to reflect the range of epileptiform discharges, normal activities, and artifacts and to contain both awake and sleep EEG. Not all records contained epileptiform activity. In addition to the seizure files, we identified 30 files in a preliminary study in which the ANN had incorrectly identified seizures. From these 30 files, we selected six for the training set. These were used to identify to the neural network events that we did not wish it to select as representing seizures. In our method, the first stage of the detector then divides each channel of EEG data into two second epochs, each containing 400 samples. In the case of the seizure detector, we used 8,000 epochs divided into ten sets of 800 epochs each. The network trained on the first set of 800 patterns for ten iterations of training, the next set of 800 for ten iterations, and so on. The network utilized 2,700 presentations of the 8,000 patterns. The first stage then parameterizes these data looking at 31 features reflecting amplitude, duration, and sharpness of the waveform. Because the amplitude of EEG can vary among patients, all amplitude measures are expressed relative to a baseline in the same patient, which helps to normalize the data for the network. Similar normalization factors are used for all the other inputs to the network. The second or "hidden" layer of the neural network has 30 nodes. We assessed the performance of the network using 10, 20, and 60 hidden nodes. Performance improved when going from 10 to 20 to 30 nodes, but there was no performance improvement when going to 60 nodes. The third stage uses rules to assess the output of the second stage and to determine whether an event of interest has occurred. The ANN reduces the original 31 parameters to eight in the case of seizure detection, and to one in the case of interictal epileptiform discharge detection.

Initially, the artificial network had only two output nodes in this third layer, seizure or no seizure. When we found that this did not classify the data satisfactorily, we changed this to eight nodes: *large seizure* of 300 microvolts or greater amplitude, *small seizure* of less than 300 microvolts' amplitude, theta activity, alpha activity, *miscellaneous normal* activity, chewing artifact, and noise. The detector was designed so as to "find" both definite seizure patterns and paroxysmal patterns that might possibly be of interest to a clinician. Our concept was that we wish to have the algorithm provide output that the human reviewer could assess. The reviewer then would make a final decision regarding the significance of selected events.

To test the ANN, we used ten test EEG files in the case of the spike detector, each of which contained no, some, or many epileptiform discharges as well as a variety of normal patterns. The EEGer marked events as *definite* or *possible* EDS. This was done to reflect the practice of many clinicians who will find some events definitely to be epileptiform in character and others to be possibly but not definitely epileptiform in character. Our goal was to reflect this potential ambiguity in the performance of the network. To test the seizure detector, we used ten separate files

that contained a variety of seizure patterns, including repetitive spikes and ictal delta, theta, alpha, or beta.

In the case of interictal epileptiform discharges, the first stage of the detector found 5,995 events that included 95% (878) of the definite epileptiform discharges and 94% (1,261) of the definite and possible epileptiform discharges. The second stage, the ANN, rejected 4,646 of these 5,995 events. In other words, the first stage found most of the events marked by the EEGer but found many other events not marked by the EEGer. This problem of false-positives is familiar to many clinicians who use programs that detect epileptiform activity and helps to define the problem. One wants to find as many of these EDs as possible and to miss as few as possible, but also to look at as few events as possible that are not going to be of final interest. How can one improve the performance of the computer program so that the important events are presented to the EEGer and the unimportant ones are not? This problem falls back to the issue of sensitivity and selectivity, already discussed.

The ANN assigned low output values to most of the candidate waveforms rejected by RPL. For example, 91% were below an output threshold of 0.2 and 98% below a threshold of 0.7. Of the waveforms identified as EDs, 55% had output values of 0.9 or greater, 75% above 0.7, and 85% above 0.5. Possible EDs were evenly distributed over a range of output thresholds. Ideally, one would want definite events to have output thresholds of, say, 0.9 or greater, possible events to have thresholds of 0.8 or greater, and so on; however, the clustering of definite events at the upper end of output thresholds and the possible events throughout the range of output thresholds would suggest that further analysis, such as those that use a clustering technique, might help to characterize mathematically the kinds of events of interest to humans.

The performance of the seizure detector was checked in records obtained from 50 patients. The detector found seizures in 26 of 34 seizure files and in 4 of 44 baseline files, a sensitivity of 76% and selectivity of 87%. The combined duration of the baseline files was 4.1 hours, giving a false detection rate of 1 per hour. These false detections were due to noise in the record but were not classified as such by the ANN.

These results can be compared with those of rule-based detectors. For example, Gotman and colleagues reported sensitivities in the range of 76% to 81% (39,40), similar to 76% measured in our study. This method (41,42) achieved a false alarm rate of 1.26 seizures per hour. Another study (43) found sensitivities in the range of 86%–95% and a false alarm rate of 0.7 per hour using this method. Another found no false-positives and no false-negatives (44). These last two studies used data from patients with implanted electrodes, whereas we studied scalp data. One would expect data from implanted electrodes to be easier for a detector to analyze, particularly because of the reduced number of artifacts.

To improve the method of seizure detection further, Klatchko et al. (45) used a clustering algorithm. This algorithm reflected the idea that seizures propagate both over time and in space. An analysis method that could reflect the propagation in space and time might be able to analyze those features of the record that the EEGer instinctively uses to identify a seizure and thus improve the accuracy of the detection. The study used a clustering algorithm (46) that was built into the detector already described. Several EEGers scored the points of onset and ending of the seizures in ten records lasting a total of 245 minutes and containing 25 seizures ranging from 6 to 90 seconds long (plus an additional seizure pattern occurring 15 seconds after the beginning of the record, within the baseline used by the method to determine overall amplitudes of data). The method constructed a Laplacian synthetic channel from the acquired data and assigned a score of 0 to 1 to each of the eight nodes of an artificial neural network for each 2-second epoch. These results then were presented to the clustering algorithm, which was updated continuously and separately for the left and right hemispheres and for the mid-

line. The algorithm looked for merging clusters of events occurring within regions of interest and across time. When a sufficient number of scores of a sufficient value was found, a seizure was declared. A seizure was identified if events were found at three or four electrodes for more than 6 seconds. Clusters that were as far as 30 seconds apart were merged into a single cluster if they met other criteria with respect to output scores. Of course, this meant that shorter events, those less than 6 seconds' duration, would not be detected by this method, although the selectivity of the method improved considerably. Additional approaches would be needed to identify these short events as might occur, for example, in the case of myoclonic seizures.

Using this method, 24 of 24 seizures were matched by cluster, but only 23 of these clusters met the criteria of being at least 6 seconds long and occurring over 3 or more channels. The algorithm had a temporal overlap of 0.59 ± 0.19 with what had been identified by humans and a combined spatiotemporal overlap of 0.34 ± 0.16. The algorithm also found 8 clusters of 6 seconds or longer, which were thought to be false-positives. Of interest was that these usually were the result of fewer events found on fewer channels. (There were 9 ± 3 clusters on 5 ± 2 channels versus 23 ± 14 clusters on 11 ± 4 channels in the case of the true events; 19 channels of digitized data were presented.) Although false-positives, these appeared to be coherent events that were sustained over time and space, suggesting that further implementations of the underlying neural network might improve the detection algorithm. It also suggested that criteria related to number of clusters and number of channels could improve accuracy. There was one false-negative as well. In this case, the algorithm found a 4-second-long portion of an 8-second-duration seizure pattern with 10 events firing on 6 channels. The ANN algorithm without the clustering had missed two events. One was the event just described. In the other case, the single-channel–based ANN did not declare a seizure because no single channel detection occurred over 3 consecutive epochs, the criteria for this method. By comparison, when the clustering algorithm assessed the seizure, it found 36 events over 12 channels during the 35-second-long seizure. This is an example of how assessment over multiple channels with merging of the data potentially could improve the results of single-channel–based detection. It is similar in many ways to the approach actually used by humans, who decide on the presence of a seizure by looking at all the data, not simply the data on a single channel.

COMMENTS

These considerations suggest that it is possible for computer-based detection algorithms to begin to approximate the results that can be obtained from humans. In assessing the quality of a detector, one still will be left with the problem that there is no precise agreement with regard to what kinds of activity should be detected. Practically speaking, one can acquire a set of data, establish criteria for what is to be identified, improve the ability of the method to detect as many events (as defined by these criteria) as possible and to reject as much of the rest of the record as possible. ANNs have a particular advantage when using this kind of approach in that they can "learn" automatically. In other words, one can improve the underlying accuracy of the method and then ask the ANN to adapt to the particular types of events that a particular EEGer wishes to find. Theoretically, ANN could "learn" a different set of criteria for each person.

At the same time, workers can continue to decide how best to characterize the underlying background EEG, whether it be that obtained with the subject awake or asleep, with implanted electrode, or with scalp data. Methods could be used to tell the underlying detector what the clinical "state" of the patient is with the detector tuning differently for different states of alertness (47). In addition, however, detectors can be used to automate and systematize the analysis of EEG even further. As we can more precisely quantitate EEG, we

will begin to be able to characterize more fully and accurately the nature of the events that we wish to find—and do this in a more objective manner. In turn, this will help us to decide better what we wish the detector to do and eventually allow a greater convergence in interpretation styles among EEGers.

ACKNOWLEDGMENTS

We have received research funding from and are entitled to sales royalty from Biologic Systems, Inc., which is developing products related to the research described in this review. Dr. Robert Webber is also a consultant to the company. The terms of this arrangement have been reviewed and approved by The Johns Hopkins University in accordance with its conflict of interest policies.

REFERENCES

1. Barlow J. Computerized clinical electroencephalography in perspective. *IEEE Trans Biomed Eng* 1979;26: 377–391.
2. Blum R. A note on the reliability of electroencephalographic judgments. *Neurology* 1954;4:143–146.
3. Gevins A, Yeager C, et al. Automated analysis of the electrical activity of the human brain (EEG): a progress report. *Proceedings of the Institute of Electronic and Electrical Engineering* 1975;63;1382–1399.
4. Gotman J, Gloor P, Schaul N. Comparison of traditional reading of the EEG and automatic recognition of interictal epileptic activity. *Electroencephalogr Clin Neurophysiol* 1978;44:48–60.
5. Hostetler WE, Doller HJ, Homan RW. Assessment of a computer program to detect epileptiform spikes. *Electroencephalogr Clin Neurophysiol* 1992;83:1–11.
6. Houfek E, Ellingson R. On the reliability of clinical EEG interpretation. *J Nerv Ment Dis* 1959;128:425–437.
7. Little S, Raffel S. Intra-rater reliability of EEG interpretations. *J Nerv Ment Dis* 1962;135;77–81.
8. Rose S, Perry J, et al. Reliability and validity of visual EEG assessment in third grade children. *Clin Electroencephalogr* 1973;4:197–205.
9. Struve FA, Becka DR, Green MA, et al. Reliability of clinical interpretation of the electroencephalogram. *Clin Electroencephalogr* 1975;6:54–60.
10. Volavka J, Matousek M, Feldstein ST. Die Zuverlassigkeit der EEG-Beurteilung. *ZEEG-EMG* 1973;4:123–130.
11. Volavka J, Matousek M, Roubicek J, et al. The reliability of visual EEG assessment. *Electroencephalogr Clin Neurophysiol* 1975;31:294.
12. Williams G, Lesser R, et al. Clinical diagnosis and EEG interpretation. *Cleve Clin J Med* 1990;57:437–440.
13. Williams GW, Lüders HO, Brickner A, et al. Interobserver variability in EEG interpretation. *Neurology* 1985;35:1714–1719.

14. Woody R. Inter-judge reliability in clinical electroencephalography. *J Clin Psychol* 1968;24:251–256.
15. Woody R. Inter-judge reliability in clinical electroencephalography. *J Clin Psychol* 1966;22:150–154.
16. de Oliveira PG, Queiroz C, Lopes da Silva FH. Spike detection based on a pattern recognition approach using a microcomputer. *Electroencephalogr Clin Neurophysiol* 1983;56;97–103.
17. Webber WRS, Litt B, Lesser RP, et al. Automatic EEG spike detection: what should the computer imitate? *Electroencephalogr Clin Neurophysiol* 1993;87:364–373.
18. Ehrenberg B, Penry J. Computer recognition of generalized spike-wave discharges. *Electroencephalogr Clin Neurophysiol* 1976;41:25–36.
19. McClelland JL, Rumelhart DE. *Explorations in parallel distributed processing.* Cambridge, MA: MIT Press, 1988.
20. Rumelhart DE, McClelland JL. In: Feldman AJ, Hayes PF, Rumelhart DE, eds. *Parallel distributed processing.* Cambridge, MA: MIT Press, 1988.
21. Wasserman PD. *Neural computing:* theory and practice. New York: Van Nostrand Reinhold, 1989.
22. Eberhart RC, Dobbins RW. Case study. I. Detection of electroencephalogram spikes. In: Eberhart RC, Dobbins RW, eds. *Neural network PC tools.* San Diego: Academic Press, 1990:215–234.
23. Zurada JM. *Introduction to artificial neural systems.* St. Paul, MN: West Publishing, 1992:455–559.
24. Murro AM, King DW, Smith JR, et al. Computerized seizure detection of complex partial seizures. *Electroencephalogr Clin Neurophysiol* 1991;79;330–333.
25. Sharma A, Wilson SE, Roy R. EEG classification for estimating anesthetic depth during halothane anesthesia. Proceedings of the 14th Annual International Conference IEEE Engineering in Medicine and Biology Society. *IEEE Trans Biomed Eng* 1992;2409–2410.
26. Mirbagheri MM, Badie K, Golpayegani RMH, et al. A neural network approach to EEG classification for the purpose of differential diagnosis between epilepsy and normal EEG. Proceedings 14th Annual International Conference IEEE Engineering in Medicine and Biology Society. *IEEE Trans Biomed Eng* 1992;2649–2650.
27. Jando J, Siegel RM, Horvath Z, et al. Pattern recognition of the electroencephalogram by artificial neural networks. *Electroencephalogr Clin Neurophysiol* 1993;86:100–109.
28. Anderer P, Saletu B, Kloppel B, et al. Discrimination between demented patients and normals based on topographic EEG slow wave activity: comparison between Z statistics discriminant analysis and artificial neural network classifiers. *Electroencephalogr Clin Neurophysiol* 1994;91:108–117.
29. Veselis RA, Reinsel R, Wronski M. Analytical methods to differentiate similar electroencephalographic spectra: neural network and discriminant analysis. *J Clin Monit* 1994;9:257–267.
30. Pritchard WS, Duke DW, Coburn KL, et al. EEG-based, neural-net predictive classification of Alzheimer's disease versus control subjects is augmented by non-linear EEG measures. *Electroencephalogr Clin Neurophysiol* 1994;91:118–130.
31. Eberhart RC, Dobbins RW, Webber WRS. EEG waveform analysis using CaseNet. In: *Proceedings of the Annual International Conference IEEE Engineering in Medicine and Biology Society.* Seattle: 1989, II:637.
32. Webber WRS, Wilson K, Lesser RP, et al. On-line detection of epileptic spikes using a patient independent neural network. *Epilepsia* 1990;31:687.
33. Ozdamar O, Yaylali I, Jayakar P, et al. Multilevel neural network system for EEG spike detection. In: Bankman IN, Tsitlik JE, eds. *Computer-based medical systems. Proceedings of the Fourth Annual IEEE Symposium.* Washington: IEEE Computer Society Press, 1991: 272–279.
34. Wilson K, Webber WRS, Lesser RP, et al. Detection of epileptiform spikes in the EEG using a patient-independent neural network. In: Bankman IN, Tsitlik JE, eds. *Computer-based medical systems. Proceedings of the Fourth Annual IEEE Symposium.* Washington: IEEE Computer Society Press, 1991:264–271.
35. Gabor AJ, Seyal M. Automated interictal EEG spike detection using artificial neural networks. *Electroencephalogr Clin Neurophysiol* 1992;83:271–280.
36. Yaylali I, Jayakar P, Ozdamar O. Detection of epileptic spikes using artificial multilevel neural networks. American Electoencephalographic Society Annual Meeting, San Francisco, 1982:82(abs).
37. Webber WRS, Litt B, Wilson K, et al. Practical detection of epileptiform discharges (EDs) in the EEG using an artificial neural network: a comparison of raw and parameterized EEG data. *Electroencephalogr Clin Neurophysiol* 1994;91:194–204.
38. Webber WRS, Lesser RP, Richardson RT, et al. An approach to seizure detection using an artificial neural network (ANN). *Electroencephalogr Clin Neurophysiol* 1996;98:250–272.
39. Gotman J. Automatic seizure detection: improvements and evaluation. *Electroencephalogr Clin Neurophysiol* 1990;76:317–324.
40. Pauri F, Pierelli F, Chatrian GE, et al. Long-term EEG-video-audio monitoring: computer detection of focal EEG seizure patterns. *Electroencephalogr Clin Neurophysiol* 1992;82:1–9.
41. Hao Q, Gotman J. Improvement in seizure detection performance by adaptation to the EEG of each patient. *Electroencephalogr Clin Neurophysiol Suppl* 1993;86: 79–87.
42. Gotman J. Automatic recognition of epileptic seizures in the EEG. *Electroencephalogr Clin Neurophysiol* 1982;54:530–540.
43. Harding GW. An automated seizure monitoring system for patients with indwelling recoding electrodes. *Electroencephalogr Clin Neurophysiol* 1993;86:428–437.
44. Osorio I, Frei MG, Wilkinson SB. Real-time automated detection and quantitative analysis of seizures and short-term prediction of clinical onset. *Epilepsia* 1998;39:615–627.
45. Klatchko A, Raviv G, Webber WRS, et al. Enhancing the detection of seizures with a clustering algorithm. *Electroencephalogr Clin Neurophysiol* 1998;106:52–63.
46. Knuth DE. Fundamental algorithms. In: Anonymous. *The art of computer programming.* Reading, MA: Addison-Wesley, 1968:233–234.
47. Gotman J. Automatic recognition of interictal spikes. *Electroencephalogr Clin Neurophysiol Suppl* 1985;37: 93–114.

Neocortical Epilepsies.
Advances in Neurology, Vol. 84,
edited by P.D. Williamson, A.M. Siegel,
D.W. Roberts, V.M. Thadani, and M.S. Gazzaniga.
Lippincott Williams & Wilkins, Philadelphia © 2000.

24

Value of Nonlinear Time Series Analysis of the EEG in Neocortical Epilepsies

C.E. Elger, G. Widman, R. Andrzejak, M. Dümpelmann, *J. Arnhold,
*P. Grassberger, and K. Lehnertz

Department of Epileptology, Medical Center, University of Bonn, D-53105 Bonn, Germany;
*John von Neumann Institute for Computing, Research Center Jülich, D-52425 Jülich, Germany

In contrast to the well-defined syndrome mesiotemporal lobe epilepsy (MTLE) (1), neocortical epilepsies (NE) comprise numerous inhomogeneous syndromes in which the threshold for epileptic seizures is lowered as a result of alterations in the neocortex. If these alterations are located in a circumscribed region of the brain, surgical treatment of NE is possible, provided that neurological deficits induced by the surgical intervention are kept at minimum. Epileptogenic functional alterations often coincide with marked structural alterations; therefore, imaging techniques such as magnetic resonance imaging (MRI), functional MRI (fMRI), positron emission tomography (PET), single-photon emission computed tomography (SPECT), or computed tomography (CT) are considered helpful for coarse localization of epileptogenic areas. Even if a neocortical lesion can be detected by these techniques, however, the corresponding so-called lesional zone (2) is not necessarily identical to the primary epileptogenic area in NEs, although in the great majority of patients both areas are related (3). Especially in cases with dual pathology or presumed widespread lesions associated with cortical dysplasia, invasive electroencephalographic (EEG) recordings still are required for an accurate localization of seizure origin.

Thus, the current "gold standard" for the localization of the primary epileptogenic area is to record the patient's spontaneous habitual seizures using chronic subdural or intrahippocampal depth electrodes. Present techniques are not sufficient, however. The seizure outcome of surgery for NE is still unsatisfactory compared with MTLE. Even in the case of extratemporal neocortical lesions, only 67% of the patients who have surgery become seizure free (4), which might have biological reasons, such as multiple dysplasias or misdevelopments, which constitute multiple epileptic foci; however, it also could be that the evaluation techniques to delineate the epileptogenic zone are insufficient or unsuccessful in these cases. To bring as many patients as possible into the successful outcome group, new localization techniques should be developed and evaluated.

In this context, looking at the basic processes of epilepsy could be interesting. Neurons discharging at high frequencies are considered to be the primary neuronal basis of the epileptogenic process. In the neuronal network, these high-frequency discharges are responsible for changes of signal properties in a way that stochastic processes are reduced and deterministic processes are increased in number. This phenomenon can be described and quantified using methods from the field of *nonlinear time series analysis* (NTSA, colloquially often termed *chaos theory*) to analyze field potentials [EEG/electrocorticography (ECoG)/stereo-electroencephalography (SEEG)]. Because capturing seizure events necessitates long-term recordings over many days, a huge amount of interictal data is collected during presurgical evaluation. This interictal data, however, also can contribute to defining the primary epileptogenic area. For example, automatic spike detection systems can provide quantitative parameters, such as spike rates, amplitudes, duration, and temporal variances of discharge rates at different recording sites and allow one to extract diagnostically relevant information from interictal electrophysiological long-term recordings (5–7). Especially in invasive recordings, it is problematic to differentiate between widespread steep potentials of normal physiological character and specific epileptiform events because exact definitions are still lacking. A recent publication reported on an insufficient spike density during intraoperative ECoG to guide the extent of surgical resection in 10% to 15% of their patients (8). Because chronic ECoG also might fail to detect spikes, sensitive analysis methods are necessary to allow one to estimate reliably the spatial extent of the primary epileptogenic area during the interictal state without referring to spikes.

During the last few years, NTSA has become a growing field of research. Within this physical–mathematical framework, methods are available that allow one to characterize highly complex dynamic systems (see ref. 9 for a comprehensive overview). Because of its versatility, NTSA already has gone beyond the physical sciences and is being applied successfully in a variety of disciplines, including neurology, epileptology, and psychiatry. In contrast to methods of analysis that rely solely on single interictal epileptiform events, spontaneous or induced, NTSA provides a means to analyze *integratively* long-lasting recordings of the brain's electric activity. Methods from the field of NTSA (e.g., the correlation dimension or the largest Lyapunov exponent) as well as other nonlinear measures provide additional and relevant information about the spatiotemporal dynamics of the primary epileptogenic area (10–14).

By extracting the so-called neuronal complexity loss L^* from intracranial EEG recordings of 20 epilepsy patients suffering from MTLE, we showed that L^* unequivocally lateralizes the primary epileptogenic area, even during *interictal* states (10). Estimates of the stability of this lateralizing power revealed that 30 minutes of *interictal* EEG is sufficient for a reliable delineation of the primary epileptogenic area (15). The neuronal complexity loss L^* also turned out to be helpful for investigating the influence of anticonvulsant drugs on the epileptogenic process (16) and estimating possible functional disturbances in mesiotemporal structures contralateral to the seizure focus (17). L^* was shown to bear potential capabilities of extracting features from EEG activity that can be regarded as long-lasting (up to 25 minutes) precursors of impending seizures (18,19). Moreover, preliminary findings in MTLE patients indicated that during specific verbal memory tasks, L^* indexes the spatiotemporal recruitment potency of neurons within or close to the primary epileptogenic area (20).

To date, nonlinear measures were applied mainly to MTLE. This is related to the fact that major computational problems arise in NE because the number of necessary sensoring electrodes greatly exceeds the number required for evaluation of MTLE. For example, in patients suffering from lesional NE, grid electrodes as well as supplementary strip electrodes often are implanted for delineation of the primary epileptogenic area (21). Recent accelerations of the time-consuming NTSA algorithms (22,23) now make diagnostic studies more feasible.

The following section presents the ability of NTSA methods to provide information about the localization and delineation of the primary epileptogenic area beyond that obtained from the spatial distribution of spikes, conventional spectral parameters of the EEG, or seizure origin. If, from these data, spatial information can be extracted that proves to be sufficiently independent of influencing factors such as changes of the state of vigilance or different levels of anticonvulsant medication, nonlinear measures can be expected to provide additional diagnostically relevant information in the assessment of patients for surgical intervention.

LOCALIZATION OF THE EPILEPTOGENIC AREA USING INTERICTAL ELECTROCORTICOGRAMS

As mentioned, the neuronal complexity loss L* allows a lateralization of the primary epileptogenic area in MTLE. Furthermore, spatiotemporal profiles of L* allow one to condense the information content of long-term intracranial EEG recordings in MTLE as well as in NE (15). Such profiles can reflect the information content of multichannel EEG recordings lasting up to 24 hours on a single sheet of paper. This synopsis allows an observer to rate interictal and periictal changes easily. Furthermore, alterations induced by different activation methods (e.g., hyperventilation or short-term narcoses) as well as by changes in the patients' state of vigilance (e.g., different sleep stages) can be assessed. An additional data compression is achieved by computing one average L* value for each electrode contact. Figure 24.1 represents typical findings obtained for the spatial distribution of L* in lesional NE. To date, L* has been evaluated in a group of 11 patients, all of whom were implanted with a subdural 64-contact grid electrode covering the lesion (21,24). In each case, an extended lesionectomy was performed on the basis of the results of presurgical evaluation. The postoperative seizure outcome was assessed over a follow-up of at least 1 year. As demonstrated in Fig. 24.1, on each grid electrode, regions with a high neuronal complexity loss L* (termed as **a**rea of **r**educed **c**omplexity =

ARC) could be identified. The overlap between the ARC and the resected area was highest in patients who became seizure free after resection and lowest when the patients' seizure status did not improve. Hence, L* maps provide information about the extent of the epileptogenic area, which is not achieved by conventional diagnosis during presurgical evaluation.

To ensure that L*-maps indeed contribute to the planning of a neurosurgical resection, the temporal stability of these ARCs over time is required. Different levels of vigilance are known to influence the EEG as well as derived measures (25,26). Figure 24.2A shows representative findings, indicating that although an overall increase of L* can be observed when the level of vigilance is lowered, a focal ARC still can be identified.

Another factor known to influence L* is the presence of anticonvulsant drugs. For the patient shown in Fig. 24.2A, data sets were recorded with two different blood levels of carbamazepine (Fig. 24.2B). Whereas the major ARC (associated with the lesion) remained almost constant when recordings were obtained with carbamazepine levels within the therapeutic range, a further, small ARC was unmasked when the level fell below the therapeutic range (<4 µg/mL). Analysis of spike latencies (Fig. 24.3) showed that the smaller ARC was caused by propagation phenomena.

FUNCTIONAL MAPPING OF ELOQUENT BRAIN AREAS

Apart from identification of the primary epileptogenic area, epilepsy surgery also requires an exact delineation of eloquent areas of the brain. Recent studies showed that non-invasive techniques such as fMRI can contribute to the localization of such areas prior to surgical intervention (27). To date, however, the gold standard for functional mapping is electric stimulation of critical areas prior to surgical intervention (2). Additional func-

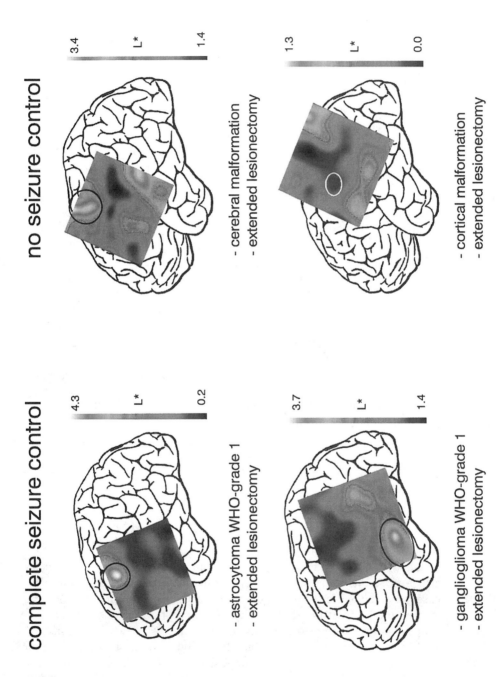

complete seizure control

4.3 — L* — 0.2

- astrocytoma WHO-grade 1
- extended lesionectomy

3.7 — L* — 1.4

- ganglioglioma WHO-grade 1
- extended lesionectomy

no seizure control

3.4 — L* — 1.4

- cerebral malformation
- extended lesionectomy

1.3 — L* — 0.0

- cortical malformation
- extended lesionectomy

FIG. 24.1. Two-dimensional plots of neuronal complexity loss L* (L*-maps). The scale was normalized for each map between maximum and minimum L*. Pixels between the contacts were interpolated using two-dimensional second-order spline functions. L*-maps were projected onto a schematic drawing of each patients' brain surface. *Circles* indicate area of resection.

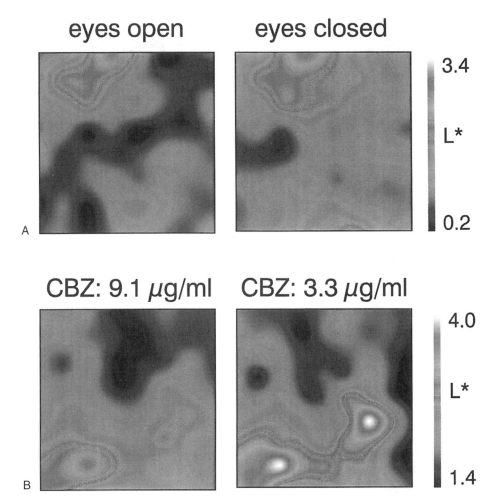

FIG. 24.2. A: L*-maps computed for two different ECoG data segments each lasting 5 minutes. During the first segment, the patient was facing a video camera; during the second segment, the patient was relaxed with the eyes closed. **B:** Same patient but computed from data sets recorded under two different blood levels of carbamazepine *(CBZ)*. Whereas the major ARC (associated with the lesion) remained almost constant, a further (small) ARC was unmasked when anticonvulsant medication fell below the therapeutic range (<4 µg/mL).

tional information can be obtained by using the neuronal complexity loss to identify eloquent areas. This is done by quantifying alterations of the *ongoing* ECoG during specific mental activation tasks. Figure 24.4 (right picture) exhibits an L*-map that was computed from 10-minute ECoG recording during rest (with the eyes opened) and compared with an L*-map computed from 10-minute ECoG recordings while the patient was reading aloud. In a circumscribed region, significant differences between the two data sets ($p < 10^{-7}$, Student's t test, two-tailed significance) can be identified. Electric stimulation of the corresponding electrode contacts was able to evoke a speech arrest.

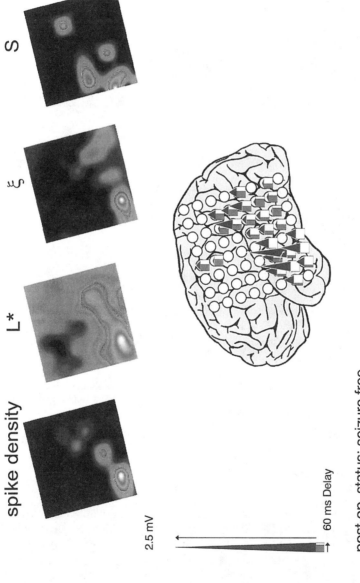

spike density   L*   ξ   S

2.5 mV

60 ms Delay

post-op. status: seizure-free

FIG. 24.3. Spike density, spike propagation time, and nonlinear measures (L*, ξ, S) indicating the same primary epileptogenic area on the temporal lobe.

322

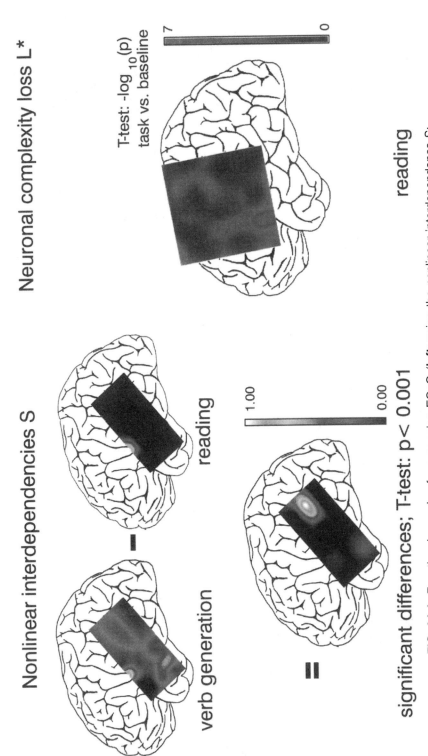

FIG. 24.4. Functional mapping from ongoing ECoG (**left:** using the nonlinear interdependence S; **right:** using L*).

EVALUATION OF POSSIBLE ADDITIONAL MESIOTEMPORAL FOCI IN NEOCORTICAL EPILEPSY

Because of the differences of histological structures, EEG signals generated in the hippocampal formation are not comparable to those generated in the neocortex. Thus, it is still an open question whether nonlinear measures extracted from these different signals reveal similar information about the spatiotemporal dynamics of the epileptogenic processes. In a group of patients suffering from lesional NE who were implanted with both subdural electrodes covering the lesion and intrahippocampal depth electrodes because of clinical hints for a mesiotemporal involvement, the neuronal complexity loss could be used as a prognostic factor for persisting mesiotemporal seizures after extended lesionectomies in the neocortex. A total of 20 patients in whom presurgical evaluation led to an extended lesionectomy were investigated. L* was computed from interictal ECoG/SEEG recordings for each contact of the implanted subdural strips, grids, and intrahippocampal depth electrodes. In 16 patients, the highest *neocortical*

L* was found at recording sites coinciding with the region of seizure onset; however, 11 of 20 patients exhibited a maximum L* throughout mesiotemporal recording sites. In this group, only one patient became seizure free after lesionectomy. In contrast, maximum L* was found at neocortical recording sites in the remaining nine patients, eight of whom became seizure free. The relationship between location of maximum L* and seizure outcome proved highly significant [chi-square, $p < 0.0004$ (28) (Fig. 24.5)]. Despite the histological differences between neocortex and hippocampus, L* seems to reveal commensurable information about the spatiotemporal dynamics of the epileptogenic process from both structures. Hence, L* can be used as an additional prognostic factor for persisting mesiotemporal seizures after extended neocortical lesionectomies.

SEIZURE PREDICTION

As mentioned, L* and other nonlinear measures allow the extraction of unequivocal alterations in the EEG up to 25 minutes before impending seizures originating in mesial tem-

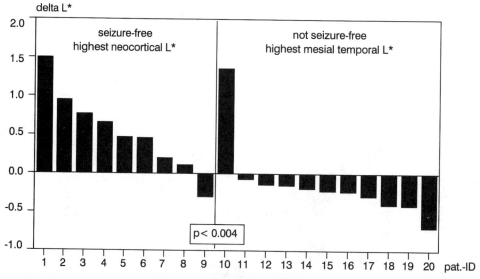

FIG. 24.5. Difference between maximum neocortical L* and maximum intrahippocampal L* in 20 patients with NE and clinical hints for MTLE. All patients underwent an extended lesionectomy. L* difference separates the two outcome groups significantly (two false allocations, chi-square: $p < 0.004$).

poral structures (18,19). These alterations are possibly caused by increasing synchronization phenomena within the primary epileptogenic area. Analogous findings in NE are hitherto less reliable, however. A possible reason might be that in MTLE the sensing electrode (i.e., the hippocampal depth electrode) is within the primary epileptogenic area. In contrast, because only a third of the neocortical neurons are located in gyri, subdural grid and strip electrodes at best cover portions of the primary epileptogenic area in NE.

Fraction of Nonlinear Determinism and Nonlinear Interdependence

Until now, most studies have been performed using measures like the largest Lyapunov exponent λ (a measure for the dependence of the development of a system from its initial conditions) or the neuronal complexity loss L*, which is based on the correlation dimension (29) and describes the number of degrees of freedom of an underlying dynamic. Two other measures from NTSA (describing additional and independent aspects of the underlying dynamic of a time series) are presently under investigation.

The *fraction of nonlinear determinism* (termed ξ) is based on the assumption that neurons in an epileptogenic tissue produce a more deterministic EEG, whereas the activity of a normal neuronal tissue can be expected to be of such a high complexity that it should hardly be separable from random noise. Another measure, the *nonlinear interdependence* (termed S) is able to detect interactions between EEG signals, not restricted to spectral similarities as known from common cross-correlation analyses. Preliminary findings concerning the localization of the primary epileptogenic area are described in Fig. 24.6.

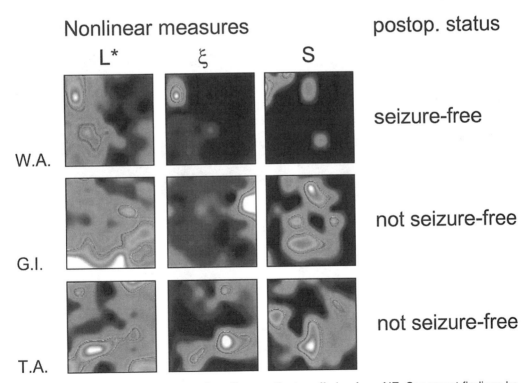

FIG. 24.6. Nonlinear measure maps from three patients suffering from NE. Congruent findings between nonlinear measures were found only in the patient who became seizure free, in contrast to the two patients with poor seizure outcome.

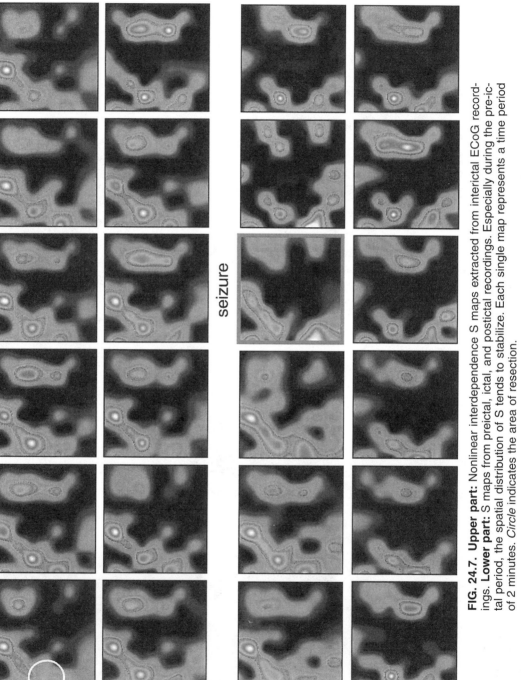

seizure

FIG. 24.7. Upper part: Nonlinear interdependence S maps extracted from interictal ECoG recordings. **Lower part:** S maps from preictal, ictal, and postictal recordings. Especially during the pre-ictal period, the spatial distribution of S tends to stabilize. Each single map represents a time period of 2 minutes. *Circle* indicates the area of resection.

Concordant findings of the three measures (L*, ξ, and S) can indicate a good surgical outcome, whereas discordant findings seem to indicate that seizures may persist postoperatively. The structure of nonlinear interdependencies in particular seems to reorganize itself in NE, about 10 minutes prior to an impending seizure (Fig. 24.7). Furthermore, functional mapping using differential plots between different mental tasks, for example, to localize Wernicke's area, becomes possible (Fig. 24.4, left).

COMPARISON OF NTSA AND "CONVENTIONAL" ANALYSIS OF INTERICTAL ELECTROENCEPHALOGRAPHY

To prove that L*- as well as ξ- and S-maps provide additional information, a comparison with conventional EEG measures was performed. In Figs. 24.3 and 24.8, L*, ξ, and S maps as well as *spike densities* (7) of three patients with a seizure-free outcome are shown. In all three patients, the major ARC is within the resected area; however, only in the patient shown in Fig. 24.3 did the maximum spike density match the major ARC. In the corresponding data set, a total of 2,310 spikes were detected within a time frame of 20 minutes. In another data set of the same patient, no spikes were detected. Nonetheless, the area of reduced complexity was nearly identical as compared to the first epoch. In conclusion, the findings derived from L* maps (as well as ξ and S maps) are independent of the occurrence of spikes and remain stable even when spike foci are variable and misleading.

It is still an open question whether nonlinear measures provide information beyond what is obtained from linear measures (30–32). However, it has been demonstrated that analysis of nonlinearity provides information about the spatial distribution of the primary epileptogenic area when one is analyzing intracranial recordings of epilepsy patients (13,14). Our present results confirm these findings. A comparison with EEG bands and "surrogate data" (33,34) revealed that the neuronal complexity loss L* as well as ξ and S extract information from ECoG signals different from linear measures, i.e., *power spectrum related properties* (Fig. 24.9).

CONCLUSION

In NE, presurgical evaluation aims to design a surgical intervention that achieves complete freedom of seizures while keeping neurological deficits as small as possible. Because epilepsy is known to be a *functional* disorder, possibly induced by *structural* alterations, the current gold-standard for identifying the primary epileptogenic area is to record the patients' spontaneous seizures. Even the interictal data recorded during the invasive phase of presurgical evaluation can be used to delineate epileptogenic areas. In contrast to conventional analysis methods (e.g., spike densities or measures derived from the power spectrum), nonlinear time series analyses like L* can be used to condense long-term recordings of multicontact electrodes into one single value per contact, representing a measure of the degree of epileptiform activity in the interictal EEG at each recording site. The integrative nonlinear measures of local brain electric activity can provide additional information. This information can be used as a diagnostic indicator for a possible persistence of an epileptogenic area (e.g., located in mesial temporal structures) after resection of a neocortical lesion. Furthermore, differential analyses between different mental states using nonlinear measures can contribute to functional mapping of eloquent brain areas and thus corroborate the information obtained by conventional techniques like electrical stimulation.

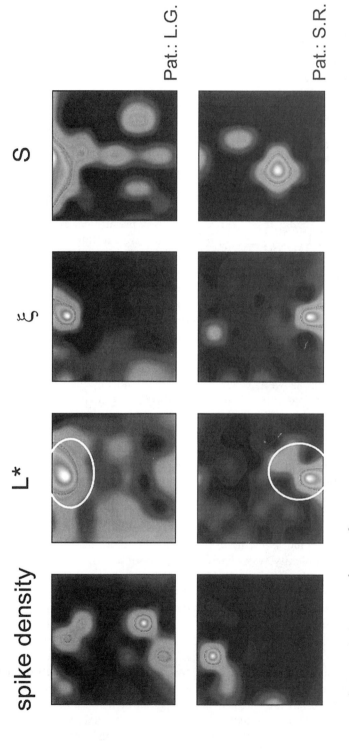

FIG. 24.8. Misleading spike foci in two patients with NE who became seizure free after extended lesionectomy within the marked area (*white circle*). Nonlinear measures indicate the epileptogenic zone.

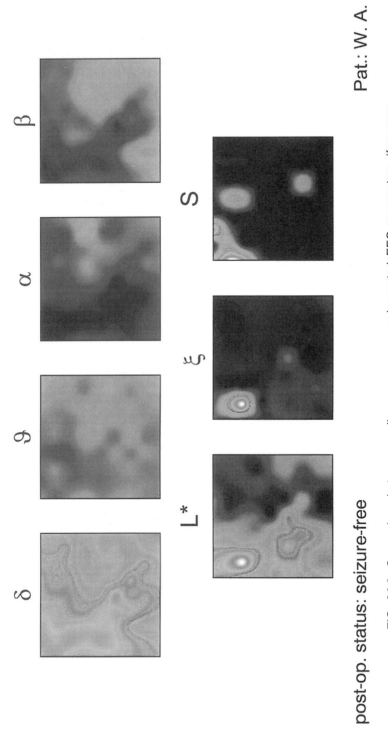

post-op. status: seizure-free   Pat.: W. A.

FIG. 24.9. Comparison between nonlinear measures and spectral EEG parameters (frequency bands in Hz: delta, 0.1–4; theta, 4–8; alpha, 8–13; beta, 13–30).

329

ACKNOWLEDGMENTS

We thank our neurosurgical colleagues J. Schramm, J. Zentner, D. Van Roost, and E. Behrens, who implanted the intracranial electrodes. This study was supported by the Deutsche Forschungsgemeinschaft (grant no. EL122/3-1).

REFERENCES

1. Gloor P. Mesial temporal sclerosis: historical background and an overview from modern perspective. In: Lüders HO, ed. *Epilepsy surgery.* New York: Raven Press, 1991:689–703.
2. Lüders HO, Awad I. Conceptual considerations. In: Lüders HO, ed. *Epilepsy surgery.* New York: Raven Press, 1991:51–62.
3. Wieser HG. Epilepsy surgery. *Baillieres Clin Neurol* 1996;5:849–875.
4. Engel J Jr, Van Ness PC, Rasmussen TB, et al. Outcome with respect to epileptic seizures. In: Engel J Jr, ed. *Surgical treatment of the epilepsies,* 2nd ed. New York: Raven Press, 1993:609–622.
5. Gotman J, Wang LY. State dependent spike detection: concepts and preliminary results. *Electroencephalogr Clin Neurophysiol* 1991;81:11–19.
6. Gotman J, Wang LY. State dependent spike detection: validation. *Electroencephalogr Clin Neurophysiol* 1992;83: 12–18.
7. Dümpelmann M, Elger CE. Automatic detection of epileptiform spikes in the electrocorticogram: a comparison of two algorithms. *Seizure* 1998;7:145–152.
8. Tran TA, Spencer SS, Javidan M, et al. Significance of spikes recorded on intraoperative electrocorticography in patients with brain tumor and epilepsy. *Epilepsia* 1997;38:1132–1139.
9. Kantz H, Schreiber T. *Nonlinear time series analysis.* Cambridge: Cambridge University Press, 1997.
10. Iasemidis LD, Sackellares JC, Zaveri HP, et al. Phase space topography and the Lyapunov exponent of electrocorticograms in partial seizures. *Brain Topogr* 1990;2:187–201.
11. Lehnertz K, Elger CE. Spatio–temporal dynamics of the primary epileptogenic area in temporal lobe epilepsy characterized by neuronal complexity loss. *Electroencephalogr Clin Neurophysiol* 1995;95:108–117.
12. van der Heyden MJ, Diks C, Pijn JP, et al. Time reversability of intracranial human EEG recordings in mesial temporal lobe epilepsy. *Phys Rev A* 1996; 216:283–288.
13. Pijn JP, Velis DN, van der Heyden MJ, et al. Nonlinear dynamics of epileptic seizures on basis of intracranial EEG recordings. *Brain Topogr* 1997;9:249–270.
14. Casdagli MC, Iasemidis LD, Savit RS, et al. Nonlinearity in invasive EEG recordings from patients with temporal lobe epilepsy. *Electroencephalogr Clin Neurophysiol* 1997;102:98–105.
15. Lehnertz K, Widman G, Elger CE. Spatio–temporal neuronal complexity loss: a condensed information content of long-term intracranial EEG recordings. *Epilepsia* 1997;38(Suppl 8):63(abst).
16. Lehnertz K, Elger CE. Neuronal complexity loss in temporal lobe epilepsy: effects of carbamazepine on the dynamics of the epileptogenic focus. *Electroencephalogr Clin Neurophysiol* 1997;103:376–380.
17. Lehnertz K, Elger CE. Neuronal complexity loss of the contralateral hippocampus in temporal lobe epilepsy: a possible indicator for secondary epileptogenesis. *Epilepsia* 1995;36(Suppl 4):21(abst).
18. Lehnertz K, Elger CE. Can epileptic seizures be predicted? evidence from nonlinear time series analysis of brain electrical activity. *Phys Rev Lett* 1998;80: 5019–5022.
19. Elger CE, Lehnertz K. Seizure prediction by nonlinear time series analysis of brain electrical activity. *Eur J Neurosci* 1998;10:786–789.
20. Lehnertz K, Weber B, Helmstaedter C, et al. Alterations in neuronal complexity during verbal memory tasks index recruitment potency in temporo–mesial structures. *Epilepsia* 1997;38(Suppl 3):238(abst).
21. Appendix II: Presurgical evaluation protocols. In: Engel J Jr, ed. *Surgical treatment of the epilepsies,* 2nd ed. New York: Raven Press, 1993:740–742.
22. Widman G, Lehnertz K, Elger CE. CPLXMON, a system for real-time, on-line monitoring of neuronal complexity loss in the ECoG of patients with temporal lobe epilepsy. *Epilepsia* 1995;36(Suppl 4):5(abst).
23. Widman G, Lehnertz K, Jansen P, et al. A fast general purpose algorithm for the computation of auto- and cross-correlation integrals from single channel data. *Physica D* 1998;121:65–74.
24. Widman G, Lehnertz K, Elger CE. Spatio–temporal distribution of neuronal complexity loss in neocortical epilepsy. *Epilepsia* 1997;38(Suppl 3):46(abst).
25. Röschke J, Aldenhoff JB. A nonlinear approach to brain function: deterministic chaos and sleep EEG. *Sleep* 1992;15:95–101.
26. Pradhan N, Sadasivan PK, Chatterji S, et al. Patterns of attractor dimensions of sleep EEG. *Comput Biol Med* 1995;25:455–462.
27. Duncan JS. Imaging and epilepsy. *Brain* 1997;120: 339–377.
28. Widman G, Elger CE, Lehnertz K. Neuronal complexity loss in lesional neocortical epilepsy: estimating the temporo–mesial involvement in the epileptogenic process. *Epilepsia* 1997;38(Suppl 8):71(abst).
29. Grassberger P, Procaccia I. Measuring the strangeness of strange attractors. *Physica D* 1983;9:189–208.
30. Pijn JP, Van Neerven J, Noest A, et al. Chaos or noise in EEG signals: dependence on state and brain site. *Electroencephalogr Clin Neurophysiol* 1991;79: 371–381.
31. Palus M. Nonlinearity in normal human EEG: cycles, temporal asymmetry, nonstationarity, and randomness, not chaos. *Biol Cybern* 1996;75:389–396.
32. Theiler J, Rapp PE. Re-examination of the evidence for low-dimensional, nonlinear structure in the human electroencephalogram. *Electroencephalogr Clin Neurophysiol* 1996;98:213–222.
33. Theiler J, Eubank S, Longtin A, et al. Testing for nonlinearity in time series: the method of surrogate data. *Physica D* 1992;58:77–92.
34. Schreiber T, Schmitz A. Improved surrogate data for nonlinearity tests. *Phys Rev Lett* 1996;77:635–638.

Neocortical Epilepsies.
Advances in Neurology, Vol. 84,
edited by P.D. Williamson, A.M. Siegel,
D.W. Roberts, V.M. Thadani, and M.S. Gazzaniga.
Lippincott Williams & Wilkins, Philadelphia © 2000.

25

Preoperative Functional Mapping Using Intracranial EEG Activation Methods

T.M. Darcey, *H.C. Hughes, H.I. Barkan, and A.J. Saykin

Dartmouth–Hitchcock Medical Center, Lebanon, New Hampshire 03756;
*Department of Psychological and Brain Sciences, Dartmouth College,
Hanover, New Hampshire 03755

In the context of epilepsy surgery, preoperative functional mapping involves the localization of cortical functions to ensure that the surgical plan spares critical but individually variable functional areas while allowing maximal resection of the seizure focus. This is especially important in cases of suspected neocortical epilepsy, which may, for instance, impinge on language or motor areas and is also useful for predicting postoperative deficits of a less profound, but potentially significant, nature. The "gold standard" for preoperative localization of cortical functions is electrical stimulation, which has been widely used both in the operating room and at the bedside via implanted electrode grids (1–4). Electrical stimulation has the advantage of having established protocols for sensorimotor and language mapping, and there is a large database of stimulation findings and surgical effects. Most users of this technique are well aware of its practical and interpretive limitations, including the laborious nature of obtaining unequivocal mapping data, the limited number of specific functions that can be practically tested for, and the risk of producing afterdischarges or seizures that nullify the results and delay the testing. In addition, no well-established protocols exist for testing other than sensorimotor and language functions, and uncertainties remain as to the localization of stimulation current owing to volume conduction.

Emerging alternatives to electric stimulation for functional mapping (reviewed in ref. 5) are positron emission tomography (PET), functional magnetic resonance imaging (fMRI), electroencephalographic (EEG) activation methods, and new methods based on magnetic and optical technologies [magnetoencephalography (MEG), transcranial magnetic stimulation, intrinsic optical imaging of exposed brain, and transcranial monitoring using near infrared light]. Although echo-planar fMRI has a great deal of promise for preoperative functional localization in that it is completely noninvasive and capable of sampling the whole brain, it has a number of disadvantages, including the limited number of brain functions that can practically be tested for, the risk of injury if a seizure occurs in the magnet, and questions (6) as to its present spatial accuracy for surgical planning. In patients with invasively placed grid electrodes, EEG-based activation methods, including event-related potentials (ERPs) and event-related spectra (ERS), are a viable alternative or adjunct to electric stimulation for functional localization (7). Advantages of the EEG-based approaches are their efficiency (all electrodes can be tested at once for each task or stimulus condition), their superior time resolution (on the order of milliseconds), the negligible risk of inducing seizures, and the simplicity of the equipment required (EEG activation testing can be performed in parallel with video/EEG monitoring and using the same EEG equipment). EEG activation techniques also have the advantage that functional testing may be tailored to the results of seizure recording and electric stimulation and then used to plan a resection that will be performed at the time the electrodes are removed (standard procedure at many centers using subdural grid implantation for the diagnosis of medically intractable neocortical epilepsies).

EEG ACTIVATION METHODS

Although more sophisticated signal processing methods may be applied, ERPs generally are obtained by synchronous, time-domain averaging of the EEG with respect to the repeated occurrence of a stimulus (e.g., a shock to the median nerve or checkerboard-pattern reversal) or a motor response (e.g., a button press to a target stimulus). Typically, digital filtering and artifact rejection also are applied. The averaging process enhances the portion of the EEG that is phase-locked to the stimulus or response relative to the background EEG (or "noise") that is unrelated. The signal-to-noise ratio (SNR) improvement will be proportional to the square root of the number of trials averaged, assuming that the background EEG arises from a gaussian random process. In practical terms, the latter condition is never met, the number of trials needed to achieve a particular SNR is greater, and there is a point at which the SNR is not improved by additional trials. In the case of intracranial recording, the EEG is virtually uncontaminated by noise and artifacts common to scalp recording such as EMG, eye blinks, and eye movements, and the number of trials needed to obtain high-quality intracranial ERPs is much less than the number needed for comparable scalp ERPs. Intracranial ERPs in epilepsy patients may be substantially contaminated by the epileptiform discharges (spikes and sharp waves) that accompany the seizure disorder, however, and

trials containing these discharges must be eliminated. It is also a major challenge to identify and localize ERPs that are specific to definable cortical functions.

Whereas ERPs assume that there is a fixed phase relationship or timing between stimulus and EEG activation, it is clear that there is no biologic requirement that there be a precise time relationship between the delivery of a stimulus and the evoked brain response, especially at higher cognitive levels. It is reasonable to expect synchronization to decrease as more synapses are traversed. This is reflected in the ERP literature and clinical applications, in which responses from early stages of sensory representation predominate (8). There is clear evidence of phase loss in responses that exceed 200 ms, and components in this latency range are typically slow waves with durations on the order of hundreds of milliseconds, the prime example being the P300 response. The logical approach to examining brain responses without requiring phase synchronization is to analyze the data in the frequency domain using spectral methods, which discard phase and assess the power as a function of frequency. The ERS approach was pioneered by Pfurtscheller and colleagues (9–11) for scalp EEG studies of cognitive processing and was used by Crone and colleagues (12) (see Chapter 26) for intracranial EEG studies of motor and language activation tasks. In its simplest form, one uses windowed fast Fourier transform (FFT) measures to compute average prestimulus and poststimulus power spectra in each recording channel. These measurements then can be assessed for stimulus- or task-related spectral changes, for example, alpha-band desynchronization (less alpha-band power following stimulus) or synchronization (more alpha-band power following stimulus). Within the limits of time-frequency resolution inherent to FFT-based spectral analysis, one can also compute a peristimulus time sequence of average spectra to assess for dynamic changes over time.

Activation paradigms may be categorized as either discrete trial or block-design approaches. Discrete or single-trial activation typically has been used for EEG activation and more recently for fMRI activation (13). It involves the presentation of sequences of identical or varying discrete stimuli or tasks. Examples of discrete trial activation would be the median nerve sensory-evoked potential (SEP), checkerboard-pattern reversal visual-evoked potential (VEP), auditory oddball P300, and self-paced voluntary movement. Discrete trial activation data can be analyzed using either time-domain averaging or frequency domain spectral methods, and such paradigms are highly flexible in that they can be used to study cognitive tasks involving stimulus categorization, decision making, and selective attention. Block design, continuous performance, or steady-state paradigms typically have been used for fMRI activation studies, but they also have been used for EEG activation purposes. Block designs consist of alternating or interleaved blocks of repetitive task performance or stimulation, examples of which would be alternating 30-second blocks of left and right finger tapping, sinusoidally modulated checkerboard-pattern reversal, and alternating blocks of words to be remembered or to be attended to passively. Block-design experiments typically are analyzed using frequency-domain methods with or without taking phase into account and looking for significant differences between conditions. Block designs are conceptually simple and often give robust results, but they are limited to the study of steady-state differences between repetitive conditions.

The following sections present examples of intracranial EEG-based localization of sensorimotor and primary visual areas and from less conventional activation tasks to illustrate the potential of the EEG activation approach for mapping a wide variety of sensory and cognitive functions preoperatively. All the EEG data for these analyses were obtained by using a standard low-bandwidth video/EEG telemetry system (Telefactor Corporation Beehive System with 70-Hz antialiasing, 200-Hz sampling) at the bedside concurrent with seizure monitoring and analyzed offline using the Matlab (The Mathworks, Inc.) data analysis and visualization package.

EEG-based Sensorimotor Localization

Localization of the sensorimotor strip is often important in cases of neocortical epilepsy involving the frontal or parietal lobe, and techniques exist for localizing both the sensory and motor representations of different portions of the body. The most common approach (14–17) uses the SEP, which is elicited by repetitive shocks or mechanical stimulation of the peripheral nerve, for example, the median, tibial, or trigeminal nerve, and certain early and middle latency cortical responses can be used to localize the S1 representation. From this, localization of the central or rolandic sulcus can be determined and the posterior boundary of the motor-strip or M1 inferred. More direct approaches to motor-strip localization are the Bereitschaftspotential (18,19), which is a negative slow potential preceding self-paced voluntary movement, and α or β band desynchronization, which is associated with sustained muscle contractions (7) (see Chapter 26). Here we illustrate a simplified method that we developed for somatosensory localization based on low-bandwidth SEPs and that does not rely on the standard approach of analyzing specific components in the 20- to 30-ms range that in any case are not resolved completely at low bandwidth. Instead, we assess the overall localization of somatosensory activation in the first 200 ms poststimulus, which relies on the fact that several early and midlatency components of the SEP in the awake patient colocalize in the postcentral somatosensory cortex (15,16,20). We confirmed the validity of this approach by comparison with high-bandwidth commercial ERP recording equipment (Nicolet Viking) and the results of sensorimotor mapping by electric stimulation.

Figure 25.1 summarizes right median nerve SEP and electric stimulation findings involving the right hand on a 4 × 8 subdural grid assembly (POG) straddling the left sensorimotor strip. The approach we used here was to obtain EEG recordings concurrent with 100 median-nerve stimuli and then analyze these recordings over the first 200 ms poststimulus for each

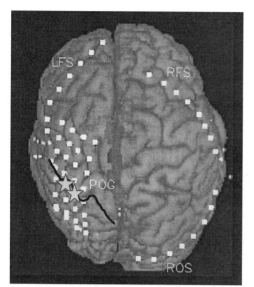
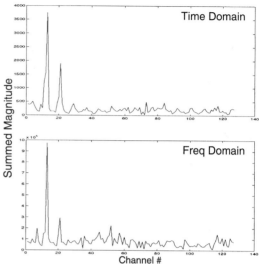

FIG. 25.1. Example of intracranial EEG-based sensorimotor localization in a patient based on low-bandwidth recordings from 127 subdural electrodes, including a 4 × 8 grid assembly over the left frontoparietal convexity. **Left:** Right median nerve SEP and electrical stimulation findings at grid contacts superimposed on cortical surface renderings. **Right:** Results of time and frequency bin summation (see text) for each of 127 contacts and illustrate concentrated response at two contacts indicated by stars and just posterior to the central sulcus. Electrical stimulation of contacts just anterior to these elicited right hand finger movement, whereas contacts just posterior elicited right hand numbness. The electrode visualizations shown in this and subsequent figures are based on preimplant high-resolution MRI corregistered with electrode contacts extracted from postimplant CT (21).

recording channel (127 subdural contacts versus an extracranial reference in this case). Both time and frequency domain results are shown in Fig. 25.1, including time (over 40 time samples of average poststimulus ERP) and frequency (over all frequencies of average poststimulus ERS) bin summation for each of the 127 recording channels. This illustrates the finding in this case that the right-hand somatosensory activation is concentrated in two electrode sites over the left hemisphere just posterior to the central sulcus, and in agreement with the results of electric stimulation. The fact that the time and frequency domain results are in close agreement with one another, indicates that the somatosensory response is highly synchronous with the stimulus in this time range.

EEG-based Visual Area Localization

In the context of presurgical mapping, localization of visual functions is important for predicting field cuts and other more specific visual deficits when occipital or parietal surgeries are contemplated. The checkerboard-pattern reversal VEP is widely used in clinical neurophysiology for the assessment (via latency and amplitude norms) of visual system integrity when demyelination or other lesions of the visual pathways are suspected (8). Babb et al. (22) used hippocampally recorded, short-latency VEPs to predict visual-field deficits resulting from compromise of the geniculostriate pathway in the course of temporal lobectomy. Although it is generally agreed that pattern reversal VEP components in the 70- to 150-ms range have their origin in V1, V2, and perhaps other extrastriate areas, there is unresolved controversy about the details. In fact, it is likely that multiple areas are active with significant spatiotemporal overlap. Despite these issues, pattern stimuli elicit highly reproducible, retinotopically organized, and focal responses in the calcarine and extracalcarine occipital lobe, and that are useful for the localization of V1, V2, and possibly other extrastriate visual areas (23). It is also the case that the components of VEPs are well resolved with the low-bandwidth EEG system used for seizure monitoring.

Figure 25.2 illustrates upper and lower right-quadrant pattern reversal VEPs recorded from a patient with 95 electrodes sampling the left parietal and occipital lobes, including the left mesial occipital lobe in the vicinity of the calcarine sulcus. In this case, highly focal responses were found on electrodes near the calcarine sulcus in the vicinity of the occipital pole at 90-ms latency and corresponding to points where simple visual phosphenes were elicited by electric stimulation. In patients in whom we have recorded from the lateral and mesial occipital pole, we observed spatially distinct but temporally overlapping components that appear to involve V1 and V2. These responses are similarly evident in the frequency domain as focal desynchronization in the α band. Although not illustrated here, we also had considerable success in recording visual responses specific to words, motion, color, and other visual submodalities. In some cases, particularly in higher cognitive tasks, these responses are best seen using frequency domain analysis. Because it has been estimated (24) that up to 60% of the neocortex is involved in vision at some level, the development of tests for mapping areas involved in specialized visual submodalities and visually

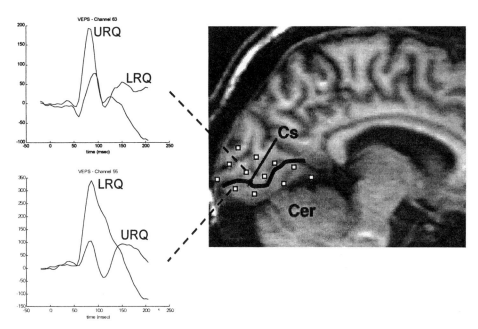

FIG. 25.2. Partial-field checkerboard-pattern reversal VEPs showing primary visual cortical responses in a patient based on intracranial EEG recordings from 95 subdural electrodes, including a 3 × 8 grid assembly covering the left mesial and basal occipital lobe. Highly focal responses with retinotopic dependence were recorded in the vicinity of the calcarine sulcus near the occipital pole, where simple visual phosphenes were elicited by electrical stimulation. *URQ,* response to upper right quadrant stimulation; *LRQ,* response to lower right quadrant stimulation; *Cs,* calcarine sulcus.

mediated cognitive functions has obvious clinical importance for the prediction of deficits resulting from parietal, temporal, and frontal lobe as well as occipital lobe resections.

EEG-based Language Area Localization

The mapping of eloquent brain areas, that is, Brocca's and Wernicke's areas, is often critical when resection is contemplated in the dominant hemisphere, especially because these areas are highly variable across patients (4,25). Typically, electrical stimulation is used for this purpose, with Broca's area identified by induced disruption of motor speech output (e.g., speech arrest when the patient is asked to count) and with Wernicke's area localized by induced errors in comprehension (e.g., paraphasic errors in visual naming). A basal temporal speech area also has been identified and is discussed in the literature (26). Promising approaches for EEG-based localization of speech areas include repetitive motor speech for Broca's area identification (e.g., by triggering off a voice-activated microphone) and visually mediated tasks involving naming or reading for Wernicke's and Broca's area identification (27) (see Chapter 26, our unpublished results). The latter is best analyzed using frequency-domain techniques because one cannot assume precise timing between item presentation and language area responses. Here we present a simple auditory technique that appears to localize auditory association cortex in the posterior perisylvian area overlapping Wernicke's area and to predict areas that produce disruption of speech comprehension when stimulated electrically. This approach is based on the analysis of middle-latency components elicited by the auditory oddball paradigm, which involves listening to sequences of tones differing in frequency and probability. These responses are distinct from primary auditory responses that might be recorded from within the sylvian fissure.

The simplest version of the paradigm would be a randomized sequence of tone bursts with 80% of the tones at 1,000 Hz and 20% at 1,200 Hz, with the patient either listening passively or counting the less frequent tones (this does not seem to matter for the purpose of localizing auditory association cortex). Sites in the dominant hemisphere that give a significantly larger response to the infrequent tone in the 150- to 250-ms range appear to be closely correlated with sites that produce naming deficits when stimulated electrically. This concept is illustrated in Fig. 25.3, which shows auditory oddball responses and electric stimulation findings in a patient with grid electrodes placed over the dominant left hemisphere.

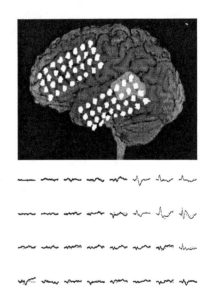

FIG. 25.3. Auditory oddball responses showing auditory association cortical responses in a patient based on intracranial EEG recordings from 72 electrode contacts. Responses *(solid curves)* to rare (1,200 Hz, $p = 0.2$) tones are overplotted on responses *(dashed curves)* to frequent (1,000 Hz, $p = 0.8$) tones for a 4×8 subdural grid assembly covering the dominant left temporal lobe. *Shaded areas* indicate where there was a significant difference between the two responses at intermediate latencies (150–250 ms poststimulus) and where visual naming was disrupted by electrical stimulation.

EEG-based Assessment of Medial Temporal Lobe Function

In cases of suspected neocortical temporal lobe epilepsy, there is often a question of whether the medial temporal lobe is involved in the seizure disorder and should be included in the therapeutic resection. To this end, the invasive study often includes electrodes in the hippocampal formation. In this context, another potentially useful application of the auditory oddball paradigm is to examine the task-dependent potentials that may be recorded from the hippocampus. In previous studies (28,29), it has been demonstrated that large, slow-wave responses may occur in the hippocampus bilaterally when the patient is asked to count the less frequent tone. This effect is modality nonspecific because it also can be observed with similarly designed visual, somatic paradigms and omit oddball paradigms. It also has been suggested (30–32) that significant hippocampal asymmetries or the absence of these responses in one hippocampus correlates well with hippocampal pathology and seizure onset. We are pursuing the utility of this test for

assessing hippocampal dysfunction and routinely obtain task-dependent oddball responses when the implant includes the hippocampus.

Figure 25.4 shows task-dependent hippocampal responses in a patient with bilateral hippocampal depth electrodes and asymmetric hippocampal slow waves and correlating well with lateralization of seizure onset.

EEG-based Assessment of Memory Function

The possible compromise of memory function is a major concern when surgery is contemplated. Although historically the intracarotid amytal or Wada test has been relied on to assess for potential memory deficits, this test is crude in that it can only indicate whether the unoperated hemisphere *could* support memory functions that *might* be compromised by nonspecific surgery in the contralateral hemisphere. Therefore, much effort has been put into the development and validation of more specific tests for localizing

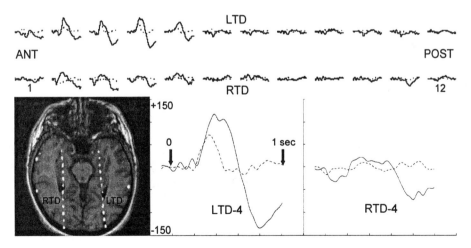

FIG. 25.4. Task-dependent auditory oddball responses recorded bilaterally from 12-contact temporal–occipital depth electrodes with contacts along the length of the hippocampal formation showing marked asymmetry of hippocampal slow-wave response with greatly diminished responses in the affected right hemisphere.

memory functions. This is particularly evident in the PET and fMRI literature. We have begun to investigate EEG-based localization of memory functions by using paradigms that are being used for ongoing parallel fMRI studies and thus far have focused on two relatively simple tasks.

The first (Fig. 25.5) is a block-design memory-encoding task consisting of eight alternating 30-second intervals in which the patient is asked to remember or to listen passively to a spoken word list for subsequent retrieval (i.e., the patient is asked to pick words from a list after testing). Difference spectra then are computed between the "listen and remember" conditions and also with respect to a rest condition. In comparing the "remember" with the "listen" condition, we found a number of band-specific left versus right hippocampal asymmetries in addition to focal α-band de-synchronization in the "remember" relative to the "listen" condition in the posterior superior temporal gyrus (Fig. 25.5), which is probably indicative of the involvement of these areas in memory encoding.

The second task (Fig. 25.6) with which we have been working is a single trial design memory retrieval task in which the patient listened to a 50-word list, including ten memorized words (learned 1 hour before) and 40 novel words. These data were analyzed by computing average difference spectra between the poststimulus and prestimulus intervals for each class of words. In this case, we found marked left–right asymmetries between both mesial and lateral temporal lobe structures for the memorized words compared with the novel words, which we believe indicates differential involvement of these structures in memory retrieval as

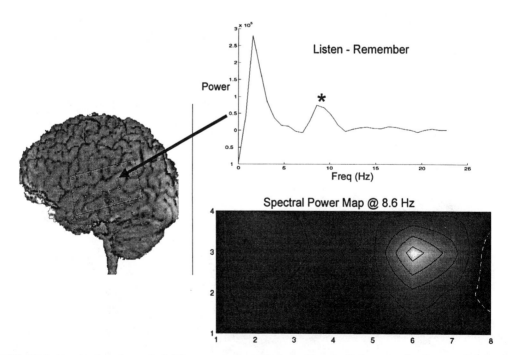

FIG. 25.5. Focal α-band spectral differences measured over the posterior superior temporal gyrus in a patient with a 4 × 8 subdural electrode grid placed over the dominant left temporal lobe. In this case, spectral analysis was applied to EEG from a block design in which the patient was asked either to remember (encode in memory) or listen to a block of spoken words.

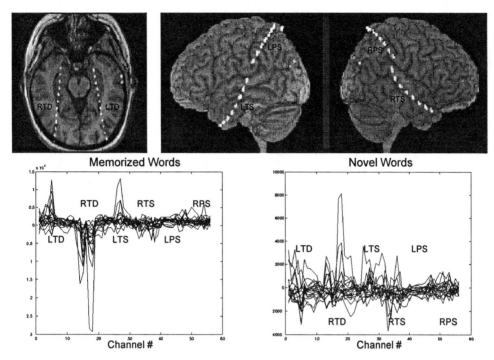

FIG. 25.6. Spectral analysis of subdural and depth electrode EEG recorded in two conditions of a single trial paradigm in which the patient listened to a sequence of spoken words that were previously memorized or not, showing dramatic medial and lateral temporal lobe asymmetries between the two conditions in multiple frequency bins up to 20 Hz.

opposed to encoding. Although we have yet to establish the generality and utility of these memory-related findings, they demonstrate the possibilities for obtaining useful localization of specific memory-related functions using EEG-activation methods.

CONCLUSION

Intracranial EEG activation methods show considerable promise as an alternative or adjunct to functional mapping by electric stimulation due to their efficiency, superior time resolution, safety, and technical simplicity. A major but surmountable obstacle to their acceptance for routine use is the need for a sufficient database of activation findings, confirmed by electrical stimulation and functional outcome following surgery to validate specific tests. No doubt, additional valida-

tion data could be obtained from fMRI activation studies using the same stimuli and tasks as those used for EEG activation. As with scalp EEG, the analysis of intracranial EEG also requires attention to issues of field analysis and source localization because volume currents may reach the recording electrodes from distant sites. Although these problems can be mitigated somewhat by analyzing the EEG data by using closely spaced bipolar or laplacian derivations (33), a more general approach would involve quantitative source localization procedures such as those that have been developed for the localization of equivalent dipoles sources from scalp-recorded EEG (32) (see Chapters 22, 27, and 28). Further, although intracranial EEG activation generally has exceptionally favorable SNR characteristics, consideration must be given to statistical issues and the appropriate quantification of EEG activation data, similar to the statistical parametric mapping approaches that have been developed for the quantification of fMRI activation data (35). Finally, it may be hoped that tests that are validated by intracranial EEG and fMRI activation mapping eventually could be done with scalp EEG recording and analyzed using quantitative source localization techniques to provide noninvasive functional localization in epilepsy surgery candidates.

ACKNOWLEDGMENTS

Supported by NIH NS17778.

REFERENCES

1. Penfield W, Jasper H. *Epilepsy and the functional anatomy of the brain.* Boston: Little, Brown, 1954.
2. Ojemann GA. Brain organization for language from the perspective of electrical stimulation mapping. *Behav Brain Sci* 1983;2:189–230.
3. Uematsu S, Roberts DW, Lesser R, et al. Motor and sensory cortex in humans—topography studied with chronic subdural stimulation. *Neurosurgery* 1992;31:59–72.
4. Lesser R, Gordon B, Uematsu S. Electrical-stimulation and language. *J Clin Neurophysiol* 1994;11:191–204.
5. Toga AW, Mazziotta JC, eds. *Brain mapping: the methods.* San Diego: Academic Press, 1996:471.
6. Cohen MS. Rapid MRI and functional applications. In: Toga AW, Mazziotta JC, eds. *Brain mapping: the methods.* San Diego: Academic Press, 1996:223–255.
7. Lesser RP, Arroyo S, Crone N, et al. Motor and sensory mapping of the frontal and occipital lobes. *Epilepsia* 1998;39(Suppl):569–580.
8. Chiappa KH. *Evoked potentials in clinical medicine.* New York: Raven Press, 1983.
9. Pfurtscheller G, Aranibar A. Evaluation of event-related desynchronization (ERD) preceding and following voluntary self-paced movement. *Electroencephalogr Clin Neurophysiol* 1979;46:138–146.
10. Pfurtscheller G. Functional topography during sensorimotor activation studied with event-related desynchronization mapping. *J Clin Neurophysiol* 1989;6:75–84.
11. Pfurtscheller G, Klimesch W. Event-related desynchronization during motor behavior and visual information processing. In: Brunia CHM, Mulder G, Verbaten MN, eds. *Event-related brain research.* New York: Elsevier, 1991:58–65.
12. Crone NE, Lesser RP, Kraus GL, et al. Topographic mapping of human sensorimotor cortex with electrocortical spectra. *Epilepsia* 1993;34:122–123.
13. Friston KJ, Fletcher P, Josephs O, et al. Event-related fMRI: characterizing differential responses. *Neuroimage* 1998;7:30–40.
14. Wood CC, Spencer DD, Allison T, et al. Localization of human sensorimotor cortex during surgery by cortical surface recording of somatosensory evoked-potentials. *J Neurosurg* 1988;68:99–111.
15. Allison T, McCarthy G, Wood CC, et al. Human cortical potentials evoked by stimulation of the median nerve. I. Cytoarchitectonic areas generating short-latency activity. *J Neurophysiol* 1989b;62:694–710.
16. Allison T, McCarthy G, Wood CC, et al. Human cortical potentials evoked by stimulation of the median nerve. II. Cytoarchitectonic areas generating long-latency activity. *J Neurophysiol* 1989b;62:711–722.
17. McCarthy G, Allison T, Spencer DD. Localization of the face area of human sensorimotor cortex by intracranial recording of somatosensory-evoked potentials. *J Neurosurg* 1993;79:874–884.
18. Ikeda A, Lüders HO, Burgess RC, et al. Movement-related potentials recorded from the supplementary motor area and primary motor area. *Brain* 1992;115:1017–1043.
19. Yazawa S, Ikeda A, Terada K, et al. Subdural recording of the Bereitschaftspotential is useful for functional mapping of the epileptogenic motor area: a case report. *Epilepsia* 1997;38:245–248.
20. Allison T, McCarthy G, Wood CC. The relationship of human long-latency somatosensory evoked potentials recorded from the cortical surface and scalp. *Electroencephalogr Clin Neurophysiol* 1992;84:301–314.
21. Darcey TM, Battistion JJ, Roberts DW, et al. Computer-assisted localization of implanted electrode assemblies for multimodal image fusion and electroanatomical localization. *Epilepsia* 1996;37(Suppl):201(abst).
22. Babb TL, Wilson CL, Crandall PH. Asymmetry and ventral course of the human geniculostriate pathway as determined by hippocampal visual evoked potentials and subsequent visual field defects after temporal lobectomy. *Exp Brain Res* 1982;47:317–328.
23. Arroyo S, Lesser RP, Poon WT, et al. Neuronal generators of visual evoked potentials in humans: visual processing in the human cortex. *Epilepsia* 1997;38:600–610.
24. Gulyas B. Functional organization of human visual cortical areas. In: Rockland KS, Kaas J, Peters A, eds. *Cerebral cortex,* vol 12. *Extrastriate cortex in primates.* New York: Plenum Press, 1997:743–775.
25. Ojemann GA. Individual variability in cortical localization of language. *J Neurosurg* 1979;50:164–169.
26. Lüders HO, Lesser RP, Dinner DS, et al. Language deficits elicited by electrical stimulation of the fusiform gyrus. In: Engel J Jr, ed. *Fundamental mechanisms of human brain function.* New York: Raven Press, 1987:83–90.
27. Fried I, Ojemann GA, Fetz EE. Language-related potentials specific to human language cortex. *Science* 1981;212:353–356.
28. McCarthy G, Wood CC, Williamson PD, et al. Task-dependent field potentials in the human hippocampal formation. *J Neurosci* 1989;9:4253–4268.
29. Halgren E, Baudena P, Clarke JM, et al. Intracerebral potentials to rare target and distractor auditory and visual stimuli. II. Medial, lateral, and posterior temporal lobe. *Electroencephalogr Clin Neurophysiol* 1995;94:229–250.
30. McCarthy G, Darcey TM, Wood CC, et al. Asymmetries in scalp and intracranial endogenous ERPs in patients with complex partial epilepsy. In: Engel J Jr, ed. *Fundamental mechanisms of human brain function.* New York: Raven Press, 1987:51–59.
31. Meador KJ, Loring DW, King DW, et al. Limbic evoked

potentials predict site of epileptic focus. *Neurology* 1987;37:494–496.

32. Meador KJ, Loring DW, King DW, et al. Spectral power of human limbic evoked potentials: relationship to seizure onset. *Ann Neurol* 1988;23:145–151.

33. Nunez PL, Pilgreen KL. The spline-Laplacian in clinical neurophysiology: a method to improve EEG spatial resolution. *J Clin Neurophysiol* 1991;8:397–413.

34. Fender DH. Source localization of brain electrical activity. In: Gevins A, Remond A, eds. *Handbook of electroencephalography and clinical neurophysiology.* Amsterdam: Elsevier, 1987:355–403.

35. Friston KJ. Statistical parametric mapping and other analyses of functional imaging data. In: Toga AW, Mazziotta JC, eds. *Brain mapping: the methods.* San Diego: Academic Press, 1996:363–386.

Neocortical Epilepsies.
Advances in Neurology, Vol. 84,
edited by P.D. Williamson, A.M. Siegel,
D.W. Roberts, V.M. Thadani, and M.S. Gazzaniga.

26

Functional Mapping with ECoG Spectral Analysis

Nathan E. Crone

Department of Neurology, The Johns Hopkins University School of Medicine,
Baltimore, Maryland 21287-7247

HISTORICAL PERSPECTIVE

In many patients undergoing surgery for intractable localization-related epilepsy, the epileptogenic zone is in close proximity to neocortical regions responsible for language and other critical cognitive functions. Because of the great interindividual variability in the functional anatomy of language, it is difficult for the surgeon to rely strictly on general guidelines drawn from historical studies of strokes and other accidental lesions. The traditional solution to this problem has been to perform electric stimulation mapping of the cortical surface in each patient prior to resection of the epileptogenic zone. This can be done in the operating room, as pioneered by Penfield and his collaborators. However, the time available for testing is limited, the patient must be awake to map language and other cognitive functions, and only a limited number of functions can be tested within these constraints. An alternative approach is to implant subdural arrays of electrodes, through which stimulation mapping can be done over the course of several days as the epileptogenic zone is more clearly defined through ictal electrocorticogram (ECoG) recordings (1). This method has allowed more refined mapping of a variety of cognitive functions both for clinical and for research purposes.

Over the past 25 years, new methods have been developed for noninvasively mapping the functional anatomy of the human brain. Each of these methods, particularly positron emission tomography (PET) and functional magnetic resonance imaging (fMRI), have raised hopes that eventually invasive functional mapping with cortical electric stimulation could be replaced. fMRI has been particularly promising because it does not require expensive isotopes or expose the patient to ionizing radiation. It is safe, inexpensive, and accessible. In addition, functional–anatomic images may be obtained within fractions of a second, making it possible to test the same subject repeatedly, using a variety of functional tasks under varying conditions. Despite the speed of its image acquisition, however, fMRI, like PET, must rely on a change in regional cerebral blood flow (rCBF), which is only an indirect index of increased neuronal activity (2). Furthermore, this change in rCBF takes time, introducing a delay of one or more seconds and dramatically reducing the temporal resolution of functional imaging. For most clinical purposes, this does not pose any critical limitation, but more refined functional–anatomic distinctions may require better temporal resolution. For example, sub-second temporal resolution is critical for studying how different brain regions, serving different functions, are coordinated as they are called into play in the execution of cognitive tasks. By identifying which brain regions are activated during the different stages of a cognitive task, we can better define the function of these regions and therefore make better predictions about the clinical consequences of losing these functional brain regions.

Electrophysiologic recordings such as electroencephalography (EEG), ECoG, and magnetoencephalography (MEG) have always offered a means for measuring the activity of cortical neuronal populations more directly and with instantaneous temporal resolution; however, it has been difficult to identify unambiguously the neuronal sources of these signals, particularly when recorded noninvasively from the scalp surface. A variety of techniques have been developed for solving the inverse problem of source localization, with varying degrees of success. Beyond the solution of this problem remains the problem of interpreting the functional significance of the signals themselves, that is, the question of what constitutes an index of cortical processing.

Signal averaging has been the most widely used method by which the functional information in electrophysiological recordings is translated. Event-related potentials (ERPs) have been used extensively to study a variety of brain functions. The technique is limited only by the requirement that the timing of the "event," either internal or external, is localizable in time so that time-locked signals can be extracted. In addition to signal averaging in the time domain (ERPs), analyses of electrophysiologic signals have also focused on event-related changes in the frequency domain. Since the discovery of EEG by Hans Berger in 1939, its component frequencies have been analyzed in order to deduce the functional state of its neuronal generators. Berger's description of alpha desynchronization during eye opening was the first correlation between a change in the power spectrum of the EEG and activation of a functionally specific brain region. Although the success of signal averaging techniques eventually led to a reduction of interest in this

aspect of EEG signal analysis, EEG frequency analysis has been revived in recent years by computer-based algorithms for EEG frequency analysis and by basic neurophysiologic investigations in animals suggesting the functional relevance of oscillatory neuronal activity.

ALPHA EVENT-RELATED DESYNCHRONIZATION

Classic observations of reactivity in the occipital alpha (3,4) and central mu (5–7) rhythms laid the foundation for the hypothesis that rhythmic activity in the alpha band (~8–13 Hz, which includes the mu rhythm) is generated by cortex that is resting, and that when cortex is active, this activity is reduced or suppressed. The neurophysiologic mechanisms underlying these EEG rhythms and their reactivity have been only partially understood (8,9). Nevertheless, scalp EEG studies have consistently demonstrated power suppression in the alpha band, dubbed *event-related desynchronization* (ERD), under a variety of task conditions (10). So far, most scalp EEG studies of alpha ERD have focused on activation of sensorimotor cortex (11,12).

Electrocorticographic recordings with subdural electrodes also have demonstrated alpha ERD in association with sensorimotor activation (13–16). Subdural ECoG overcomes some of the important technical limitations of scalp EEG. ECoG has superior spatial resolution as a result of its closer electrode spacing (usually 1 cm) and the absence of spatial blurring from the scalp, skull, and dura mater (17,18). Because ECoG electrodes lie directly on the cortical surface, and because cranial myogenic potentials are attenuated by the same barriers that usually attenuate scalp EEG potentials, the signal-to-noise ratio of ECoG recordings is also better than scalp EEG, particularly for frequencies higher than the alpha band (19).

To investigate the utility of alpha ERD as an index of cortical activation, we have examined its topographic and temporal patterns in ECoG recordings during a visual–motor task designed to activate somatotopically the sensorimotor cortex (15). We ask our patients to make sustained voluntary muscle contractions in different body parts (tongue, arm, or leg) in response to visual stimuli that consist of black-and-white line drawings depicting different motor actions: tongue protrusion, fist-clenching, or dorsiflexion of one foot. The patients are instructed to begin the action depicted as quickly as possible and to sustain the muscle contraction for the duration of the visual stimulus—a fixed interval of three seconds.

Prior to spectral analysis, ECoG signals are segmented into 200-ms epochs that overlap in time by 50% (100 ms). Prior to statistical analysis, absolute-power spectral density values are calculated using the fast Fourier transform, and these values are transformed by the natural logarithm to approximate a gaussian (normal) distribution (20,21). To determine whether the spectral density values in poststimulus epochs differ significantly from those in prestimulus (baseline) epochs, we first calculate a measure of the change in log power for each poststimulus epoch within each trial. A separate mixed-effects analysis of variance (ANOVA) model then is fitted for each channel and each frequency using the change value as the dependent variable and the poststimulus epoch as the independent variable. Further details of the statistical model used can be found elsewhere (15).

For each body part tested, statistically significant alpha ERD usually occurs in a wide region in and around sensorimotor cortices. Simply the presence of any significant alpha ERD is therefore not a sufficient criterion to distinguish a somatotopically distinct pattern for different body parts. However, examination of the time course of ERD usually reveals more specific patterns for each body part. In particular, we observed two different temporal patterns of gamma ERD—*sustained* and *transient*—which appear to define relatively distinct spatial patterns observed during early and late stages, respectively, of task execution (Fig. 26.1).

When alpha ERD occurs continuously from its onset to the end of the muscle contraction, we call it *sustained*. This temporal pattern corresponds to the continuous performance of the motor task. Typically, the spatial pattern of *sustained alpha ERD* is concentrated over somatotopically specific regions of sensorimotor cortex. Alpha ERD also occurs in a *transient* temporal pattern that ends before the end of the muscle contraction; this occurs in spatial patterns that typically involve cortical regions immediately adjacent to and outside of precentral and postcentral gyri, or regions within them corresponding to body parts not involved in the motor task. In addition to the temporal congruence between alpha ERD and motor performance, the magnitude of alpha ERD provides another means of examining the functional specificity of alpha ERD. When its magnitude is mapped with a two-dimensional array, it is typically maximal in the same regions where it is sustained, that is, in somatotopically defined regions near the central sulcus (Fig. 26.1).

We consistently observed alpha ERD in all our patients, suggesting that it is a relatively sensitive index of task-related cortical activity, particularly when recorded from the cortical surface. However, the topographic pattern of alpha ERD fulfills traditional expectations of somatotopy only if its temporal profile closely approximates that of the motor response, that is, if it is sustained. The topographic patterns of beta (15–25 Hz and 20–30 Hz) ERD are often more discrete and somatotopically specific than those of alpha ERD, but beta ERD is often transient and sometimes absent altogether, suggesting that it may be a less sensitive index of cortical activation.

Comparison of ESA maps with cortical stimulation maps usually reveals a good deal of congruence between these two methods of functional brain mapping. Sustained alpha and beta ERD are usually recorded from electrodes at which cortical stimulation produces some kind of disruption of motor function in the same body part; however, transient alpha and beta ERD often occur in patterns that do not meet conventional expectations of soma-

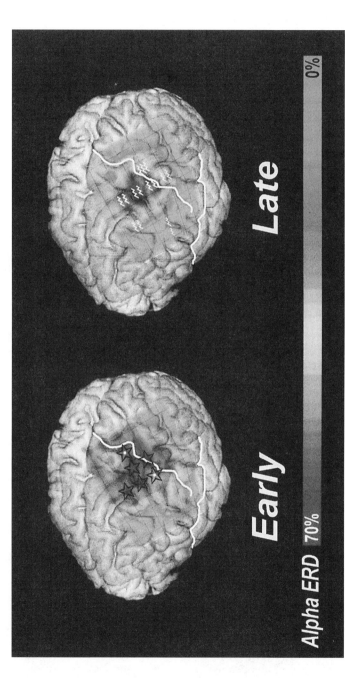

FIG. 26.1. Cortical topography of alpha ERD and gamma ERS over left frontoparietal cortex during right (contralateral) fist-clenching. Brain is tilted so that the interhemispheric fissure can be seen. Central sulcus and sylvian fissures are traced in white. *Black stars* denote low gamma ERS, and *white dots* denote high gamma ERS. Gray-scale surface plots of alpha ERD illustrate the distinction between transient (early) and sustained (late) power changes. Early ERD was calculated by averaging the percentage (geometric mean) ERD for three 200-ms poststimulus epochs centered at 600, 700, and 800 ms. Late ERD was calculated by averaging the percentage ERD in the 1,700-, 1,800-, and 1,900-ms epochs. Late ERD corresponds to ERD that was sustained; that is, after its onset, it continued through the end of the 2-second poststimulus period of analysis. Alpha ERD measures at each electrode (original values at thin line crossings) were interpolated using an inverse-distance weighting algorithm to produce a smooth gray-scale map. Lightning-bolt icons denote electric stimulation-induced disruption of motor function in the right arm: one bolt = slowing or cessation of ongoing motor activity (wriggling tongue, fingers, or toes); two bolts = involuntary motor response (e.g., posturing); and three bolts = clonic muscular contractions. *Faded X,* electrode sites in which ECoG could not be reliably recorded.

totopy. For example, transient alpha ERD may occur in tongue regions at the onset of fist-clenching. In addition, unilateral limb movements may be associated with transient, sometimes sustained, alpha and beta ERD over bilateral sensorimotor cortices. There are several possible interpretations for these findings (15), but overall they suggest that alpha and beta ERD reflect the activation of a network of neuronal resources that are participating in, but are not necessarily critical to, execution of a particular functional task.

GAMMA EVENT-RELATED SYNCHRONIZATION

In addition to changes in the alpha and beta bands, changes in higher frequencies, collectively known as the *gamma band* (> 30 Hz), have also been associated with cortical activation (22,23) with special attention being paid to changes in the 40-Hz band. Typically, these changes have consisted of an *increase,* or augmentation, of spectral power, which has been called *event-related synchronization (ERS).*

Over the past 20 years, neurophysiologic investigations in animals have suggested the relevance of gamma band activity (24–26). In cat visual cortex, oscillatory neuronal firing at 40 to 60 Hz can become synchronized during visual stimulation between spatially separate columns (27), between areas 17 and 18 (28), and even between areas 17 of the two hemispheres (29). High-frequency local field activity (25–35 Hz and 15–50 Hz, respectively) also may be recorded in the sensorimotor cortex of awake monkeys during hand movements (30,31). Bursts of single-unit firing are commonly synchronized with local field potential oscillations, suggesting that gamma band activity facilitates or is facilitated by the synchronization of neuronal firing between spatially segregated but functionally related neurons. Synchronization of neuronal firing could form the temporal coding by which temporary assemblies of neurons represent higher-order, or global, stimulus properties. Von der Malsburg (32) proposed such a mechanism as the solution to the binding problem associated with psychological phenomena such as sensory segmentation, invariant object recognition, and language parsing. Gamma band activity has also figured prominently in recent theories of visual awareness and consciousness (33,34).

Fewer studies of gamma band activity have been done in humans, and until recently these studies were limited to extracranial recordings. Using scalp EEG, Pfurtscheller et al. (22) demonstrated a lateralized 40-Hz ERS during finger movements in three subjects, and in one of these subjects they showed a somatotopic pattern of gamma ERS during movements of the tongue, finger, and toes. MEG recordings also demonstrated evoked gamma band oscillations in response to auditory stimulation (35,36).

To study more fully the validity of gamma band ERS as an index of cortical activation and its utility for human functional brain mapping, we studied this phenomenon in subdural ECoGs recorded during a visual-motor task (using the same methods described under the preceding section entitled "Alpha Event-related Desynchronization"). Taking an exploratory approach with respect to gamma frequencies, we studied ERS in 10-Hz-wide bands (overlapping by 5 Hz) ranging from 30 to 100 Hz and compared our findings in these bands with changes (i.e., ERD) in the alpha (8–13 Hz) and beta (15–25 Hz) bands.

During putative activation of sensorimotor cortex, there is a significant augmentation of power in the 35- to 50-Hz range, which includes the widely studied 40-Hz band (35–45 Hz in our case). In addition, there is augmentation of power in a higher-frequency range (75–100 Hz), which is still within the broadly defined gamma band (> 30 Hz). Whenever augmentation of either low or high gamma power is observed, it occurs in a spatial pattern that is somatotopically specific for the body part used. In particular, tongue protrusion is associated with gamma ERS over inferior–lateral perirolandic cortex, fist-clenching is associated with gamma ERS over more superior perirolandic cortex, and foot dorsiflexion is associated with gamma ERS over parasagittal perirolandic cortex. This localization is usually consistent with the results of cortical electric stimulation using the same subdural electrodes.

Although alpha and beta ERD are often observed over bilateral sensorimotor cortices during unilateral limb movements (15,37), gamma ERS is usually observed only over contralateral sensorimotor cortex (38), a finding which is more consistent with the majority of lesion studies in both animals and humans. Maps of gamma ERS are also more consistent with those derived from PET and functional MRI (39,40), in which activation of sensorimotor cortex has been more discrete and more consistently contralateral than that observed with alpha or beta ERD.

We now have observed gamma ERS in seven of nine patients. Scalp recordings in humans detected 40-Hz ERS in only a few subjects (22). Gamma band activity may be more difficult to record with scalp EEG because of the low-pass filtering effect of the skull and because the frequency spectrum of myogenic potentials from cranial muscles overlaps that of cortically generated gamma activity. In some of our patients, we have not been able to detect gamma ERS during the visual–motor task. It is possible that in these patients the generators for gamma activity were too small or oriented incorrectly, were spatially distributed with insufficient density, or were insufficiently coherent for summation and detection at the cortical surface. Our ECoG recordings used subdural electrodes with 1-cm interelectrode distances. The spatial patterns of gamma ERS were usually quite discrete, often involving noncontiguous electrodes. Perhaps subdural electrode arrays with interelectrode distances of 5 mm or less will be necessary to consistently capture gamma band activity.

LANGUAGE MAPPING

We also used ESA to study the functional anatomy of language. For this purpose, we used tasks such as visual object naming, single-word reading, auditory repetition of single words, and auditory discrimination of two syllables. These tasks require the coordination of different combinations of functional and anatomic subunits. By comparing the spatiotemporal patterns of ECoG spectral changes associated with these different tasks, we attempted to identify their constituent functional/anatomic subunits and to examine how they are dynamically allocated to perform complex cognitive functions. To date, both alpha ERD and gamma ERS have been observed in patterns consistent with cortical stimulation maps and with prior lesion-based studies of the functional–anatomic components of language.

For example, we studied the functional anatomy of naming using a task in which the patient was presented a series of pictured objects and asked to name each one (Fig. 26.2). Using this task, we observed alpha ERD over temporal–occipital regions during the early stages of task execution, presumably corresponding to object identification. This was followed by alpha ERD over superior temporal gyrus and surrounding regions of the temporal and parietal lobes, presumably corresponding to activation of semantic and phonological representations of the object. Simultaneously or soon thereafter, we observed alpha ERD over posterior inferior frontal gyrus (i.e., Broca's area) and over inferior perirolandic cortex, presumably corresponding to word production and articulation. Late in the task, as the patient was still speaking the word response, there was activation of both supra and infrasylvian cortices, presumably resulting from speech production and auditory monitoring of the patient's own speech.

We have also observed gamma ERS during the same language tasks, but its occurrence has not been as consistent as that of alpha ERD. Again, this could be due to the technical limitations of our recording apparatus. Nevertheless, we observed robust language-induced gamma ERS in several patients (41–44).

We recently presented an interesting case of a professional sign language interpreter with normal hearing, in whom we recorded subdural ECoG during picture naming, word

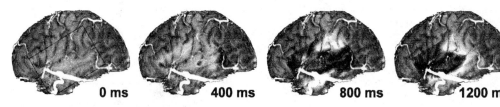

FIG. 26.2. EcoG activation. (*Dark blobs*, alpha desynchronization = activation) during picture naming (0 ms = stimulus onset; ~800 ms = response onset.)

reading, and word repetition, using both spoken and signed responses (45). We studied the spatiotemporal patterns of alpha ERD and gamma ERS during these tasks and found further evidence for conceptual distinctions between these two indices of cortical activation (see preceding). Maps of gamma ERS showed that spoken responses produced discrete activation of tongue regions of sensorimotor cortex and signed responses produced activation of hand regions. Maps of alpha ERD, however, showed a good deal of overlap between tongue and hand regions during both types of responses. Furthermore, we observed that during the early (input) stages of the language tasks, gamma ERS occurred over superior temporal gyrus (STG) in the word-repetition task (auditory input), but not in the word-reading and picture-naming tasks (visual inputs). During later (output) stages of the tasks, we observed gamma ERS over STG when the responses were spoken but not when they were signed, suggesting that this activation corresponded either to self-monitoring or involvement in spoken word production.

CONCLUSION

Our preliminary studies suggest the potential utility of ESA for quickly obtaining complete functional maps of several cognitive functions, perhaps within the time constraints of a single surgical procedure done with the patient awake part of the time. In patients requiring only functional mapping (e.g., dominant temporal lobe neoplasms and vascular malformations), this conceivably could eliminate the need for two operations, as currently required to (1) implant the electrode array for extraoperative cortical stimulation and (2) to remove the array and the diseased brain. In patients with epilepsy who require both seizure localization and functional mapping, cortical stimulation mapping often artificially induces seizures that have suspect localizing validity. The clinician then may have to postpone functional mapping until after a sufficient number of spontaneous seizures have been recorded for seizure localization. ESA could provide a preliminary map of several different cortical functions within the first few days after subdural electrode implantation. Cortical stimulation could thus be postponed until after seizure localization and could focus on the regions that are relevant to the resection and that have been identified by ESA as participating or critical to function. Before ESA can be used clinically, however, its validity and reliability must be tested more extensively. In particular, it will be important to compare the maps generated by ESA with those generated by cortical stimulation and fMRI and to study the effects of resection of those regions identified by different ESA indices of cortical activation.

REFERENCES

1. Lesser RP, Lüders HO, Klem G, et al. Extraoperative cortical functional localization in patients with epilepsy. J Clin *Neurophysiology* 1987;4:27–53.
2. Magistretti PJ, Pellerin L, Rothman DL, et al. Energy on demand. *Science* 1999;283:496–497.
3. Adrian ED, Matthews BHC. The Berger rhythm: potential changes from the occipital lobes in man. *Brain* 1934;57:355–385.

4. Berger H. Über das elektrenkephalogramm des menschen. II. *J Psychol Neurol (Leipzig)* 1930;40:160–179.
5. Chatrian GE, Petersen MC, Lazarte JA. The blocking of the rolandic wicket rhythm and some central changes related to movement. *Electroencephalogr Clin Neurophysiol* 1959;11:497–510.
6. Gastaut H. Étude electrocorticographique de la reactivite des rythmes rolandique s. *Rev Neurol (Paris)* 1952;87:176–182.
7. Jasper HH, Andrews HL. Electro-encephalography. III. Normal differentiation of occipital and precentral regions in man. *Arch Neurol Psychiatry* 1938;39: 96–115.
8. Lopes da Silva F. Neural mechanisms underlying brain waves: from neural membranes to networks. *Electroencephalogr Clin Neurophysiol* 1991;79:81–93.
9. Steriade M, Gloor P, Llinas R, et al. Basic mechanisms of cerebral rhythmic activities. *Electroencephalogr clin Neurophysiol* 1990;76:481–508.
10. Pfurtscheller G, Aranibar A. Evaluation of event-related desynchronization (ERD) preceding and following voluntary self-paced movement. *Electroencephalogr Clin Neurophysiol* 1979;46:138–146.
11. Pfurtscheller G, Flotzinger D, Neuper C. Differentiation between finger, toe, and tongue movement in man based on 40 Hz EEG. *Electroencephalogr Clin Neurophysiol* 1994;90:456–460.
12. Pfurtscheller G, Neuper C. Event-related synchronization of mu rhythm in the EEG over the cortical hand area in man. *Neurosci Lett* 1994;174:93–96.
13. Arroyo S, Lesser RP, Gordon B, et al. Functional significance of the mu rhythm of human cortex: an electrophysiologic study with subdural electrodes. *Electroencephalogr Clin Neurophysiol* 1993;87:76–87.
14. Crone NE, Lesser RP, Kraus GL, et al. Topographic mapping of human sensorimotor cortex with electrocortical spectra. *Epilepsia* 1993;34:122–123.
15. Crone NE, Miglioretti DL, Gordon B, et al. Functional mapping of human sensorimotor cortex with electrocorticographic spectral analysis. I. Alpha and beta event-related desynchronization. *Brain* 1998b;121: 2271–2299.
16. Toro C, Deuschl G, Thatcher R, et al. Event-related desynchronization and movement-related cortical potentials on the ECoG and EEG. *Electroencephalogr Clin Neurophysiol* 1994;93:380–389.
17. Cooper R, Winter AL, Crow HJ, et al. Comparison of subcortical, cortical, and scalp activity using chronically indwelling electrodes in man. *Electroencephalogr Clin Neurophysiol* 1965;18:217–228.
18. Gevins A, Cutillo B, Desmond J, et al. Subdural grid recordings of distributed neocortical networks involved with somatosensory discrimination. *Electroencephalogr Clin Neurophysiol* 1994;92:282–290.
19. Pfurtscheller G, Cooper R. Frequency dependence of the transmission of the EEG from cortex to scalp. *Electroencephalogr Clin Neurophysiol* 1975;38:93–96.
20. Gasser T, Bächer P, Möcks J. Transformations towards the normal distribution of broad band spectral parameters of the EEG. *Electroencephalogr Clin Neurophysiol* 1982;53:119–124.
21. Oken BS, Chiappa KH. Short-term variability in EEG frequency analysis. *Electroencephalogr Clin Neurophysiol* 1988;69:191–198.
22. Pfurtscheller G, Neuper C, Kalcher J. 40-Hz oscillations during motor behavior in man. *Neurosci Lett* 1993;164: 179–182.
23. Spydell JD, Ford MR, Sheer DE. Task dependent cerebral lateralization of the 40 Hertz EEG rhythm. *Psychophysiology* 1979;16:347–350.
24. Bouyer JJ, Montaron MF, Vahnée JM, et al. Anatomical localization of cortical beta rhythms in cat. *Neuroscience* 1987;22:863–869.
25. Bressler SL, Freeman WJ. Frequency analysis of olfactory system EEG in cat, rabbit, and rat. *Electroencephalogr Clin Neurophysiol* 1980;50:19–24.
26. Freeman WJ. Spatial properties of an EEG event in the olfactory bulb and cortex. *Electroencephalogr Clin Neurophysiol* 1978;44:586–605.
27. Gray CM, König P, Engel AK, et al. Oscillatory responses in cat visual cortex exhibit inter-columnar synchronization which reflects global stimulus properties. *Nature* 1989;338:334–337.
28. Eckhorn R, Bauer R, Jordan W, et al. Coherent oscillations: a mechanism of feature linking in the visual cortex? multiple electrode and correlation analyses in the cat. *Biol Cyber* 1988;60:121–130.
29. Engel AK, König P, Kreiter AK, et al. Interhemispheric synchronization of oscillatory neuronal responses in cat visual cortex. *Science* 1991;252:1177–1179.
30. Murthy VN, Fetz EE. Coherent 25- to 35-Hz oscillations in the sensorimotor cortex of awake behaving monkeys. *Proc Natl Acad Sci USA* 1992;89:5670–5674.
31. Sanes JN, Donoghue JP. Oscillations in local field potentials of the primate motor cortex during voluntary movement. *Proc Natl Acad Sci USA* 1993;90: 4470–4474.
32. Von der Malsburg C. Bindings in models of perception and brain function. *Curr Opin Neurobiol* 1995;5: 520–526.
33. Crick F, Koch C. Some reflections on visual awareness. [Review]. *Cold Spring Harb Symp Quant Biol* 1990; 55:953–962.
34. Llinas RR, Pare D. Of dreaming and wakefulness [Review]. *Neuroscience* 1991;44:521–535.
35. Pantev C, Makeig S, Hoke M, et al. Human auditory evoked gamma-band magnetic fields. *Proc Natl Acad Sci USA* 1991;88:8996–9000.
36. Ribary U, Ioannides AA, Singh KD, et al. Magnetic field tomography of coherent thalamocortical 40-Hz oscillations in humans. *Proc Natl Acad Sci USA* 1991; 88:11037–11041.
37. Pfurtscheller G, Klimesch W. Event-related desynchronization during motor behavior and visual information processsing. In: Brunia CHM, Mulder G, Verbaten MN, eds. *Event-related brain research.* New York: Elsevier, 1991:58–65.
38. Crone NE, Miglioretti DL, Gordon B, et al. Functional mapping of human sensorimotor cortex with electrocorticographic spectral analysis. II. Event-related synchronization in the gamma band. *Brain* 1998;121: 2301–2315.
39. Grafton ST, Woods RP, Mazziotta JC, et al. Somatotopic mapping of the primary motor cortex in humans: activation studies with cerebral blood flow and positron emission tomography. *J Neurophysiol* 1991;66: 735–743.
40. Kim S, Ashe J, Georgopoulos AP, et al. Functional imaging of human motor cortex at high magnetic field. *J Neurophysiol* 1993;69:297–302.

41. Crone NE, Boatman D, Hart J, et al. Electrocortico-graphic gamma band augmentation: an index of cortical activation in humans. *Soc Neurosci Abst* 1995;21: 274.

42. Crone NE, Hart J Jr, Boatman D, et al. Regional cortical activation during language and related tasks identified by direct cortical electrical recording. *Brain Lang* 1994;47:466–468.

43. Crone NE, Hart J, Lesser RP, et al. Spectral changes associated with regional cerebral processing: results of direct cortical recording in humans. *Epilepsia* 1994;35(Suppl):103.

44. Crone NE, Nathan S, Lesser RP, et al. Patterns of change in electrocorticographic spectra during human language processing. *Am Electroencephalography Society Annual Meeting* 1993;34:122–123.

45. Crone NE, Hart J, Hao L, et al. Functional mapping of word production in human sign language using electrocorticographic spectral analysis. *Neurology* 1999;52 (Suppl 2):A233.

Neocortical Epilepsies.
Advances in Neurology, Vol. 84,
edited by P.D. Williamson, A.M. Siegel,
D.W. Roberts, V.M. Thadani, and M.S. Gazzaniga.
Lippincott Williams & Wilkins, Philadelphia © 2000.

27

Sublobar Localization of Temporal Neocortical Epileptogenic Foci by Source Modeling

John S. Ebersole

Epilepsy Program, University of Chicago, Chicago, Illinois 60637

Until recently, temporal lobe epilepsy and classic mesial temporal limbic epilepsy (MTLE) have been synonymous. It is now recognized that neocortical temporal lobe epilepsy (NTLE) is relatively common. In fact, distinguishing between the two forms of temporal lobe epilepsy now consumes much of our presurgical diagnostic efforts. This distinction is important because NTLE may not be cured by surgery unless the epileptogenic cortex is removed, and most lateral temporal neocortex is usually not resected in standard lobectomies.

Similarly, descriptions of electroencephalographic (EEG) abnormalities in temporal lobe epilepsy until recently have not attempted to distinguish between those associated with MLTE versus NTLE. Anterior temporal sharp waves and spikes, particularly if detected from inferior or sphenoidal electrodes, are often thought to be good indicators of MTLE. In the same manner, an ictal buildup of temporal theta rhythms has been considered a marker of MTLE. It was shown, however, that neither of these interictal or ictal potentials are actually generated in mesial temporal structures (1,2); rather, both are products of propagated temporal neocortical activity. More sophisticated analyses of the source character and propagation patterns of spikes and seizures are necessary, therefore, if we are to distinguish between these two types of temporal lobe epilepsy.

TEMPORAL LOBE INTERICTAL SPIKES

Ebersole and Wade (3,4) first noted that the voltage topography of anterior temporal spikes was not consistent, even among those with a similar frontotemporal negative field maximum. They showed that the corresponding positive field maximum varied in location from near the vertex to the contralateral temporal region. They called the former distribution with vertex positivity a *type 1* spike field, and the latter pattern with contralateral temporal positivity a *type 2* spike field (Figs. 27.1 and 27.2) (5–7). Patients with predominantly type 1 spikes tended to have unilateral hippocampal atrophy, intracranial EEG seizures that began in mesiotemporal structures, and an increased likelihood of seizure elimination following standard anteromedial temporal resection. Patients with type 2 spikes were less likely to have hippocampal atrophy, commonly had seizures originating from nonmesial temporal structures on intracranial EEG, and were less likely to be surgical successes.

It also was learned that the location and, in particular, the orientation of the discharging cortical area determined the resultant spike voltage topography. Type 1 spikes with an inferior temporal negative maximum and a vertex positive maximum were generated princi-

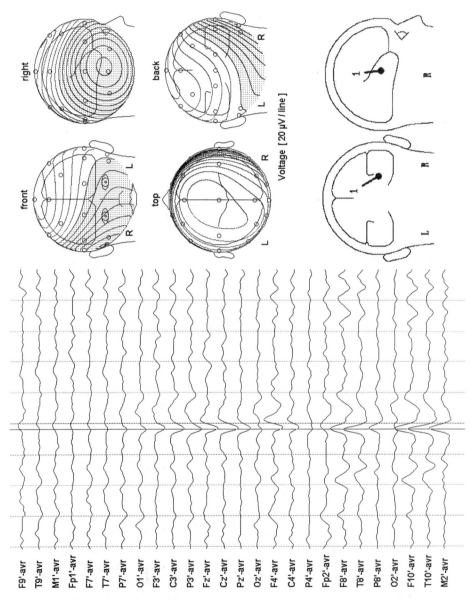

FIG. 27.1. Left: Right temporal type 1 spike. In this and subsequent figures, the EEG is depicted in a common average reference montage. **Right top:** Voltage topography of spike at cursor. In this and subsequent figures, the scalp voltage fields are illustrated by isopotential lines; negative field is speckled. **Right bottom:** Single dipole model of spike field at cursor and in voltage map. Dot denotes location; vector denotes source orientation. Note the subtemporal negative field maximum and vertex positive field maximum that is characteristic of type 1 spikes. Dipole model has an elevated orientation. Both field and dipole suggest a temporal basal cortex source.

354

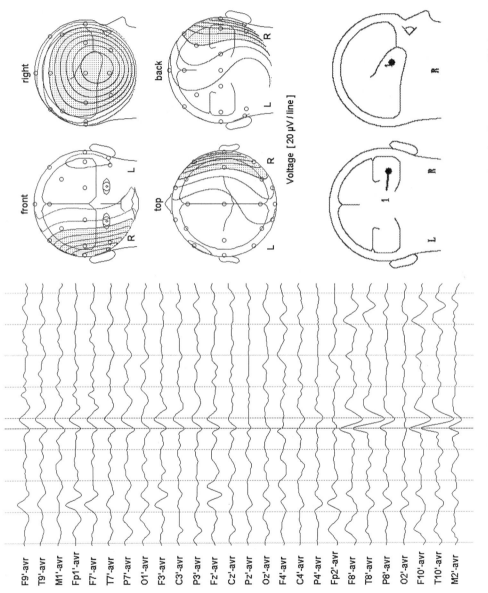

FIG. 27.2. Left: Right temporal type 2 spike. **Right top:** Voltage topography of spike at cursor. **Right bottom:** Single dipole model of spike field at cursor and in voltage map. Note the lateral temporal negative field maximum and contralateral positive field maximum that is characteristic of type 2 spikes. Dipole model has a horizontal and radial orientation. Both field and dipole suggest a lateral temporal cortex source.

355

pally by basal and inferolateral cortex, whereas type 2 spikes were generated by lateral temporal cortex. When these spike fields were modeled by equivalent dipoles, type 1 spikes resulted in a dipole having an elevated, sometimes vertical, orientation; type 2 spikes resulted in dipoles with a horizontal and radial orientation (5–7) (Figs. 27.1 and 27.2). Soon thereafter, several laboratories around the world confirmed these basic findings (8–13). In general, the consensus was that dipole orientation revealed more information than dipole localization in distinguishing among sublobar temporal sources. A close association between spike voltage topography and dipole models with cortical spike and seizure origins was confirmed by intracranial EEG and surgical outcome.

It should be emphasized that the type 1 spike field does not directly reflect hippocampal or amygdalar activity. Spikes confined to these structures do not generate scalp-recordable voltage fields due to the small source area and curved source shape, which favors voltage cancellation. Rather, it is the common, preferred propagation of this epileptiform activity into the entorhinal, fusiform, and other basal cortex that results in a generator of sufficient area to produce scalp EEG potentials (1,2). In general, some degree of propagation commonly occurs before either spike and seizure potentials are recordable at the scalp. Because voltage fields are orthogonal to the net orientation of their source cortex, a temporal lobe base spike is seen as subtemporal negativity and vertex positivity, which in turn is modeled by a dipole with elevated orientation.

Spikes that originate in basal temporal cortex may produce a similar voltage field. Alternatively, these spikes frequently propagate into temporal tip cortex by the time sufficient cortex is activated to produce a scalp EEG field. Temporal tip cortex has a net anterior facing orientation. Accordingly, spike sources in this cortex result in a voltage field with a frontotemporal to frontopolar negative maximum and a posterior positive maximum. Di-

pole models of the temporal tip spikes have a horizontal, tangential, anteroposterior (AP) orientation (2,14) (Fig. 27.3).

Spikes originating in the lateral temporal cortex commonly propagate in the AP direction along the lateral convexity. The net vertical orientation of this temporal cortex results in a lateral negative maximum and a positive maximum over the contralateral temporal area. Dipole models of this voltage field are thus horizontal and radial in orientation. Occasionally, lateral temporal spikes will propagate mesially into basal cortex, which causes the later portions of its voltage field to change. It is therefore always important to consider the evolution of each spike voltage field. Because propagation is common, one cannot conclude that the voltage field of the spike peak best represents the character of the spike source. This is true only if the contours of the voltage field do not change over the course of the spike potential. Otherwise, the voltage topography and dipole model of the earliest portion of the spike potential should be regarded as being associated most closely with the spike origin (2,7).

In summary, temporal spikes whose earliest voltage fields are modeled by vertical dipoles are likely to be seen in patients with MTLE or primary basal temporal neocortical epilepsy. Patients with spikes modeled by horizontal tangential AP dipoles likely have entorhinal, basal, or primary temporal tip neocortical epilepsy. In any of these cases, the epileptogenic focus will be removed by standard anteromesial temporal lobectomy. Accordingly, patients with these spikes are good candidates for surgery without invasive EEG monitoring. To the contrary, patients with spikes modeled by radial horizontal dipoles are likely to have lateral neocortical sources. Such foci may not be removed by standard temporal lobectomy. Invasive monitoring probably will benefit these patients by defining the exact location and extent of the focus and its encroachment on language areas, if on the dominant hemisphere. Tailored resections may increase the surgical success rate in such patients.

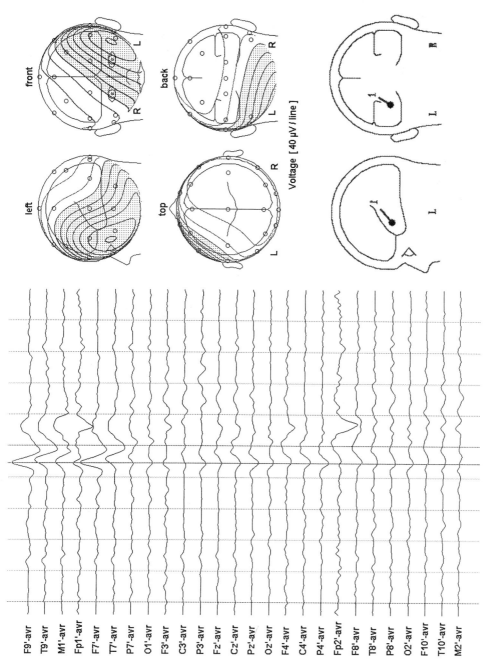

FIG. 27.3. Left: Left temporal tip spike. **Right top:** Voltage topography of spike at cursor. **Right bottom:** Single dipole model of spike field at cursor and in voltage map. Note the inferior frontotemporal negative field maximum and the contralateral posterior positive field maximum that is characteristic of temporal tip spikes. Dipole model has mostly a horizontal and AP orientation. Both field and dipole suggest a temporal tip cortex source.

front

left

back

top

Voltage [40 μV / line]

R

L

R

L

L

R

L

R

L

F9'-avr
T9'-avr
M1'-avr
Fp1'-avr
F7'-avr
T7'-avr
P7'-avr
O1'-avr
F3'-avr
C3'-avr
P3'-avr
Fz'-avr
Cz'-avr
Pz'-avr
Oz'-avr
F4'-avr
C4'-avr
P4'-avr
Fp2'-avr
F8'-avr
T8'-avr
P8'-avr
O2'-avr
F10'-avr
T10'-avr
M2'-avr

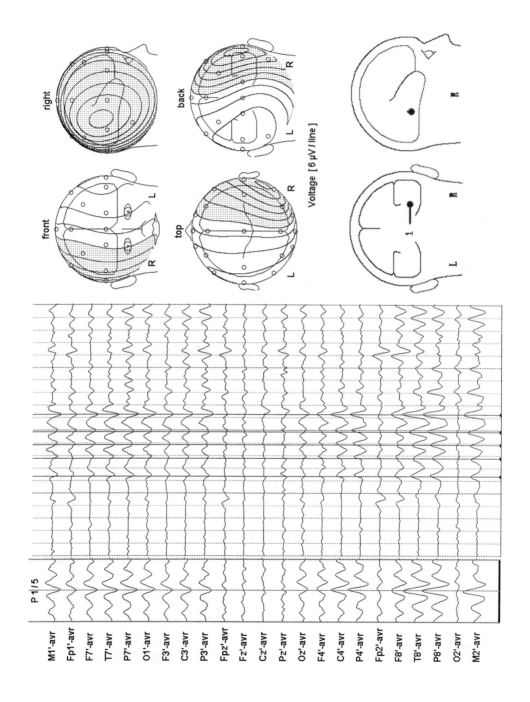

Temporal Lobe Seizures

The ictal EEG patterns of temporal lobe epilepsy have been described by a number of investigators (15–18). Only recently has there been an attempt to define patterns that distinguish seizures of neocortical origin from those of hippocampal or amygdalar origin (19,20). Ebersole and Pacia (19) defined three categories of temporal lobe ictal EEGs. Their type 2 and 3 ictal patterns were highly correlated with nonhippocampal temporal lobe seizure onsets. An ictal onset of slow frequency (<5 Hz) was the most prominent feature (Fig. 27.4). At times, these slow-frequency potentials took the form of regular, periodic discharges. Later in the seizure, more typical theta frequency rhythms could develop. These were typical of the onset of mesial temporal seizures (Fig. 27.5).

Subsequent simultaneous intracranial and scalp EEG in a subpopulation of these patients revealed that the slow ictal rhythms were intrinsic to temporal neocortex and the theta rhythms required, or at least were associated with, hippocampal seizure activity at the same frequency (1). These studies also showed that most temporal lobe neocortical seizures began with high-frequency, low-voltage discharges that were not evident on scalp EEG. The slower ictal frequencies developed some seconds later.

Although this schema identified EEG seizure patterns that were likely to be of temporal neocortical origin, it could not further differentiate the sublobar origins of these seizures. Dipole modeling also can be applied to seizure rhythms with some modifications in the protocol used for spikes (7,9–11). The earliest recognizable seizure potentials should be preferentially modeled because they are more likely to reflect the seizure origin than are later rhythms, which may develop only after significant propagation. Because ictal-onset rhythms are typically of low amplitude and commonly are confounded with movement and muscle artifact, averaging successive potentials may be necessary to increase the signal to noise. The key is to average seizure waveforms with a similar voltage topography (Fig. 27.4); only these reflect the same source configuration. Ictal EEG voltage fields are usually spatially stable for only a few seconds, however. Tight bandpass filtering is also useful in ictal dipole modeling. Most temporal lobe seizure frequencies are less than 12 Hz. A high-frequency filter of 13 to 20 Hz is therefore reasonable to reduce muscle artifact. Similarly, a low linear filter of 1 to 2 Hz will minimize low-frequency artifact secondary to movement of the patient or electrode leads.

The orientation of dipole models of ictal waveforms carries the same significance as those of spikes in that it is most useful in identifying sublobar temporal lobe sources (7,9–11, 21–23). Temporal lobe seizures modeled by dipoles with dominant vertical, horizontal tangential AP, or horizontal radial orientations are most likely associated with hippocampal/basal, temporal tip, and lateral temporal seizures, respectively (Fig. 27.4, 27.5, and 27.6). Additionally, many temporal lobe seizures are modeled best by dipoles that have an anterior oblique orientation that is a combination of all three previous orientations (Fig. 27.7). In this case, the ictally active cortical region includes inferior, tip, and lateral temporal cortex.

Source characteristics of both spikes and seizures also may be obtained from a multiple fixed dipole model, which attempts simply to determine the relative contribution of activity in various cortical surfaces to the measured

---

FIG. 27.4. Left: Right temporal type 2 seizure onset pattern. Cursors mark ictal potentials that were averaged to improve signal to noise. Averaged ictal waveform is at far left. **Right top:** Voltage topography of averaged ictal waveform at cursor. **Right bottom:** Single dipole model of ictal field at cursor and in voltage map. Note the lateral, midposterior negative field maximum and the contralateral positive field maximum that is characteristic of type 2 seizures. Dipole model has a horizontal and radial orientation. Both field and dipole suggest a lateral temporal cortex source.

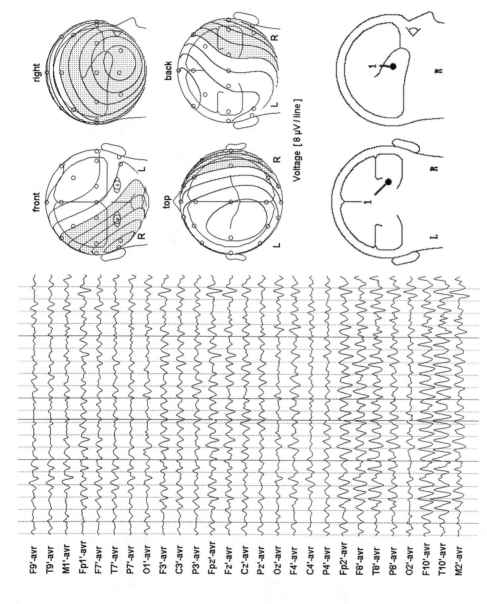

FIG. 27.5. Left: Right temporal type 1 seizure onset pattern. **Right top:** Voltage topography of ictal waveform at cursor. **Right bottom:** Single dipole model of ictal field at cursor and in voltage map. Note the anterior subtemporal field maximum and the vertex positive field maximum that is characteristic of type 1 seizures. Dipole model has an elevated orientation. Both field and dipole suggest a temporal basal cortex source.

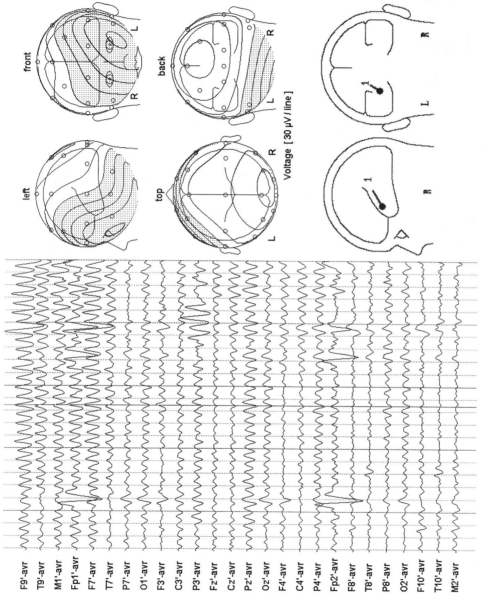

FIG. 27.6. **Left:** Left temporal tip seizure onset pattern. **Right, top:** Voltage topography of ictal waveform at cursor. **Right bottom:** Single dipole model of ictal field at cursor and in voltage map. Note the inferior frontal negative field maximum and the posterior positive field maximum, which are characteristic of temporal tip seizures. Dipole model has mostly a horizontal and AP orientation. Both field and dipole suggest a temporal tip cortex source.

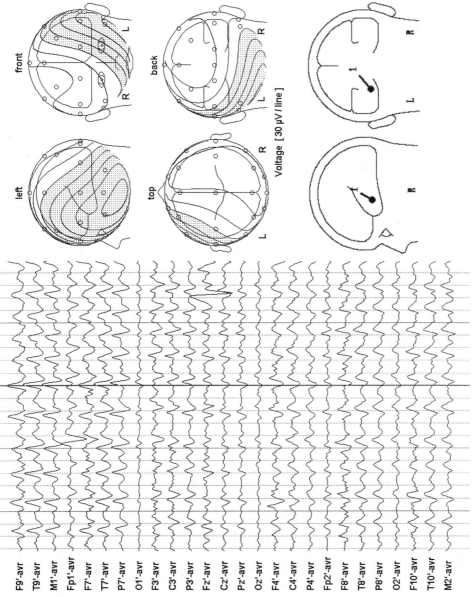

FIG. 27.7. Left: Left temporal, "oblique dipole" seizure onset pattern. **Right top:** Voltage topography of ictal waveform at cursor. **Right bottom:** Single dipole model of ictal field at cursor and in voltage map. Note the anterior subtemporal negative field maximum and the posterior vertex positive field maximum, which are characteristic of these temporal seizures. Dipole model has an anterior oblique orientation. Both field and dipole suggest a temporal source involving the anterior basal, tip, and inferolateral cortex.

waveform. This technique was used more recently to determine temporal lobe seizure origins and to predict surgical outcome following standard temporal lobectomy (21–24).

Ictal EEG dipole models have been correlated with intracranial EEG and surgical outcome (7,9–11,21–23). The results are similar to those found with spike dipole modeling. Patients with seizures modeled by horizontal radial dipoles, which suggest a lateral cortex origin, do less well following a standard anteromesial resection and should be considered candidates for invasive monitoring and possibly tailored temporal lobe resections. Patients whose seizures are modeled best by dipoles with a vertical, horizontal AP, or anterior oblique orientation have seizures that probably originated in mesial structures, basil, entorhinal, or temporal tip cortex, respectively. All these patients do well following surgery because these cortices are customarily removed in the standard temporal lobe resection.

CONCLUSION

Neocortical temporal lobe epilepsy represents an increasingly large fraction of the epilepsy surgery candidate population. EEG analysis, particularly using advanced techniques such as voltage topography and dipole modeling, can help to differentiate patients with this disorder from those with MTLE, even in the absence of structural lesions. Sublobar temporal lobe localization of epileptogenic foci can be achieved, which should add significantly to surgical decision making. Patients with NTLE can be excellent surgical candidates if their foci reside in basal and tip cortex that is customarily resected. To the contrary, patients with lateral cortical foci may do better after invasive EEG monitoring and tailored neocortical resection.

REFERENCES

1. Pacia SV, Ebersole JS. Intracranial EEG substrates of scalp ictal patterns from temporal lobe foci. *Epilepsia* 1997;38:642–653.
2. Ebersole JS. Defining epileptogenic foci: past, present, and future. *J Clin Neurophysiol* 1997;14:470–483.
3. Ebersole JS, Wade PB. Spike voltage topography and equivalent dipole localization in complex partial epilepsy. *Brain Topogr* 1990;3:21–34.
4. Ebersole JS, Wade PB. Spike voltage topography identifies two types of fronto-temporal epileptic foci. *Neurology* 1991;41:1425–1433.
5. Ebersole JS. EEG dipole modeling in complex partial epilepsy. *Brain Topogr* 1991;4:113–123.
6. Ebersole JS. Equivalent dipole modeling: a new EEG method for epileptogenic focus localization. In: Pedley TA, Meldrum BS, eds. *Recent advances in epilepsy*, vol 5. Edinburgh: Churchill Livingstone, 1991:51–72.
7. Ebersole JS. Noninvasive localization of the epileptogenic focus by EEG dipole modeling. *Acta Neurol Scand Suppl* 1994;152:20–28.
8. Baumgartner C, Lindinger G, Ebner A, et al. Propagation of interictal epileptic activity in temporal lobe epilepsy. *Neurology* 1995;45:118–122.
9. Boon P, D'Havé M. Interictal and ictal dipole modeling in patients with refractory partial epilepsy. *Acta Neurol Scand* 1995;92:7–18.
10. Boon P, D'Havé M, Adam C, et al. Dipole modeling in epilepsy surgery candidates. *Epilepsia* 1997;38:208–218.
11. Boon P, D'Havé M, Vandekerckhove T, et al. Dipole modeling and intracranial EEG recording: correlation between dipole and ictal onset zone. *Acta Neurochir* 1997;139:643–652.
12. Lantz G, Holub M, Ryding E, et al. Simultaneous intracranial and extracranial recording of interictal epileptiform activity in patients with drug resistant partial epilepsy: patterns of conduction and results from dipole reconstructions. *Electroencephalogr Clin Neurophysiol* 1996;99:69–78.
13. Merlet I, Garcia-Larrea L, Gregoire MC, et al. Source propagation of interictal spikes in temporal lobe epilepsy. *Brain* 1996;119:377–392.
14. Thompson JL, Ebersole JS. Dipole modeling of scalp-recorded interictal EEG spikes in mesial vs. nonmesial temporal lobe epilepsy. *J Clin Neurophysiol* 1995;12:501.
15. Anziska B, Cracco RQ. Changes in frequency and amplitude in electrographic seizure discharges. *Clin Electroencephalogr* 1977;8:206–210.
16. Geiger LR, Harner RN. EEG patterns at the time of focal seizure onset. *Arch Neurol* 1978;35:276–286.
17. Blume WT, Young GB, Lemieux JF. EEG morphology of partial epileptic seizures. *Electroencephalogr Clin Neurophysiol* 1984;57:295–302.
18. Risinger MW, Engel J, Van Ness PC, et al. Ictal Localization of temporal lobe seizures with scalp/sphenoidal recordings. *Neurology* 1989;39:1288–1293.
19. Ebersole JS, Pacia SV. Localization of temporal lobe foci by ictal EEG patterns. *Epilepsia* 1996;37:386–399.
20. Vossler DG, Kraemer DLA, Knowlton RC, et al. Temporal ictal electroencephalographic frequency correlates with hippocampal atrophy and sclerosis. *Ann Neurol* 1998;43:756–762.
21. Thompson JL, Assaf BA, Ebersole JS. Multiple fixed dipole analysis of scalp-recorded interictal spikes and seizures in temporal lobe epilepsy. *Epilepsia* 1996;37 (Suppl 5):89.
22. Assaf BA, Ebersole JS. Continuous source imaging of scalp ictal rhythms in temporal lobe epilepsy. *Epilepsia* 1997;38:1114–1123.
23. Assaf BA, Ebersole JS. Visual and quantitative ictal EEG predictors of outcome after temporal lobectomy. *Epilepsia* 1999;40:52–61.
24. Scherg M, Ebersole JS. Brain source imaging of focal and multifocal epileptiform EEG activity. *Neurophysiol Clin* 1994;24:51–60.

Neocortical Epilepsies.
Advances in Neurology, Vol. 84,
edited by P.D. Williamson, A.M. Siegel,
D.W. Roberts, V.M. Thadani, and M.S. Gazzaniga.
Lippincott Williams & Wilkins, Philadelphia © 2000.

28

Interictal and Ictal Source Localization in Neocortical Versus Medial Temporal Lobe Epilepsy

P. Boon, M. D'Havé, G. Van Hoey, B. Vanrumste, K. Vonck, *C. Adam, and †T. Vandekerckhove

*Department of Neurology, EEG Laboratory–Epilepsy Monitoring Unit, University Hospital Gent, B-9000 Gent, Belgium; *Department of Neurology, Clinique Paul Castaigne, Hôpital Pitié-Salpêtrière, Paris, France; †Department of Neurosurgery, University Hospital Gent, B-9000 Gent, Belgium*

The main purpose of performing electroencephalography (EEG) in the presurgical evaluation of patients with refractory epilepsy is to identify the "epileptic focus" (1). Intracranial EEG, however, has remained the gold standard of presurgical localization in epilepsy (2). Invasive EEG procedures require large resources, they are expensive and time consuming, they carry a risk, and they have limitations. In 10% to 20% of patients who undergo intracranial EEG monitoring, seizures cannot be localized, which leads to the decision not to perform resective surgery (2).

Recently, dipole analysis of epileptic potentials has emerged and has rapidly become one of the most investigated noninvasive EEG techniques (3). Several authors have tried to define criteria for different types of epileptic spikes in different epileptic syndromes, such as medial temporal lobe epilepsy and benign epilepsy of childhood with centrotemporal spikes (3–12).

Intracranial EEG recording in epilepsy surgery candidates with underlying structural lesions is considered redundant in most cases because the lesion is most likely the cause of the seizures (13,14). When discrepancies between noninvasive examinations are found,

the etiologic relationship of lesion and seizures must be further documented (14). We previously presented dipole modeling in patients with refractory seizures and structural lesions (15–17). Previous dipole modeling was based on the assumption that (a) electrodes were in standard positions, and (b) a spherical head model could be used to calculate the underlying brain source. This method resulted in considerable localization errors (16,18). The aim of this work is to demonstrate the usefulness of source localization in distinguishing between medial temporal and neocortical epilepsy using a more sophisticated dipole analysis technique.

PATIENTS AND METHODS

Between October 1990 and June 1998, a population of 850 patients were evaluated at the University Hospital of Gent Epilepsy Monitoring Unit and the Clinique Paul Castaigne at the Salpêtrière Hospital in Paris. From that larger series, 51 patients (Gent: n = 37; Paris: n = 14) with long-standing refractory complex partial seizures (CPS) and a structural lesion on magnetic resonance imaging (MRI) were selected. All patients underwent a comprehensive presurgical workup that has been previously described, and included clinical neurologic and neuropsychological examination, video–EEG monitoring with prolonged interictal and ictal recording, and 1.5 T MRI according to an optimum MR protocol (1,14) and interictal fluorodeoxyglucose (FDG)–positron emission tomography (PET).

Additional invasive video–EEG monitoring was performed in 13 patients because of discrepancies between the results of noninvasive examinations. These included noncongruency between the location of the lesion and the EEG abnormality and the clinical semiology of the seizures or the absence of lateralized ictal scalp EEG recruitment in patients with a medial temporal lobe structural lesion. The appropriate set of depth electrodes (ADTECH, SD-12 Spencer probes) or subdural strips and grids (ADTECH, T-WS-4; T-WS-8; T-WG-20; T-WG-64 Wyler subdural electrodes) was determined for each patient. Both centers used semirigid, 12-contact depth electrodes that were placed in a sagittal plane according to the occipitotemporal approach. The proximal part of the electrodes was situated in the occipital cortex, the distal part in the amygdala. In 12 of 13 patients, an additional combination of different types of silicone embedded strips (4- and 8-contact) or a subdural grid (20- and 64-contact) was placed in the subdural space to sample near the suspected lesion (1,19).

Besides the presence of refractory CPS and the detection on MRI of a structural lesion, patient selection was based on the availability of high-quality EEG data. Our methodology of EEG recording and dipole modeling strategy has been described previously (16,17). Patients with bilateral independent spikes were excluded. For the purpose of the present study, 32-channel scalp EEG was recorded continuously for 48 to 72 hours at a 200 Hz sampling rate in digital-multiplexed format using a TELEFACTOR-Beehive (Gent) or BMSI (Paris) monitoring system (20). Twenty-one scalp electrodes were placed in International 10–20 system positions. To enhance coverage from the basal cortex and allow EEG registration below the equator of the spherical model, three supplementary inferior temporal electrodes on each side (in respectively, zygomatic: F9-F10; preauricular: T9-T10; and mastoid: Tp9-Tp10 positions) were placed on the scalp in most patients. Spherical fat markers were attached to the electrodes to visualize their positions on the MRI. Subsequently a set of rapid-acquisition MRIs (MPRAGE) was acquired. The markers showed up as high-intensity discs on MRI and were automatically localized using a custom-designed MATLAB program (18). Subsequently, the marker positions were matched with the appropriate electrode labels.

Data were recorded to a common reference electrode on the mastoid contralateral to the spike focus. Periods of active interictal epileptiform spiking were visually located during sleep stages 1, 2, and 3. The electrode sites where spikes had maximum negativity were statistically determined (Student's t test; unilateral confidence level: $p <0.05$). Only channels where spikes had a negative maximum superior to (mean + estimated standard error $\times t_{0.05}$) were taken into consideration. Epochs of 1,345 ms VHS recorded digital EEG, each containing one manually selected epileptiform transient (sharp wave, spike, spike and wave), were sliced and converted to a TELEFACTOR-Beekeeper format by means of a customer-designed software program (Gent) or FOCUS (MEGIS; Paris). The binary Beekeeper files were converted to raw ASCII files for BESA (brain electromagnetic source analysis; MEGIS) software package. The conversion also performed a filtering of "glitches." These are high-amplitude, high-frequency artifacts that probably result from switching noise at the time of acquisition. The raw ASCII files were read, baseline corrected, and filtered in BESA using a digital zero phase shift low-pass filter at 20 Hz and 24 dB/Oct slope and a digital zero phase shift high-pass filter at 2 Hz and 12 dB/Oct slope. Between 3 and 39 filtered spike files were averaged for each patient. An averaged file then was saved as a BESA (.avr) file.

Spatiotemporal multiple dipole modeling was performed according to the following strategy. A first fitting with a regional source was performed on each individual file to determine the quality of the EEG background activity and the spike for the dipole modeling. The exact time when the spike had maximum amplitude for temporal alignment of different files was determined automatically by the use of a customer-designed software program (Gent). A second conversion of the selected raw ASCII files was made with temporal alignment of the spikes. Files were again read in BESA with adding and averaging to enhance amplitude and improve the signal-to-noise (S/N) ratio. A second fitting was made with a regional source. This was first done for the whole epoch (895 ms) and for location and orientation; finally, a third fitting restricted to the epoch of the spike itself was performed. A total residual variance over all channels for the selected epoch of ≤15% was empirically considered as an appropriate fit. To import the electrode positions into BESA, which uses a spherical head model, the best-fitting sphere was calculated based on the localized marker positions. Projecting the marker positions on this sphere permitted calculation of the theta and phi coordinates of each electrode; these calculations were used to specify its position in BESA (.elp-file). First, the electrode positions as a whole were rotated with respect to the sphere's center so that simultaneously Cz was positioned on the vertical axis through the center and Fz was in the sagittal plane. This rotation corrected for a possible tilted position of the patient's head in the MRI scanner and allowed objective interpretation of the dipole orientation parameters acquired through dipole analysis. The calculated dipole in the spherical model was transformed to the coordinates of the best-fitting ellipsoid through the electrodes. Finally, the real positions offered a framework according to which the calculated dipole (BESA .pux-file) was mapped back on the MRIs. For each patient, interictal dipoles were visualized on the appropriate sagittal, axial, and coronal images,

providing a combination of source localization and anatomical information (21).

Although ictal EEG was recorded in all patients, it was available for review in only 46 patients. In 6 of 46 patients, the presence of movement artifact did not allow meaningful analysis. Hence, in 40 patients, ictal EEG files were available for dipole modeling. For each seizure, a 20-second epoch was manually sampled at the onset of the first visible ictal scalp EEG changes using narrow-band (1–14 Hz) digital filtering to minimize movement and muscle artifact. Each such epoch was sliced in smaller consecutive epochs of 1,345 ms. The data then were read, baseline corrected, and filtered in BESA. This was done in the same way as the interictal spike files but using a low-pass filter at 14 Hz. Because of the rapid frequency changes of ictal discharges, averaging was limited to too few epochs (2–5) and did not significantly improve the S/N ratio. As a result, original, nonaveraged ictal files were further processed according to this strategy. Much like the interictal dipoles, ictal dipoles were visualized on the MRI of individual patients.

RESULTS

Patient Population

Fifty-one patients (26 male, 25 female) with a mean age of 32 years (range: 12–57 years) and mean duration of epilepsy of 17 years (range: 2–41 years) were included in the study (Table 28.1). All patients had refractory CPS and were candidates for epilepsy surgery. They were included in a presurgical evaluation protocol after a structural lesion was detected by computed tomography (CT) or MRI. In 16 of 51 patients, the structural lesion appeared as space occupying; in 32 of 50 patients, an atrophic lesion was suspected; in 3 of 51 patients, a limited area of cortical dysplasia was present. Lesions were in the temporal lobe in 41 patients (confined to the medial temporal structures in 37 patients; in the medial and a limited part of the lateral temporal neocortex, 3 pa-

TABLE 28.1. *Clinical patient characteristics*

No.	Sex	Age (yr)	Seizure dur. (yr)	Lesion location	Inv. EEG	Neuroimaging	Pathology	Outcome F.U. (mo)
1	M	33	30	LF orbital	Yes	Space-occupying	Oligodendroglioma grade I	Ia(46)
2	M	15	10	LT med + lat	Yes	Atrophic	MTS	Ia(28)
3	F	42	35	RF parasellar	Yes	Space-occupying	Gliosis	IVb(46)
4	F	31	20	RT med + lat	Yes	Atrophic	MTS	Ia(37)
5	M	15	9	RT medial	No	Space-occupying	Astrocytoma grade III	Ia(34)
6	F	20	17	RT medial	No	Atrophic	MTS	Ia(22)
7	F	54	25	RF convex	No	Space-occupying	Cav. hemangioma	Ia(31)
8	M	33	5	RT medial	No	Space-occupying	Epiderm. cyst + MTS	Ia(31)
9	M	45	5	LT medial	No	Space-occupying	?	
10	F	28	25	RT medial	No	Space-occupying	Oligodendroglioma grade I	Ia(28)
11	F	40	2	LP convex	No	Space-occupying	Astrocytoma grade II	IIIa(24)
12	F	25	11	RT medial	No	Atrophic	MTS	Ia(22)
13	F	39	26	RT medial	No	Atrophic	?	
14	M	53	20	LT medial	No	Space-occupying	Cav. hemangioma	Ia(26)
15	M	37	19	RT medial	No	Atrophic	Astrocytoma grade I	Ia(18)
16	M	30	29	RT medial	Yes	Atrophic	MTS	Ia(12)
17	F	26	15	RT medial	Yes	Atrophic	MTS	Ia(12)
18	M	36	20	RT medial	No	Atrophic	?	
19	F	30	16	RT medial	Yes	Atrophic	MTS	Ia(12)
20	F	38	30	RF convex	No	Atrophic	?	
21	F	42	18	LP convex	No	Space-occupying	?	
22	F	27	14	RT medial	Yes	Atrophic	MTS	Ia(12)
23	M	22	8	LT medial	No	Atrophic	?	
24	F	57	7	RF convex	No	Space-occupying	Astrocytoma grade I	Ia(6)
25	F	22	14	RT medial	Yes	Atrophic	MTS	Ia(30)
26	F	29	28	RT bas + med	Yes	Dysplasia + heterotop.	Dysplasia	Ia(25)
27	F	18	7	RT medial	No	Atrophic	MTS	Ia(45)
28	F	33	8	RT medial	Yes	Atrophic	MTS	Ia(6)
29	M	46	27	RTO medial	No	Dysplasia	?	
30	M	30	15	LT medial	No	Space-occupying	Oligodendroglioma grade I	Ia(27)
31	F	28	27	RO medial	Yes	Atrophic	Dysplasia	IIIa(21)
32	M	45	41	RT medial	No	Atrophic	MTS	Id(37)
33	F	25	13	RT medial	No	Atrophic	MTS	Ib(48)
34	F	26	16	LT medial	No	Atrophic	MTS	Ib(42)
35	M	25	10	RF convex	No	Atrophic	Gliosis	IIc(34)
36	M	32	24	LT medial	No	Atrophic	MTS	Ia(50)
37	M	30	4	RT medial	No	Space-occupying	Astrocytoma grade I	Ia(10)
38	F	39	30	LT medial	No	Space-occupying	Astrocytoma grade I	IIIa(15)
39	M	35	10	RT medial	No	Atrophic	?	
40	M	22	9	RT medial	No	Space-occupying	?	
41	F	25	9	RT med + lat	No	Atrophic	?	
42	M	26	19	LT medial	No	Atrophic	MTS	Ia(7)
43	M	25	22	LT medial	No	Atrophic	MTS	Ia(14)
44	M	39	18	RT medial	No	Atrophic	MTS	Ia(17)
45	M	30	13	RT medial	No	Atrophic	?	
46	F	37	14	LT medial	No	Atrophic	?	
47	F	40	30	LT medial	Yes	Dysplasia	?	
48	M	29	17	RT medial	No	Atrophic	MTS	Ia(7)
49	M	22	10	RT medial	No	Space-occupying	Astrocytoma grade I	Ia(9)
50	M	28	27	RT medial	No	Atrophic	MTS	Ia(9)
51	M	12	6	RT medial	No	Atrophic	?	

LF, left frontal; MTS, medial temporal structures; LT, left temporal; RF, right frontal; RT, right temporal. Outcome: Engel scale.

tients; limited to the lateral neocortex only, 1 patient); in the frontal lobe in 6 patients; in the postcentral area of the parietal lobe in 2; and in the medial occipital lobe in 2 patients. Video–EEG monitoring documented CPS in all patients.

Thirty-seven patients underwent complete surgical resection of the lesion with a cura-

tive purpose. In 20 of these patients, histologic examination of the resected specimen showed mesial temporal sclerosis (MTS). A cavernous angioma was found in two patients. Low-grade oligodendrogliomas were found in three patients, grade I/II astrocytomas in six patients. A grade III astrocytoma, an epidermoid cyst, and gliosis were found in one patient each. Finally, in two patients, cortical dysplasia +/− heterotopia was demonstrated. One additional patient with an inaccessible, parasellar lesion underwent a hippocampectomy on the basis of depth EEG findings. Pathological examination in this patient revealed only mild gliosis. No tissue of the space-occupying parasellar lesion was available. According to the Engel outcome scale, postoperative seizure control was rated I in 32 patients, II in 1, III in three patients, and IV in one patient; average follow-up was 25 months (range: 6–50 months).

Interictal and Ictal EEG

In all patients, a unilateral or predominantly (>90% of ipsilateral discharges) unilateral spike or sharp wave focus was demonstrated. All patients with medial temporal lobe lesions had amplitude maxima in anterior, mid, or inferior temporal electrode positions, as did all three patients with combined medial and lateral neocortical structural lesions and the patient with a neocortical temporal lesion. Five of six patients with frontal lobe lesions also presented with an anterior to midtemporal spike; one patient with a parietal lobe lesion and both patients with an occipital lobe lesion had a broad spike field over the posterior temporal and parietal area. One patient with a parasellar lesion and the second patient with a parietal lesion had a spike with a mid to posterior temporal and parietal distribution.

Ictal scalp EEG was recorded in all patients but could be analyzed only in 40 patients. Characteristics of ictal scalp EEG, based on visual analysis, are described in Table 28.2.

Intracranial EEG

Invasive EEG monitoring was performed only when discrepancies were found between the results of different noninvasive tests. Thirteen patients underwent such invasive recordings. Two of these patients had small space-occupying lesions in the *frontal orbital*

and parasellar area. In one patient with a small, parasellar lesion, unequivocal hippocampal seizure onset was demonstrated. A set of four frontal depth electrodes in the immediate vicinity of the lesion and frontal subdural strips recorded frontal EEG abnormalities only seconds after the initial ictal hippocampal discharge. This patient, in whom the frontal lesion was hardly accessible, underwent a hippocampectomy based on the findings of the intracranial recording. After a short seizure-free period, complex partial seizures resumed at the presurgical frequency. The other patient with a left *frontal–orbital* lesion underwent implantation of hippocampal depth electrodes and two subdural frontal strips overlying the lesion. Simultaneous left-sided anterior hippocampal and posterior frontal orbital seizure onset was demonstrated. The electrode contacts in the immediate vicinity of the lesion remained relatively silent, but posterior contacts that approached the tip of the temporal lobe were active. In this patient, the surgical procedure included complete lesionectomy with margins and resection of the left temporal tip and the anterior 2 cm of the left hippocampus. The patient has been entirely seizure free since the procedure was done. Two other patients of these 13 had atrophic structural abnormalities involving both *medial temporal structures and limited parts of the lateral temporal neocortex*. In these last two patients, clear-cut ipsilateral hippocampal seizure onset was demonstrated. Seven patients who had *medial–temporal* atrophic structural lesions also underwent implantation of bilateral hippocampal depth electrodes with or without combined subdural electrodes; in all these patients, unilateral anterior to mid hippocampal seizure onset was demonstrated. Two patients with dysplastic lesions underwent invasive EEG recording, one of whom who had a *hippocampal* dysplastic lesion was shown to have an anterior hippocampal onset; the other patient with a *medial occipital lobe* lesion had six seizures recorded with ictal onset zone in the posterior margin of the lesion.

TABLE 28.2. *Ictal scalp EEG data and interictal and ictal dipole analysis*

Patient No.	2a Ictal scalp EEG	2b Ictal intracranial EEG	2c Type dipole	2c Elevated interictal	2c Elevated ictal
1	L frontotemporal recruitment	R frontobasal-anterior temp onset	2	13.9	10.7
2	L > R temporal recruitment	L anterior hippocampal onset	1	24.8	
3	R paroxysmal activity	R hippocampal onset	2	4.5	5.8
4	R temporal recruitment	R hippocampal onset	1	24.1	
5	R temporal recruitment		1	30.7	35.6
6	R temporal recruitment		1	45.4	25.6
7	Normal		2	3.0	
8	R temporal recruitment		1	41.4	35.1
9	Not available		1	38.2	
10	R temporal recruitment		1	23.7	28.6
11	Normal		2	3.6	
12	R temporal recruitment		1	41.2	53.6
13	R = L recruitment		1	42.3	
14	L temporal recruitment		1	39.6	
15	R temporal recruitment		1	48.4	42.0
16	R temporal recruitment	R anterior hippocampal onset	1	44.7	33.6
17	R > L temporal recruitment	R midhippocampal onset	1	45.4	21.9
18	R frontotemporal recruitment		1	39.9	39.0
19	R temporal recruitment	R hippocampal onset	1	36.1	27.1
20	Not available		2	6.4	
21	L > R frontotemp. recruitment		2	3.0	
22	R temporal recruitment	R hippocampal onset	1	31.3	56.7
23	R > L temporal recruitment		1	37.6	54.0
24	R temporal recruitment		2	7.8	12.9
25	Bilateral recruitment	R hippocampal onset	1	29.2	76.5
26	R > L temporal recruitment	R hippocampal onset	1	62.1	69.1
27	Bilateral recruitment		1	21.2	75.7
28	R = L paroxysmal activity	R anterior hippocampal onset	1	33.8	
29	R temporal recruitment	R post. occipital onset	1	27.0	47.5
30	L temporal recruitment		1	36.3	43.7
31	R temporal recruitment		1	66.4	71.1
32	R > L temporal recruitment		1	36.1	39.0
33	R temporal recruitment		1	23.0	22.3
34	L recruitment		1	27.9	61.8
35	Bilateral recruitment		2	4.4	9.4
36	Bilateral recruitment		1	79.4	23.5
37	R > L posterior recruitment		1	24.1	61.9
38	L temporal recruitment		1	88.2	25.9
39	R temporal recruitment		1	30.9	54.3
40	R temporal recruitment		1	30.0	26.2
41	R temporal recruitment		1	45.0	25.2
42	Bilateral temporal recruitment		1	45.0	24.1
43	L temporal recruitment		1	76.7	77.7
44	R frontotemporal recruitment		1	44.6	31.3
45	L temporal recruitment		1	21.0	30.5
46	L temporal recruitment		1	23.1	45.7
47	L > R temporal recruitment	L anterior hippocampal onset	1	52.3	38.8
48	R temporal recruitment		1	36.4	49.1
49	R temporal recruitment		1	31.4	43.5
50	R temporal recruitment		1	27.5	29.1
51	R temporal recruitment		2	3.5	9.4

EEG, electroencephalographic; L, left; R, right.

Interictal Dipole Modeling

All patients with structural lesions in the medial temporal lobe (n = 40) had a voltage field pattern with the following characteristics: ipsilateral, well delineated, negative voltage field, and occupying less than 50% of the scalp with a contralateral positive voltage field that extended well beyond the midline. The negative voltage field had a steeper gradient than the positive field. The corresponding dipole had an average elevation of 39.4 degrees (range: 21.0–88.2 degrees; SD = 15.8 degrees) relative to the axial plane. All patients with lateral temporal involvement associated with a medial temporal lobe structural abnormality and both patients with medial occipital lobe lesions also presented with this spike type. Figure 28.1 shows an example of a mapped interictal dipole in patient 46.

Nine patients presented with a different spike voltage field and dipole. All but one had extratemporal lesions (frontal orbital, n = 1; parasellar, n = 1; frontal convexity, n = 4; parietal convexity, n = 2); the remaining patient had a neocortical temporal lesion. The spike voltage field showed a less well-delineated negativity with a smoother gradient toward a less pronounced positivity. The corresponding dipole had an average elevation relative to the axial plane of 5.57 degrees (range: 2.97–13.90 degrees; SD = 3.52 degrees) (Fig. 28.2; patient 51).

Dipole Modeling of Ictal Discharges

In 41 patients, dipoles were calculated from early epochs of ictal paroxysmal scalp EEG activity. Thirty-three patients with a medial temporal lobe lesion, one with a medial + lateral temporal lobe lesion, and two with a medial occipital lesion were found to have an ictal dipole with an average elevation of 43.0 degrees (range: 21.9–77.7 degrees: SD = 17.1 degrees) relative to the axial plane. This finding corresponded to the interictal dipole pattern found in each of these patients (see Fig. 28.3 for the ictal dipole of patient 46). Four patients with extratemporal lesions (parasagittal frontal orbital, n = 1; parasellar, n = 1; frontal convexity, n = 2) and the patient with a neocortical temporal lesion presented with a different dipole pattern. The calculated ictal dipole had an elevation of 9.63 degrees (range: 5.77–12.90 degrees; SD = 2.59 degrees), similar to the patients' interictal dipole configuration (see Fig. 28.4; patient 51).

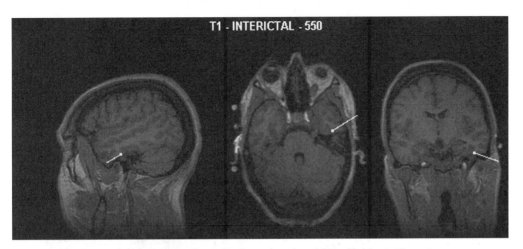

FIG. 28.1. Interictal dipole mapped on MRI of patient 46.

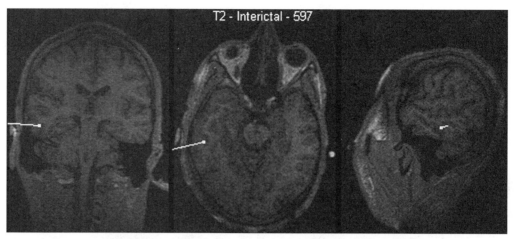

FIG. 28.2. Interictal dipole mapped on MRI of patient 51.

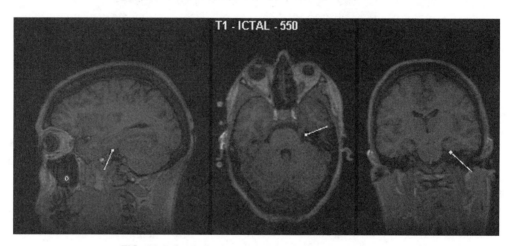

FIG. 28.3. Ictal dipole mapped on MRI of patient 46.

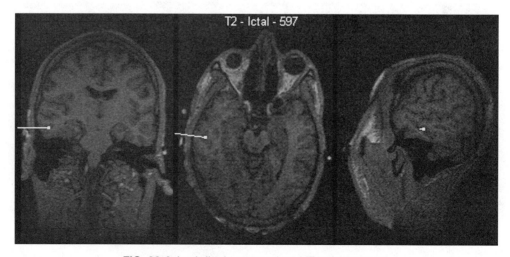

FIG. 28.4. Ictal dipole mapped on MRI of patient 51.

DISCUSSION

This study evaluated focal interictal and ictal EEG abnormalities, measured at the scalp, in patients with known intracranial structural and, presumably epileptogenic, lesions. Additionally, in 13 patients, invasive EEG recordings from bilateral hippocampal depth electrodes +/− subdural electrodes show seizure origin congruent with lesion location. Postsurgical seizure freedom further confirmed the epileptogenicity of the structural abnormality in 32 of 37 patients who underwent the operation. Spatiotemporal multiple dipole modeling identified different types of *interictal* spikes. All patients with a lesion confined to the medial temporal lobe (n = 40) and both patients with a medial occipital lobe lesion had a stable dipole that had a high degree of elevation relative to the axial plane. All three patients with lesions involving medial temporal structures and parts of the lateral temporal neocortex also had this type of dipole, which may seem contradictory to the findings of Ebersole and Wade, who would predict a different spike pattern in these patients (8). In two of three patients, however, a clear-cut hippocampal seizure onset was demonstrated by invasive EEG recording. This finding confirmed the previous finding that medial temporal lobe foci are highly correlated with an oblique dipole that remains relatively stable on spatiotemporal modeling (3,8).

The fact that both patients with a medial occipital lobe lesion also presented with a type 1 dipole is not surprising. The presence of a primarily tangential dipole in these patients is a reflection rather of a *medial* and *basal* origin of the underlying source than of an extratemporal location. All but two (medial occipital) patients with extratemporal (frontal orbital area, frontal convexity, parietal convexity) lesions and the single patient with a lateral (neocortical) temporal lesion had a predominantly radial (type 2) dipole that was also less stable on spatiotemporal modeling, which was reflected by a higher residual variance.

We did not find dipoles of different types in a single patient. Only few reports in the literature describe *ictal* dipole modeling in epilepsy surgery candidates (3,15,16). We analyzed brief epochs of ictal scalp EEG discharges in 41 patients. In this group, all patients with medial and combined medial and lateral temporal lobe lesions and both patients with a medial occipital lobe lesion presented with an ictal dipole with a high degree of elevation, in agreement with their interictal findings. Four patients with an extratemporal lesion and the neocortical temporal patient, in whom we were able to analyze ictal data, did not show this type of ictal dipole; rather, they showed a type 2 configuration, similar to their interictal dipole. Unlike interictal spikes that were easily recognizable and could be averaged to improve S/N ratio, ictal data were much more difficult to manage. Narrow band filtering of raw ictal data was necessary in trying to establish the earliest rhythmic changes of the scalp EEG trace. The S/N ratio of ictal data was less favorable because averaging could not be performed.

In the subgroup of patients in whom ictal dipoles were calculated, localization of the ictal dipole could be correlated with localization based on intracranial EEG findings. We found complete congruency between proven medial temporal lobe ictal EEG onset and the presence of a type 1 ictal (and interictal) dipole. In two patients with a frontal orbital and a parasellar lesion but with clear intracranially documented hippocampal seizure onset, a type 2 ictal (and interictal) dipole was found. Only the patient in whom a parasellar lesion could not be resected and who presented a type 2 dipole is not seizure free, suggesting that hippocampal localization by intracranial EEG recording may have been misleading. The other frontal patient in whom a type 2 dipole was calculated but in whom complete resection of the lesion was achieved has been entirely seizure free. This study confirms our preliminary results, although numbers are fairly small in the type 2 dipole category (15–17).

Presently available dipole modeling techniques have different limitations. The most important conceptional limitation is that calculating the inverse problem has no unique solution unless a series of constraints are introduced (22). Among the most important constraints are that (a) the three-shell spherical head model that is used is not physiological; (b) the model is based entirely on volume conduction principles; and (c) EEG electrodes are assumed to be in standard International 10–20 system positions. Because of inaccuracies in the calculations induced by the spherical model and the standard coordinates, localization of dipoles is less accurate than orientation (16,18); however, dipole calculations in the present study were performed by using an enhanced methodology. The localization of electrode coordinates by automatic detection on MRIs of markers on the scalp is easy and reliable (18). The custom-designed software does not require task-specific equipment such as a digitizer. Since MRIs are required in any patient who undergoes a presurgical evaluation, the use of this expensive imaging modality for electrode localization as well is justified. Moreover, mapping of the dipole on the actual MRI of the individual patients facilitates the clinical interpretation of the EEG data compared with the schematic representation that was previously used.

The clinical implications of interictal and ictal dipole mapping seem obvious. Dipole mapping may provide an additional and reliable means of measuring the underlying brain source. It remains unclear why in one patient with a parasellar lesion seizure onset in that area could not be demonstrated, despite the presence of several frontal intracerebral and subdural electrodes. Sampling error resulting in false-negative findings has been well recognized in the literature and is a major concern whenever intracranial studies are planned in the frontal and parietal lobe (2). Another patient with a frontal orbital lesion who was also demonstrated to have early ictal changes in the hippocampus, whereas the area around the lesion remained relatively silent, presented with a radial dipole suggesting extratemporal spike origin. The surgical approach was based on the find-

ing of a hippocampal seizure onset, but seizure cure probably was achieved because the entire lesion was removed. In this patient, the rationale for performing a hippocampectomy could be challenged. In the previous two patients as well as in the patient with a neocortical temporal lesion, dipole mapping provided additional evidence that the medial temporal structures were not primarily involved. Our findings suggest that in future lesional patients presenting with similar data, intracranial EEG recording possibly could be avoided. It is tempting but probably preliminary to speculate that, in selected patients, surgical decisions could be based on the results of dipole modeling instead of intracranially recorded EEG. To improve the anatomic accuracy of our methodology, the use of realistic head models, based on individual anatomic data, is needed. Present research is aimed at developing algorithms based on either the boundary element method (BEM), finite element method (FEM), or finite difference method (FDM) (21,23). Whereas BEM allows calculating potentials at a discrete set of nodes arranged in triangles located on the surface of the brain, FEM uses a grid composed of nodes located on tetrahedrons on the cortex. FDM is based on calculations of potentials on nodes of a cubic grid throughout the brain volume. Several pilot studies addressed the difficulties and advantages of these newer methods (21,24). Validation and application of these methods in an extended number of patients studied with intracranial EEG recordings are ongoing.

ACKNOWLEDGMENTS

This study was supported by grants BOZF-01104495 and 011A0996 from the University of Gent, by a grant from the Fund for Scientific Research-Flanders (F.W.O.), and by the Clinical Epilepsy Grant 1998–1999. The EEG technicians of the EEG laboratory at the Departments of Neurology in Gent and Paris are gratefully acknowledged for their continuous dedication.

REFERENCES

1. Boon PA, Williamson PD. Presurgical evaluation of patients with intractable partial seizures, indications, and evaluation techniques for resective surgery. *Clin Neurol Neurosurg* 1989;91:3–11.
2. Spencer SS, So NK, Engel J Jr, et al. Depth electrodes. In: Engel J Jr, ed. *Surgical treatment of the epilepsies,* 2nd ed. New York: Raven Press, 1993:359–375.
3. Ebersole JS. Equivalent dipole modeling, a new EEG method for localisation of epileptogenic foci. In: Pedley TA, Meldrum BS, eds. *Recent advances in epilepsy.* New York: Churchill Livingstone, 1992:51–71.
4. Gregory DL, Wong PK. Clinical relevance of a dipole field in rolandic spikes. *Epilepsia* 1992;33:36–44.
5. Lesser RP, Lüders HO, Morris HH, et al. Extracranial EEG evaluation. In: Engel J Jr, ed. *Surgical treatment of the epilepsies.* New York: Raven Press, 1987:173–181.
6. Wong PK, Gregory DL. Rolandic dipole discharges in children. *Am J EEG Technol* 1988;28:243–250.
7. Lüders HO, Dinner DS, Morris HH, et al. EEG evaluation for epilepsy surgery in children. *Cleve Clin J Med* 1989;56(Suppl):53–61.
8. Ebersole JS, Wade PB. Spike voltage topography identifies two types of frontotemporal epileptic foci. *Neurology* 1991;41:1425–1433.
9. Ebersole JS. EEG dipole modeling in complex partial epilepsy. *Brain Topogr* 1991;4:113–123.
10. Gregory DL, Wong PK. Topographical analysis of the centrotemporal discharges in benign rolandic epilepsy of childhood. *Epilepsia* 1984;6:705–711.
11. Laxer KD, Rowley AR, Novotny EJ, et al. Experimental technologies. In: Engel J Jr, ed. *Surgical treatment of the epilepsies,* 2nd ed. New York: Raven Press, 1993: 291–307.
12. Ebner A, Hoppe M. Non-invasive electroencephalography and mesial temporal sclerosis. *J Clin Neurophysiol* 1995;12:23–31.
13. Boon PA, Williamson PD, Fried I, et al. Intracranial, intraaxial, space-occupying lesions in patients with intractable partial seizures: an anatomoclinical, neuropsychological, and surgical correlation. *Epilepsia* 1991;32: 467–476.
14. Boon PA, De Reuck J, Calliauw L, et al. Clinical and neurophysiological correlations in patients with refractory partial epilepsy and intracranial structural lesions. *Acta Neurochir* 1994;128:68–83.
15. Boon P, D'Havé M. Interictal and ictal dipole modeling in patients with refractory partial seizures and an underlying intracranial structural lesion. *Acta Neurol Scand* 1995;92:7–18.
16. Boon P, D'Havé M, Adam C, et al. Dipole modeling in epilepsy surgery candidates. *Epilepsia* 1997;38: 208–218.
17. Boon P, D'Havé M, Vandekerckhove T, et al. Dipole modeling and intracranial EEG recording: correlation between dipole and ictal onset zone. *Acta Neurochir* 1997;139:643–652.
18. Van Hoey G, Vanrumste B, Van de Walle R, et al. Automatic marker recognition on MR images for EEG electrode localization. In: Veen JP, ed. *Proceedings of the ProRISC Workshop on Circuits, Systems, and Signal Processing.* The Netherlands: Mierlo, 1997:625–630.
19. Ojemann GA, Engel J. Acute and chronic intracranial recording and stimulation. In: Engel J Jr, ed. *Surgical treatment of the epilepsies.* New York: Raven Press, 1987:263–288.
20. Boon P, De Reuck J, Drieghe C, et al. Long-term video-EEG monitoring revisited: the value of interictal and ictal video-EEG recording, a follow-up study. *Eur Neurol* 1994;34:33–39.
21. Vanrumste B, Van Hoey G, Boon P, et al. Dipole mapping om magnetic resonance images of patients with epilepsy. In: Veen JP, ed. *Proceedings of the ProRISC Workshop on Circuits, Systems, and Signal Processing.* The Netherlands: Mierlo, 1997:643–645.
22. Scherg M. Fundamentals of dipole source potential analysis. In: Hoke M, ed. *Advances in audiology.* Basel: Karger, 1990:40–69.
23. Waberski TD, Buchner H, Lehnertz K, et al. Properties of advanced headmodelling and source reconstruction for the localization of epileptiform activity. *Brain Topogr* 1998;10:283–290.
24. Vanrumste B, Van Hoey G, Boon P, et al. The need for realistically shaped head models in EEG source analysis. In: *Proceedings ACOMEN, International Conference on Advanced Computational Methods in Engineering* 1998:527–535.

Neocortical Epilepsies.
Advances in Neurology, Vol. 84,
edited by P.D. Williamson, A.M. Siegel,
D.W. Roberts, V.M. Thadani, and M.S. Gazzaniga.
Lippincott Williams & Wilkins, Philadelphia © 2000.

29

Neuroimaging in Neocortical Epilepsies: Structural Magnetic Resonance Imaging

Gregory D. Cascino

Department of Neurology, Mayo Medical School, Division of Epilepsy, Mayo Clinic, Rochester, Minnesota 55905

Partial or localization-related epileptic syndromes in patients being considered for surgical treatment have been separated into three domains: medial temporal lobe epilepsy (MTLE), lesional epilepsy, and neocortical (extrahippocampal) epilepsy (1). This last epileptic syndrome includes patients with extratemporal and lateral temporal neocortical seizures (1). Mesial temporal sclerosis is the hallmark pathological finding in patients with MTLE (2,3). Intraaxial foreign-tissue lesions [i.e., tumors, vascular malformations, and disorders of cortical development (DCD)] represent the epileptogenic structural alteration in patients with a lesional epileptic syndrome (4).

Magnetic resonance imaging (MRI) has been demonstrated to be the most sensitive and specific structural neuroimaging procedure in patients with localization-related epilepsy who are being considered for surgical treatment (5–10). The diagnostic yield of MRI in patients with partial epileptic syndromes has obviated the routine use of radiographic computed tomography (CT). The results of structural neuroimaging have proved useful in identifying potential surgical candidates and tailoring the presurgical evaluation (11). MRI allows the acquisition of multiplanar anatomic data without bony artifact or the use of ionizing radiation (10). MRI has no known biological toxicity. MRI

findings are also of prognostic importance in patients undergoing epilepsy surgery (5,8,10,12,13).

The diagnostic yield of MRI depends on the underlying surgical pathology and localization of the ictal onset zone in patients with partial epilepsy (14). The high diagnostic yield of MRI in patients with MTLE and lesional epilepsy has been confirmed (2,6,7,13,15). MRI is a reliable indicator of mesial temporal sclerosis and foreign-tissue lesions (13,16–19). Surgical treatment in patients with MTLE and lesional epilepsy is typically substrate directed (11). The operative strategy in these patients includes excision of the underlying pathology associated with the partial seizure disorder. There is less information regarding the use of structural MRI in patients with neocortical epilepsy that is not substrate directed. The rationale for surgical therapy in these patients is to excise the epileptogenic zone completely.

The appropriate methodology for MRI studies, the relationship of structural neuroimaging procedures to pathology, and the potential applications of this neuroimaging procedure in patients with neocortical epilepsy undergoing surgical treatment for partial epilepsy are considered herein. A new development in MRI that allows multimodality imaging and coregistration of single photon emission tomography (SPECT) is also introduced.

MAGNETIC RESONANCE IMAGING: METHODOLOGY

The methodology used for a MRI study depends on the pathological finding underlying the epileptic brain tissue and the site of seizure onset. Coronal and sagittal images are performed routinely using the MRI head-seizure protocol at the Mayo Clinic (13,16,20). Axial images are useful to identify the central sulcus and evaluate perirolandic lesions in patients with neocortical epilepsy (Fig. 29.1). Coronal images are important in patients with suspected MTLE to evaluate the amygdalohippocampal complex (17,21). MRI reveals a reduction in the hippocampal formation volume or size in these patients, with images acquired using a short repetition time/echo time (TR/TE) pulse sequence that enhances the differences in the Tl relaxation times of different substances, that is, Tl-weighted (7,10,13,14,16,21,22). A Tl-weighted image allows the gray matter to be separated easily from the surrounding white matter. A short TR/TE scan in the coronal plane is optimal to evaluate the volume of the hippocampus and amygdala in patients with MTLE (21). Images acquired with a long TR/TE pulse sequence enhance the differences in the T2 relaxation time of different substances, that is, T2-weighted. Tissue characterization is based on the differences in the Tl and T2 relaxation time.

Lesional pathology is associated with an increase in the TI and T2 relaxation times of tissue (Figs. 29.1 and 29.2) (6,8). The most useful imaging sequence for identifying a neocortical structural abnormality is a T2-weighted sequence in the coronal plane (10). Proton-density scans using a long TR and short TE may prove useful in differentiating brain pathology from cerebrospinal fluid

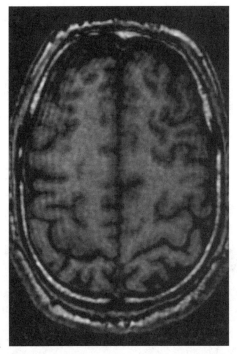 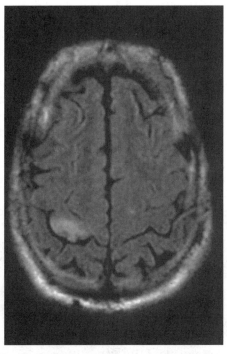

A   B

FIG. 29.1. MRI head in the axial plane in a patient with neocortical epilepsy associated with a somatomotor and somatosensory aura. T1-weighted image **(A)** and FLAIR sequence **(B)** show a left precentral lesion. A low-grade glial neoplasm was resected subsequently, and the patient experienced an excellent operative outcome. (*Note: The left cerebral hemisphere is on the left side of the figures.*)

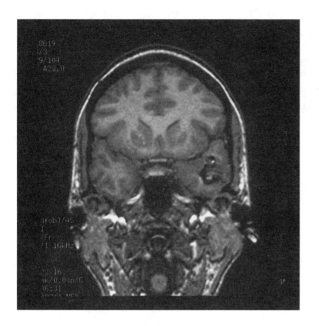

FIG. 29.2. MRI head in a patient with left temporal lobe neocortical epilepsy. A cavernous hemangioma was identified in the right anterior temporal lobe. A T1-weighted image in the oblique–coronal plane shows the lesion with evidence of remote hemorrhage. The patient was rendered seizure free by a lesionectomy and cortical margin excision. (*Note: The left cerebral hemisphere is on the right side of the figure.*)

(CSF). A fluid-attenuated inversion recovery (FLAIR) pulse sequence appears to improve the contrast between lesions and CSF further (Fig. 29.1). Gadolinium-DPTA is a paramagnetic contrast agent that produces predominantly a T1 shortening effect and is used with a Tl-weighted image sequence (20). An enhanced MRI study may be useful to "reveal" intracranial lesions associated with breakdown of the blood–brain barrier. Gadolinium does not improve the sensitivity of MRI in patients with partial epilepsy (20). An enhanced study may be useful to increase the specificity of MRI in patients with lesional epileptic syndromes. Enhancement of an imaging alteration may suggest the specific underlying pathological substrate associated with partial epilepsy.

NEOCORTICAL EPILEPSY: SUBSTRATE DIRECTED

Magnetic Resonance Imaging

Patients with lesional epileptic syndromes may be highly favorable candidates for epilepsy surgery; that is, these patients are likely to experience a reduction in seizure frequency without significant neurologic mor-

bidity (Figs. 29.1–29.3) (4,14,23). MRI plays an essential role in the identification of neocortical lesions and in the tailoring of the operative resection (24). The pathology of the foreign-tissue lesion and localization of the epileptic brain tissue are the primary determinants of the surgical outcome. About 30% of patients undergoing epilepsy surgery have pathologically verified lesional pathology (25). MRI has been confirmed to be a reliable and accurate indicator of foreign-tissue pathology, that is, vascular malformation, tumor, tuberous sclerosis, DCD, posttraumatic encephalomalcia, and remote cerebral infarction (Figs. 29.1–29.5) (6,26). The sensitivity of MRI approaches 100% in patients with tumors and vascular malformations (Figs. 29.1–29.5) (10,27,28). The diagnostic yield of MRI in DCDs depends on the specific pathological finding (5). The introduction of MRI has been associated with an increased recognition of focal cortical dysplasias (FCD) in patients with intractable partial epilepsy. Radiographic CT may be unremarkable in patients with FCD (26).

The most frequent neocortical tumors associated with partial epilepsy include primary glial neoplasms, gangliogliomas, and dysem-

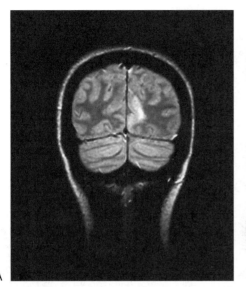
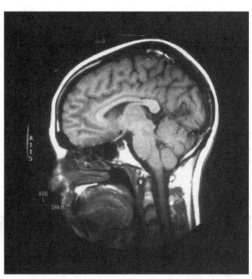

A   B

FIG. 29.3. MRI head in a patient with left occipital lobe seizures. An oblique–coronal T2-weighted image **(A)** revealed the medial occipital lobe lesion. A sagittal T1–weighted image **(B)** demonstrated the anterior-to-posterior extent of the intraaxial abnormality. A region of probable cortical dysplasia was surgically excised. The patient was rendered seizure free. (*Note: The left cerebral hemisphere is on the right side of the figure*).

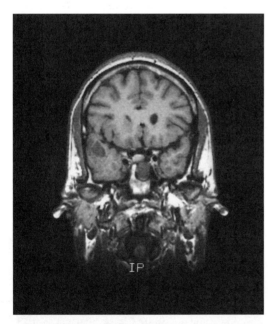

FIG. 29.4. MRI head in a patient with right temporal lobe neocortical seizures. The T1-weighted image in the oblique–coronal plane revealed the lesional pathology. A low-grade oligodendroglioma was completely excised. The patient had an excellent seizure outcome. (*Note: the right cerebral hemisphere is on the left side of the figure.)*

bryoplastic neuroepitheliomas (DNETs) (Figs. 29.1, 29.3–29.5) (4,6,10,27,29). Most glial neoplasms in patients with chronic seizure disorders are low-grade gliomas (10,27). Neoplasms characteristically produce a prominent increase in Tl and T2 relaxation times of tissue. T2-weighted images are most sensitive in revealing foreign-tissue lesions. Variably, there may be pathological contrast enhancement. Gadolinium-DTPA enhanced MRI scans may be useful to differentiate edema from tumor. Most tumors associated with a chronic partial seizure disorder are low-grade glial neoplasms that are associated with little edema and variable mass effect.

The most important neocortical cerebral vascular malformations in patients with medically refractory partial epilepsy are the arteriovenous malformations (AVMs), including the angiographically occult lesions, and cavernous hemangiomas or cavernomas (Fig. 29.2) (24,28). Seizures may be the only clinical manifestation associated with an AVM or cavernous hemangioma. Other neurologic symptoms in these patients include headache and

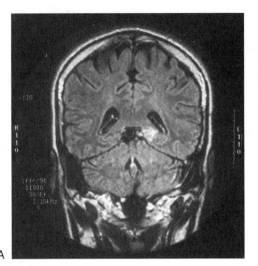
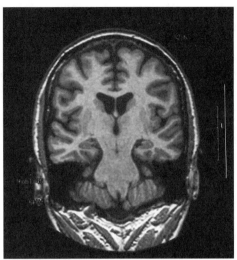

A B

FIG. 29.5. MRI head in a patient with complex partial seizures refractory to antiepileptic drug medication. The FLAIR sequence in the oblique–coronal plane **(A)** revealed a left posterior medial temporal lobe lesion. T1-weighted image in the oblique–coronal plane **(B)** shows left anterior hippocampal atrophy (confirmed with volumetric studies). (*Note: The left cerebral hemisphere is on the right side of the figures.*)

intracerebral hemorrhage. On MRI, AVMs may be associated with a flow signal. The cavernomas have a characteristic MRI appearance on the T2-weighted scans, with a region of increased T2 signal intensity surrounded by an area of decreased signal produced by hemorrhage associated with methemoglobin deposition in macrophages. Multiple vascular malformations may occur in patients who have familial cavernous hemangiomas.

The developmental lesions have been classified according to the MRI findings by Kuzniecky as *generalized, unilateral hemispheric,* and *focal* malformations (10). The high diagnostic yields of MRI in patients with generalized and unilateral hemispheric lesions have been confirmed (Fig. 29.6) (5). The generalized DCDs include lissencephaly, pachygyria, band or laminar heterotopia, and subependymal heterotopias. Hemimegalencephaly and Sturge–Weber syndrome are the predominant types of unilateral hemispheric abnormality. Hemimegalencephaly is characterized by an enlargement of one hemisphere with pachygyria or polymicrogyria. The MRI in Sturge–Weber syndrome reveals cerebral

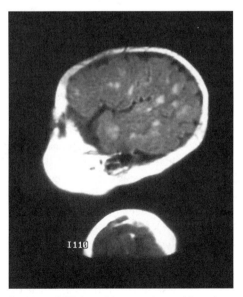

FIG. 29.6. MRI head in a patient with seizures and tuberous sclerosis. A FLAIR sequence in the sagittal plane shows the multiple cortical tubers.

atrophy, intracranial calcifications and the leptomeningeal angiomatosis. Anatomically restricted or focal forms of DCDs include FCD, polymicrogyria, focal subependymal heterotopias and schizencephaly. These DCDs are usually associated with MRI alterations, but there may be exceptions (Fig. 29.3). In FCD, the Tl-weighted image may identify a region of abnormal cortical white matter organization (5,26). The T2-weighted image in these patients shows a signal intensity alteration that may be difficult to differentiate from a neoplasm. Typically, the imaging abnormality associated with FCD is a high-intensity lesion without mass effect or pathological gadolinium enhancement. Finally, the spectrum of DCDs includes patients with pathologies that appear at present to be uncommonly associated with a specific MRI alteration. The surgically excised tissue in these patients may reveal cortical microdysgenesis (30). The pathological findings associated with cortical microdysgenesis include disruption of cortical lamination, a localized protrusion of neurons in deeper cortical regions, and single-neuron heterotopias. Microdysgenesis may have no macroscopic correlation and may not be imaged by MRI.

Surgical Outcome

Complete or total resection of the neocortical lesional pathology is the most important factor in determining a favorable operative outcome (23,27,28,31). About 80% to 90% of patients with intractable lesional epilepsy are rendered seizure free or near seizure free following resection of the epileptogenic zone and the lesional pathology (Figs. 29.1–29.5) (23,27,28,31). Resection of the lesion alone stereotactically produces less favorable results with about 50% of patients who become seizure free (24). MRI is used during the data-acquisition phase to delineate the limits of the lesion prior to the stereotactic lesionectomy. The extent of resection of the epileptic brain tissue is of less prognostic importance (31). Resection of the epileptogenic zone alone has yielded dismal results, even if chronic in-

tracranial EEG monitoring is used preoperatively (31). A high correlation exists between the site of the neuroimaging-identified epileptogenic lesion and the epileptogenic zone. Prior to surgery, the patient should undergo a comprehensive presurgical evaluation to determine the relationship between the mass lesion and the site of the epileptic brain tissue (32). Potential epileptogenic lesions may be demonstrated to be remote from the site of seizure onset (23). Selected patients with non-medically refractory lesional epilepsy even may be considered for surgical treatment (e.g., patients who are unable to tolerate antiepileptic drug medication or are interested in pursuing a pregnancy). MRI should be performed early in the course of treatment for partial epilepsy to avoid unnecessary medication trials in patients with intracranial mass lesions.

The choice of operative procedure may be affected by the MRI study. Patients with localized pathology, such as foreign-tissue lesions, intimately associated with the epileptogenic zone, may be rendered seizure free following resection of the lesion and the epileptic brain tissue. Patients with widespread unilateral pathology, for example, hemimegalencephaly or Sturge–Weber syndrome, may require a multilobar resection or a hemispherectomy to reduce seizure tendency significantly, regardless of the ictal semiology and preoperative electrophysiologic studies. Patients with bihemispheric pathology, for example, congenital bilateral perisylvian syndrome, may be candidates for a corpus callosotomy because a focal cortical resection is usually unsuccessful.

Illustrated Case Presentations

Case 1

A 32-year-old patient experienced a single secondarily generalized tonic–clonic seizure 5 years earlier. Subsequently, the patient developed recurrent, unprovoked seizures associated with left arm somatomotor and somatosensory aura and speech arrest. There was no impairment in consciousness. The seizures were refractory to antiepileptic drug medication. EEG showed left central region spike activity. MRI revealed a lesion in the left precentral gyrus (Fig. 29.1). Neurologic examination was normal interictally. Postictally, the patient had a mild right hemiparesis and dysphasia. Scalp-recorded EEG monitoring suggested left frontotemporal seizure activity. The patient underwent chronic intracranial EEG monitoring and functional mapping. The ictal onset zone was immediately posterior to the lesional pathology. A lesionectomy and a focal cortical resection were performed. A grade I–II oligodendroglioma was excised. There was mild, transient right lower facial weakness postoperatively without any dysphasia. The patient has been seizure free and asymptomatic for 4 years following surgery. Postoperative MRI studies have not revealed any residual or recurrent tumor.

Comment: This patient has lesional epilepsy associated with a neoplastic lesion in the left frontal lobe (33). MRI was used preoperatively to tailor the presurgical evaluation and provide a target for intracranial EEG electrode placement. After surgery, MRI confirmed the extent of tumor resection.

Case 2

A 32-year-old patient presented with complex partial seizures characterized by a behavioral arrest, staring, and confusion. There was variable posturing of the right upper extremity and occasional secondarily generalized tonic–clonic seizures. EEG showed left frontotemporal spiking. MRI revealed a left temporal lobe neocortical lesion consistent with a cavernous hemangioma (Fig. 29.2). The medial temporal lobe structures appeared normal. No hippocampal formation atrophy was present. Long-term EEG monitoring confirmed the diagnosis of left temporal lobe epilepsy. The patient underwent a focal cortical resection that included the lesional pathology. Postoperative MRI confirmed the complete excision of the neocortical lesion. This patient has been seizure free during a 12-

month period following surgery except for occasional nondisabling auras.

Comment: This patient had temporal lobe epilepsy related to a neocortical lesion (33). The pathological finding underlying the epileptogenic zone proved to be a cavernous hemangioma. The operative strategy was limited to a lesionectomy with a limited cortical margin. The prognostic importance of the extent of lesion excision has been shown (26).

Case 3

A 33-year-old patient developed recurrent, unprovoked complex partial seizures at 22 years of age. The patient experienced prominent ictal dysphasia. Ictal behavior included staring and right upper extremity dystonic posturing. EEG revealed bitemporal, independent spike activity, maximal on the left. MRI head-seizure protocol revealed a left posterior temporal neocortical lesion consistent with a low-grade glioma (Fig. 29.5). The patient underwent a tumor biposy and resection. A grade II fibrillary astrocytoma was resected. The patient was seizure-free for 6 months. Subsequently, he developed recurrent seizures similar to the initial seizure type. MRI revealed no recurrent or residual tumor. Subtle left hippocampal formation atrophy was present. Scalp-recorded EEG showed bitemporal spike discharges. The patient underwent chronic intracranial EEG monitoring with bitemporal depth electrodes. The diagnosis of left MTLE was confirmed. The patient is seizure free 4 years following an anterior temporal lobectomy. He has been withdrawn from antiepileptic drug medication. Pathological examination of the left medial temporal lobe revealed gliosis and mild hippocampal neuronal loss.

Comment: This patient had dual pathology associated with symptomatic partial epilepsy (3). There was evidence for a neocortical lesion in the posterior temporal lobe and mesial temporal sclerosis. The initial operative strategy involved tumor surgery. The lesion was remote from the amygdalohippocampal complex. The patient was not rendered seizure-free and successfully withdrawn from antiepileptic drug therapy until an anterior temporal lobe neocortical resection and amygdalohippocampectomy were performed.

NEOCORTICAL EPILEPSY: NOT SUBSTRATE DIRECTED

Magnetic Resonance Imaging

Unfortunately, an unremarkable structural MRI study is not uncommon in a patient with neocortical epilepsy (29). The ictal behavior may be sufficiently vague and does not allow appropriate lateralization or localization of the epileptogenic zone based on semiology alone (33). Physicians directly caring for these patients should review the structural MRI carefully. Subtle alterations that may not be easily recognized include changes associated with a DCD. The most common pathological finding in patients with a normal MRI is gliosis with variable neuronal loss. The purpose of structural neuroimaging in patients with neocortical (nonlesional) epilepsy is to exclude a pathological substrate coexistent with the epileptogenic zone as well as to identify a potentially epileptiform subtle nonlesional cortical alteration. Lateralized or localized atrophy or alteration in the gyral pattern may represent a marker for the site of seizure onset. Potential imaging options in patients with a "normal" MRI and intractable partial epilepsy include reimaging the area of interest using contiguous slices less than 2 mm thick by using additional sequences (such as FLAIR) that were not incorporated in the initial MRI protocol or by using contrast studies. Three-dimensional surface cortical mapping using MRI may delineate an anatomic change that may suggest localization of the epileptogenic brain tissue in neocortical epilepsy. Altered gyral morphology, including increased gyral complexity, may be a reliable marker of the site of seizure onset and may serve as a target for placement of intracranial EEG electrodes (29). Fractal analysis and "cortical volume–surface area relationships" are cur-

rently under investigation as potential MRI techniques for patients with "normal" structural MRI studies being considered for epilepsy surgery (29).

Subtraction Ictal SPECT Coregistered to MRI

Subtraction ictal SPECT coregistered to MRI (SISCOM) is a recent development that increases the diagnostic yield of functional neuroimaging in patients with partial epilepsy (1,34). The rationale for ictal SPECT is the identification of region(s) of increased or decreased cerebral blood flow that may be a reliable marker of the ictal onset zone. The high sensitivity and specificity of ictal SPECT in patients with temporal lobe epilepsy have been shown by multiple groups. The value of these studies in patients with nonlesional extratemporal seizures is less clear. Ictal SPECT scans are superior in sensitivity and specificity to interictal studies. The significance of baseline blood flow changes that are unrelated to partial seizure activity may not be recognized. Interictal SPECT studies may not be a reliable marker of the ictal onset zone. There are concerns regarding both sensitivity and specificity with interictal blood flow measurements alone. There are also significant limitations associated with nonsubtracted interictal and ictal SPECT. A subtle ictal perfusion alteration may not be obvious by the traditional side-by-side viewing of the ictal and interictal images.

The current SISCOM protocol at Mayo Foundation was developed by O'Brien and colleagues (34,35). The rationale for this procedure is to demonstrate a blood flow alteration related to partial seizure activity and to display the change on a volumetric high-resolution structural MRI. Therefore, there is the merging of functional and structural imaging alterations. These studies were intended specifically for patients with pharmacoresistant partial epilepsy being considered for surgical treatment. The SISCOM studies are currently available 7 days per week from 7:00 a.m. to 11:00 p.m. at Mayo, Rochester. The patient is admitted to the epilepsy monitoring unit for ictal long-term EEG recordings. Prior to admission for EEG monitoring, the patients have a volumetric structural MRI using a designed seizure protocol that was previously described. At admission, a patient is identified as being an appropriate candidate for a SISCOM study.

The radioisotope is injected at seizure onset by an EEG technician who has been observing the patient on closed-circuit television. The technician may remain in the room prior to the ictal injection if the patient has frequent or brief seizure episodes. The timing of the injection in relation to ictal onset is determined by a review of the electroclinical correlation. The diagnostic yield is highest when the radioisotope is injected within 45 seconds of seizure onset (34). The seizure duration should be at least 10 seconds for a valid functional imaging study (34). The seizure type does not appear to be of predictive value. An interictal SPECT scan is performed at a time the patient has been seizure-free for a minimum of 24 hours, if possible. Subsequently, the ictal and interictal cerebral blood flow changes are subtracted and coregistered to the volumetric structural MRI.

The use of structural MRI to demonstrate the anatomic region of ictal hyperperfusion or hypoperfusion has several advatanges. First, the relationship between the lesional zone and the SPECT imaging alteration can be shown in patients with a lesional epileptic syndrome. Second, the anatomic landmarks underlying the localized blood flow change can be determined. Third, the SISCOM data may determine the site of intracranial EEG electrode placement in patients requiring chronic intracranial EEG monitoring.

The diagnostic yield of SISCOM studies in patients with medically refractory partial epilepsy has been evaluated (34). This study would serve as a validation of the SISCOM technique in patients being considered for epilepsy surgery. SISCOM was compared by three blinded investigators to the side-by-side ictal and interictal SPECT scans in 51 patients (34). The sensitivity and specificity of the

functional neuroimaging studies are improved significantly by the coregistration with MRI. The interobserver agreement also favored the SISCOM technique. There were significant errors in interpretation, that is, both false-positive and false-negative studies, associated with the nonsubtracted ictal and interictal SPECT scans. The prognostic importance of SISCOM also was assessed in patients who underwent a focal cortical resection (34). A significant difference in operative outcome was found when two groups were compared: localized SISCOM alteration that was concordant with the ictal onset zone versus nonlocalized SISCOM alteration (p <0.05). About 60% of the former group of patients had an excellent operative outcome; that is, they may be able to operate a motor vehicle. About 20% of the patients with a nonlocalized SISCOM experienced an excellent outcome.

A subsequent study compared the predictive value of SISCOM operative outcome in patients with nonlesional extratemporal seizures. These patients do not have a substrate-directed partial epilepsy and have a higher risk for surgical failure. The prognostic importance of the SISCOM studies was once again demonstrated. About 70% of the patients with a localized SISCOM alteration had an excellent outcome compared with 17% of patients with nonlocalized SISCOM studies (p <0.05).

Illustrated Case Presentations

Case 1

A 24-year-old patient had a history of recurrent, unprovoked seizures since 6 months of age. The patient had a high fever and a prolonged generalized tonic–clonic seizure at 3 months of age. The patient has a coexistent chronic, global, static encephalopathy. For the past 30 years, the patient has had multiple daily seizures associated with sleep. The clinical episodes last less than 1 minute and are associated with yelling, facial grimacing, and posturing of both upper extremities. There is no postictal confusion. The patient believes he remains awake during seizure activity. The seizures had been refractory to multiple antiepileptic drug regimens. Routine EEG revealed generalized spike-and-wave discharges that are maximal in the anterior head region. Multiple scalp-recorded seizures have failed to demonstrate a localized electrographic seizure pattern. The patient was presumed to have a symptomatic generalized epilepsy. MRI head-on multiple occasions have been normal. Neurologic examination was unremarkable except for mild developmental delay. A SISCOM study was performed by allowing the patient to sleep during the daytime in the epilepsy monitoring unit. No definite electrographic seizure discharge was observed during a typical spell. The SISCOM study revealed a localized left anterior frontal lobe alteration (Fig. 29.7). Chronic intracranial EEG monitoring confirmed the relationship between the site of seizure onset and the SISCOM change. A cortical resection was performed and revealed focal cortical dysplasia. There was no neurological morbidity. The patient has remained completely seizure-free 6 months following surgery. The antiepileptic drug medication has been reduced.

Comment: The SISCOM procedure not only localized the ictal onset zone but also suggested the diagnosis of partial epilepsy.

The blood flow change provided a "target" for implanting the intracranial electrodes.

Case 2

A 33-year-old patient had multiple, bihemispheric cavernous hemangiomas and a partial seizure disorder. The seizures were predominantly secondarily generalized tonic–clonic type. Several of the vascular malformations had evidence of recent or remote hemorrhage as determined by MRI. EEG revealed bilateral, independent spike activity. Ictal EEG suggested the right hemisphere origin of seizures. There were multiple right extratemporal and a right neocortical temporal lobe cavernous hemangiomas. The SISCOM revealed a localized right frontal lobe alteration in blood flow (Fig. 29.8). The patient underwent a right frontal lobectomy with resection of the vascular malformation. The patient was rendered seizure free and successfully tapered off antiepileptic drug medication.

Comment: The SISCOM study was useful to identify the pathological substrate underlying the epileptogenic zone in a patient with multiple lesions. The scalp-recorded EEG suggested only the lateralization and not localization of the epileptic brain tissue.

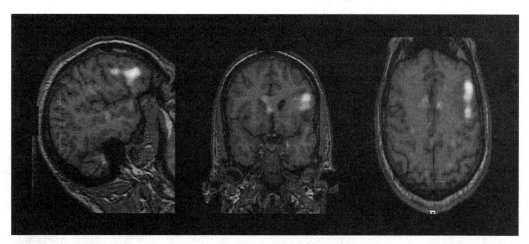

FIG. 29.7. A subtraction periictal SPECT study coregistered to a volumetric MRI, revealed a localized region of cerebral hyperperfusion in the left anterior frontal lobe (sagittal, oblique–coronal, and axial planes). The structural MRI study was normal. (*Note: The left cerebral hemisphere is on the right side of the figures.*)

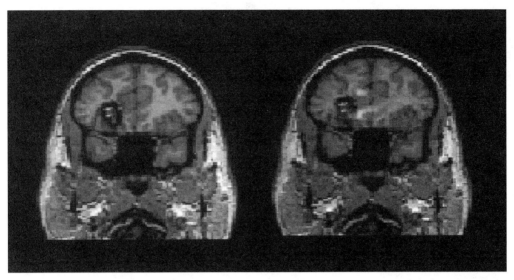

FIG. 29.8. A subtraction periictal SPECT study coregistered to a volumetric MRI revealed a localized region of cerebral hyperperfusion in the right frontal lobe. The structural MRI revealed multiple cavernous hemangiomas including in the right temporal lobe. (*Note: The right cerebral hemisphere is on the left side of the figures.*)

Case 3

A 54-year-old patient had a 5-year history of partial seizures of probable right perirolandic origin. The most frequent type of seizure was associated with a sensorimotor aura involving predominantly the left arm without altered mentation. These clinical episodes were occurring several times per day. Variably the patient had a secondarily generalized tonic-clonic seizure. The seizures were refractory to antiepileptic drug medication. Neurologic examination was normal. The patient had a mild left hemiparesis and hemisensory deficit subsequent to the simple partial seizures. Interictal EEG revealed right central region spikes. MRI head-seizure protocol was unremarkable except for nonspecific white matter changes in both hemispheres suggesting "small-vessel disease." Scalp-recorded ictal EEG did not reveal a definite electrographic alteration during the simple partial seizures. A SISCOM study revealed a localized region of cerebral hyperperfusion in the right postcentral gyrus (Fig. 29.9). Chronic intracranial EEG monitoring was performed using a subdural plate of electrodes for localizing the ictal onset zone and the mapping of the functional cortex. The epileptogenic zone was concordant with the SISCOM alteration. A focal cortical resection was performed that revealed gliosis. The patient has been seizure free subsequent to surgery (approximately 2.5 years) and did not experience any significant morbidity.

Comment: The SISCOM provided a potential "target" for placement of intracranial EEG electrodes in this patient with neocortical epilepsy of perirolandic origin. The functional neuroimaging study was important in counseling the patient prior to the neurosurgical procedure. The abnormal SISCOM study predicted an excellent operative outcome in the patient. The ictal semiology confirmed the lateralization of the ictal onset zone. Intracranial EEG monitoring was necesssary in this patient to define the anatomical boundaries of the ictal onset zone and for functional cortical mapping.

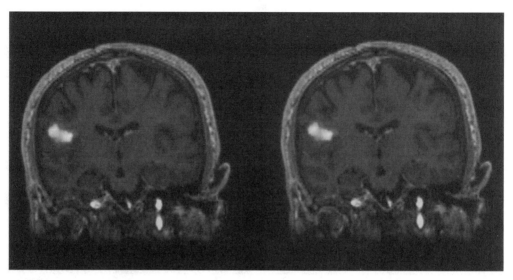

FIG. 29.9. A subtraction periictal SPECT study coregistered to a volumetric MRI revealed a localized region of cerebral hyperperfusion in the right perirolandic region. The structural MRI study was normal. (*Note: The right cerebral hemisphere is on the left side of the figures.*)

REFERENCES

1. Cascino GD. Neuroimaging in partial epilepsy: structural magnetic resonance imaging. *J Epilepsy* 1998; 11:121–129.
2. Cascino GD, Jack CR, Parisi J, et al. Magnetic resonance imaging-based hippocampal volumetric studies in temporal lobe epilepsy: pathological correlation. *Ann Neurol* 1991;30:31–36.
3. Cascino GD, Jack CR, Parisi JE, et al. Operative strategy in patients with MRI identified dual pathology and temporal lobe epilepsy. *Epilepsy Res* 1993a;14: 175–180.
4. Boon PA, Williamson PD, Fried I, et al. Intracranial, intra-axial, space-occupying lesions in patients with intractable partial seizures: an anatomoclinical, neuropsychological, and surgical correlation. *Epilepsia* 1991;32: 467–476.
5. Barkovitch A, Chuang S, Norman D. MR of neuronal migration anomalies. *AJNR Am J Neuroradiol* 1987; 8:1009–1017.
6. Bergen D, Bleck T, Ramsey R, et al. Magnetic resonance imaging as a sensitive and specific predictor of neoplasms removed for intractable epilepsy. *Epilepsia* 1989;30:310–321.
7. Berkovic S, Andermann F, Olivier A, et al. Hippocampal sclerosis in temporal lobe epilepsy demonstrated by MM. *Ann Neurol* 1991;29:175–182.
8. Brooks B, King D, El Gammal T, et al. MRI in patients with intractable complex partial seizures. *AJNR Am J Neuroradiol* 1990;11:93–99.
9. Cascino GD. Commentary: How has neuroimaging improved patient care? *Epilepsia* 1994;35(Suppl 6): S103–S107.
10. Kuzniecky R, Cascino G, Palmini A, et al. Structural neuroimaging. In: Engel J Jr, ed. *Surgical treatment of the epilepsies,* 2nd ed. New York: Raven Press, 1993: 197.
11. Spencer DD. Strategies for focal resection in medically intractable epilepsy. *Epilepsy Res* 1992(Suppl 5);157–168.
12. Cascino GD, Trenerry MR, So EL, et al. Routine EEG and temporal lobe epilepsy: relation to quantitative MRI and operative outcome. *Epilepsia* 1996;36:692–696.
13. Jack CR, Sharbrough FW, Cascino GD, et al. Magnetic resonance imaging-based hippocampal volumetry: correlation with outcome after temporal lobectomy. *Ann Neurol* 31,138–146.
14. Cascino GD, Jack CR, Parisi JE, et al. MRI in the presurgical evaluation of patients with frontal lobe epilepsy and children with temporal lobe epilepsy: pathologic correlation and prognostic importance. *Epilepsy Res* 1992a;11:51–59.
15. Jackson GD, Berkovic SF, Tress BM, et al. Hippocampal sclerosis can be reliably detected by magnetic resonance imaging. *Neurology* 1990;40:1869–1875.
16. Jack CR, Sharbrough FW, Twomey CK, et al. Temporal lobe seizures: lateralization with with MR volume measurements of hippocampal formation. *Radiology* 1990; 176:205–209.
17. Spencer SS, McCarthy G, Spencer DD. Diagnosis of medial temporal lobe seizure onset: relative specificty and sensitivity of quantitative MRI. *Neurology* 1993;43: 2117–2124.
18. Trenerry MR, Jack CR, Ivnik RJ, et al. Memory is correlated with presurgical MRI hippocampal volumes before and after temporal lobectomy for intractable epilepsy. *Epilepsia* 1991;32:73(abstr).
19. Trenerry MR, Jack CR, Cascino GD, et al. MRI hippocampal volumes: association with onset and duration of epilepsy, and febrile convulsions in temporal lobectomy patients. *Epilepsy Res* 1993;15:247–252.

20. Cascino GD, Hirschorn KA, Jack CR, et al. Gadolinium-DTPA enhanced MRI in intractable partial epilepsy. *Neurology* 1989;39:1115–1118.

21. Lencz T, McCarthy G, Bronen R, et al. Quantitative MRI of the hippocampus in temporal lobe epilepsy. *Ann Neurol* 1992;31:629–637.

22. Cascino GD, Jack CR, Sharbrough FW, et al. MRI assessments of hippocampal pathology in extratemporal lesional epilepsy. *Neurology* 1993b;43:2380–2382.

23. Awad IA, Rosenfeld J, Ahl H, et al. Intractable epilepsy and structural lesions of the brain, mapping, resection strategies, and seizure outcome. *Epilepsia* 1991;32:179–186.

24. Cascino GD, Kelly PJ, Sharbrough FW, et al. Long-term follow-up of stereotactic lesionectomy in partial epilepsy: predictive factors and electroencephalographic results. *Epilepsia* 1992b;33:639–644.

25. Brown WJ, Babb TL. Neuropathological changes in the temporal lobe associated with complex partial seizures. In: Hopkins A, ed. *Epilepsy.* New York: Demons, 1987.

26. Palmini A, Andermann F, Olivier A, et al. Focal neuronal migrational disorders and intractable partial epilepsy: a study of 30 patients. *Ann Neurol* 1991;30:741–749.

27. Britton J, Cascino GD, Sharbrough FW, et al. Low-grade glial neoplasms and intractable partial epilepsy: efficacy of surgical treatment. *Epilepsia* 1994;35:1130–1135.

28. Dodick D, Cascino GD, Meyer FB. Vascular malformations and intractable epilepsy: outcome after surgical treatment. *Mayo Clin Proc* 1994;69:741–745.

29. Cook M, Sisodyia SM. Magnetic resonance imaging in epilepsy surgery. In: Shorvon S, Dreifuss F, Fish D, Thomas D, eds. *The treatment of epilepsy.* London: Blackwell Science, 1996:589.

30. Meencke HJ. Minimal developmental disturbances in epilepsy and MRI. In: Bydder GM, Stefan H, eds. New York: Plenum Press, 1994:127.

31. Fish DR, Andermann F, Olivier A. Complex partial seizures and posterior temporal or extratemporal lesions: surgical strategies. *Neurology* 1991;41:1781–1784.

32. Dreifuss FE. Goals of surgery for epilepsy. In: Engel J Jr, ed. *Surgical treatment of the epilepsies.* New York: Raven Press, 1987:31

33. Williamson PD, Weiser HG, Delgado-Escueta AV. Clinical characteristics of partial seizures. In: Engel J Jr, ed. *Surgical treatment of the epilepsies.* New York: Raven Press, 1987:101

34. O'Brien TJ, So EL, Mullan BP, et al. Subtraction ictal SPECT co-registered to MRI improves clinical usefulness of SPECT in localizing the surgical seizure focus. *Neurology* 1998;50:445–454.

35. O'Brien TJ, So EL, Mullan BP, et al. Subtraction SPECT co-registered to MRI improves postictal SPECT localization of seizure foci. *Neurology* 1999;52:137–146.

Neocortical Epilepsies.
Advances in Neurology, Vol. 84,
edited by P.D. Williamson, A.M. Siegel,
D.W. Roberts, V.M. Thadani, and M.S. Gazzaniga.
Lippincott Williams & Wilkins, Philadelphia © 2000.

30

The Use of fMRI in Neocortical Epilepsy

William D. Gaillard, *Susan Y. Bookheimer, and *Mark Cohen

*The George Washington University School of Medicine, Director, Comprehensive
Pediatric Epilepsy Program, Children's National Medical Center,
Washington, D.C. 20010;*Department of Neurology, Brain Mapping Division,
UCLA School of Medicine, Los Angeles, California 90095-1769*

The goal of epilepsy surgery is to resect the epileptogenic focus while preserving normal neuronal function. This chapter reviews new techniques for identifying eloquent cortex that the prudent epilepsy surgeon seeks to spare. This task is particularly relevant to the neocortical epilepsies. The injection of amytal is traditionally used to identify the hemisphere for language dominance and to ascertain whether the contralateral hemisphere can sustain memory (1–4). Until recently, localization of function was possible only with cortical stimulation, either in the operating room or through subdural grids (5–7). A number of new techniques, namely transcranial magnetic stimulation, O-15 positron emission tomography (PET), and, the subject of this review, functional magnetic resonance (fMRI), make possible the noninvasive identification and localization of cortical function. These may be "simple" cortical functions, such as primary motor and sensory cortex—touch, sight, and hearing—or "higher-ordered" cortical function, such as that involved in language and memory.

This chapter reviews the work on which fMRI is based and also reviews fMRI and image analysis principles. Then we examine the application of fMRI in lateralizing and localizing cortical functions. Finally, this chapter closes with considering the advantages and limitations of fMRI.

BACKGROUND: PET STUDIES

Roy and Sherrington first made the observation that increased cortical activity is associated with increased cerebral blood flow (CBF) and that the physiologic phenomena is cortically localized (8). In a series of elegant landmark studies in the 1980s, investigators at Washington University pioneered the use of O-15 water PET to map cerebral function. Injections of O-15 water were made to tag blood flow during performance of tasks. The cortical regions involved with a chosen task exhibited increased activity and hence blood flow identified by PET. The first studies identified primary visual and motor cortex; subsequent studies, using a subtraction technique, identified receptive and expressive language cortex (9–12). In the course of their studies, they found that the oxygen content in activated cortex increased rather than decreased as expected (10–13). This last observation is the basis for most fMRI techniques. As signal with O-15 water PET studies is low compared with noise, group studies involving many patients were necessary to map cerebral function. The need for group studies necessitated the warping of individual data into a standard space or atlas. The most common current atlases used are that by Talaraich and Tournoux (14) and that from the Montreal Neurologic Institute.

Although PET is most often used for group studies, advances in PET technology allow repeated runs on patients with less radiation exposure, which may be used to identify language cortex in individual subjects (15–20). Bookheimer et al. (21) compared individual activation patterns with PET and subdural grid stimulation and found excellent correlation between the disruption elicited by cortical stimulation and the CBF activation elicited by task performance. Theirs was the first study to confirm the assumed reciprocal relationship between activation as defined by local increase in blood flow and the disruption of function elicited by cortical stimulation.

fMRI PRINCIPLES

Most current techniques make use of the MR signal properties which differ in oxy- versus deoxyhemoglobin, known collectively as blood oxygen level dependent, or BOLD, techniques. As observed by Fox et al. (10,13). Increased blood flow during neural activity exceeds the metabolic demand for oxygen. Because increased blood flow brings more oxyhemoglobin into the capillary bed than is extracted by neurons, the concentration of oxygenated, as opposed to deoxygenated blood, increases in the venous side of the vascular system during brain activity. Since oxyhemoglobin and deoxyhemoglobin differ in their magnetic susceptibility, the local magnetic field gradient lessens during neural activity. A more homogeneous magnetic field leads to higher MRI signal intensity during increased blood flow, which diminishes as blood flow returns to baseline. Thus, during increased neural activity, the MRI signal intensity increases at a rate congruent with the blood flow response and likewise decreases as blood flow does. The magnitude of these signal increases is quite small—on the order of a few percent—but because the baseline fluctuations in signal intensity are also small, change is readily detected with multiple observations.

Optical imaging studies of cortical response to visual stimulation in the cat demonstrate an increase in deoxygenated hemoglobin (hence increased oxygen extraction) immediately following stimulus outset and followed by in-

creased blood flow and an accompanying increase in oxyhemoglobin (22,23). The change in blood flow and absolute and relative increase in oxyhemoglobin concentration does not occur until 1 to 2 seconds after stimulus onset, reaching its peak in 5 to 7 seconds. The reasons underlying this hemodynamic response are unknown. For example, increased blood flow and oxyhemoglobin may represent a means to provide for possible increased need and to assure that active brain tissue will not exhaust metabolic stores; alternatively, increased blood flow may serve as a means to remove metabolic waste products. It is the epiphenomena of postactivation luxury perfusion that forms the basis of BOLD fMRI.

The delay in the vascular response to increased neural activity has several implications. First, it suggests that increased blood flow may not occur to fill the brain's immediate need for oxygen, as blood flow increases exceed the apparent need for oxygen. Second, the delayed rise and fall of CBF limit the temporal resolution of blood flow imaging techniques. Whereas the temporal resolution of fMRI is rapid compared with PET, it is slow by neural-firing standards. Because the dependent variable in fMRI, signal intensity, is measured in arbitrary units unrelated to actual biologic characteristics, absolute measures of blood flow are impossible. fMRI, unlike PET, is a purely relative measure of blood flow: One condition, an activation condition, must be compared with a second, control condition. There is no "resting fMRI" measure of blood flow at present.

Conventional MRI sequences, such as spoiled gradient recall (SPGR), can provide functional MRIs, typically with longer repetition times (TRs) and a small field of view. Fast MRI techniques, such as echoplanar or spiral imaging, allow detection in signal change continuously over time; these sequences allow acquisition of whole brain in as little as 2 to 5 seconds. The spatial resolution of most fMRI techniques spans from 2 to 5 mm. Studies also can be performed with contrast injection or spin tagging blood with a magnetic pulse in the carotids (24).

By definition, fMRI experiments must include an activation and a control or comparison task. The stimulus must be sufficient to increase neuronal activity, which subsequently elicits a hemodynamic response, and the control task should not elicit alterations in blood flow in the brain regions of interest. This set of requirements is met with less facility than might be imagined; for example, control tasks involving passive presentations of stimuli (no response is required of the subject) can certainly produce "automatic" engagement of cortical regions that may elicit a blood flow response. Tasks that are overrehearsed may produce a reduced blood flow response or an alteration in the pattern of blood flow (25). Tasks that the subject cannot perform also may not produce a blood flow response in the target brain regions. In patients with epilepsy, cognitive deficits may affect the pattern of fMRI activation, and patients should be evaluated carefully before mapping studies that may affect surgical plans.

Several types of experimental designs are available for functional activation studies. Blocked designs use at least two conditions in which one task is presented over a period during which the subject continuously performs the task in alternation with the comparison task (usually 20–60 seconds for each condition). Most studies use more than one blocked presentation; typically, they use three to six repetitions or cycles to distinguish signal from noise in activated brain regions and to mitigate the effects of signal drift unrelated to the task, which could influence results in significance tests of signal intensity. Single trial designs, relatively new in fMRI studies, present a single stimulus, followed by a delay sufficient for the blood flow to return to baseline, with multiple repetitions of trials. Images taken during each TR in the predicted blood flow rise and fall are averaged and then evaluated statistically. Parametric designs present multiple levels of the same variable in different blocks. For instance, subjects may perform a finger-opposition task at a slow, medium, and fast rate in separate blocks. The analysis searches for brain regions showing a predicted blood flow response over the different levels (perhaps a monotonic increase with rate of movement).

In each of these designs, maps of statistically significant signal-intensity change depend on the relative changes of blood flow across conditions. The choice of activation and control conditions is critical, therefore, to activation patterns seen. For example, if a task is reading single words (e.g., "stop") and the control task is pseudowords (e.g., "glih"), a significant difference may not be seen in the left middle and superior temporal gyrus because the same cortex necessary to comprehend words is used to determine whether a pseudoword is a real word (26,27). On the other hand, a language task such as word generation also activates areas not critical to language, such as areas involved in motor planning [supplementary motor area (SMA)] and attention (cingulate) (21,28).

Numerous statistical methods have been used to identify brain areas, or *voxels*, "activated" during test conditions, including t statistics, usually with a Bonferroni correction, nonparametric maps, and statistical parametric mapping (SPM) (ultimately displayed as z maps), correlation maps with reference or idealized signal-response patterns (29), and linear regression tests (30,31). The truly significant threshold is unclear because many are overly strict for practical purposes and underestimate true activation in location and extent. Some strategies include a cluster analysis, maintaining that adjacent pixels activated are less likely to be spurious or secondary to physiologic noise. Most fMRI analyses are performed on individual brains because of the difficulties that continue to be encountered in group studies; significant data are lost when individual variability in activation is warped into a standard space (32,33). For the purposes of mapping patients prior to surgery, within-subject analysis is essential, and so the choice of both experimental design and statistical test is critical. For most purposes, multiple tasks, multiple repetitions of tasks, and well-characterized task and control conditions are prerequisite, as is neuropsychologic testing on the tasks planned for activation paradigms.

Functional MRI studies are subject to motion artifact. Although post hoc mathematical image alignment helps, keeping patients still in the magnet is essential. In most cases, the need to minimize any motion requires having the subject perform tasks silently (such as covert word generation). Concurrent acquisition of behavioral data, such as a key-press response, can ensure that the subject has performed the task; an additional cognitive component is then added to the task but does not guarantee that the subject is not preoccupied with other matters. Thus, for individual studies of mapping patients, if patterns typical from normative data are not found, the task should be repeated to ascertain replicability. Activation maps that cannot be rationally interpreted should be considered nondiagnostic and require confirmation by repeat fMRI studies or by other means, such as intra-carotid amytal test (IAT) or cortical stimulation.

fMRI APPLICATIONS

Functional MRI has been used to identify reliably, primary sensory and motor cortex as well as cortical language areas. Memory studies are in their infancy and are not yet reliable for patient evaluation and management. fMRI has also been used in rare patients to identify the seizure focus.

Motor and Sensory Mapping

Functional MRI studies have been successful identifying primary motor and sensory cortex (34–39). Signal changes in the primary motor and sensory modalities are near 5% on a 1.5 T scanner, whereas higher-ordered cognitive activation is closer to a 0.5% to 1.5% signal change. Operations on neocortex in parietal or frontal lobe epilepsy often require identification of the sensory or motor cortex. In practice, such cases usually entail resection of lesions: tumor, vascular malformation, or dysplasia.

Several small studies comprising nearly 70 patients demonstrated the capacity of fMRI to identify these areas (40–50). Most of these series used fMRI for identifying these areas in preparation for tumor or vascular malformation surgery; a minority of patients had atrophy or encephalomalacia. Motor cortex representing tongue, hand, finger, arm, and foot areas are readily identified with tongue movement, finger tapping, and toe wiggling; analogous

sensory areas are identified with brushing or an air puff. In all cases, the precentral or postcentral gyrus was identified. Correlation at the time of resection as confirmed by corticography or evoked potential mapping in more than 50 of these patients has been excellent. Cortical stimulation and fMRI activation typically lie within 3 to 5 mm of each other (45).

Activation showing motor or sensory cortex are in areas adjacent to tumor and may be compressed or displaced (43,44). Activation is robust, and so it is rare not to elicit motor or sensory activation in patients with mass lesions (43). Activation has been identified in edematous tissue (43). Few studies have examined the ability of dysplastic tissue to sustain BOLD activation; Schwartz et al. (51) used a finger-tapping task to identify motor cortex in dysplastic cortex in a patient with schizencephaly and polymicrogyria.

Language Lateralization and Localization

Functional MRI of language processing has focused predominantly on language lateralization and, to a lesser extent, on localization. Epilepsy is associated with altered cerebral representation of language functions. Neuronal insult before the age of 3 to 6 years may result in shifted language dominance to the right hemisphere (2,52), and insult to the brain in middle childhood (5–9 years of age) may result in intrahemispheric redistribution of language function (53). Cortical mapping studies have readily shown variability of language function (7,53,54).

Numerous studies demonstrate fMRI to identify language hemispheric dominance reliably. Most studies have relied on tests of verbal fluency: *phonetic,* based on word generation to letters or generating a rhyming word; or *semantic,* word generation to categories or verb generation from nouns (43,47,48, 55–60). These paradigms reliably activate inferior and midfrontal cortex (dorsolateral prefrontal cortex, or DLPF). Other investigators have used tests involving semantic decision (61–64) that activate DLPF regions. Most tasks demonstrate some degree of bilateral activation, but significant activity is predomi-

TABLE 30.1. *Normal fMRI studies*

Study	MRI	Task	Brodmann's areas
Hinke et al. (65)	4.0 T[a]	Verbal fluency (letters)	44,45,47
Rueckert et al. (66)	1.5 T[a]	Verbal fluency (letters)	44,45,4,6 (39,22)
McCarthy et al. (67)	1.5 T[a]	Verb generation (noun-verb)	47
Cuenod et al. (56)	1.5 T[a]	Verbal fluency (letters)	44,47,46,9,6 (37,39)
Grandin et al. (28,68)	1.5 T	Verbal fluency (letters)	44,45,9,6 (22)
		Verbal fluency (categories)	44,45,9,6 (22)
Demb et al. (61)	1.5 T[a]	Semantic encoding (abstract-concrete)	45,47,46,8
Binder et al. (21,39,37)	1.5 T	Auditory semantic category	44,45,47,46,9,8
Shaywitz et al. (55)	2.1 T[a]	Phonemic rhyme	44
Xiong et al. (69)	1.5 T	Verb generation (noun-verb)	44,45,46,47,21,22,37,38
Schlosser et al. (70)	1.5 T	Auditory comprehension (listen)	22 (37,39)
Spitzer et al. (71)	1.5 T	Object name (semantic categories)	22,44,9
Small et al. (72)	1.5 T	Read words	22,39
Phelps et al. (73)	2.1 T	Verbal fluency (letters)	45,8
Just et al. (74)	1.5 T	Read comprehension (sentences)	21,22,44,45
Booth et al. (75)	1.5 T	Auditory comprehension (sentences)	21,22,44,45
Bevalier et al. (76)	4.0 T	Read comprehension (sentences)	21,22,44,45,9

[a]Some studies were single or limited slice studies. Parentheses denote areas with inconstant findings.
fMRI, functional magnetic resonance imaging.

nantly on the dominant hemisphere. All these have more marked activation in frontal cortex and are limited in extent and presence in temporal regions (28). Table 30.1 summarizes normal volunteer studies; Fig. 30.1 identifies the corresponding Brodmann's areas.

Desmond et al. (62) used a semantic decision task (i.e., determining whether a word pair is abstract or concrete) to examine laterality of language dominance in seven postoperative temporal lobectomy partial epilepsy patients. They included three patients with

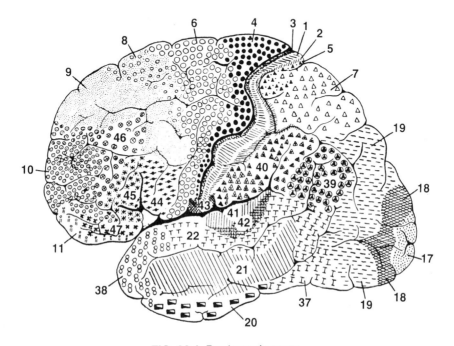

FIG. 30.1 Brodmann's areas.

IAT-demonstrated right-hemisphere dominance. Studies were limited to a single coronal slice in frontal lobes (35 mm to anterior commissure), but all studies agreed with IAT. There was more bilateral and displaced activity in the patients who were right hemisphere dominant.

Hertz-Pannier et al. (57) studied 11 children preoperatively with fMRI of the frontal lobe using a test of verbal fluency. They, too, found excellent agreement with the seven patients who had IAT or electrocorticography, including one child with bilateral activation (IAT confirmed). Several other investigators found similar results in small clusters of adults with tests of verbal fluency (43,48, 58–60), thus adding an additional 47 patients with IAT or cortical stimulation confirmation in 33 of these 47 patients. All authors, except Worthington et al. (60), described excellent agreement with fMRI and language laterality.

Binder et al. (62) used a semantic decision task similar to that of Desmond and colleagues (64) (to determine whether an animal is indigenous to the North American continent and of use to humans). They used whole-brain acquisition, with an auditory task and included controls for attention and tone (for primary auditory cortex activation). Their series of 22 patients, which included four patients with bilateral or right-hemispheric language representation, showed excellent correlation with a fMRI and IAT lateralization index.

In our studies (W.D.G.) of verbal fluency encompassing 30 adults, all normal subjects demonstrated activation of frontal head regions, but only 50% show temporal activation (28,68). Binder and colleagues also noted reliable activation of frontal cortex but inconsistent activation of temporal cortex. In the studies reviewed so far, the bulk of activated pixels for determining the laterality index arose from the frontal lobe. Such tasks are useful in lateralization in frontal head regions, but they are not reliable for investigating temporal language areas. Paradigms designed to identify receptive language fields use stronger auditory and visual language stimuli.

Reading single words activates, to a modest degree, superior and midtemporal gyrus when appropriate control conditions are used (72,77,78). Reading paradigms using sentences readily activate dominant superior and middle temporal cortex at 4T (76). Just et al. (74) demonstrated activation in superior temporal gyrus (BA 22, 42, and occasionally 21) when patients read a series of sentences with increasing syntactic complexity (control: consonant strings). The more complex sentences activate homologous regions in nondominant cortex. Schlosser et al. (70), using listening to sentences (with control task of listening to Turkish sentences), found activation of the left superior temporal gyrus with minor activation in right regions. Booth et al. (75), using an auditory form of the Just et al. (74) paradigm, found similar results.

A series at the Children's National Medical Center and the Epilepsy Research Branch, National Institutes of Neurologic Disorders Stroke (NINDS) (W.D.G.) examined auditory responsive naming (79) and reading tasks in normal volunteer adults and children. Listening to a description of an object and then naming the described object activates both bilateral primary auditory cortex and also cortex in posterior temporal cortex dominant lobe. A reading paradigm using similar stimuli activates dominant middle temporal cortex (6 to 8 times more activation in the left than right temporal cortex). For both paradigms, there is activation in left DLPF cortex and Broca's area. More complex reading tasks, such as reading fables, is a more robust activator of left temporal cortex. The receptive language paradigms were used to identify dominant temporal cortex in 15 adult and pediatric epilepsy patients, confirmed in ten by IAT, including three patients (one child, two adults) with the right hemisphere dominant for language (Fig. 30.2). Fitzgerald et al. (47) (using single-word reading and listening) found similar results confirmed by cortical stimulation in 11 in patients with tumors. They found activation adjacent to stimulation in most patients and nearly all within 1 cm of fMRI activation.

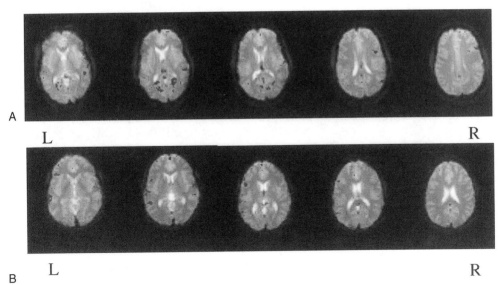

FIG. 30.2. Functional MRI of auditory responsive naming. **A:** A 26-year-old right-handed woman with refractory complex partial epilepsy with a left temporal focus. fMRI shows predominant activation in right temporal neocortex, right DLPFC and right Broca's area. IAT and subsequent resection of the left temporal lobe confirmed these findings. **B:** A 24-year-old normal woman showing typical activation of left temporal neocortex, DLPF cortex, and Broca's area. There is a small degree of bilateral activation in primary auditory cortex. (*Note: Left image is left brain.*)

Sufficient evidence has been found that fMRI can be used to lateralize language dominance. The data and methods of Worthington et al. (60) are not presented in detail, and without outcome from surgery, it is difficult to ascertain the reasons for these investigators' discrepant observations. In total, 13 patients with right or bilateral hemisphere dominance have been reported in the literature with concordant IAT and fMRI results, thereby making chance the unlikely identifier of dominant left cortex.

Recent work from the University of California Los Angeles (UCLA) studies (S.Y.B., M.C.) emphasizes potential errors in fMRI localization of language cortex where tumors are infiltrative (80). Examples of such patients are shown in Fig. 30.3. Large tumors compressing Broca's area may disrupt the normal blood flow response and result in false-negative activation in dominant cortex; homologous activation in the nondominant hemisphere may be interpreted incorrectly. Results are further complicated in left-

handed patients, who are more likely to have mixed or right-hemisphere speech dominance (Fig. 30.4). In two such patients with left-hemisphere tumors, fMRI suggested bilateral speech representation, whereas the IAT showed left-hemisphere speech, which was confirmed with direct cortical stimulation.

It remains unclear, however, how exact the correspondence is between cortical stimulation and fMRI activation. Most evidence suggests that it is good but not completely overlapping (21,45,47). The error of coregistration programs, BOLD identification of draining veins rather than capillaries, and the loss of true positives with overly stringent thresholds may account for some of these differences, adding up to millimeters (usually < 5 mm). Fitzgerald et al. (47) and Ojemann (54) stress the need to perform several different language tasks during mapping because different aspects of language are expressed differentially, a phenomena especially noted in multilingual patients (47,54,81). The imaging experience

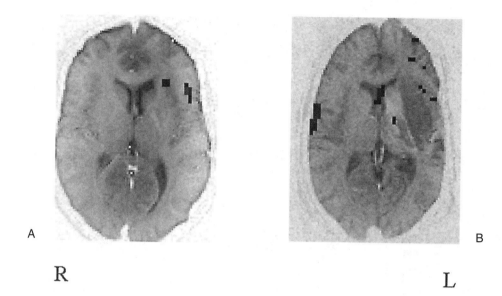

R   L

FIG. 30.3. fMRI slices through Broca's area on two patients with gliomas. **Left:** Patient A has a superior frontal tumor, not seen on this slice, and shows a typical activation in the opercular portion of BA 44 and the left anterior insula. **Right:** Patient B has a perisylvian tumor and shows minimal activation of the same regions, with additional activity in the right inferior frontal gyrus and the left middle frontal gyrus anterior to Broca's area. (*Note: Left image is right brain.*)

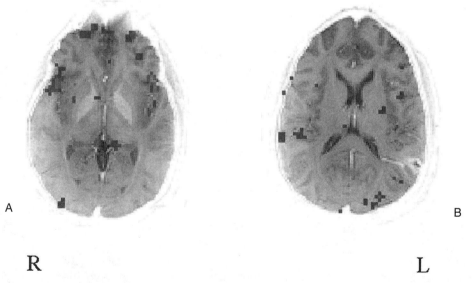

R   L

FIG. 30.4. Two slices through the brain of a patient with an arteriovenous malformation near Wernicke's area. fMRI shows bilateral activation on an auditory responsive naming task in the perisylvian region **(A)** (insula and Broca's area), and right hemisphere activation in Wernicke's area **(B)** contralateral to the lesion. IAT and electric stimulation confirmed left hemisphere expressive and receptive speech. (*Note: Left image is right brain.*)

supports these observations (71,81). Although there are similarities in the fMRI studies discussed, there may be considerable differences in the ability of each paradigm to activate different cortical regions; these differences are particularly marked for tests of fluency and semantic decision making for anterior regions and reading or listening paradigms for posterior language areas. The appropriate tasks need to be selected for studying the appropriate area.

Memory

Memory has been more difficult to identify in hippocampal structures. Although a number of PET and fMRI studies have been performed exploring working memory involving the frontal lobes, the effect of epilepsy and surgery on these areas is not well understood (30,31,82,83). From a practical perspective, the ability to assess the integrity of hippocampal function is desired, primarily for surgery on mesial structures. Most PET and fMRI studies have resulted in conflicting and confusing results arising in part from differences in paradigm design, the difficulty in task design for the study of memory, and because almost everything we do uses memory, and presumably the hippocampus, in some capacity (84)

No studies have found activation in the hippocampus proper, and only recently has activation of regions adjacent to hippocampus been demonstrated reliably by tests of encoding and retrieval. These demonstrated activation of posterior and bilateral hippocampus and parahippocampal gyrus during encoding (85,86). These tasks relied on encoding of complex pictures. Asymmetry indices were not performed. Retrieval, using verbal identifiers of encoded memory for pictures, appears to involve anterior subiculum bilaterally. These tasks have involved both visual spatial and verbal components joined. Encoding of stimuli—especially novel items, subsequently recalled, is associated with activation of posterior mesial temporal regions, namely parahippocampus (87,88). Verbal encoding appears to activate preferentially the left parahippocampal gyrus; nonverbal stimuli, such as faces, preferentially activate the right parahippocampus. Complex pictures, which also may involve verbal encoding as well as visual imagery encoding, activate bilateral parahippocampal regions (87–89). Insufficient numbers of normal volunteers have been studied to establish normative data, application of these techniques has not been employed evaluating patients, and paradigms that will be predictive have not yet been designed. Two small series have explored the application of memory techniques (90,91).

Detre et al. (90) found bilateral activation in a visual-encoding paradigm similar to that used by Stern and colleagues (85). They found a slightly greater activation in the right posterior parahippocampus in their normal population. Reported asymmetry in the posterior hippocampal formation region of interest fMRI matched IAT lateralization and asymmetries in patients with temporal lobe complex partial seizures (90). Bellowagan et al. (91) described activation of the middle left parahippocampal gyrus and hippocampus during verbal encoding of the semantic decision task described already (39) in the right temporal lobe seizure focus patients. As the analysis is reported as a group study, however, individual variation may have been lost. No clinical difference in performance was found between right- and left-sided temporal lobe epilepsy patient groups, suggesting that the left temporal lobe patients maintained the capacity to perform the task. These two studies revealed the potential promise for fMRI to assess capacity for and the ability to sustain memory function in epilepsy patients.

Ictal Localization

Three reports have described the use of fMRI to identify an ictal focus. The first involved a 4-year-old child with Rasmussen's encephalitis with frequent facial twitching. The child was anaesthetized and placed in a MRI scanner, and seizures were noted clinically by the occurrence of facial twitching. Time-course analysis was examined to look for regional increases in the MR signal during clinical seizures. Ictal onset was identified in lateral cortex that matched ictal SPECT compared with interictal SPECT. Moreover, the time course analysis demonstrated the anatomic distribution of seizure propagation (92). In this instance, the time resolution was superior to single-photon emission (SPECT) or PET CBF-based studies.

A second patient had simple partial seizures arising from posterior inferior left frontal lobe. A fMRI study of 11 minutes duration, without clinically apparent seizures, was screened for signal change. Two periods of identical increase in signal were identified that occurred in a restricted region in posterior inferior left frontal lobe, later confirmed to be the ictal origin by chronic subdural electrode recording. As with the previous study, the seizure propagation could be mapped (93). The circumstantial evidence, without clinical change and in the absence of EEG, suggested the events captured were subclinical seizures.

A third case, also serendipitous, has added to the ictal fMRI experience; this case involved a 16-year-old patient with refractory sensorimotor seizures arising from a right central dysplastic cleft with polymicrogyri. fMRI sensory mapping identified sensory cortex in the anterior side of the cleft, and a clinical seizure occurring during further fMRI studies allowed identification of the ictal focus as being from the posterior margin of the cleft. Intraoperative cortical mapping confirmed the site of sensory cortex; excision of posterior margin resulted in complete seizure control (51).

These three cases are unusual; all were neocortical and serendipitous. All patients had frequent simple partial seizures and remained sufficiently free of motion artifact to obtain successful mapping. These cases are instructive because they are rare. The ability to follow seizure propagation exceeds the ability of radiolabeled perfusion techniques, O-15 PET and SPECT, and the limitations of electrode placement during invasive mapping. Significant advancements in MR technology will be necessary before this can become clinically useful given the current limitations of ictal SPECT.

CONCLUSION: fMRI ADVANTAGES AND LIMITATIONS

Functional MRI has a number of strengths. Unlike PET, the technology is common and relatively inexpensive. Studies are done with little risk and no radiation and at considerably less risk than IAT or grid mapping. Consequently, studies can be repeated if no or unusual activation patterns are found for confirmation. We (W.D.G.) have repeated studies in five children when initial studies were unrevealing and whenever activation patterns are unexpected. fMRI can be used to study children at age 7 years and possibly as young as 5 years. A number of different paradigms can be performed to map different aspects of language, often more than can be performed in the operating room. Additionally, fMRI identifies language areas deep in sulci, often inaccessible to cortical stimulation.

Functional MRI also has limitations. It is restricted to patients who are medically safe in the scanner. Patients must be awake and cooperative to be studied successfully, and they must remain still. Motion correction is limited to a few millimeters and degrees of rotation, and motion artifact remains the principal origin of failed studies. This is challenging in young or cognitively impaired patients, although usually training, behavioral training, and repeat studies can surmount this obstacle. Similarly, speech areas may not be activated for a variety of reasons. Activation is dependent on both tasks but also on control, and one can identify only that for which one tests. The task may not be optimal for identifying the regional cortex of interest. The task may be too simple such that the response is automatic in the neuronal work involved and is insufficient to trigger the hemodynamic response detected by fMRI techniques. The differences between task and control conditions may not be appropriate:

They may share features that do not allow distinction between them. Cortex also may participate in the task but not sufficiently to exceed the statistical threshold. A variety of factors may contribute to error in measurement and activation, for example, errors in motion and registration correction (1–4 mm) and spatial resolution of the technique (1–5 mm). The hemodynamic responses are best detected in draining veins and venules millimeters distal to the capillary site of activation.

Functional MRI may be unreliable when there is a vascular steal or significant compression from mass to distort the activation response. Memory paradigms are not well established, although this limitation is likely to be surmounted within the next few years. Application for seizure mapping is limited with current technology, is almost entirely fortuitous and cannot be used reliably except in rare circumstances.

As a clinical tool, fMRI can be used reliably to lateralize language function and to identify the motor or sensory strip in anticipation of surgery. It also can also localize language function. For resection-sparing surgery, fMRI is best viewed as a guide. Areas activated are likely to be real, although not all activated areas are critical for language function. Similarly, language areas may not be activated for a variety of reasons already discussed. Also, the statistical threshold used may underestimate the extent of the area that is activated.

Most fMRI studies are based on PET paradigms and are performed in only a few normal volunteers. Greater experience is necessary with most paradigms to appreciate the natural variability neuronal activation. The penchant for group studies and the use of rigid thresholds tend to obscure this variability. Common sense dictates that a panel of tests needs to be used to assess the capacity of brain regions to sustain language and that the appropriate task be used to map the area of clinical interest. For instance, it is not appropriate to use a verbal fluency task when mapping temporal neocortex.

In sum, fMRI has been as reliable and more versatile than IAT in identifying language dominance. fMRI can localize eloquent areas preoperatively and can be used to direct surgery and cortical mapping necessary for anatomic confirmation. fMRI's value as a research tool for understanding the neural networks involved in cortical activity is obvious, let alone as a means to understand how disease affects cortical function, adaptatation, and reorganization.

ACKNOWLEDGMENTS

The work of William Davis Gaillard is supported by NINDS K08-NS01663 the Epilepsy Research Branch, NINDS, National Institutes of Health.

REFERENCES

1. Wada JA, Rasmussen T. Intracarotid injection of sodium amytal for the lateralization of cerebral speech dominance. *J Neurosurg* 1960;17:266–282.
2. Rasmussen T, Milner B. The role of early left-brain injury in determining lateralization of cerebral speech functions. *Ann NY Acad Sci* 1977;299:355–369.
3. Loring DW, Meador KJ, Lee GP, et al. Cerebral language lateralization: evidence from intracarotid amobarbital testing. *Neuropsychologia* 1990;28:831–838.
4. Helmstaedter C, Kurthen, Linke DB, et al. Patterns of language dominance in focal left and right hemisphere epilepsies: relation to MRI findings, EEG, sex, and age at onset of epilepsy. *Brain Cogn* 1997;33:135–150.
5. Penfield W, Roberts L. *Speech and brain mechanisms.* Princeton: Princeton University Press, 1959.
6. Lesser RP, Lüders HO, Dinner DS, et al. The location of speech and writing functions in the frontal language area: results of extraoperative cortical stimulation. *Brain* 1984;107:275–291.
7. Ojemann G, Ojemann J, Lettich E, et al. Cortical language localization in left dominant hemisphere: an electrical stimulation mapping investigation in 117 patients. *J Neurosurg* 1989;71:316–326.
8. Roy CS, Sherrington CS. On the regulation of blood flow to the brain. *J Physiol* 1890;11:85–108.
8. Silbersweig DA, Stern E, Frith CD, et al. Detection of thirty-second cognitive activations in single subjects with positron emission tomography: a new low-dose 15-O water regional cerebral blood flow three-dimensional imaging technique. *J Cereb Blood Flow Metab* 1993;13:617–629.
9. Fox PT, Mintun MA, Raichle ME, et al. Mapping human visual cortex with positron emission tomography. *Nature* 1986;323:806–809.
10. Fox PT, Raichle ME. Focal physiological uncoupling of cerebral blood flow and oxidative metabolism during somatosensory stimulation of human subjects. *Proc Natl Acad Sci USA* 1986;83:1140–1144.

11. Peterson S, Fox, P, Posner M, et al. Positron emission tomographic studies of the cortical anatomy of single word processing. *Nature* 1988;331:585–589.

12. Peterson S, Fox P, Posner M, et al. Positron emission tomographic studies of processing of single words. *J Cogn Neurosci* 1989;1:153–170.

13. Fox PT, Raichle ME, Mintun MA, et al. Nonoxidative glucose consumption during focal physiologic neuronal activity. *Science* 1988;241:462–464.

14. Talairach J, Tournoux P. *Co-planar stereotaxic atlas of the human brain.* New York: Thieme, 1988.

15. Pardo JV, Fox PT. Preoperative assessment of the cerebral dominance for language with CBF PET. *Human Brain Mapping* 1993;1:57–68.

16. Vinas FC, Zamorano L, Mueller RA, et al. [15-O]–Water PET and intraoperative brain mapping: a comparison in the localization of eloquent cortex. *Neurol Res* 1997; 19:601–608.

17. Duncan JD, Moss SD, Bandy DJ, et al. Use of positron emission tomography for presurgical localization of eloquent brain areas in children with seizures. *Pediatr Neurosurg* 1997;26:144–156.

18. Henry TR, Buchtel HA, Koeppe RA, et al. Absence of normal activation of the left anterior fusiform gyrus during naming in left temporal lobe epilepsy. *Neurology* 1998;50:787–790.

19. Mueller R-A, Rothermel RD, Behen ME, et al. Determination of language dominance by O-15 water positron emission tomography in pediatric patients: a comparison with the WADA test. *Arch Neurol* 1998;55: 1113–1119.

20. Hunter KE, Blaxton TA, Bookheimer SY, et al. 15-O water positron emission tomography in language localization: a study comparing rater evaluations and computerized region of interest analysis of PET studies with the WADA test. *Ann Neurol* 2000;45:662–665.

21. Bookheimer SY, Zeffiro T, Blaxton T, et al. A direct comparison of PET activation and electrocortical stimulation mapping for language localization. *Neurology* 1997;48:1056–1065.

22. Malonek D, Grinvald A. Interactions between electrical activity and cortical microcirculation revealed by imaging spectroscopy: implications for functional brain mapping. *Science* 1996;272:551–554.

23. Malonek D, Dirnagl U, Lindauer U, et al. Vascular imprints of neuronal activity: relationships between the dynamics of cortical blood flow, oxygenation, and volume changes following sensory stimulation. *Proc Natl Acad Sci USA* 1997;94:14826–14831.

24. Belliveau J, Kennedy D, McKinstry R, et al. Functional mapping of the human visual cortex by magnetic resonance imaging. *Science* 1991;254:716–719.

25. Raichle ME, Fiez JA, Videen TO, et al. Practice-related changes in human brain functional anatomy during nonmotor learning. *Cereb Cortex* 1994;4:8–26.

26. Wise R, Chollet F, Hadar U, et al. Distribution of cortical neural networks involved in word comprehension and word retrieval. *Brain* 1991;114:1803–1817.

27. Warburton E, Wise RJS, Price CJ, et al. Noun and verb retrieval by normal subjects. *Brain* 1996;119:159–179.

28. Grandin CB, Gaillard WD, Whitnah JR, et al. Gender related differences in activated brain areas for language processing: an fMRI study. *Neuroimage* 1998;7;S159.

29. Bandettini PA, Jesmanowitz A, Wong EC, et al. Processing strategies for time-course data sets in functional MRI of the human brain. *Magn Reson Imaging* 1993; 30:161–173.

30. Courtney SM, Ungerleider LG, Kell K, et al. Transient and sustained activity in a distributed neural system for human working memory. *Nature* 1997;386:608–611.

31. Courtney SM, Petit L, Maiog JM, et al. An area specialized for spatial working memory in human frontal cortex. *Science* 1998;270:1347–1351.

32. Steinmetz H, Rudiger JS. Functional anatomy of language processing: neuroimaging and the problem of individual variability *Neuropsychologia* 1991;29:1149–1161.

33. Clark VP, Parasuraman R, Keil K, et al. *Human Brain Mapping* 1995;3(suppl 1):32.

34. Kim SG, Ashe J, Georgopoulos AP, et al. Functional imaging of human motor cortex at high magnetic field. *J Neurophysiol* 1993;69:297–302.

35. Rao SM, Binder JR, Bandettini PA, et al. Functional magnetic resonance imaging of complex human movements. *Neurology* 1993;43:2311–1328.

36. Hammeke TA, Yetkin FZ, Mueller WM, et al. Functional magnetic resonance imaging of somatosensory stimulation. *Neurosurgery* 1994;35:677–681.

37. Ogawa S, Tank DW, Menon R, et al. Intrinsic signal changes accompanying sensory stimulation: functional brain mapping with magnetic resonance imaging. *Proc Natl Acad Sci USA* 1992;89:5951–5955.

38. Kwong K, Belliveau J, Chesler D, et al. Dynamic magnetic resonance imaging of human brain activity during primary sensory stimulation. *Proc Natl Acad Sci USA* 1992;89:5675–5679.

39. Binder JR, Rao SM, Hammeke TA, et al. Lateralized human brain language systems demonstrated by task subtraction functional magnetic resonance imaging. *Arch Neurol* 1995;52:593–601.

40. Jack CR, Thompson RM, Butts RK, et al. Sensory motor cortex: correlation of presurgical mapping with functional MR imaging and invasive cortical mapping. *Radiology* 1994;190:85–92.

41. Latchaw RE, Hu X, Ugurbil K, et al. Functional magnetic resonance imaging as a management tool for cerebral arteriovenous malformations. *Neurosurgery* 1995; 37:619–626.

42. Yousry TA, Schmid UD, Jassoy AG, et al. Topography of the cortical motor hand area: prospective study with functional MR imaging and direct motor mapping at surgery. *Radiology* 1995;195:23–29.

43. Mueller WM, Yetkin Z, Hammeke TA, et al. Functional magnetic imaging mapping of the motor cortex in patients with cerebral tumors. *Neurosurgery* 1996;39: 515–521.

44. Atlas SW, Howard RS, Maldjian J, et al. Functional magnetic resonance imaging of regional brainactivity in patients with intracerebral gliomas: findings and implications for clinical management. *Neurosurgery* 1996; 38:329–338.

45. Cosgrove GR, Buchbinder BR, Jiang H. Functional magnetic resonance imaging for intracranial navigation. *Clinical Frontiers of Interactive Image-guided Neurosurgery* 1996;7:1042–3680.

46. Maldjian J, Atlas SW, Howard RS, et al. Functional magnetic resonance imaging of regional brain activity in patients with intracerebral arteriovenous malformations before surgical or endovascular therapy. *J Neurosurg* 1996;84:477–483.

47. Fitzgerald DB, Cosgrove GR, Ronner S, et al. Location

of language in the cortex: a comparison between functional MR imaging and electrocortical stimulation. *Am J Neuroradiol* 1997;18:1529–1539.

48. Stapleton SR, Kiriakipoulos E, Mikulis D, et al. Combined utility of functional MRI, cortical mapping, and frameless stereotaxy in the resection of lesions in eloquent areas of brain in children. *Pediatr Neurosurg* 1997;26:68–82.

49. Schulder M, Maldjian JA, Liu W-C, et al. Functional image-guided surgery of intracranial tumors located in or near the sensorimotor cortex. *J Neurosurg* 1998; 89:412–418.

50. Buchbinder BR, Cosgrove GR. Cortical activation MR studies in brain disorders. *Magn Reson Imaging Clin N Am* 1998;6:67–93.

51. Schwartz TH, Resor SR, De La Paz R, et al. Functional magnetic resonance imaging localization of ictal onset to a dysplastic cleft with simultaneous sensorimonitor mapping: intraoperative electrophysiological confirmation and postoperative follow-up: technical note. *Neurosurgery* 1998;43:639–645.

52. Woods RP, Dodrill CB, Ojemann GA. Brain injury, handedness, and speech lateralization in a series of amobarbital studies. *Ann Neurol* 1988;23:510–518.

53. Devinsky O, Perrine K, Llinas R, et al. Anterior temporal language areas in patients with early onset temporal lobe epilepsy. *Ann Neurol* 1993;34:727–732.

54. Ojemann GA. Cortical organization of language. *J Neurosci* 1991;11:2281–2287.

55. Shaywitz BA, Shaywitz SE, Pugh KR, et al. Sex differences in functional organization of the brain for language. *Nature* 1995;373:607–609.

56. Cuenod CA, Bookheimer SY, Hertz-Pannier L, et al. Functional MRI during word generation, using conventional equipment. *Neurology* 1995;45:1821–1827.

57. Hertz-Pannier L, Gaillard WD, Mott S, et al. Assessment of language hemispheric dominance in children with epilepsy using functional MRI. *Neurology* 1997; 48:1003–1012.

58. Bahn MM, Lin W, Silbergeld DL, et al. Localization of language cortices by functional imaging compared with intracarotid amobarbital hemispheric sedation. *AJR AM J Roentgenol* 1997;169:575–579.

59. van der Kallen BFW, Morris GL, Yetkin FZ, et al. Hemispheric language dominance studied with functional MR: preliminary study in healthy volunteers and patients with epilepsy. *Am J Neuroradiol* 1998;19:73–77.

60. Worthington C, Vincent DJ, Bryant AE, et al. Comparison of functional magnetic resonance imaging for language localization and intracarotid speech amytal testing in presurgical evaluation for intractible epilepsy. *Tereotactic and Functional Neurosurgery* 1997;69: 197–201.

61. Demb JB, Desmond JE, Wagner AD, et al. Semantic encoding and retrieval in the left inferior and prefrontal cortex: a functional MRI study of task difficulty and process specificity. *J Neurosci* 1955;15:5870–5878.

62. Desmond JE, Sum JM, Wagner AD, et al. Language lateralization in WADA-tested patients using functional MRI. *Brain* 1995;118:1411–1419.

63. Benson RR, Kwong KK, Buchbinder BR, et al. Noninvasive evaluation of language dominance using functional MRI. *Proc Soc Magn Reson Med* 1994:684.

64. Binder JR, Swanson SJ, Hammeke TA, et al. Determination of language dominance using functional MRI: a comparison with the WADA test. *Neurology* 1996; 46:978–984.

65. Hinke RM, Hu X, Stillman AE, et al. Functional magnetic resonance imaging of Broca's area during internal speech. *Cogn Neurosci Neuropsychol* 1993;4:675–678.

66. Rueckert L, Appollonio I, Graffman J, et al. Magnetic resonance imaging functional activation of left frontal cortex during covert word production. *J Neuroimag* 1994;4:67–70.

67. McCarthy G, Blamire AM, Rothman DL, et al. Echo-plannar magnetic resonance imaging studies of frontal cortex activation during word generation in humans. *Proc Natl Acad Sci USA* 1993;90:4952–4956.

68. Grandin CB, Gaillard WD, Whitnah JR, et al. Comparison of phonological and semantic verbal fluency tasks: an fMRI study. *Neuroimage* 1998;7:S133.

69. Xiong J, Rao S, Gao JH, et al. Evaluation of hemispheric dominance for language using functional MRI: a comparison with positron emission tomography. *Human Brain Mapping* 1998;6:42–58.

70. Schlosser MJ, Aoyagi N, Fulbright RK, et al. Functional MRI studies of auditory comprehension. *Human Brain Mapping* 1998;6:1–13.

71. Spitzer M, Kwong KK, Kennedy W, et al. Category-specific brain activation in fMRI during picture naming. *Neuroreport* 1995;6:2109–2112.

72. Small S, Noll DC, Perfetti CA, et al. Localizing the lexicon for reading aloud: replication of a PET study using MRI. *Neuroreport* 1996;7:961–965.

73. Phelps EA, Hyder F, Blamire A, et al. fMRI of the prefrontal cortex during overt verbal fluency. *Neuroreport* 1997;8:561–565.

74. Just MA, Carpenter PA, Keller TA, et al. Brain activity modulated by sentence comprehension. *Science* 1996; 274:114–116.

75. Booth JR, Feldman HM, Macwhinney B, et al. Functional activation patterns in adults, children, and pediatric patients with brain lesions. *Prog Neuropsychopharmacol Biol Psychiatry* 1999;23:669–682.

76. Bavelier D, Corina D, Jezzard P, et al. Sentence reading: a functional MRI study at 4 Tesla. *J Cogn Neurosci* 1997;9:664–686.

77. Howard D, Patterson K, Wise R, et al. The cortical localization of the lexicons. *Brain* 1992;115:1769–1782.

78. Price CJ, Wise RJS, Watson JDG, et al. Brain activity during reading: the effects of exposure and duration of task. *Brain* 1994;117:1255–1269.

79. Bookheimer SY, Zeffiro TA, Blaxton TA, et al. Regional cerebral blood flow during auditory responsive naming: evidence for cross-modality neural activation. *Neuroreport* 1998;9:2409–2413.

80. Bookheimer SY, Dapretto M, Black K, et al. fMRI of language in patients with aggressive brain tumors. *Soc Neurosci Abst* 1997;23:1060.

81. Kim KH, Relkin NR, Lee KM, et al. Distinct cortical areas associated with native and second languages. *Nature* 1997;388:171–174.

82. Underleider LG. Functional brain imaging studies of cortical mechanisms for memory. *Science* 1995;270: 769–775.

83. Cohen JD, Peristein WM, Braver TS, et al. Temporal dynamics of brain activation during a working memory task. *Nature* 1997;386:604–607.

84. Gabrieli JDE. Cognitive neuroscience of human memory. *Annu Rev Psychol* 1998;49:87–115.

85. Stern CE, Corkin S, Gonzalez RG, et al. The hippocampal formation participates in novel picture encoding: evidence from functional magnetic resonance imaging. *Proc Natl Acad Sci USA* 1996;93:8660–8665.
86. Gabrieli JDE, Brewer JB, Desmond JE, et al. Separate neural bases of two fundamental memory processes in the human medial temporal lobe. *Science* 1997;276:264–266.
87. Brewer JB, Zhao Z, Desmond JE, et al. Making memories: brain activity that predicts how well visual experience will be remembered. *Science* 1998;281:1185–1187.
88. Wagner AD, Schacter DL, Rotte M, et al. Building memories: remembering and forgetting of verbal experiences as predicted by brain activity. *Science* 1998;281: 1188–1191.
89. Kelley WM, Miezin FM, McDermott KB, et al. Hemispheric specialization in human dorsal frontal cortex and medial temporal lobe for verbal and nonverbal memory encoding. *Neuron* 1998;20:927–936.
90. Detre JA, Maccotta L, King D, et al. Functional MRI lateralization of memory in temporal lobe epilepsy. *Neurology* 1998;50:926–932.
91. Bellowagan PSF, Binder JR, Swanson SJ, et al. Side of seizure focus predicts left medial temporal lobe activation during verbal encoding. *Neurology* 1998;51: 479–484.
92. Jackson GD, Connelly A, Cross JH, et al. Functional magnetic resonance imaging of focal seizures. *Neurology* 1994;44:850–856.
93. Detre JA, Sirven JI, Alsop DC, et al. Localization of subclinical ictal activity by functional magnetic resonance imaging: correlation with invasive monitoring. *Ann Neurol* 1995;38:618–624.

Neocortical Epilepsies.
Advances in Neurology, Vol. 84,
edited by P.D. Williamson, A.M. Siegel,
D.W. Roberts, V.M. Thadani, and M.S. Gazzaniga.
Lippincott Williams & Wilkins, Philadelphia © 2000.

31

Magnetic Resonance Spectroscopy in Neocortical Epilepsies

Kenneth D. Laxer

*Department of Neurology, University of California, San Francisco,
San Francisco, California 94143-0138*

The best surgical results are obtained when the various preoperative localizing examinations, such as video/electroencephalographic (EEG) telemetry, magnetic resonance imaging (MRI), positron emission tomography (PET), single-photon emission computed tomography (SPECT), and others, are concordant, implicating the same brain region. Temporal lobe epilepsy (TLE) patients with unilateral hippocampal atrophy or increased signal on MRI concordant with the ictal EEG have as great as a 95% chance of becoming seizure free following temporal lobectomy (1,2). In patients without MRI abnormalities (i.e., nonconcordant), however, the prognosis for seizure-free outcome drops to about 50% (1). Similar findings are seen in neocortical epilepsy (NE), but non-lesional patients having an even poorer outcome (3). There remains a large population of medically refractory patients in whom imaging (e.g., MRI, SPECT, PET) fails to confirm the epileptogenic region as defined by EEG. Therefore, better imaging techniques for MRI-negative partial epilepsy need to be developed, and this was the impetus for investigating the use of spectroscopy in the evaluation of medically refractory epilepsy.

Magnetic resonance spectroscopy (MRS) is the only noninvasive technique capable of measuring chemicals within the body. In addition, the nuclear magnetic resonance signals from many compounds can be detected simultaneously in one MRS experiment. Because the same instrument can be used for both MRI and MRS, the recent overwhelming proliferation of MRI units throughout the world has allowed this new technique to flourish as well. MRS exploits the principle that every chemically distinct nucleus in a compound resonates at a slightly different frequency, allowing the detection of a wide variety of metabolites [for review, see Matson and Weiner (4)]. The resonant frequency of a nucleus is linearly proportional to the magnetic field strength experienced by that nucleus. The magnetic field seen by the nucleus is dominated by the external static magnetic field (typically 1.5 T) plus the applied magnetic field gradients. The external magnetic field also affects the electrons surrounding the nuclei, causing them to produce a local magnetic field opposite to the applied field. Because the effective field at the nucleus is dependent on the surrounding environment, the resonant frequency will vary slightly. In spectroscopy, this shift in frequency *(chemical shift)* provides information about chemical structure. The size of the signal at a particular frequency is proportional to the number of spins producing the signal and is measured by the area under the peak on a frequency versus signal intensity curve. Because differentiation of the various nuclei depends on extremely subtle differences in resonant frequency, there is a need for extremely homogeneous magnetic fields in performing spectroscopic measurements compared with MRI. Nuclei with nonzero nuclear-spin angular momentum that have been used in medicine include ^{1}H, ^{31}P, ^{13}C, ^{19}F, and ^{23}Na, but as a result of low relative sensitivities and low natural abundances, only ^{1}H and ^{31}P have clinical utility in the study of in vivo metabolites (5).

Many of the metabolites involved in energy metabolism can be measured by ^{31}P MRS. Figure 31.1 shows a spectrum obtained from normal brain, revealing peaks for phosphocreatine (PCr), the three peaks for the nucleotide triphosphates, predominantly adenosine triphosphate (ATP), inorganic phosphate (Pi), phosphomonoesters (PME), largely phosphorylcholine and phosphorylethanolamine, and phosphodiesters (PDE), largely glycerophosphorylcholine, glycerophosphorylethanolamine, and mobile phospholipids (6). The area under each peak is proportional to the concentration of the species producing the peak, and the resonance frequency for the peak is specific for the chemical being detected. The resonant frequency of Pi is dependent on the relative contributions of HPO_4^{2-} and $H_2PO_4^-$, depending on the equilib-

rium concentration of H^+; therefore, the chemical shift of the Pi frequency can be used to measure intracellular pH (5). Similarly, free Mg^{2+} can be measured from the chemical shift of ATP. PCr, ATP, Pi, and pH provide information about bioenergetics. PDE and PME provide information about lipid metabolism.

Proton (^{1}H) MRS is now available on most commercial MRI equipment, and unlike ^{31}P MRS, does not require any special instrumentation above that needed for MRI; however, proton studies are difficult to perform as a result of the large interfering signals from water and lipids. Furthermore, interference from lipids, areas of magnetic susceptibility artifact, and the need for homogeneous magnetic fields limit the intracranial regions that can be studied. For these reasons, ^{1}H MRS is not capable of performing a "whole-brain" study. Typically, a region of interest (ROI) or a single slice is defined within which these artifacts can be kept to a minimum (5).

Figure 31.2 demonstrates such a slice with the point resolved spectral selection (PRESS)

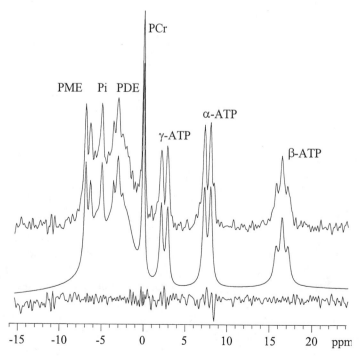

FIG. 31.1. ^{31}P MRSI spectrum from normal cerebral cortex. **Top:** The unprocessed spectrum is shown. **Middle:** The fitted spectrum. **Bottom:** The difference between the two.

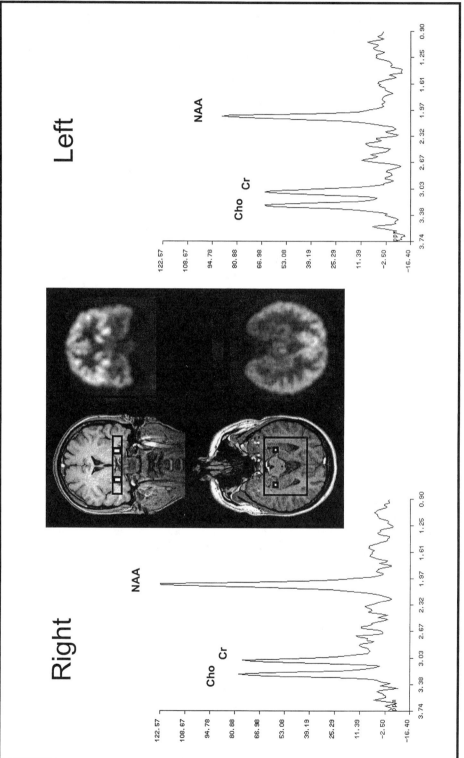

FIG. 31.2. ¹H MRS from a TLE patient with the PRESS volume placed along the long axis of the hippocampus. A typical ¹H spectrum is shown from the right (normal) hippocampus. The epileptogenic (left) hippocampus reveals decreased NAA. Corresponding PET images on right.

volume placed along the long axis of the hippocampus. The anterior border of the PRESS volume is placed to exclude the sinuses, and the lateral boundaries do not include the cortical mantle so as to avoid lipid contamination from the scalp and skull. The spatial resolution in this volume is approximately 1 cc in volume. A typical ^{1}H spectrum is also shown (Fig. 31.2) from the hippocampus, revealing peaks for N-acetyl compounds, largely N-acetylaspartate (NAA), creatine (Cr), and PCr, and choline-containing compounds (Cho). NAA has been of special interest because it is located primarily in neurons and is decreased in conditions associated with neuron loss or dysfunction, including amyotrophic lateral sclerosis (ALS) (7), tumors (8), and strokes (9). Cr and Cho are found in both neurons and glia. Correlating the signal amplitudes with absolute metabolite concentrations is difficult; therefore, most laboratories report their results in ratios of peak areas between resonances within the spectrum rather than molar concentration. The ratios typically reported are NAA/Cr, NAA/Cho, or NAA/Cr+Cho.

[31]P MAGNETIC RESONANCE SPECTROSCOPY

Changes in energy metabolism have been demonstrated interictally by PET scanning. The seizure foci of epileptic patients have shown decreased glucose uptake and decreased perfusion interictally (10–13). These data suggested that metabolic abnormalities, such as an asymmetry of high-energy phosphates or pH, might be detected by MRS interictally in patients with epilepsy.

Many of the metabolites involved in energy metabolism can be measured by ^{31}P MRS, including ATP, phosphocreatine, and inorganic phosphate, thus allowing interictal detection of altered metabolism associated with the seizure focus. Utilizing ^{31}P MRS in a single voxel study in which the region of interest included the medial temporal lobes, patients with TLE demonstrated increased Pi and increased pH as well as de-

creased PME, on the side of the seizure focus (14). Whole-brain MRSI simultaneously obtains spectra from multiple regions throughout the field of view with effective voxel sizes of 16–25 ml. From these spectra, metabolite images can be reconstructed (15,16). By using spectroscopic imaging, similar results were found in TLE (17). The epileptogenic hippocampal region again demonstrated interictal increases in Pi and pH and decreased PME. The pH and Pi changes were not related to the patients' age, seizure duration, seizure frequency, or neuroimaging findings. Kuzniecky et al. found similar results in patients with TLE using both medium- and high-field magnets (4.1T) (18). Chu et al., using a high-field magnet (4.1T), found decreases in the PCr:Pi and gamma-ATP:Pi ratios in the ipsilateral anterior medial temporal lobe in TLE (19). They found a 30% reduction in these two ratios and were able to lateralize 70%–73% of their patients correctly by using these data, including the accurate lateralization of some patients with nonlocalizing MRI. These authors, however, did not find an alteration in pH (20). Thus, whether pH alterations are associated with the epileptogenic region remains controversial. [31]P SI studies are limited by poor spatial resolution, with typical ROI of approximately 30 mL with medium-strength magnets (1.5 and 2.0 T) and 12 mL at 4.1 T.

In the only published study of ^{31}P MRS in NE, Garcia et al. investigated frontal lobe epilepsy (FLE) (21). In this study of eight patients with nonlesional FLE, the epileptogenic frontal lobe demonstrated changes similar to those found in TLE. Alkalosis was found in the epileptogenic frontal lobe compared with the contralateral lobe in all patients (7.10 ± 0.05 versus 7.00 ± 0.06, $p < 0.001$). Seven of eight patients also exhibited decreased PME in the epileptogenic frontal lobe (16.0 ± 6.0 v. 23.0 ± 4.0 $p < 0.01$). In contrast to TLE, inorganic phosphate was not increased in the epileptogenic frontal lobe. These patients were chosen because they had well-defined frontal epileptogenic foci without evidence of focal pathology on neuroimaging. Despite the absence of concordant imaging data (MRI or PET), the ^{31}P MRS was able to predict the correct *lateralization*. Of special note is that the patients in this study had normal MRI and PET scans, suggesting that ^{31}P MRS may have clinical utility when other imaging modalities fail in the lateralization of FLE.

Virtually all the studies to date focused on the ability of MRS to lateralize the seizure focus. The question to be answered is whether this technique can be used for localization of the epileptogenic region; that is, is the region of maximal metabolic derangement indicative of the epileptogenic focus? Van der Grond and colleagues, using ^{31}P MRS, found the focus in TLE to have the most abnormal values of all regions studied, but changes were seen diffusely throughout the brain both ipsilateral and contralateral to the seizure focus (22). There have been no published reports of the ability of ^{31}P to localize FLE, although an abstract by Garcia et al. reported such a capability (23). FLE/NE epilepsies can be so difficult to localize that even the poor spatial resolution of ^{31}PMRS, if lobar specificity could be obtained, would be considered a major advancement.

[1]H MAGNETIC RESONANCE SPECTROSCOPY

^{1}H MRS is the spectroscopy technique most frequently used in the evaluation of focal epilepsy. Several centers (more than ten published series to date) have reported decreased NAA or NAA ratios in the epileptogenic hippocampus in TLE (e.g., 24–31). NAA has been proposed as a specific neuronal cell marker, and the decreased NAA has been suggested as a measure of cell loss. These TLE series have reported significant NAA decreases in the epileptogenic hippocampus in 60% to 90% of the patients studied. Of note, in studies in which comparison to a control population was made, 20% to 50% of the patients had evidence of bilateral decreases in hippocampal NAA

(30). ^{1}H MRS could accurately identify the epileptogenic hippocampus when the side with the lowest hippocampal NAA or NAA ratio was used for lateralization. Many of these patients had normal-appearing hippocampi on MRI or hippocampal volumetry; thus, it appears that ^{1}H measurement of NAA is a more sensitive measure of neuronal dysfunction than MRI (31,32).

Few studies have used ^{1}H MRS in NE, in part because of the increased technical difficulties of studying cortical regions close to the inner table of the skull and the sinuses. Typically in ^{1}H MRSI, only a small portion of the frontal lobes is included in the volume of brain in which the water signal can be adequately suppressed (PRESS volume). Garcia et al. summed all the voxels in the PRESS volume that contained frontal lobe tissue in a population of patients with nonlesional FLE; thus, the spectra were obtained only from the available frontal lobe tissue (33). In each patient studied, the frontal lobe containing the seizure focus demonstrated decreased NAA signal compared with the contralateral side, but the values for Cho and Cr were unchanged. The mean NAA/Cr was decreased in the epileptogenic frontal lobe by about 30%, similar to TLE. This finding was present in all patients studied, regardless of the pathology present, and implied that neuronal loss is a common feature to all localization-related epilepsies. These results were particularly striking given that the protocol was optimized to study patients with TLE and only a small portion of the frontal lobe was available for spectral analysis; therefore, the neuronal cell loss and concomitant NAA decrease must be widespread.

Kuzniecky et al. studied patients with NE resulting from malformations of cortical development using ^{1}H MRSI at 4.1 T (34). Focal cortical dysplasias were associated with significant metabolic abnormalities that corresponded to the lesion. Patients with heterotopia and polymicrogyria demonstrated no subcortical MRSI abnormalities. The metabolic abnormalities correlated with the frequency of seizures but not with the degree of interictal EEG discharges. Quantitative neuronal and glial cell counts revealed no significant correlation between cell loss and the abnormal metabolic ratios.

Using a two-dimensional MRSI technique, with the ROI including both frontal lobes and the precentral/postcentral regions, Stanley et al. investigated patients with nonlesional extratemporal epilepsy (35). To limit the artifacts, the ROI was positioned to exclude the most lateral and anterior portions of the frontal lobes. The ROI was further divided into hemispheric divisions, quadrants, and 16 "focal" subdivisions. The focal subdivision was chosen to reflect the best spatial resolution possible when comparing the MRS results with the epileptogenic region as defined by EEG. For all three subdivisions, the intensity ratios (NAA/Cr, NAA/[Cho + Cr], and NAA/Cho) were significantly decreased in the patients compared with controls. In the focal subdivision scheme, the ratios with the greatest reductions occurred in the epileptogenic region compared with the nonepileptogenic regions. These findings again suggested that the epileptogenic focus was associated with widespread neuronal damage or dysfunction but that the greatest change in NAA or NAA ratios occurred in the epileptogenic focus. Therefore, MRS has the potential to provide localizing information in patients with extratemporal epilepsy.

The inability of ^{1}H techniques to provide data on the entire brain has limited its use in epilepsies other than TLE. These studies are limited to either single voxels or multiple voxels within a single slice that typically does not include cortical regions close to the inner table of the skull. Multiple slice techniques, in which these slices are "stacked," are just beginning to be used, and again the epileptogenic focus has abnormally low NAA (36,37).

Similarly, improved techniques for removing lipid contamination will allow larger volumes of the brain to be studied, including the cortical ribbon. An example of such a multi-ple-slice technique with improved lipid suppression and automated curve fitting in a patient with TLE is shown in Fig. 31.3. Other than unilateral decreased NAA in the epileptogenic hippocampus, the images reveal symmetric extrahippocampal distributions. Figure 31.4 demonstrates proton multislice NAA and (Cr+Ch) metabolite images from a NE patient with a lesion in the right posterior parietal lobe. The lesion is clearly visible in the NAA image (reduced signal) and in the (Cr + Ch) image (increased signal). Accordingly, the spectrum from this region (Ib) showed decreased NAA compared with the contralateral homologous region (Ia). In addition, the spectrum derived from a voxel in the right lateral parietal lobe with normal-appearing MRI (IIb) also showed reduced NAA compared with the contralateral spectrum (IIa). It is this voxel position that coincided with the EEG localization of the seizure focus.

Almost all of the studies to date have focused on the ability of MRS to lateralize the seizure focus, with few demonstrating localizing ability. As described for ^{31}P, the question that needs to be fully answered is whether the focus is the area with the most abnormal metabolite. Preliminary reports suggest similar findings for ^{1}H MRS. Two abstracts have reported the use of ^{1}H MRSI in NE with the focus having the most abnormal NAA values (38,39).

CONCLUSION

Preliminary studies using ^{1}H and ^{31}P MRS demonstrated metabolic abnormalities in the epileptogenic zone, including decreased NAA and PME and increased Pi. The metabolite changes in the seizure focus were found in TLE and NE, and these abnormalities can be used to lateralize the seizure focus accurately. These studies also demonstrated that the changes can be used to predict with accuracy the side of seizure onset, even in the setting of normal MRIs. Whether MRS also can predict seizure localization accurately still needs to be ascertained, but preliminary evidence suggests that will be the case.

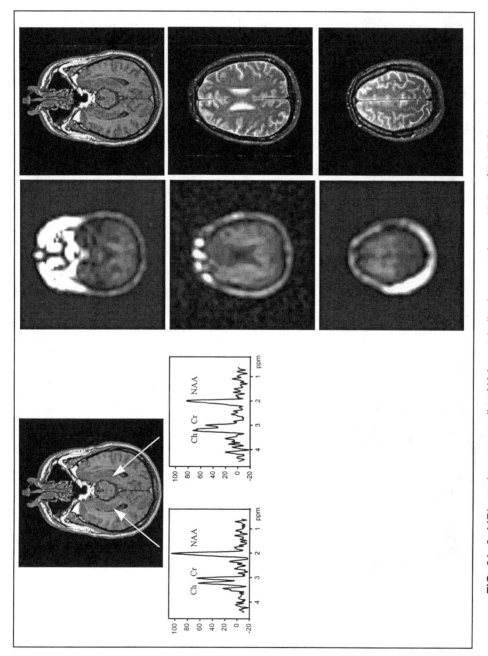

FIG. 31. 3. MRIs and corresponding NAA metabolite images of a multislice ¹H MRSI study on a mTLE patient; spectra from left (ipsilateral) and right hippocampus.

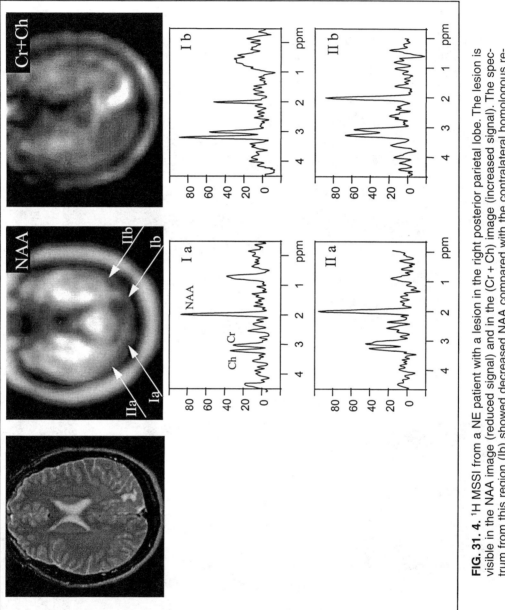

FIG. 31. 4. ¹H MSSI from a NE patient with a lesion in the right posterior parietal lobe. The lesion is visible in the NAA image (reduced signal) and in the (Cr+Ch) image (increased signal). The spectrum from this region (Ib) showed decreased NAA compared with the contralateral homologous region (Ia). The spectrum derived from a voxel in the right lateral parietal lobe with normal-appearing MRI (IIb) also showed reduced NAA.

ACKNOWLEDGMENTS

This work was supported by National Institutes of Health (NIH) grant RO1-NS31966.

REFERENCES

1. Garcia PA, Laxer KD, Barbaro NM, et al. The prognostic value of qualitative MRI hippocampal abnormalities in patients undergoing temporal lobectomy for medically refractory seizures. *Epilepsia* 1994;35:520–524.
2. Jack CR, Sharbrough FW, Cascino GD, et al. Magnetic resonance image-based hippocampal volumetry: correlation with outcome after temporal lobectomy. *Ann Neurol* 1992;31:138–146.
3. Bergen D, Bleck T, Ramsey R, et al. Magnetic resonance imaging as a sensitive and specific predictor of neoplasms removed for intractable epilepsy. *Epilepsia* 1989;30:318–321.
4. Matson GB, Weiner MW. Spectroscopy. In: Stark DD, Bradley WG, eds. *MRI*. St. Louis: Mosby Yearbook, 1992:438–478.
5. Salibi N, Brown MA. *Clinical MR spectroscopy: first principles*. New York: Wiley-Liss, 1998:1–19.
6. Hugg JW, Matson GB, Twieg DB, et al. ^{31}Phosphorus MR spectroscopic imaging (MRSI) of normal and pathological human brains. *Magn Reson Imaging* 1992;10:227–243.
7. Ellis CM, Simmons A, Andrews C, et al. A proton magnetic resonance spectroscopic study in ALS. *Neurology* 1998;51:1104–1109.
8. Arnold DL, Shoubridge EA, Villemure JG, et al. Proton and phosphorus magnetic resonance spectroscopy of human astrocytomas in vivo: preliminary observations on tumor grading. *Nuclear Magnetic Resonance in Biomedicine* 1990;3:184–189.
9. Hugg JW, Duijn JH, Matson GB, et al. Elevated lactate and alkalosis in chronic human brain infarction observed by ^{1}H and ^{31}P MR spectroscopic imaging. *J Cereb Blood Flow Metab* 1992;12:734–744.
10. Engel J, Henry TR, Risinger MW, et al. Presurgical evaluation for partial epilepsy: relative contributions of chronic depth–electrode recordings versus FDG–PET and scalp–sphenoidal ictal EEG. *Neurology* 1990;40:1670–1677.
11. Duncan JS. Positron emission tomography studies of cerebral blood flow and glucose metabolism. *Epilepsia* 1997;38(Suppl):42–47.
12. Ryvlin P, Philippon B, Cinotti L, et al. Functional neuroimaging strategy in temporal lobe epilepsy: a comparative study of ^{18}FDG-PET and ^{99m}Tc-HMPAO-SPECT. *Ann Neurol* 1992;31:650–656.
13. Theodore WH. Positron emission tomography in the evaluation of epilepsy. In: Cascino GD, Jack CR, eds. *Neuroimaging in epilepsy*. Boston: Butterworth–Heinemann, 1996:165–176.
14. Laxer KD, Hubesch B, Sappey-Marinier D, et al. Increased pH and inorganic phosphate in temporal seizure foci, demonstrated by ^{31}P MRS. *Epilepsia* 1992;33:618–623.
15. Maudsley AA, Lin E, Weiner MW. Spectroscopic imaging display and analysis. *Magn Reson Imaging* 1992;10:471–485.
16. Haupt CI, Schuff N, Weiner MW, et al. Removal of lipid artifacts in ^{1}H spectroscopic imaging by data extrapolation. *Magn Reson Med* 1996;35:678–687.
17. Hugg JW, Laxer KD, Matson GB, et al. Lateralization of human focal epilepsy by ^{31}P magnetic resonance spectroscopic imaging. *Neurology* 1992;42:2011–2018.
18. Kuzniecky R, Elgavish GA, Hetherington HP, et al. In vivo ^{31}P nuclear magnetic resonance spectroscopy of human temporal lobe epilepsy. *Neurology* 1992;42:1586–1590.
19. Chu WJ, Hetherington HP, Kuzniecky RI, et al. Lateralization of human temporal lobe epilepsy by ^{31}P NMR spectroscopic imaging at 4.1 T. *Neurology* 1998;51:472–479.
20. Chu WJ, Hetherington HP, Kuzniecky RJ, et al. Is the intracellular pH different from normal in the epileptic focus of patients with temporal lobe epilepsy? a ^{31}P NMR study. *Neurology* 1996;47:756–760.
21. Garcia PA, Laxer KD, van der Grond JR, et al. Phosphorus magnetic resonance spectroscopic imaging in patients with frontal lobe epilepsy. *Annals Neurol* 1994;35:217–221.
22. van der Grond J, Gerson JR, Laxer KD, et al. Regional distribution of interictal ^{31}P metabolic changes in patients with temporal lobe epilepsy. *Epilepsia* 1998;39:527–536.
23. Garcia PA, Laxer KD, van der grond J, et al. Multiregional analysis of ^{31}P magnetic resonance spectroscopic imaging (MRSI) in patients with extratemporal complex partial seizures. *Epilepsia* 1994;35(Suppl 8):19.
24. Hugg JW, Laxer KD, Matson GB, et al. Neuron loss localizes human temporal lobe epilepsy by in vivo proton magnetic resonance spectroscopic imaging. *Ann Neurol* 1993;34:788–794.
25. Connelly A, Jackson GD, Duncan JS, et al. Magnetic resonance spectroscopy in temporal lobe epilepsy. *Neurology* 1994;44:1411–1417.
26. NG T, Comair Y, Xue M, et al. Temporal lobe epilepsy: presurgical localization with proton chemical shift imaging. *Radiology* 1994;193:465–471.
27. Vainio P, Usenius JP, Vapalahti M, et al. Reduced N-acetylaspartate concentration in temporal lobe epilepsy by quantitative ^{1}H MRS in vivo. *Neuroreport* 1994;5:1733–1736.
28. Cendes F, Andermann F, Preul MC, et al. Lateralization of temporal lobe epilepsy based on regional metabolic abnormalities in proton magnetic resonance spectroscopic images. *Ann Neurol* 1994;35:211–216.
29. Garcia PA, Laxer KD, van der Grond J, et al. The relationship of partial epilepsy severity to neuronal loss as determined by proton magnetic resonance spectroscopic imaging (^{1}H MRSI). *Neurology* 1995;45(Suppl 4):A404.
30. Ende G, Laxer KD, Knowlton RC, et al. Proton MRSI reveals bilateral hippocampal metabolite changes in temporal lobe epilepsy. *Radiology* 1996;202:809–817.
31. Knowlton RC, Laxer KD, Ende G, et al. Presurgical multimodality neuroimaging in EEG lateralized temporal lobe epilepsy. *Ann Neurol* 1997;42:829–837.
32. Kuzniecky R, Hugg JW, Hetherington H, et al. Relative utility of ^{1}H spectroscopic imaging and hippocampal volumetry in the lateralization of mesial temporal lobe epilepsy. *Neurology* 1998;51:66–71.
33. Garcia PA, Laxer KD, van der Grond J, et al. Proton mag-

netic resonance spectroscopic imaging in patients with
frontal lobe epilepsy. *Ann Neurol* 1995;37:279–281.

34. Kuzniecky R, Hetherington H, Pan J, et al. Proton spectroscopic imaging at 4.1 tesla in patients with malformations of cortical development and epilepsy. *Neurology* 1997;48:1018–1024.

35. Stanley JA, Cendes F, Dubeau F, et al. Proton magnetic
resonance spectroscopic imaging in patients with extratemporal epilepsy. *Epilepsia* 1998;39:267–273.

36. Vermathen P, Laxer KD, El Din M, et al. Hippocampal
NAA loss in mesial temporal lobe epilepsy is not accompanied by changes in other brain regions. Society
of Magnetic Resonance (SMR). *Proceedings of the 5th
Society of Magnetic Resonance, Vancouver, Canada*
1997;36.

37. Vermathen P, Laxer KD, Schuff N, et al. Simultaneous
detection of reduced NAA in hippocampal and other
brain regions in mesial temporal lobe epilepsy using
multislice proton MRSI. Society of Magnetic Resonance (SMR). *Proceedings of the 6th Society of Magnetic Resonance, Sydney, Australia,* 1998;1729.

38. Barker PB, Smith BJ, Hearshen DO. Multi-slice proton
spectroscopic imaging in frontal lobe epilepsy. Society of
Magnetic Resonance (SMR), *Proceedings of the 5th Society of Magnetic Resonance, Vancouver, Canada,* 1997;37.

39. Vermathen P, Laxer KD, Schuff N, et al. Reduced NAA
localizes the seizure focus in neocortical epilepsy: a multislice MR spectroscopic imaging study. Society of Magnetic Resonance (SMR). *Proceedings of the 6th Society
of Magnetic Resonance, Sydney, Australia,* 1998;1728.

Neocortical Epilepsies.
Advances in Neurology, Vol. 84,
edited by P.D. Williamson, A.M. Siegel,
D.W. Roberts, V.M. Thadani, and M.S. Gazzaniga.
Lippincott Williams & Wilkins, Philadelphia © 2000.

32

Magnetoencephalography in Neocortical Epilepsy

Don W. King, Yong D. Park, *Joseph R. Smith,
and †James W. Wheless

Department of Neurology, Medical College of Georgia, Augusta, Georgia 30912;
Department of Surgery, Section of Neurosurgery, Medical College of Georgia, Augusta,
Georgia 30912; †Department of Neurology, University of Texas–Houston, Houston, Texas 77030

Localization of the epileptogenic zone in patients with intractable neocortical epilepsy presents a major challenge for the epileptologist. Localization is especially difficult in patients with neocortical epilepsy who have a normal magnetic resonance imaging (MRI) or an MRI showing a structural lesion extending over a broad area of cortex. Noninvasive studies that may assist localization in these patients include interictal electroencephalography (EEG), ictal EEG, positron emission tomography (PET), interictal single-photon emission tomography (SPECT), ictal SPECT, magnetic resonance spectroscopy, and source localization of scalp-recorded EEG. These studies are covered in other chapters of this text. One additional technique that has received considerable attention is magnetoencephalography (MEG). This chapter briefly reviews a few of the principles and methods used in recording the MEG and provides an overview of the major studies of MEG in patients with intractable epilepsy.

MAGNETOENCEPHALOGRAPHY: BASIC PRINCIPLES AND METHODS

Magnetoencephalography refers to the measurement of extracranial magnetic fields produced by electric currents generated within the brain. One of the basic principles of magnetism is that an electric current produces a magnetic field at a right angle to the flow of current. The direction of the magnetic field follows the "the right-hand rule"; that is, if the current is in the direction of the extended right thumb, the magnetic field follows the curled fingers of the right hand (Fig. 32.1). As demonstrated in Fig. 32.1, intracranial currents that are radial to the surface of the scalp do not generate magnetic fields that can be measured extracranially. On the other hand, intracranial currents that are tangential to the scalp will give rise to magnetic fields that can be detected by a sensor placed over the scalp surface (Fig. 32.1). The basic concepts underlying MEG and the use of MEG in patients with intractable epilepsy have been described in a number of reviews (1–7).

Just as scalp EEG measures electric activity that is generated by pyramidal cells in the cerebral cortex, MEG measures magnetic flux generated by the electric activity of cortical pyramidal cells. Unlike EEG, which measures extracellular or "volume" current, MEG detects magnetic flux, which is generated by intracellular current, also called

RIGHT HAND RULE

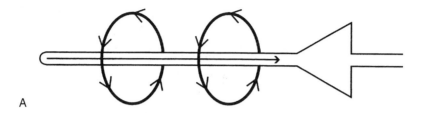

A

TANGENTIAL & RADIAL SOURCES

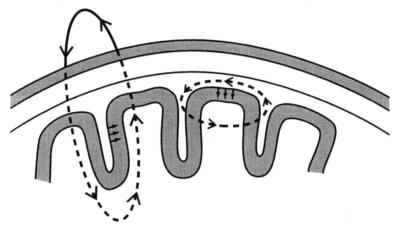

B

FIG. 32.1. A: Schematic diagram showing intracellular current within a pyramidal cell resulting in a magnetic field that follows the right hand rule. **B:** Schematic diagram demonstrating how tangential electrical currents will produce magnetic fields that can be recorded from the scalp, whereas radial electric currents cannot be recorded from the scalp. The diagram is used for illustration purposes only. The magnetic fields measured in patients with intractable epilepsy result from currents generated by a larger population of neurons covering a much broader area of cortex than is demonstrated in this diagram.

source current. The currents measured by both EEG and MEG are generated by the synchronous activity of thousands of cortical neurons extending over a broad area of cortex (1–7).

Background magnetic fields generated by intracranial electric activity are small, on the order of a few hundred femto-Tesla. High-voltage epileptiform discharges produce larger magnetic fields, but they are still only a few thousand femto-Tesla. These fields are much smaller than both the earth's steady magnetic field and the magnetic fields produced by distant moving metal objects. Differentiating the small intracranially generated magnetic fields from the background magnetic "noise" requires a gradiometer, consisting of a set of oppositely wound induction coils, linked to a superconducting quantum interference device (SQUID). One set of coils plus one SQUID constitutes one sensor, or "channel" of MEG activity. A *biomagnetometer* consists of one or more of these sensors bathed in liquid helium within a cryogenic vessel called a *dewar* (1–7).

Early studies of MEG in epilepsy were performed using one or a few sensors arrayed over a small area of scalp (8–15). Both extremes of a given magnetic field cannot be recorded simultaneously with such limited coverage (Fig. 32.1); therefore, it was necessary in these early studies to perform serial recordings to encompass the entire magnetic field produced by a single epileptiform transient. As a result, these recordings were time consuming. More importantly, because epileptiform transients often vary in waveform from one transient to another, one could never be certain that the waveforms recorded in one location were identical to those recorded in another location at a different time.

Most recent studies of MEG in epilepsy have been carried out using larger biomagnetometers (16–34). Most of the large studies described in this chapter used single or dual 37-channel systems that cover an area of scalp up to 15 cm in diameter. Although representing a significant advance, these 37-channel systems also require multiple recordings from each side of the head for complete coverage. Whole-head units, composed of up to 148 channels, have now become available (5,20,24,25). Whole-head biomagnetometers allow recording of epileptiform transients simultaneously from all areas of the scalp, considerably improving localization of the neural source from which the recorded magnetic fields arise.

Numerous studies have shown that MEG can detect interictal spikes or "epileptiform discharges" in patients with intractable epilepsy (8–34). As with EEG, one can develop a topographic display of MEG waveforms and a voltage map using the MEG signals recorded from multiple locations over the scalp (3–7).

For the recorded MEG signals to be useful, it is necessary to estimate the location of the cortical generator or intracranial electric source responsible for the recorded magnetic field. This requires mathematical modeling. The most commonly used method for source modeling is the single equivalent current dipole (ECD) method. The single ECD method assumes that the source is a single electric dipole. The search algorithm specifies the location, orientation, and strength of a single dipole source that accounts for the measured magnetic field at a given point in time. The single ECD method can be applied to each time point throughout the course of the epileptiform discharge. Most recent investigators have used the ECD solution at the time point of the highest correlation between the forward-calculated magnetic field and the measured magnetic field. The ECD location is considered valid only if the correlation coefficient is greater than 0.98 (21,22, 26,30).

Although somewhat simplistic, the single ECD method provides useful clinical information in many patients who have epilepsy, and most studies in patients with intractable epilepsy have used this model (21,22,26,30). The single ECD method is not adequate for electric events in which the electric generator involves different sets of cortical neurons that interact over space and time to produce complex waveforms. These problems can be addressed by using spatiotemporal multiple dipole modeling. Spatiotemporal multiple dipole modeling employs various strategies to determine the location, orientation, and amplitude of an epileptiform discharge throughout its entire course (1).

After calculating the presumed electric source of a measured magnetic field, one then can coregister this calculated source with an anatomic image of the brain (2–5). This is sometimes called *magnetic source imaging* (MSI). Coregistration of the calculated source with MRI is now used routinely in the evaluation of patients with partial epilepsy, including those with neocortical epilepsy (Fig. 32.2).

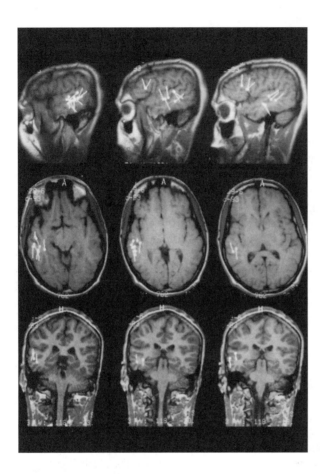

FIG. 32.2. Sagittal, axial, and coronal views of MSI in a 16-year-old boy with intractable complex partial seizures. MRI showed no structural abnormality. MSI shows spike dipoles clustered over the right posterior temporal region. The patient underwent a right posterior temporal neocortical resection and was seizure free at 1-year follow-up.

EARLY STUDIES OF MEG IN EPILEPSY

A number of investigators in the 1980s, using either a single sensor or a small array of sensors, showed that patients with epilepsy often have epileptiform discharges or "spikes" recorded by MEG similar to and often simultaneous with those recorded by EEG (8–15). In addition, early investigators were able to show that MEG could record rhythmic electrographic seizures during ictal events (15). Early investigators also demonstrated that MEG spike localization correlated with localization by noninvasive EEG (8–15), intracranial EEG (11–15), and imaging studies (14,15). As noted previously, these early studies suffered from the disadvantages inherent in small sensor arrays.

Studies of MEG in Epilepsy Using Large-Array MEG

During the 1990s, numerous MEG studies have been performed in patients with epilepsy using large array biomagnetometers (16–35). In most instances, these studies were performed in patients with intractable epilepsy who were being evaluated for epilepsy surgery. Paetau et al. studied the MEG in 13 children with intractable epilepsy using either a 7- or 24-channel biomagnetometer system (27). Patients' ages ranged from 7 to 19 years. MEG spikes were obtained in 10 of the 13 patients, and the MEG spikes were focal or regional, and therefore useful in localization, in 7 of the 13 patients. In the three patients who underwent surgery, source localization of MEG spikes correlated with the ECOG in each patient (27).

Stefan et al. studied 22 patients with temporal lobe epilepsy using a 37-channel biomagnetometer (33). Eleven patients had hippocampal atrophy, and 11 patients had temporal lobe structural lesions. Of the 11 patients with hippocampal atrophy, 9 showed MEG spikes in the ipsilateral temporal lobe, one showed MEG spikes in the ipsilateral temporal and frontal lobes, and one showed ipsilateral frontal lobe MEG spikes. Of the 11 patients with structural lesions, all showed MEG spikes in the ipsilateral temporal region. The proximity of the spikes to the structural lesion was less than 1.0 cm in eight patients; 1.0 to less than 2.0 cm in one patient; 2.0 to less than 3.0 cm in one patient; and greater than 3.0 cm in one patient. Eight of the patients with structural lesions underwent surgery; and seven of those patients had demonstrated MEG spikes less than 1.0 cm from the lesion, and one had demonstrated MEG spikes between 1 and 2 cm from the lesion. Following surgery, five of the eight patients were class I, and three were class II (33). These data suggest that MEG is capable of localizing epileptiform activity in proximity to an epileptogenic structural lesion.

Ebersole and Smith in 1995 studied the MEG in 30 patients with intractable complex partial seizures (17). Each patient was recorded using a single or dual 37-channel MEG system and 21 to 32 channels of EEG. Single ECD modeling and spatiotemporal multiple dipole modeling were used for both MEG and EEG. When MEG spikes were present, patients with temporal lobe epilepsy demonstrated one of the following patterns. Five patients had basal horizontal dipoles, all of whom had mesial temporal seizure onset. One patient had anterior vertical dipoles. This patient also had mesial temporal seizure onset. Seven patients had mid to posterior temporal vertical dipoles, six of whom had lateral temporal or unlocalized seizure onset. These data suggest that MEG may be a useful tool in differentiating medial temporal lobe epilepsy from lateral temporal or neocortical temporal lobe epilepsy. In this study, MEG spike

dipoles resulting from source localization were more clearly defined and more consistently localized than the EEG spike dipoles using similar methodology (17).

Eliashiv and colleagues reported seven patients with intractable complex partial seizures who underwent bilateral 37 channel MEG recording prior to implantation of intracranial electrodes (19). Interictal MEG localization was generally concordant with interictal intracranial recording. In one patient, MEG defined an intracranially confirmed ictal onset zone not suspected by standard phase I evaluation. In two patients, one with seizure onset in the orbital frontal region and one with seizure onset in the mesial temporal region, MEG did not reveal the intracranially demonstrated ictal onset zone (19).

Smith and associates studied 50 patients with intractable epilepsy who were being evaluated for epilepsy surgery (30). A single- or dual-probe 37-channel biomagnetometer system was used. Multiple 6-second epochs of data were obtained from two to five sites on each side of the head. MEG localization was compared with "standard" localization of the epileptogenic zone as determined by MRI, noninvasive EEG, and invasive EEG. Of the 50 patients studied, there was complete agreement between MEG localization and standard localization in 56% of the patients, partial agreement in 12%, no agreement in 10%, no MEG spikes in 16%, and inadequate data in 6%. Of the 20 patients with convexity localization by standard preoperative testing, MEG showed complete agreement in 17 patients, partial agreement in two patients, and no spikes in one patient. On the other hand, of the 18 patients with medial temporal lobe epilepsy, there was complete agreement in 56% of the patients, partial agreement in 11%, no agreement in 11%, and no EEG spikes in 22%. Patients with localization in the orbital frontal region and those with poorly localized epileptogenic zones by standard testing were not well localized with MEG. These data suggest that MEG may be more useful in patients with epileptogenic zones involving the cerebral convexity than in those with epileptogenic zones deep to the surface of the brain (30).

Knowlton et al. performed MEG in 22 patients with intractable epilepsy who were being evaluated for possible surgery (22). Sixteen of the 22 patients had both MEG and EEG spikes. Eleven of 12 patients with neocortical epilepsy, but only 5 of 10 patients with mesial temporal lobe epilepsy (MTLE), had spike discharges. These data, similar to those reported by Smith et al., suggest that the yield of MEG may be higher in patients with neocortical epilepsy than in those with MTLE. In five of six patients with structural abnormalities, the calculated source of the MEG spike was immediately adjacent to the structural abnormality, confirming the findings previously reported by Stefan et al. (33).

Fourteen of the 22 patients studied by Knowlton et al. had an MRI scan which was unlocalized; that is, either no abnormality was present, or a diffuse abnormality was present. Twelve of these 14 patients had both MEG and EEG spike discharges. In 11 of the 12 patients with spike discharges, the MEG discharges were localized to the epileptogenic zone as determined by standard preoperative evaluation. Seven of the 11 patients who had surgery were class I, and 2 were class II. These data suggest that MEG may be a useful method of localization in patients with unlocalized MRI (22).

Knowlton and colleagues also compared interictal MEG with scalp ictal EEG in localizing the epileptogenic zone. In the 12 patients with localized MEG spikes, the MEG spikes were concordant with the epileptogenic zone in 92%. In only 55% of 11 patients with well-recorded scalp ictal EEG were the scalp-recorded electrographic seizures concordant with the epileptogenic zone (22).

Wheless et al. compared MEG, MRI, interictal scalp video/EEG (VEEG ii), ictal scalp video/EEG (VEEG i), interictal subdural video/EEG (SD-VEEG ii), and ictal subdural video/EEG (SD-VEEG i) in determining the epileptogenic zone in 58 patients with intractable epilepsy (33). In patients who were

either seizure free (class I) or had rare seizures (class II), MEG was second only to SD-VEEG i in predicting the epileptogenic zone. MEG was superior to MR, VEEG ii, VEEG i, AND SD-VEEG ii. MEG was also superior to these four modalities in patients who underwent anterior temporal lobectomy. In patients who underwent extratemporal resection, MEG was superior only to MRI, VEEG i, and VEEG ii (35). These data suggest that, except for intracranial ictal EEG, MEG is as effective or more effective than standard methods for localizing the epileptogenic zone (33).

Park and associates studied 16 children with intractable epilepsy using a single- or dual-probe 37-channel biomagnetometer system (26). MEG spikes were recorded in 15 patients. There was complete agreement between MEG data localization and standard localization in 53% of the patients, partial agreement in 27%, and disagreement in 20%. Of the eight patients who underwent surgery, 75% were seizure free, and 25% had greater than 90% reduction in seizure frequency at 1 year follow-up (26).

Merlet et al. compared MEG and EEG spikes in four children with partial epilepsy (24). The MEG peak preceded the EEG peak from 9 to 40 ms in seven of ten spike averages. A small positive EEG spike coincided with the negative MEG spike in six of the seven asynchronous spikes. Synchronous spikes were separated by 5 to 23 ms. Asynchronous spikes were separated by 12 to 67 ms. These investigators concluded that nonidentical neuron currents generate MEG and EEG spikes (24).

We recently reviewed MEG data on 48 patients with intractable seizures who were being evaluated for epilepsy surgery (21), including 18 male patients and 20 female patients. Age ranged from 7 to 48 years. MEG studies were reviewed blindly by two investigators. The following patterns of MEG spikes were present in the 48 patients: focal, 23; regional, 4; multifocal, 13; scattered, 4; and none, 4. Based on localization and orientation of the primary focus of MEG spike dipoles, patients were divided into the following groups: anterior/midtemporal (horizontal orientation), 14; mid/posterior temporal ± parietal, 13; extratemporal, 13; and scattered or no spikes, 8 (21).

Thirty-six patients underwent surgery for the control of epilepsy. Based on the modified Engel classification, outcome at 1 year follow-up was as follows: class I, 47%; class II, 19%; class III, 14%; and class IV, 19%. Of the 19 patients who had a complete or almost complete resection of the primary MEG spike focus, 74% were class I, 21% were class II, 5% were class III, and no patients were class IV. Of the 17 patients who had only a partial resection of the primary spike focus or resection of tissue that demonstrated no MEG spike dipoles, only 18% were class I, 18% were class II, 24% were class III, and 41% were class IV. These data suggest that resection of the primary MEG spike focus correlates strongly with excellent outcome (21).

Comparison of MEG Source Localization to Scalp EEG Source Localization

Ebersole, Scherg, and colleagues demonstrated in a number of studies that source localization can be applied to the electric fields detected by scalp EEG (36–40). Although no large studies have been done directly comparing source localization of MEG signals to source localization of scalp recorded EEG, there are theoretic reasons to suggest that MEG may provide superior information. MEG is sensitive solely to tangential currents, whereas EEG is sensitive to a combination of radial and tangential currents. In addition, magnetic fields are not distorted by the skull and soft tissues as is the case with EEG. For both these reasons, MEG source localization should be more precise and accurate than EEG source localization. In addition, the newer whole-head MEG units allow recording from up to 148 separate scalp sites simultaneously, a feat not easily accomplished with our present EEG recording methods. As noted previously, simultaneous recording over a broad area allows more accurate source localization.

On the other hand, EEG source localization has potential advantages. Because EEG records both radial and tangential currents, EEG theoretically provides a more complete picture of intracranially generated epileptiform transients. In addition, EEG is widely available, is much less expensive, and can be used more easily for prolonged monitoring of ictal events.

Ebersole and colleagues provided some data showing direct comparisons between MEG source localization and EEG source localization. Based on these limited data, MEG source location does appear to provide more consistent and well-localized spike dipoles (2). Additional comparison studies are necessary to determine whether source localization of EEG signals can be used as effectively as source localization using MEG.

CONCLUSION AND FUTURE DIRECTIONS

Magnetoencephalography is an effective method for detecting interictal and ictal epileptiform activity in patients with epilepsy. Localization using interictal MEG combined with source localization and coregistration with MRI has been shown to agree with "standard" localization provided by scalp EEG, invasive EEG, MRI, PET, and the convergence of these tests. In addition, interictal MEG has been shown to correlate with outcome following epilepsy surgery. Based on theoretic considerations as well as published observations, it appears that MEG and EEG provide complementary, nonredundant information, and that MEG offers significant advantages over scalp interictal EEG, ictal EEG, and source localization based on scalp EEG. The data thus far suggest that MEG may be more useful in patients with neocortical epilepsy than in those with medial temporal lobe epilepsy, especially in patients with epileptogenic zones over the convexity.

The primary clinical use of MEG thus far has been in localization of the epileptogenic zone in patients who are being evaluated for epilepsy surgery. MEG will likely be unnecessary in patients whose epileptogenic zone is easily determined on standard noninvasive evaluation. On the other hand, MEG may provide important information in at least two major categories of patients with intractable epilepsy, that is, those with normal MRI's and those with widespread MRI abnormalities. Most centers using MEG now use the MEG in such patients to determine the location for intracranial electrode placement, and this should continue to be a major use of MEG. Based on the data provided by Smith et al. (30) and a review of our recent data (21), it is possible that in some patients MEG localization also may help to define the extent of surgery, with or without prior intracranial recording. In other patients, MEG may provide evidence of a widespread epileptogenic zone or no epileptiform activity, thus preventing surgery in some patients who might otherwise be considered for surgery.

At this time, MEG is an expensive procedure not available to most epilepsy surgery centers. To define more fully the types of patients in whom MEG may be indicated, additional studies are needed. These include studies comparing the sensitivity and specificity of MEG to other presurgical tests, studies defining the use of MEG in predicting outcome following epilepsy surgery, and studies comparing source localization using MEG to source localization using EEG to determine if MEG offers significant advantages over EEG.

REFERENCES

1. Ebersole JS. New applications of EEG/MEG in epilepsy evaluation. In: Leppik IE, ed. *Rational polypharmacy.* New York: Elsevier, 1996:227–237.
2. Ebersole JS. Magnetoencephalography/magnetic source imaging in the assessment of patients with epilepsy. *Epilepsia* 1997;38(Suppl 4):S1–S5.
3. Ebersole JS, Squires KC, Eliashiv SD, et al. Applications of magnetic source imaging in evaluation of candidates for epilepsy surgery. In: Kucharczyk J, Mosely ME, Roberts T, Orrison WW, eds. *Neuroimaging Clin N Am* 1995;5:267–288.
4. Gallen GC, Hirschkoff EC, Buchanan DS. Magnetoencephalography and magnetic source imaging: capabilities and limitations. In: Kucharczyk J, Mosely ME,

5. Roberts T, Orrison WW, eds. Functional neuroimaging. *Neuroimaging Clin N Am* 1995;5:227–249.
5. Lewine JD, Orrison WD. Spike and slow wave localization by magnetoencephalography. In: Latchaw R, Jack C, eds. Epilepsy: clinical evaluation, neuroimaging, surgery. *Neuroimaging Clin N Am* 1995;5:575–596.
6. Rose DF, Smith PD, Sato S. Magnetoencephalography and epilepsy research. *Science* 1987;238:329–335.
7. Sato S, Smith PD. Magnetoencephalography. *J Clin Neurophysiol* 1985;2:173–192.
8. Barth DS, Sutherling W, Engel J, et al. Neuromagnetic localization of epileptiform spike activity in the human brain. *Science* 1982;218:891–894.
9. Barth DS, Sutherling W, Engel J, et al. Neuromagnetic evidence of spatially distributed sources underlying epileptiform spikes in the human brain. *Science* 1984;223:293–296.
10. Modena I, Ricci GB, Barbanera S, et al. Biomagnetic measurements of spontaneous brain activity in epileptic patients. *Electroencephalogr Clin Neurophysiol* 1982; 54:622–628.
11. Ricci GB, Romani GL, Salustri C, et al. Study of focal epilepsy by multichannel neuromagnetic measurements. *Electroencephalogr Clin Neurophysiol* 1987;66: 358–368.
12. Rose DF, Sato S, Smith PD, et al. Localization of magnetic interictal discharges in temporal lobe epilepsy. *Ann Neurol* 1987;22:348–354.
13. Sutherling WW, Barth DS. Neocortical propagation in temporal lobe spike foci on magnetoencephalography and electroencephalography. *Ann Neurol* 1989;25: 373–381.
14. Sutherling WW, Crandall PH, Cahan LD, et al. The magnetic field of epileptic spikes agrees with intracranial localizations in complex partial epilepsy. *Neurology* 1988;38:778–786.
15. Sutherling WW, Crandall PH, Engel J, et al. The magnetic field of complex partial seizures agrees with intracranial localizations. *Ann Neurol* 1987;21:548–558.
16. Aung M, Sobel DF, Gallen CC, et al. Potential contribution of bilateral magnetic source imaging to the evaluation of epilepsy surgery candidates. *Neurosurgery* 1995;37:1113–1121.
17. Ebersole JS, Smith JR. MEG spike modeling differentiates baso-mesial from lateral cortical temporal epilepsy. *Electroencephalogr Clin Neurophysiol* 1995;95:20P.
18. Eisenberg HM, Papanicolaou AC, Baumann SB, et al. Magnetoencephalographic localization of interictal spike sources. *J Neurosurg* 1991;74:660–664.
19. Eliashiv SD, Velasco AL, Wilson CL, et al. Magnetic source imaging as a predictor of invasive-electrode–defined irritative and ictal onset zones. *Electroencephalogr Clin Neurophysiol* 1995;95:20P.
20. Hari R, Ahonen A, Forss N, et al. Parietal epileptic mirror focus detected with a whole-head neuromagnetometer. *Neuroreport* 1993;5:45–48.
21. King, DW, Park YD, Smith JR, et al. Unpublished data.
22. Knowlton R, Laxer K, Aminoff M, et al. Magnetoencephalography in partial epilepsy: clinical yield and localization accuracy. *Ann Neurol* 1997;42:622–631.
23. Ko D, Kufta C, Scaffidi D, et al. Source localization determined by magnetoencephalography and electroencephalography in temporal lobe epilepsy: comparison with electrocorticography—technical case report. *Neurosurgery* 1998;42:414–421.

24. Merlet I, Paetau R, Garcia-Larrea L, et al. Apparent asynchrony between interictal electric and magnetic spikes. *Neuroreport* 1997;8:1071–1076.

25. Mikuni N, Nagamine T, Ikeda A, et al. Simultaneous recording of epileptiform discharges by MEG and subdural electrodes in temporal lobe epilepsy. *Neuroimage* 1997;5:298–306.

26. Park YD, Hu C, Smith JR. Magnetoencephalographic/magnetic source imaging evaluation of patients with intractable epilepsy. Unpublished data.

27. Paetau R, Hämäläinen M, Hari R, et al. Magnetoencephalographic evaluation of children and adolescents with intractable epilepsy. *Epilepsia* 1994;35:275–284.

28. Paetau R, Kajola M, Hari R. Magnetoencephalography in the study of epilepsy. *Neurophysiol Clin* 1990;20: 169–187.

29. Paetau R, Kajola M, Karhu J, et al. Magnetoencephalographic localization of epileptic cortex—impact on surgical treatment. *Ann Neurol* 1992;32:106–109.

30. Smith JR, Schwartz BJ, Gallen C, et al. Utilization of multichannel magnetoencephalography in the guidance of ablative seizure surgery. *J Epilepsy* 1995;8:119–130.

31. Stefan H, Schneider S, Abraham-Fuchs K, et al. Magnetic source localization in focal epilepsy. *Brain* 1990;113:1347–1359.

32. Stefan H, Schneider S, Feistel H, et al. Ictal and interictal activity in partial epilepsy recorded with multichannel magnetoencephalography: correlation of electroencephalography/electrocorticography, magnetic resonance imaging, single photon emission computed tomography, and positron emission tomography findings. *Epilepsia* 1992;33:874–887.

33. Stefan H, Schüler P, Abraham-Fuchs K, et al. Magnetic source localization and morphological changes in temporal lobe epilepsy: comparison of MEG/FEG, ECoG, and volumetric MRI in presurgical evaluation of operated patients. *Acta Neurol Scand* 1994(Suppl 1);52:83–88.

34. Tiihonen J, Hari R, Kajola M, et al. Localization of epileptic foci using a large-area magnetometer and functional brain anatomy. *Ann Neurol* 1990;27: 283–290.

35. Wheless JW, Willmore LJ, Dreier JI, et al. A comparison of magnetoencephalography, MRI, and V-EEG in patients evaluated for epilepsy surgery. *Epilepsia* 2000 (in press).

36. Ebersole JS. EEG dipole modeling in complex partial epilepsy. *Brain Topography* 1991;4:113–123.

37. Ebersole JS. Non-invasive localization of the epileptogenic focus by EEG dipole modeling. *Acta Neurol Scand* 1994(Suppl 1);52:20–28.

38. Ebersole JS, Wade PB. Spike voltage topography identifies two types of frontotemporal epileptic foci. *Neurology* 1991;41:1425–1433.

39. Scherg M, Ebersole JS. Models of brain sources. *Brain Topogr* 1993;5:419–423.

40. Scherg M, Ebersole JS. Brain source imaging of focal and multifocal epileptiform EEG activity. *Neurophysiol Clin* 1994;24:51–60.

Neocortical Epilepsies.
Advances in Neurology, Vol. 84,
edited by P. D. Williamson, A. M. Siegel,
D. W. Roberts, V. M. Thadani, and M. S. Gazzaniga.
Lippincott Williams & Wilkins, Philadelphia © 2000.

33

SPECT in Neocortical Epilepsies

Vijay M. Thadani, Alan H. Siegel, Petra Lewis, Adrian M. Siegel,
Karen L. Gilbert, Terrance M. Darcey, David W. Roberts,
and Peter D. Williamson

*Section of Neurology, Dartmouth Medical School, Dartmouth–Hitchcock Medical Center,
Lebanon, New Hampshire 03756*

The localization of neocortical seizure foci for epilepsy surgery presents major problems. When structural lesions are present, complete removal of the lesion, with a narrow margin of normal-appearing cortex, is strongly correlated with cure of the epilepsy (1,2). Attempts to define and resect areas of electric abnormality do not appear to produce results different or better than resection of the lesion alone (3). In the absence of a structural lesion, or in the presence of a structural lesion so large or in such a position that it cannot be completely resected, resective surgery is less often successful. In these circumstances, the gold standard for localization of seizure foci has been intracranial electroencephalography (EEG) to demonstrate the regions of seizure onset and spread.

Advanced imaging techniques, including quantitative magnetic resonance imaging (MRI), MRI spectroscopy, single-photon emission computed tomography (SPECT), and positron emission tomography (PET), all have been used in attempts to identify seizure foci and guide surgical resection (4–7). It is unclear at this time which of these techniques holds the greatest promise from the theoretical viewpoint or which will prove to be most successful in practice.

Previously, interictal SPECT demonstrated hypoperfusion in the temporal lobe concordant with seizure onset; however, sensitivity has been low compared with interictal PET, MRI spectroscopy, and intracranial EEG recording (7–9). In epilepsy originating outside the temporal lobes, interictal SPECT has not given useful localizing information (10).

More recently, ictal SPECT, when the isotope is injected within seconds of seizure onset, has shown high sensitivity and specificity in demonstrating hyperperfusion of the region where the seizure began. Although the sensitivity and specificity of the technique appear to be highest in temporal lobe epilepsy, it is particularly useful in extratemporal neocortical epilepsy where other localizing techniques are less effective, particularly in the absence of a structural lesion (11,12). Use of continuous video/EEG and the recent availability of a stable isotope greatly facilitate injection at the moment of seizure onset.

Whereas ictal SPECT is sensitive and specific for identifying seizure foci, ambiguous and erroneous results are possible. We present here a series of patients who had interictal and ictal SPECT, with intracranial EEG recordings of seizures and surgical outcome used as the gold standard for localization. We could thus validate the results of interictal and ictal SPECT in a manner that has not often been done.

METHODS

Brain SPECT is a means of creating a perfusion map or an image of the blood flow that is occurring at the time of or shortly after the injection of a radioactive tracer. Estimates of partial and complete circulation times range from 15 to 60 seconds, and so the map probably reflects cerebral blood flow, as it was less than 1 minute after the time of intravenous injection (13). Radioactive tracers can be injected during seizure activity *(ictal)*, immediately after seizure activity *(postictal)*, or during a seizure-free period *(interictal)*. During the seizure, the blood flow to the electric focus may be increased by as much as 300% (14). Interictally, seizure foci may show decreased blood flow. Unfortunately, ictal SPECT (which is more sensitive and specific than interictal SPECT) is among the most difficult and demanding of the procedures performed in nuclear medicine.

There are two commonly used agents for brain-perfusion SPECT in the United States: technetium-99m hexamethylpropylamineoxime or HMPAO, Ceretec (Amersham), and Technetium-99m ethylene cysteinate dimer, or ECD Neurolite (Dupont). Although there are differences between these two agents, neither has been proven superior to the other. The localization of these agents in the brain is approximately proportional to blood flow. Their uptake and localization are rapid and stable. Imaging can be performed within a window of several hours following the injection (and should not be performed immediately because time is needed to allow for background clearance). It is important to realize that cerebral localization is an indication of blood flow at the time of injection, and not at the time of scanning.

These agents are labeled with technetium-99m, a radioisotope that emits photons that allow for imaging. The radiation dose received by the patients from these procedures is small and of relatively minor concern; however, the radioactivity leads to many issues concerning radiation safety and licensing.

Radioactive materials can be administered only by persons approved to perform this procedure. Normally, these are physicians in the nuclear medicine laboratory and technologists who act under the authority of those physicians. Because the performance of ictal SPECT requires a significant amount of dedicated time and continuous observation of the patient, the staffing necessary to perform these studies becomes a serious issue. At Dartmouth, it was necessary that additional persons be designated for patient monitoring and radiotracer injection. Several physicians and nurses were trained and approved as "adjunct nuclear medicine technologists," who are permitted to function in this capacity only when a nuclear medicine physician is on the premises, and they must follow the *Rules for the Safe Handling of Radioactive Materials* of Dartmouth–Hitchcock Medical Center. Each undergoes a training program that includes classroom lessons in radiation safety, physics, instrumentation, and quality control as well as an orientation period in the nuclear medicine section. The certified nuclear medicine technologists still perform dose calibration, room surveys, wipe tests, and cleanup (if necessary) of any spills. The program was approved by the Radiation Safety Committee at Dartmouth–Hitchcock Medical Center and the State of New Hampshire.

Shielded syringes were tested, and it was found that the exposure rate from the plunger end exceeded permissible levels. The State of New Hampshire requires that radiation doses to the continuously exposed general public be less than 100 mR per year. At 2 mR per hour through the plunger, anyone in the vicinity of the injection would be exposed to unacceptably high levels of radiation. A custom-made syringe shield consisting of an acrylic holder with a leaded plunger was brought into use (Fig. 33.1), and radiation surveys showed an exposure of only 0.08 mR per hour. These levels were satisfactory for the procedure to be performed in the epilepsy monitoring unit without additional shielding, such as leaded walls, to protect the general public. Also, the

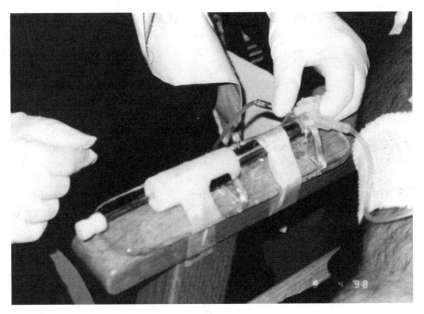

FIG. 33.1. 1 Custom-made single acrylic and lead syringe shield for minimizing radiation exposure.

radiation exposure of the adjunct technologist was thus minimized.

The patient population in this study comprised 27 patients (18 men and 9 women) with medically refractory epilepsy. Age at onset of epilepsy ranged from 4 months to 40 years. Age at time of SPECT ranged from 11 to 49 years. Some were of borderline intelligence, but none was mentally retarded, and none had progressive neurologic disease. Postsurgical follow-up was at least 2 years.

Patients were admitted to the inpatient video/EEG monitoring unit at Dartmouth–Hitchcock Medical Center and had antiepileptic medications withdrawn sequentially to precipitate seizures. Seizures were detected by direct observation and computerized detection devices. An adjunct technician supervised video/EEG recording and sat continuously with the patient. As soon as a clinical or electrographic seizure was detected, the patient was injected with either 20 mci Tc99m HMPAO (Ceretec) or 20 mci Tc99m ECD (Neurolite). Times between seizure onset and injection ranged from 16 to 40 seconds.

Brain SPECT scanning was performed using a Picker Prism 3000 three-headed camera. Sequential acquisitions were obtained, and frames were excluded in the cases of patient movement. Scans were reconstructed in sagittal, coronal, axial, and temporal lobe planes. Similar SPECT studies were performed interictally on each patient. The SPECT scans were registered to each patient's MRI scan using an automated registration method. Subtraction images also were obtained for ictal minus interictal SPECT following normalization to elucidate the region or regions of hyperperfusion. Although multiheaded cameras tend to be superior for brain SPECT, good-quality studies can be obtained with a single-headed camera.

The MRIs were obtained on a 1.5 Tesla GE scanner with T1- and T2-weighted sequences in horizontal, sagittal, and coronal planes. Three-dimensional MPGR 1.5-mm cuts also were obtained in the coronal plane and used for image registration.

Based on the results of the scalp EEG, clinical features of the seizures, and imaging studies, patients underwent intracranial EEG recording. Intracranial EEG was done with varying combinations of 12-contact depth electrodes, 1 × 8 strips, and 4 × 8 or 8 × 8 grids. A specially designed 3 × 8 two-sided grid was used for interhemispheric recording. Up to 128 channels of intracranial EEG were recorded referentially and were analyzed in referential and bipolar montages using Telefactor equipment. Occasionally, additional ictal SPECT studies were obtained in patients who were being monitored with intracranial electrodes.

RESULTS

In evaluating the accuracy of interictal and ictal SPECT for the localization of seizure foci, intracranial EEG recordings and surgical outcome were used as the gold standard. Interictal SPECT showed focal hypoperfusion consistent with intracranial EEG localization of the seizure focus in 33% of patients. In 52% of patients with seizures localized by intracranial EEG, the interictal SPECT was normal. In 7% of patients, interictal SPECT provided correct lateralization but not localization; and in 7%, it was misleading with contralateral hypoperfusion. These data are summarized in Table 33.1. This table also indicates that ictal SPECT usually showed hyperfusion corresponding to the hypoperfusion seen on the interictal studies. Furthermore, hyperfusion on the ictal studies, concordant with EEG findings, was seen in most of the patients who had normal interictal studies.

Ictal SPECT showed hyperperfusion consistent with intracranial EEG localization of the seizure focus in 74% of patients. In 7% of patients with seizures localized by intracranial EEG, the ictal SPECT was normal. In 4% of patients, the ictal SPECT provided correct lateralization but not localization; and in 15%, it was misleading with contralateral hyperperfusion. The time it took to inject the isotope after the seizure began (mean injection time) appeared to be similar for all of the subgroups of patients and could not be correlated with results (concordant or discordant) obtained with intracranial EEG and interictal SPECT (Table 33.2).

After it became clear that interictal SPECT was not a sensitive study and gave little information independent of ictal SPECT, further analysis was done correlating ictal SPECT with MRI findings and surgical results. Fifty-two percent of patients had normal MRI, and 48% had a variety of structural lesions, including low-grade astrocytoma, ganglioglioma, hamartoma, vascular malformation, and cortical scar. None had mesial temporal sclerosis. The presence or absence of structural lesions did not appear to affect the reliability of ictal SPECT data. Generally, the same correlation with intracranial EEG was found in both groups. Table 33.3 shows that in patients with normal MRI, ictal SPECT was concordant with intracranial EEG data in 86% of the patients and discordant in 14%. In patients with structural lesions, there was concordance between ictal SPECT and intracranial EEG data 62% of the time. This

TABLE 33.1. *Interictal SPECT correlated with focal intracranial EEG and ictal SPECT (27 patients)*

Interictal findings	Ictal findings
Hypoperfusion concordant with EEG (9 patients, 33%)	Hyperperfusion concordant with EEG (9 patients)
Hypoperfusion lateralized but not localized with EEG (2 patients, 7%)	Hyperperfusion concordant with EEG (2 patients)
Hypoperfusion contralateral to EEG (2 patients, 7%)	Hyperperfusion concordant with EEG (1 patient)
	Hyperperfusion contralateral to EEG (1 patient)
Normal study (14 patients, 52%)	Hyperperfusion concordant with EEG (11 patients)
	Hyperperfusion contralateral to EEG (1 patient)
	Normal study (2 patients)

EEG, electroencephalographic.

TABLE 33.2. *Correlation of SPECT with focal intracranial EEG (27 patients)*

Type of study	Concordant with EEG focus	Correct lateralization but not localization	Contralateral to EEG focus	Normal study
Ictal SPECT	20 (74%)	1 (4%)	4 (15%)	2 (7%)
Mean injection time	17 s	38 s	22.5 s	17 s
Interictal SPECT	9 (33%)	2 (7%)	2 (7%)	14 (52%)

EEG, electroencephalographic; SPECT, single-photon emission computed tomography.

TABLE 33.3. Correlation of ictal SPECT with MRI and intracranial EEG (27 patients)

MRI findings	Ictal SPECT			
	Concordant with EEG focus	Correct lateralization but not localized	Contralateral to EEG focus	Normal study
Normal (14 patients)	12 (86%)	0	2 (14%)	0
Structural lesion (13 patients)	8 (62%)	1 (8%)	2 (15%)	2 (15%)

EEG, electroencephalography; MRI, magnetic resonance imaging; SPECT, single-photon emission computed tomography.

TABLE 33.4. *Correlation of ictal SPECT, intracranial EEG, and surgical outcome (23 patients)*

EEG focus	Outcome class			
	I	II	III	IV
Temporal (7 patients)				
Concordant SPECT	6	0	0	0
Discordant/normal SPECT	0	0	0	1
Frontal (14 patients)				
Concordant SPECT	6	1	3	1
Discordant/normal SPECT	1	1	1	0
Occipital (2 patients)				
Concordant SPECT	1	0	1	0
All patients (23 patients)				
Concordant SPECT	13	1	4	1
Discordant/normal SPECT	1	1	1	1

EEG, electroencephalographic; SPECT, single-photon emission computed tomography.

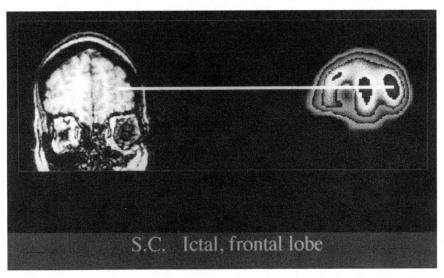

FIG. 33.2. Ictal SPECT shows hyperperfusion (dark areas) of left-sided mesial and lateral frontal cortex. MRI coregistration shows normal anatomy.

correlation did not differ significantly from the 86% concordance seen in patients without structural lesions.

Of 27 patients with seizures localized by intracranial EEG, 23 went on to surgery. Sixty-one percent had class I outcomes, 8% were class II, and 31% were class III or IV. Surgery was guided by intracranial EEG data and the boundaries of structural lesions. In this series, these were always concordant, and all resections were complete. Table 33.4 shows that when ictal SPECT data were concordant with intracranial EEG data, there was a trend toward better outcome (68% class I). Only one of four patients (25%) with discor-

dant or normal ictal SPECT data had a class I outcome. This is shown in Table 33.4, which also shows a breakdown of patients by region of localization. Outcomes were somewhat better for patients having temporal lobe surgery than those having extratemporal resections. Two typical cases are discussed here.

Patient 1 was a 36-year-old woman who had nocturnal seizures characterized by thrashing around in bed. MRI was normal. An ictal SPECT showed marked, left-sided mesial frontal and lateral frontal hyperperfusion (Fig. 33.2). An interictal study was essentially normal. Intracranial EEG showed left mesial and lateral frontal seizure onset (Fig. 33.3). Fol-

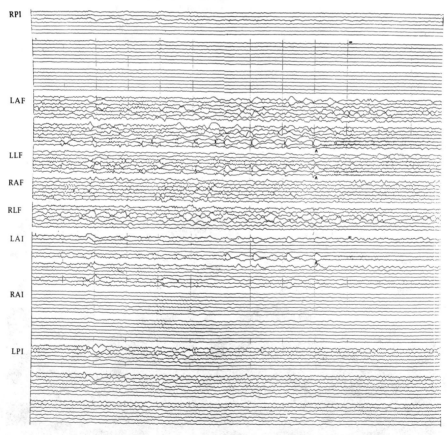

FIG. 33. 3. Electrode identification: *LAI,* left anterior interhemispheric 2 × 8 contact; *RAI,* right anterior interhemispheric 2 × 8 contact; *LPI,* left posterior interhemispheric 3 × 8 contact (double-sided); *RPI,* right posterior interhemispheric 3 × 8 contact; *LAF,* left anterior frontal 2 × 8 contact; *LLF,* left lateral frontal 1 × 8 contact; *RAF,* right anterior frontal 1 × 8 contact; *RLF,* right lateral frontal 1 × 8 contact. Intracranial ictal EEG shows rhythmic spiking in LAI, LAF, and LLF electrodes, with sudden change to low-amplitude, fast, and sharp activity *(arrowheads),* coinciding with seizure onset and SPECT hyperperfusion of left-sided mesial and lateral frontal cortex.

lowing resection of left mesial and lateral frontal cortex, the patient is seizure free. Pathological examination showed disorganization of cortical architecture.

Patient 2 was an 18-year-old woman who had complex partial seizures of temporal lobe type, with automatisms and loss of contact. MRI showed an equivocal right orbital frontal lesion consistent with scar. Ictal SPECT showed mild orbital frontal and marked right temporal hyperperfusion. Interictal SPECT was normal. Intracranial EEG studies showed right orbital frontal seizure onset with significant spread to the right temporal lobe. The patient is seizure free following a right frontal resection. Pathological examination was normal.

DISCUSSION

A vast literature now exists describing the various imaging modalities that can be used to localize seizure foci. For the detection of structural abnormalities, there is little doubt that MRI is superior to other modalities (15–17). It is not always clear, however, that the epileptic focus coincides with the structural abnormality; and when no structural abnormality is found, other modalities, such as MRI spectroscopy and PET, must be used to find the epileptic focus. Unfortunately, few studies have been done that compare the different modalities systematically, and fewer still compare several imaging modalities against a gold standard, such as intracranial EEG recording or surgical cure following focal resection (5,7–9,18,19).

There is consensus now, corroborated by the findings of this study, that interictal SPECT is of limited value in identifying epileptic foci. In temporal lobe epilepsy, interictal hypoperfusion in the epileptogenic temporal lobe is a specific finding, but sensitivity is only about 50%. Outside the temporal lobes, the sensitivity appears to be even lower (8,10). Interictal SPECT is useful only in interpreting ictal SPECT, but the computerized coregistration of interictal and ictal SPECT with MRI, as shown in this and other studies, is useful in localizing the surgical seizure focus (20).

Ictal SPECT in temporal lobe epilepsy shows striking hyperperfusion in more than 90% of cases in which the site of seizure origin has been unequivocally confirmed by temporal lobectomy (21). SPECT scans done in patients with temporal lobe epilepsy, in whom the injection was performed in the postictal period, also show lateralized abnormalities, but interpretation may be more difficult (6).

Outside the temporal lobes, localization of seizure foci with ictal SPECT has been reported for frontal, parietal, and occipital lobe epilepsy. These data again demonstrate a high rate of focal ictal hyperperfusion, but correlation with intracranial EEG data and surgical cure following focal resection is less well established (11,12,22,23).

Data comparing various imaging modalities are even harder to obtain. There is some evidence that interictal PET in temporal lobe epilepsy lateralizes with a sensitivity and specificity comparable to MRI combined with MRI spectroscopy (9). Other evidence suggests that combined ictal and interictal SPECT may be comparably precise (21). Ictal PET in principle, might localize hypermetabolic epileptic foci, but for logistical reasons, it is difficult to do such studies (24). Preliminary evidence also suggests that epileptic foci may be deficient in various receptor molecules. Injection of radiolabeled receptor ligands, followed by PET and SPECT imaging, may identify areas of benzodiazepine and other receptor deficiency, and these may prove to be regions of seizure onset (25–27).

In most series, including this one, MRI and ictal SPECT were used to guide the placement of intracranial electrodes. We showed that focal ictal hyperperfusion on SPECT is well correlated with the results of intracranial EEG studies and with successful surgical resection. We also found that in about 25% of patients, intracranial EEG showed seizure onset in a region other than that of ictal hyperperfusion. When this occurred, surgery was done on the basis of intracranial EEG and lesional MRI data, but outcomes were relatively poor. There are sufficient discrepancies here to caution anyone wishing to use ictal SPECT or intracranial EEG data as a basis for surgery, particularly when the data are discordant. In the absence of controlled comparative studies, it is unknown whether we would do better by giving greater weight to ictal SPECT.

We are also aware that because ictal SPECT data were used in this study to guide the placement of intracranial electrodes, the information provided by the two modalities was not truly independent. There is an element of circular reasoning here; that is, the intracranial electrodes placed on the basis of ictal SPECT data were likely to give localizing information that coincided with the SPECT data on which their placement was based. Because we believe the use of combined modalities gives localizing information superior to that obtainable from any single modality, it is hard to justify comparative trials in which patients would be randomized to surgery on the basis of seizure localization by one or another modality.

Even when MRI, ictal SPECT, and intracranial EEG data are concordant, true surgical success (class I outcome) is achieved only about 70% of the time, which suggests that all the aforementioned modalities may fail to show the region of seizure onset, or even if it is correctly identified, the region may not be completely resected. Ictal SPECT is only one of the ways in which we can try to localize the seizure focus more precisely and resect it more completely.

REFERENCES

1. Boon PA, Williamson PD, Fried I, et al. Intracranial, intraaxial, space-occupying lesions in patients with intractable partial seizures: an anatomoclinical, neuropsychological, and surgical correlation. *Epilepsia* 1991;32: 467–476.
2. Li LM, Cendes F, Watson C, et al. Surgical treatment of patients with single and dual pathology: relevance of lesion and of hippocampal atrophy to seizure outcome. *Neurology* 1997;48:437–444.
3. Awad AA, Rosenfeld J, Ahl J, et al. Intractable epilepsy and structural lesions of the brain: mapping, resection strategies, and seizure outcome. *Epilepsia* 1991;32: 179–186.
4. Van Paesschen W, Revesz T, Duncan JS, et al. Quantitative neuropathology and quantitative magnetic resonance imaging of the hippocampus in temporal lobe epilepsy. *Ann Neurol* 1997;42:756–766.
5. Connelly A, Van Paesschen W, Porter DA, et al. Proton magnetic resonance spectroscopy in MRI-negative temporal lobe epilepsy. *Neurology* 1998;51:61–66.
6. Rowe CC, Berkovic SF, Sia STB, et al. Localization of epileptic foci with postictal single photon emission computed tomography. *Ann Neurol* 1989;26:660–668.
7. Theodore WH, Sato S, Kufta CV, et al. FDG-positron emission tomography and invasive EEG: seizure focus detection and surgical outcome. *Epilepsia* 1997;38: 81–86.
8. Jack CR Jr, Mullan BP, Sharbrough FW, et al. Intractable nonlesional epilepsy of temporal lobe origin: lateralization by interictal SPECT versus MRI. *Neurology* 1994;44:829–836.
9. Knowlton RC, Laxer KD, Ende G, et al. Presurgical multimodality neuroimaging in electroencephalographic lateralized temporal lobe epilepsy. *Ann Neurol* 1997;42:829–837.
10. Marks DA, Katz A, Hoffer P, et al. Localization of extratemporal epileptic foci during ictal single photon emission computed tomography. *Ann Neurol* 1992;31: 250–255.
11. Harvey AS, Hopkins IJ, Bowe JM, et al. Frontal lobe epilepsy: clinical seizure characteristics and localization with ictal 99mTc-HMPAO SPECT. *Neurology* 1993;43:1966–1980.
12. Ho SS, Berkovic SF, Newton MR, et al. Parietal lobe epilepsy: clinical features and seizure localization by ictal SPECT. *Neurology* 1994;44:2277–2284.
13. Guyton AC. *Textbook of medical physiology.* Philadelphia: WB Saunders, 1956.
14. Hougaard K, Oikawa T, Sveinsdottir E, et al. Regional cerebral blood flow in focal cortical epilepsy. *Arch Neurol* 1979;33:527–535.
15. Cascino GD, Jack CR Jr, Sharbrough FW, et al. MRI assessments of hippocampal pathology in extratemporal lesional epilepsy. *Neurology* 1993;43:2380–2382.
16. Sisodiya SM, Stevens JM, Fish DR, et al. The demonstration of gyral abnormalities in patients with cryptogenic partial epilepsy using three-dimensional MRI. *Arch Neurol* 1996;53:28–34.
17. Ho SS, Kuzniecky RI, Gilliam F, et al. Temporal lobe developmental malformations and epilepsy: dual pathology and bilateral hippocampal abnormalities. *Neurology* 1998;50:748–754.
18. Cendes F, Caramanos Z, Andermann F, et al. Proton magnetic resonance spectroscopic imaging and magnetic resonance imaging volumetry in the lateralization of temporal lobe epilepsy: a series of 100 patients. *Ann Neurol* 1997;42:737–746.
19. Stanley JA, Cendes F, Dubeau F, et al. Proton magnetic resonance spectroscopic imaging in patients with extratemporal epilepsy. *Epilepsia* 1998;39(3):267–273.
20. O'Brien TJ, So EL, Mullan BP, et al. Subtraction ictal SPECT co-registered to MRI improves clinical usefulness of SPECT in localizing the surgical seizure focus. *Neurology* 1998;50:445–454.
21. Ho SS, Berkovic SF, McKay WJ, et al. Temporal lobe epilepsy subtypes: differential patterns of cerebral perfusion on ictal SPECT. *Epilepsia* 1996;37:788–795.
22. Duncan R, Biraben A, Patterson J, et al. Ictal single photon emission computed tomography in occipital lobe seizures. *Epilepsia* 1997;38:839–843.
23. Aihara M, Hatakeyama K, Koizumi K, et al. Ictal EEG and single photon emission computed tomography in a

patient with cortical dysplasia presenting with atonic seizures. *Epilepsia* 1997;38:723–727.

24. Scheyer RD, Dey HM, Spencer SS. Ictal PET in epilepsy. *Epilepsia* 1995;36:164(abst).

25. Richardson MP, Koepp MJ, Brooks DJ, et al. Benzodiazepine receptors in focal epilepsy with cortical dysgenesis: an 11C-flumazenil PET study. *Ann Neurol* 1996; 40:188–198.

26. Savic I, Svanborg E, Thorell JO. Cortical benzodiazepine receptor changes are related to frequency of partial seizures: a positron emission tomography study. *Epilepsia* 1996;37:236–244.

27. Boundy KL, Rowe CC, Black AB, et al. Localization of temporal lobe epileptic foci with iodine-123 iododexetimide cholinergic neuroreceptor single-photon emission computed tomography. *Neurology* 1996;47:1015–1020.

Neocortical Epilepsies.
Advances in Neurology, Vol. 84,
edited by P.D. Williamson, A.M. Siegel,
D.W. Roberts, V.M. Thadani, and M.S. Gazzaniga.
Lippincott Williams & Wilkins, Philadelphia © 2000.

34

Positron Emission Tomography in Neocortical Epilepsies

William H. Theodore and *William D. Gaillard

*National Institute of Neurological Disorders and Stroke, National Institute of Health,
Bethesda, Maryland 20892-1428; *Department of Neurology and Pediatrics,
Children's National Medical Center, Washington, D.C. 20010*

Positron emission tomography (PET) can be used to measure cerebral glucose metabolism (CMRglc) with fluorodeoxyglucose (FDG), cerebral blood flow (CBF), or the distribution of a variety of neurotransmitter ligands. In patients with neocortical epilepsy, potential roles for PET include localization of epileptic foci, preoperative functional mapping, and pathophysiologic studies. Several important clinical questions have been raised for PET to answer: Can mesial temporal be distinguished from temporal neocortical foci? Can extratemporal foci be localized? What can PET tell us about patients with migration anomalies, secondary generalized epilepsies, the Lennox–Gastaut Syndrome (LGS), or infantile spasms? How reliable are activation studies for cognitive and motor mapping? Does diffuse hypometabolism explain, predict, or correlate with cognitive or behavioral dysfunction? Can PET help to select patients for surgery?

The results of PET studies may be related to scanner hardware, software, the isotope used, and data analysis strategy. The images are an average of activity over a period that ranges from 1 to 2 minutes for oxygen-15 blood flow studies to 30 to 40 minutes for FDG, and more than an hour for some receptor ligand scans. Clearly, Increased activity resulting from a brief seizure will have more effect on measurement of CBF than CMRglc. Using low-resolution scanners reduces the sensitivity and probably specificity of PET (1). Engel et al. reported that detection of temporal lobe foci increased from about 50% to 80% with improved scanners (2). The patient population chosen also can affect outcome; De Reuck et al. found no focal abnormalities in CBF or CMRglc in patients over 50 years of age with new-onset seizures, although global values tended to be lower than normal (3).

Because PET CBF studies, using either inhaled O15-labelled gases or H215O, have been less useful than FDG for identification of epileptic foci or prediction of surgical outcome from temporal lobectomy, they should not be used for this purpose (4–6). The difference may be due to lower resolution or to a metabolism/perfusion mismatch. O15, however, is useful for activation studies designed to obtain preoperative functional mapping data.

The anatomic data that seem to appear on PET scans are in part illusory. To improve localization, images can be coregistered with anatomic magnetic resonance imaging

(MRI) scans via a variety of computer programs (7). The accuracy of PET is improved by using quantitative image analysis methods rather than relying on visual interpretation (8,9).

Focal FDG PET hypometabolism accurately lateralizes the hemisphere of seizure onset in temporal lobe epilepsy, but intrahemispheric localization is less reliable. There are rare reports of false localization on FDG PET scans, some of which may be related to the use of visual as opposed to quantitative analysis (1–2,10).

After a seizure, hypometabolism may be accentuated for a variable time span (11). In addition, the pattern of reduced CMRglc may be influenced by the type of most recently preceding seizure, and it is important to be careful about interpreting the localizing value of a scan when the most recent preceding seizure was "nonhabitual" (12).

MESIAL TEMPORAL VERSUS LATERAL TEMPORAL NEOCORTICAL EPILEPSY

Of the patients with temporal lobe epileptogenic (TLE) zones, 78%, whether in mesial or lateral temporal neocortex, have hypometabolism on FDG PET ipsilateral to the ictal focus, and unilateral PET hypometabolism predicts a good outcome from temporal lobectomy (13–18). Patients with temporal lobe foci and restricted lesions such as mesial temporal sclerosis, however, may have widespread hypometabolism, which can involve lateral temporal neocortex, ipsilateral thalamus, and basal ganglia as well as frontal and parietal lobes (8,19–22). Cerebellar hypometabolism, which is frequently found, may be ipsilateral, contralateral, or bilateral (23,24).

It is uncertain whether PET can be used to distinguish mesial from lateral neocortical temporal lobe seizure onset. In an early study using a relatively low-resolution scanner, patients with anterior mesial temporal foci (most had surgery or depth electrode confirmation) had greater relative lateral than mesial temporal hypometabolism (22). Subsequently, Hajek et al. attempted to differentiate presumed mesial temporal from lateral temporal neocortical epileptogenic zones using FDG PET in 25 patients, basing the classification on MRI and foramen ovale electrodes (25). Lateral temporal metabolism was equally depressed in both groups (although not at all in patients with mesial tumors), whereas the mesial temporal onset, nonlesional group had greater mean mesial than lateral hypometabolism. Unfortunately, the data range was too wide to make individual localizing judgments. Other investigators also reported equal mesial and lateral hypometabolism in mesial-onset TLE (22,26). In a dipole modeling study, the decrease in glucose uptake was not found to be more pronounced in regions containing dipoles (e.g., hippocampus) than in their presumed projection regions (e.g., lateral temporal neocortex) (26).

We found that lateral temporal hypometabolism was greater than mesial, even in patient with mesial foci; but the difference was significantly greater if a lateral temporal neocortical focus was present (Table 34.1; Figs. 34.1 and 34.2). The degree of interindividual variability makes it difficult to make the distinction on an individual basis, however, and FDG PET seems to be more useful as a lateralizing than a localizing tool. These results parallel findings from surface EEG, which also may have difficulty distinguishing mesial from lateral temporal neocortical foci (27). It is interesting that in a study of children with benign childhood epilepsy with centrotemporal spikes, interictal CMRglc was normal (28). FDG PET studies of children with Landau–Kleffner syndrome have shown both increased and decreased temporal metabolism, which may have been related to sleep stage and EEG discharges

TABLE 34.1. *Effect of Electroencephalographic (EEG) focus on mesial and lateral temporal hypometabolism*

	Mesial EEG focus	Lateral EEG focus	
Inferior lateral temporal asymmetry index	0.22 ± 0.12	0.19 ± 12	
Inferior mesial temporal asymmetry index	0.18 ± 0.13	0.13 ± .07	p <0.05

(29). Subcortical hypometabolism was present as well.

In addition to FDG, several other ligands have been used to study temporal lobe foci. Increased monoaminoxidase (MAO-B) binding may be a marker for mesial temporal gliosis rather than a physiologically important alteration in neurotransmission (30). Increased, mu and delta opiate receptor binding was more prominent in lateral temporal neocortex, even in patients with mesial foci (31–33). A study with a mixed mu and kappa receptor ligand showed increased mesial and lateral binding (34). Some studies suggested that reduced benzodiazepine receptor binding may identify focal pathology and seizure origin more reliably than FDG PET, showing reduced binding restricted to mesial temporal cortex (35–37).

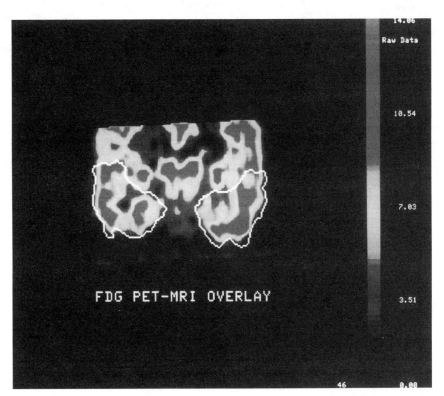

FIG. 34.1. FDG PET scan showing focal mesial temporal hypometabolism in a patient who became seizure free after a temporal lobectomy.

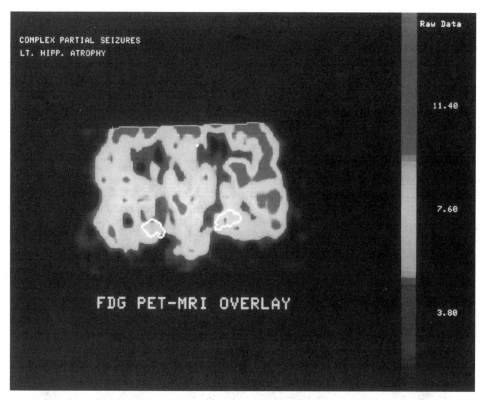

FIG. 34.2. Widespread mesial and lateral temporal hypometabolism in a patient with basal and lateral temporal epileptiform discharges.

FRONTAL LOBE EPILEPSY

In patients with frontal lobe seizures (FLE), FDG PET is less likely to show hypometabolism unless a structural lesion is present. Reported correlation with EEG is less precise than for patients with temporal lobe foci. In contrast to the general agreement of results in patients with TLE, marked differences have been found in reports of the sensitivity of FDG PET in nonlesional FLE, ranging from 20% to 80%. For example, we found that only 4 of 15 patients without structural lesions had focal hypometabolism (Fig. 34.3) (38). Even when present, hypometabolism may be bilateral or widespread in most patients (20,39–41). Interestingly, focal hypometabolism was reported in a patient with autosomal dominant nocturnal

frontal lobe epilepsy who had a normal MRI scan (42).

Some investigators have had better results. Swartz et al. (43) found that "quantitative normalized analysis" was much more accurate than visual interpretation, detecting hypometabolism congruent with the results of depth electrode studies and surgical outcome in 75% of patients with FLE, including nonlesional cases. Patients with either focal hypometabolism or normal PET scans were more likely to have a good surgical outcome than those with diffuse or multifocal hypometabolism, which could suggest poor localization of the epileptic focus (44).

Patterns of hypometabolism may reflect clinical characteristics of FLE and perhaps help in localization of epileptogenic zones. Schlaug et al. (45) reported that patients with

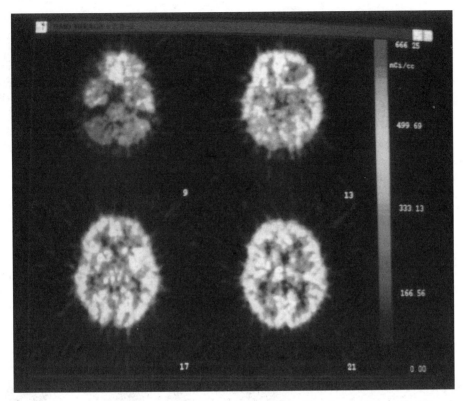

FIG. 34.3. Right frontal FDG PET hypometabolism in a patient with a frontal lobe epileptogenic zone. Note left cerebellar hypometabolism as well.

lateralized, predominantly focal, tonic seizures had unilateral frontomesial and perirolandic hypometabolism. Patients with versive seizures had mainly contralateral metabolic depression but no consistent regional pattern. "Hypermotor" seizures were associated with reduced CMRglc in frontomesial, anterior cingulate, perirolandic, and anterior insular/frontal operculum areas. All their patients had bilateral symmetric hypometabolism of the thalamus and cerebellum; however, patients with complex partial seizures of temporal origin with posturing as a clinical manifestation of a recent seizure may have frontal hypometabolism as well (12). Patients with TLE may have hypometabolism extending to the frontal lobes, although the reduction is usually less than in the temporal regions (19,46,47). When present, well-localized hypometabolism may be a positive predictor of surgical outcome in patients with FLE as well as TLE; coregistration with MRI and improved image analysis techniques may increase the specificity of these studies.

FOCAL PARIETAL AND OCCIPITAL EPILEPSY

Fewer reports of PET results in parietal and occipital lobe epilepsies have appeared, but the evidence suggests that well-circumscribed hypometabolic areas probably identify epileptogenic zones. Henry et al. (20) studied five patients with occipital foci. One had focal FDG PET hypometabolism corresponding to a focal MRI scan, and four had a multilobar/diffuse CMRglc reduction; one of these had a normal MR. FDG PET is unlikely to add localizing data to a positive MRI scan and may be more likely to lead to false localization than in patients with TLE (40).

PET NEURORECEPTOR STUDIES IN EXTRATEMPORAL EPILEPSY

Patients with "reading epilepsy" EEG who showed multifocal seizure onset bilaterally in temporal and frontocentral regions revealed periictal opioid binding decreases in both temporal lobes and the left frontal lobe on [11C]diprenorphine PET, suggesting endogenous opioid release during seizures (48). Six patients with frontal foci had reduced frontal benzodiazepine receptor binding on 11C-flumazenil scans (49). Three of four patients studied had focal FDG PET hypometabolism; however, benzodiazepine receptor binding

may show a greater reduction in patients with higher seizure frequency, and the abnormality may extend to primary projection areas of the seizure activity (50). In a larger group of patients with extratemporal foci, increased as well as decreased benzodiazepines (BZP) binding was found, which could extend to the lobe as well as the hemisphere of presumed seizure origin (51). So far, the localizing value of these findings is uncertain.

SECONDARY GENERALIZED EPILEPSY

It is difficult to interpret PET scans in multifocal disorders such as tuberous sclerosis. PET usually adds little to structural imaging, although a small number of children may have regions of focal hypometabolism not corresponding to MRI lesions,

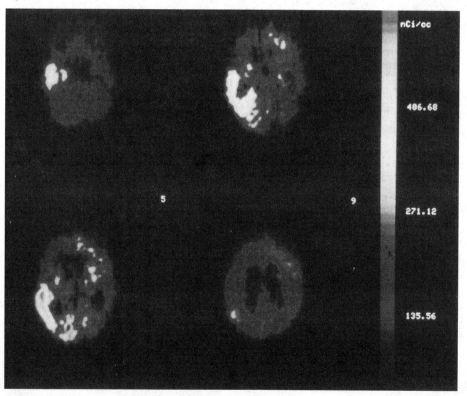

FIG. 34.4. A child with cryptogenic infantile spasms had increased left posterior quadrant metabolism on FDG PET during nearly continuous spasms.

which could indicate the presence of small tubers undetected by structural imaging (52). In children with LGS, hypometabolism can be multifocal or global; the presence of the former abnormalities may depend on underlying structural lesions or etiology (53,54). In a group of children with diffuse epileptic encephalopathies, hypometabolic regions were common (in five of six patients with LGS following infantile spasms), even if MRI was normal, and more likely to be detected by semiquantitative analysis than visual inspection (55,56). In patients with malformations of cortical development, regions of increased and decreased CMRglc are associated with structural defects, but they may extent beyond their limits. Children with cryptogenic infantile spasms may have posterior quadrant hypometabolism associated with underlying cortical dysplasia, even if structural imaging studies are normal; most have focal or lateralized EEG abnor-

malities rather than consistent generalized hypsarrythmia at some point in their course (Fig. 34.4) (57). PET in children with Sturge–Weber syndrome tended to show diffuse abnormalities with little localizing value (58). When hypometabolism contralateral to the side of the anatomic lesion is present in children with hemimegalencephaly, surgical outcome is worse (59). Ferrie et al. found a high incidence of focal hypometabolic regions unsuspected on MRI scan in a group of children with "epileptic encephalopathies."

FOCAL CORTICAL DYSPLASIA

Patients with cortical dysplasia may have regions of decreased and increased CMRglc that generally correspond to the pattern of abnormal cortical organization (Figs. 34.5 and 34.6) (60). FDG PET but not structural imaging might detect small heterotopic regions, al-

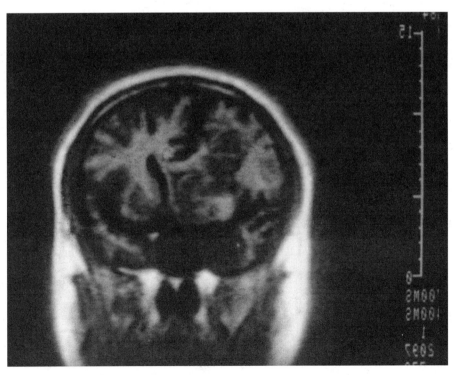

FIG. 34.5. MRI scan in a patient with agenesis of the corpus callosum and a large cortical heterotopia.

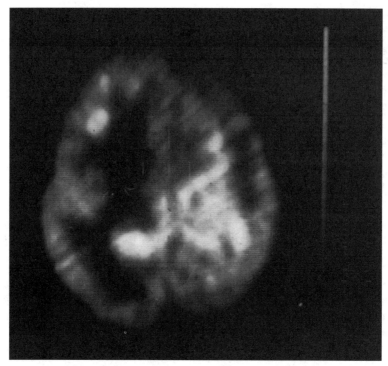

FIG. 34.6. FDG PET scan in the same patient showing relatively increased metabolism in the heterotopic gray matter.

though this will become increasingly less common with improvements in MRI technology (61).

Abnormal BZP binding may be present in an irregular pattern with an inconsistent relation to the structural anomalies. Both increased and decreased binding were found (62). Although the BZP receptor aberrations seemed out of proportion to structural anomalies, they did not distinguish clearly between epileptogenic and nonepileptogenic regions. Areas of focal cortical dysplasia had high 11C-methionine uptake, perhaps suggesting increased protein synthesis (63). In the same patients, FDG PET showed low interictal and high ictal metabolism; equivalent current dipole (ECD) single-photon emission computed tomography (SPECT) was less sensitive. Although these studies may be interesting from a pathophysiologic viewpoint, they probably do not contribute to seizure focus localization or therapeutic planning.

PET, COGNITIVE, AND BEHAVIORAL STUDIES

Frontal hypometabolism in patients with TLE may be associated with impaired neuropsychological function or depression (Fig. 34.7) (64,65). Patients with TLE and "epileptic psychoses" have been reported to have low oxygen extraction ratio in frontal as well as temporal lobes and basal ganglia (66). Impairment on verbal and performance intelligence measures, but not episodic memory or psychiatric symptoms, was predicted by prefrontal hypometabolism (67). Verbal fluency and verbal intelligence quotient (VIQ) correlated with left parietotemporal junction metabolism (22). In children with epileptic encephalopathies who had FDG PET, adaptive and maladaptive behavior showed an inverse correlation with the degree of frontal hypometabolism but was not related to the presence or absence of focal cortical PET abnormalities (55).

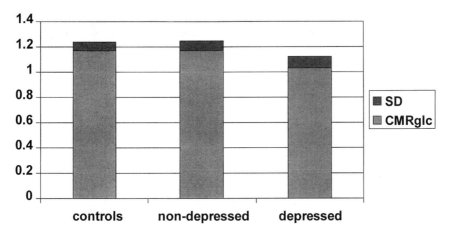

FIG. 34.7. The effect of depression on inferior frontal metabolism in patients with complex partial seizures. (Modified from Bromfield EB, Altshuler L, Leiderman DB, et al. Cerebral metabolism and depression in patients with complex partial seizures. *Arch Neurol* 1992;49:617–623, Fig. 2, with permission.)

Patients with unilateral frontal foci may fail to show normal increases in metabolism during working memory tasks in a large task-related circuit ipsilateral and contralateral to the focus (68,69). Peripheral cortical regions compensate poorly for the area of dysfunction.

Taken together, these studies suggest that, with temporal lobe foci, frontal hypometabolism may be associated with behavioral and psychiatric symptoms in patients. The extent of extratemporal hypometabolism in patients with temporal lobe foci could predict neuropsychological function. Improvement of frontal metabolism after temporal lobectomy might correlate with improved mood.

PET FUNCTIONAL MAPPING

Interictal CBF studies using PET are unreliable for seizure focus localization, but they may be used for preoperative functional mapping. In several studies, conducted mainly in patients with TLE, they have provided data

matching Wada or subdural grid stimulation results (70–73). It is important to remember that PET (or functional MRI) shows regions of activation, whereas the Wada tests and electrostimulation cortical mapping are based on inhibition (71). Although overlap in several studies between ECM and PET has been good, the procedures may not be absolutely comparable in their results. For example, task-related increases in CBF have been more widespread than the points at which ECM leads to arrest of function (71,74,75). Whereas this may be due in part to the much greater sampling afforded by PET, it could represent recruitment of regions associated with, but not necessary for, task performance. These regions, then, could be safely resected if part of the epileptogenic zone. Another possibility, at least theoretically, is that an area that is in fact critical for normal function might not, perhaps for technical reasons, appear activated on PET (or functional MRI). At this point, we know little about the functional capacity of structurally or physiologically abnormal cortex. An interesting study in patients with cortical dysplasia showed a complex pattern of correspondences and differences in activation compared with controls; focally dysgenic cortex might activate "normally," whereas regions "normal" on MRI might fail to activate (76). Activation in right "Broca's area" has been observed in a patient with a left-sided heterotopia (77). Most PET studies to date have compared groups of patients with normals, but Individual studies can be performed as higher-resolution scanners become available and lower-dose 15O-water injections become feasible.

CONCLUSION

It is possible for FDG PET to lateralize, and occasionally localize, epileptogenic zones. In patients with suspected extratemporal epilepsy, it should be performed when structural MRI is normal and other tests such as ictal SPECT or MRS have been unrevealing. Any functional imaging study should be interpreted in the context of the clinical, and particularly in the case of seizure disorders, neurophysiologic, state of the subject during the appropriate physiologic "window" for the study. The 15O-water studies are useful for language mapping, but will probably be superseded by functional MRI. Other tracers, such as benzodiazepine receptor ligands, are used appropriately in research studies. Their clinical role has not yet been established, but it is possible that they will prove to be valuable.

REFERENCES

1. Debets RMC, van Veelen CWM, Maquet P, et al. Quantitative analysis of 18FDG-PET in the presurgical evaluation of patients suffering from refractory partial epilepsy. *Acta Neurochir (Wien)* 1990;50(Suppl):88–94.
2. Engel J Jr, Henry TR, Risinger MW, et al. Presurgical evaluation for epilepsy: relative contributions of chronic depth-electrode recordings versus FDG-PET and scalp-sphenoidal ictal EEG. *Neurology* 1990;40:1670–1677.
3. De Reuck J, Santens P, Decoo D, et al. Positron emission tomographic study of late-onset cryptogenic symptomatic seizures. *Clin Neurol Neurosurg* 1995;97:208–212.
4. Theodore WH, Gaillard WD, Sato S, et al. PET measurement of cerebral blood flow and temporal lobectomy. *Ann Neurol* 36:241–244;1994.
5. Fink GR, Pawlik G, Stefan H, et al. Temporal-lobe epilepsy—evidence for interictal uncoupling of blood-flow and glucose-metabolism in temporomesial structures. *J Neurol Sci* 1996;137:28–34.
6. Gaillard WD, Fazilat S, White S, et al. Interictal metabolism and blood flow are uncoupled in temporal lobe cortex of patients with partial epilepsy. *Neurology* 1995;45:1841–1848.
7. Levin DN, Pelizzari CA, Chen GTY, et al. Retrospective geometric correlation of MR, CT, and PET images. *Radiology* 1988;169:817–823.
8. Henry TR, Mazziotta JC, Engel J Jr, et al. Quantifying interictal metabolic anatomy in human temporal lobe epilepsy. *J Cereb Blood Flow Metab* 1990;10:748–757.
9. Theodore WH, Sato S, Kufta C, et al. Temporal lobectomy for uncontrolled seizures: the role of positron emission tomography. *Ann Neurol* 1992;32:789–794.
10. Sperling MR, Alavi A, Reivich M, et al. False lateralization of temporal lobe epilepsy with FDG positron emission tomography. *Epilepsia* 1995;36:722–727.
11. Leiderman DB, Albert P, Balish M, et al. The dynamics of metabolic change following seizures as measured by positron emission tomography with 18-Fluoro-2-deoxyglucose. *Arch Neurol* 1994;51:932–936.
12. Savic I, Altshuler L, Baxter L, et al. Pattern of interictal hypometabolism in PET scans with fluorodeoxyglucose F 18 reflects prior seizure types in patients with mesial temporal lobe seizures. *Arch Neurol* 1997;54:129–136.
13. Engel J Jr, Kuhl DE, Phelps ME, et al. Comparative localization of epileptic foci in partial epilepsy by PCT and EEG. *Ann Neurol* 1982;12:529–537.
14. Engel J Jr, Kuhl DE, Phelps ME, et al. Interictal cerebral glucose metabolism in partial epilepsy and its relation to EEG changes. *Ann Neurol* 1982;12:510–517.
15. Engel J Jr, Brown WJ, Kuhl DE, et al. Pathological findings underlying focal temporal lobe hypometabolism in partial epilepsy. *Ann Neurol* 1982;12:518–529.
16. Theodore WH, Newmark ME, Sato S, et al. 18-F-Fluorodeoxyglucose positron emission tomography in refractory complex partial seizures. *Ann Neurol* 1983;14:429–437.
17. Abou-Khalil BW, Siegel GJ, Sackellares JC, et al. Positron emission tomography studies of cerebral glucose metabolism in chronic partial epilepsy. *Ann Neurol* 1987;22:480–486.
18. Wong CY, Geller EB, Chen EQ, et al. Outcome of temporal lobe epilepsy surgery predicted by statistical parametric PET imaging. *J Nucl Med* 1996;37:1094–1100.
19. Sackellares JC, Siegel GJ, Abou-khalil BW, et al. Differences between lateral and mesial temporal hypometabolism interictally in epilepsy of mesial temporal origin. *Neurology* 1990;40:1420–1426.
20. Henry TR, Sutherling WW, Engel J Jr, et al. Interictal cerebral metabolism in partial epilepsies of neocortical origin. *Epilepsy Res* 1991;10:174–182.
22. Arnold S, Schlaug G, Niemann H, et al. Topography of interictal glucose hypometabolism in unilateral mesiotemporal epilepsy. *Neurology* 1996;46:1422–1430.
23. Theodore WH, Fishbein D, Deitz M, et al. Complex partial seizures: cerebellar metabolism. *Epilepsia* 1987;28:319–323.
24. Savic I, Altshuler L, Passaro E, et al. Localized cerebellar hypometabolism in patients with complex partial seizures. *Epilepsia* 1996;37(8):781–787.
25. Hajek M, Antonini A, Leenders KL, et al. Mesiobasal

versus lateral temporal lobe epilepsy: metabolic differences in the temporal lobe shown by interictal—18F–FDG positron emission tomography. *Neurology* 1993;43:79–86.

26. Merlet I, Garcia-Larrea L, Gregoire MC, et al. Source propagation of interictal spikes in temporal lobe epilepsy: correlations between spike dipole modeling and [18F]fluorodeoxyglucose PET data. *Brain* 1996; 119:377–392.

27. Burgerman RS, Sperling MR, French JA, et al. Comparison of mesial versus neocortical onset temporal lobe seizures: neurodiagnostic findings and surgical outcome. *Epilepsia* 1995;36:662–670.

28. Van Bogaert P, Wikler D, Damhaut P, et al. Cerebral glucose metabolism and centrotemporal spikes. *Epilepsy Res* 1998;29:123–127.

29. Maquet P, Hirsch E, Dive D, et al. Cerebral glucose utilization during sleep in Landau–Kleffner syndrome: a PET study. *Epilepsia* 1990;31:778–783.

30. Kumlien E, Bergstrom M, Lilja A, et al. Positron emission tomography with 11C-deuterium-deprenyl in temporal lobe epilepsy. *Epilepsia* 1995;36:712–721.

31. Frost JJ, Mayberg HS, Fisher RS, et al. Mu-opiate receptors measured by positron emission tomography are increased in temporal lobe epilepsy. *Ann Neurol* 1988; 23:231–237.

32. Mayberg HS, Sadzot B, Meltzer CC, et al. Quantification of Mu and non-Mu opiate receptors in temporal lobe epilepsy using positron emission tomography. *Ann Neurol* 1991;30:3–11.

33. Madar I, Lesser RP, Krauss G, et al. Imaging of delta- and mu-opioid receptors in temporal lobe epilepsy by positron emission tomography. *Ann Neurol* 1997;41: 358–367.

34. Theodore WH, Carson RE, Andreasen P, et al. PET imaging of opiate receptor binding in human epilepsy using (18F) Cyclofoxy. *Epilepsy Res* 1992;13:129–140.

35. Henry TR, Frey KA, Sackellares JC, et al. In vivo cerebral metabolism and central benzodiazepine receptor binding in temporal lobe epilepsy. *Neurology* 1993;43: 1998–2006.

36. Burdette DE, Sakuri SY, Henry TR, et al. Temporal lobe central benzodiazepine binding in unilateral mesial temporal lobe epilepsy. *Neurology* 1995;45:934–942.

37. Savic I, Roland P, Sedvall G, et al. In vivo demonstration of reduced benzodiazepine receptor binding in human epileptic foci. *Lancet* 1988;2:863–866.

38. Gaillard WD, Conry JA, Weinstein S, et al. Fluorodeoxyglucose positron emission tomography in children and adolescents with frontal lobe epilepsy. *Ann Neurol* 1996;40:304.

39. Swartz BE, Halgren E, Delgado-Escueta AV, et al. Neuroimaging in patients with seizures of probable frontal origin. *Epilepsia* 1989;30:547–558.

40. Radtke RA, Hanson MW, Hoffman JM, et al. Positron emission tomography: comparison of clinical utility in temporal lobe and extratemporal epilepsy. *J Epilepsy* 1994;7:27–33.

41. da Silva EA, Chugani DC, Muzik O, et al. Identification of frontal lobe epileptic foci in children using positron emission tomography. *Epilepsia* 1997;38:1198–1208.

42. Hayman M, Scheffer IE, Chinvarun Y, et al. Autosomal dominant nocturnal frontal lobe epilepsy: demonstration of focal frontal onset and intrafamilial variation. *Neurology* 1997;49:969–975.

43. Swartz BW, Khonsari A, Vrown C, et al. Improved sensitivity of 18FDG-positron emission tomography scans in frontal and "frontal plus" epilepsy. *Epilepsia* 1995;36:388–395.

44. Swartz BE, Delgado-Escueta AV, Walsh GO, et al. Surgical outcomes in pure frontal lobe epilepsy and foci that mimic them. *Epilepsy Res* 1998;29:97–108.

45. Schlaug G, Antke C, Holthausen H, et al. Ictal motor signs and interictal regional cerebral hypometabolism. *Neurology* 1997;49:341–350.

46. Theodore WH, Fishbein D, Dubinsky R. Patterns of cerebral glucose metabolism in patients with partial seizures. *Neurology* 1988;38:1201–1206.

47. Henry TR, Mazziotta JC, Engel J Jr. Interictal metabolic anatomy of mesial temporal lobe epilepsy. *Arch Neurol* 1993;50:582–589.

48. Koepp MJ, Richardson MP, Brooks DJ, et al. Focal cortical release of endogenous opioids during reading-induced seizures. *Lancet* 1998;352:952–955.

49. Savic I, Thorell JO, Roland P. 11C-flumazenil positron emission tomography visualizes frontal epileptogenic regions. *Epilepsia* 1995;36:1225–1232.

50. Savic I, Svanborg E, Thorell JO. Cortical benzodiazepine receptor changes are related to frequency of partial seizures: a positron emission tomography study. *Epilepsia* 1996;37:236–244.

51. Richardson MP, Koepp MJ, Brooks DJ, et al. 1C-flumazenil PET in neocortical epilepsy. *Neurology* 1998;51:485–921.

52. Rintahaka PJ, Chugani HT. Clinical role of positron emission tomography in children with tuberous sclerosis complex. *J Child Neurol* 1997;12:42–52.

53. Chugani HT, Engel J Jr, Mazziotta JC, et al. The Lennox–Gastaut syndrome: metabolic subtypes determined by 2-deoxy-2-[18F]-Fluoro-D-glucose positron emission tomography. *Ann Neurol* 1987;21:4–13.

54. Theodore WH, Rose D, Patronas N, et al. Cerebral glucose metabolism in the Lennox–Gastaut Syndrome. *Ann Neurol* 1987;21:14–21.

55. Ferrie CD, Madigan C, Tilling K, et al. Adaptive and maladaptive behavior in children with epileptic encephalopathies: correlation with cerebral glucose metabolism. *Dev Med Child Neurol* 1997;39:588–595.

56. Ferrie CD, Marsden PK, Maisey MN, et al. Visual and semiquantitative analysis of cortical FDG-PET scans in childhood epileptic encephalopathies. *J Nucl Med* 1997;38:1891–1894.

57. Chugani HT, Shields WD, Shewmon DA, et al. Infantile spasms: 1. PET identifies focal cortical dysgenesis in cryogenic cases for surgical treatment. *Ann Neurol* 1990;27:406–413.

58. Dietrich RB, el Saden S, Chugani HT, et al. Resective surgery for intractable epilepsy in children: radiologic evaluation. *Am J Neuroradiol* 1991;12:1149–1158.

59. Rintahaka PJ, Chugani HT, Messa C, et al. Hemimegalencephaly: evaluation with positron emission tomography. *Pediatr Neurol* 1993;9:21–28.

60. Bairamian D, Di Chiro G, Theodore WH, et al. MR imaging and positron emission tomography of cortical heterotopia. *J Comput Assist Tomogr* 1985;9:1137–1139.

61. Lee N, Radtke RA, Gray L, et al. Neuronal migration disorders: positron emission tomography correlations. *Ann Neurol* 1994;35:290–297.

62. Richardson MP, Friston KJ, Sisodiya SM, et al. Cortical grey matter and benzodiazepine receptors in malforma-

tions of cortical development: a voxel-based comparison of structural and functional imaging data. *Brain* 1997;120:1961–1973.

63. Sasaki M, Kuwabara Y, Yoshida T, et al. Carbon-11-methionine PET in focal cortical dysplasia: a comparison with fluorine-18-FDG PET and technetium-99m-ECD SPECT. *J Nucl Med* 1998;39:974–947.

64. Bromfield EB, Altshuler L, Leiderman DB, et al. Cerebral metabolism and depression in patients with complex partial seizures. *Arch Neurol* 1992;49:617–625.

65. Victoreff JI, Benson DF, Grafton ST, et al. Depression in complex partial seizures: electroencephalography and cerebral metabolic correlates. *Arch Neurol* 1994;51: 155–163.

66. Gallhofer B, Trimble MR, Frackowiack R, et al. A study of cerebral blood flow and metabolism in epileptic psychosis using positron emission tomography and oxygen. *J Neurol Neurosurg Psychiatry* 1985;48:201–206.

67. Jokeit H, Seitz RJ, Markowitsch HJ, et al. Prefrontal asymmetric interictal glucose hypometabolism and cognitive impairment in patients with temporal lobe epilepsy. *Brain* 1997;120:2283–2294.

68. Swartz BE, Halgren E, Simpkins F, et al. Studies of working memory using 18FDG-positron emission tomography in normal controls and subjects with epilepsy. *Life Sci* 1996;58:2057–2064.

69. Swartz BE, Halgren E, Simpkins F, et al. Primary or working memory in frontal lobe epilepsy: an 18FDG-PET study of dysfunctional zones. *Neurology* 1996;46: 737–747.

70. Pardo JV, Fox PT. Preoperative assessment of the cerebral hemispheric dominance for language with CBF PET. *Human Brain Mapping* 1993;1:57–68.

71. Bookheimer SY, Zeffiro TA, Blaxton T, et al. A direct comparison of PET activation and electrocortical stimulation mapping for language localization. *Neurology* 1997;48:1056–1065.

72. Henry TR, Buchtel HA, Koeppe RA, et al. Absence of normal activation of the left anterior fusiform gyrus during naming in left temporal lobe epilepsy. *Neurology* 1998;50:787–790.

73. Hunter KE, Blaxton TA, Bookheimer SY, et al. O15 positron emission tomography in language localization: a study comparing rater evaluations of PET studies with the Wada test. *Ann Neurol* 1999;45:662–665.

74. Vinas FC, Zamorano L, Mueller RA, et al. [15O]-water PET and intraoperative brain mapping: a comparison in the localization of eloquent cortex. *Neurol Res* 1997; 19:601–608.

75. Duncan JD, Moss SD, Bandy DJ, et al. Use of positron emission tomography for presurgical localization of eloquent brain areas in children with seizures. *Pediatr Neurosurg* 1997;26:144–156.

76. Richardson MP, Koepp MJ, Brooks DJ, et al. Cerebral activation in malformations of cortical development. *Brain* 1998;121:1295–1304.

77. Calabrese P, Fink GR, Markowitsch HJ, et al. Left hemisphere neuronal heterotopia: a PET, MRI, EEG, and neuropsychological investigation. *Neurology* 1995;44: 302–305.

Neocortical Epilepsies.
Advances in Neurology, Vol. 84,
edited by P. D. Williamson, A. M. Siegel,
D. W. Roberts, V. M. Thadani, and M. S. Gazzaniga.
Lippincott Williams & Wilkins, Philadelphia © 2000.

35

New Directions in PET Neuroimaging for Neocortical Epilepsy

Diane C. Chugani and Harry T. Chugani

PET Center, Children's Hospital of Michigan, Detroit, Michigan 48201

The role of neuroimaging in neocortical epilepsy is to detect potentially epileptogenic lesions, to define their boundaries, and to predict their nature. Unlike the limited sampling available with intracranial electroencephalographic (EEG) monitoring, neuroimaging allows assessment of the entire brain to define the location and extent of all abnormal regions. Whereas gross or microscopic abnormalities of the neocortical architecture or functional alterations related to interictal and ictal epileptiform discharges may produce metabolic abnormalities shown by positron emission tomography (PET) (1–5), these alterations of cerebral function are not always related to discrete anatomical abnormalities detectable by structural neuroimaging with x-ray computed tomography (CT) or magnetic resonance imaging (MRI). PET is a form of biochemical imaging that allows the measurement of metabolic functions (for example, glucose metabolism or neurotransmitter synthesis) as well as the measurement of neurotransmitter receptor binding in specific regions of the brain by using radiolabeled tracers (6). Numerous PET tracers have been applied to the study of epilepsy (7), and 2-[^{18}F]fluoro-2-deoxy-D-glucose (FDG) for the measurement of glucose metabolism is now established in the clinical evaluation of patients with medically refractory epilepsy.

Interictal FDG PET has proven to be a reliable test for identifying dysfunctional cortical regions of hypometabolism that correspond, in general, to the location of epileptic foci (7–10). Comparative studies of interictal FDG PET and MRI indicated that regional cerebral glucose hypometabolism occurs more frequently than does focal cerebral structural abnormality in groups of patients with partial epilepsy (11–17); however, FDG PET studies report a somewhat lower sensitivity of FDG PET for the identification of epileptic foci in frontal lobe epilepsy compared with temporal lobe epilepsy, with the observation of cortical glucose hypometabolism in 45% to 60% of the cases (1,12,15). Using quantitative FDG PET data analysis, Swartz et al. (18) later reported a sensitivity of 96% (81% in nonlesional cases) and a specificity of 74% to 78% for seizure focus detection in adult patients with frontal lobe epilepsy. More recently, using a high-resolution PET scanner, we showed a sensitivity of 92% in the detection of frontal lobe epileptic foci with FDG PET in children, with a specificity of 62.5% (19). The consistent observation of large areas of glucose hypometabolism on PET extending beyond the epileptogenic region has precluded the use of FDG PET to define precisely the boundary of the epileptogenic zone for surgical resection (1,2,10).

One of the new directions in functional neuroimaging for the study of epilepsy is aimed at developing new PET tracers that are both more specific and more sensitive in the identification of epileptogenic cortex. In this chapter, we describe localization of neocortical epileptogenic regions with the PET tracers [¹¹C]flumazenil (FMZ) for the measurement of the GABA/benzodiazepine receptor complex and α[¹¹C]methyl-L-tryptophan (AMT) for the measurement of serotonin synthesis.

[¹¹C]FLUMAZENIL FOR MEASUREMENT OF THE GABA/BENZODIAZEPINE RECEPTOR COMPLEX

The PET studies with FMZ were undertaken in an attempt to apply a PET tracer more specific than FDG for accurate neuroimaging identification of epileptogenic cortex. Comparison studies of FMZ and FDG PET in patients with temporal lobe epilepsy being considered for epilepsy surgery re-ported that FMZ PET reveals a more restricted area of abnormality than FDG PET (20,21). Subsequently, Savic et al. (22) applied FMZ PET in patients with frontal lobe epilepsy and found a good correlation between location of FMZ PET abnormalities and epileptic foci identified by surface and intracranial EEG with subdural electrodes. Again, FMZ PET abnormalities were more restricted than those delineated with FDG PET. That study, however, did not provide a precise correlation between PET abnormalities and various intracranial EEG measures.

To investigate the relationship betwen functional abnormalities defined by PET and intracranial EEG, we applied recent advances in image processing that allow precise coregistration of the MRI or skull radiograph showing the positions of subdural grid electrodes with the FDG and FMZ PET data sets (23). Using this approach, which allows a highly accurate comparison of the sites of FDG and FMZ PET cortical abnormalities with intracranial EEG measures (e.g., seizure onset, seizure propagation, frequent spiking) (Fig. 35.1), we have

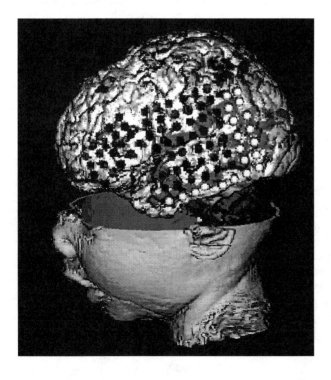

FIG. 35.1. Surface rendered MRI overlayed with FMZ PET data and subdural grid electrode locations. *Hatched gray shading* shows cortical regions with decreased FMZ binding. Subdural electrodes (one 4 × 5 and one 8 × 8 grid electrode arrays) are color coded: *white* = seizure onset (and frequent interictal spiking), *black* = normal. FMZ PET correctly detected the region of seizure onset in the left temporal and parietal lobes of this 4-year-old boy. Additional cortical regions in the frontal lobe (superior to the sylvian fissure) showed decreased FMZ without an electrographic correlate.

shown that the location of FMZ PET abnormalities *always* included the cortical region identified as the seizure onset zone by subdural EEG, whereas FDG PET was able to detect the seizure onset region in 80% of subjects (23). Receiver operating analysis demonstrated that FMZ PET was significantly more sensitive than FDG PET for the detection of cortical regions of seizure onset and frequent spiking in patients with extratemporal lobe epilepsy. Both FDG and FMZ PET showed low sensitivity in the detection of cortical areas of rapid seizure spread. Thus, functional changes in cortex resulting in facilitated seizure spread do not result in changes in measurable changes of glucose metabolism or benzodiazepine receptor binding.

Our findings are at odds with a recent prospective study in 100 patients with refractory partial epilepsy (24) (42 with extratemporal lobe epilepsy, 14 of whom underwent intracranial EEG monitoring), concluding that FMZ PET was not superior to FDG PET in assessing the extent of the ictal onset zone as defined by intracranial EEG recordings. The differences in methodology between that study and ours are numerous and significant enough to account for differing conclusions. Nonetheless, Ryvlin et al. (24) do concur with us that FMZ PET is clinically useful in patients with unilateral cryptogenic frontal lobe epilepsy.

Consistent with the findings of Savic et al. (22), we found that FMZ PET showed smaller areas of abnormalities compared with FDG PET in seven of ten patients (23); however, in contrast to previous reports, three patients showed larger cortical abnormalities with FMZ than with FDG. In two of these three subjects, additional cortical regions that were abnormal on FMZ included the location of seizure onset. Also, two of the subjects with a larger FMZ than FDG abnormality showed *increased* FMZ binding and glucose hypermetabolism. Increased FMZ binding was reported by Richardson et al. (25) in patients with cerebral dysgenesis. Cortical dysgenesis, however, was not observed in our two cases with increased FMZ binding. The MRIs were

normal in both cases, and pathological examination of the resected tissue showed gliosis. The EEG performed during these PET studies demonstrated epileptiform activity in the same location as the PET findings, but no clinical seizures were detected. Increased glucose metabolism in the presence of subclinical epileptiform activity was reported previously (26). The mechanism of increased FMZ binding under these circumstances is presently not known and warrants further investigation.

Although the sensitivity of FMZ PET in detecting the locations of seizure onset and frequent interictal spiking in extratemporal lobe epilepsy was high, the specificity was suboptimal. Additional cortical regions that showed no electrographic abnormalities were abnormal on FMZ PET in all ten patients studied (23). Infrequent interictal spiking and background slowing were not addressed in the study, however. These additional cortical regions showing abnormal FMZ binding may be due to changes in benzodiazepine receptors associated with the formation of secondary epileptic foci, but this remains to be determined. Interestingly, there is often a region of decreased FMZ binding in the parietal cortex that has no electrographic correlate. Decreased parietal and thalamic glucose metabolism has been reported in patients with temporal lobe epilepsy (27); in these cases, the parietal region rarely evolves into a seizure focus following temporal lobectomy. Furthermore, Savic et al. (28) reported that FMZ binding alterations in cortical areas outside the epileptic focus normalized following surgical removal of the epileptic focus. Regardless of the mechanism responsible for these additional regions of cortical FMZ binding abnormalities, their presence precludes the use of FMZ PET alone to define the boundaries of the area that needs to be removed for complete seizure control; however, FMZ PET should be a more effective tool than PET with FDG to guide subdural electrode placement to ensure coverage of the epileptogenic zone in patients with neocortical epilepsy.

Our use of FMZ PET in presurgical evaluation provided a unique opportunity to compare in vivo FMZ binding parameters with in vitro measures of FMZ binding (29). In vitro measures of receptor affinity (K_D), number (B_{max}), and laminar distribution of [^{3}H]-FMZ binding in the epileptic focus in 38 patients were compared with nonspiking cortex from a subgroup of 12 patients and also with tissue obtained from five nonepileptic patients who underwent surgery for traumatic brain injury. The in vitro binding parameters were compared with in vivo [^{11}C]-FMZ binding measured with PET in 19 of the patients. The B_{max} was higher in the 38 spiking tissues compared with the 12 nonspiking tissues. Paired comparison of spiking versus nonspiking binding in the 12 patients from whom nonspiking tissue was available showed statistically significant increases in both K_D and B_{max} in spiking cortex. A positive correlation was found between K_D and B_{max} values for 38 patients, the magnitude of the K_D increase being twice that of the B_{max} increase. In addition, there was a significant correlation between the asymmetry indices of the in vivo FMZ binding on PET and in vitro K_D of spiking cortex. The laminar distribution of [^{3}H]-FMZ showed increased FMZ binding in cortical layers V–VI in spiking cortex compared with nonspiking and control cortex. The increased receptor number in spiking cortical layers V–VI may be a compensatory mechanism to decreased GABAergic input; however, this increased B_{max} in spiking cortex was accompanied by a larger *decrease* in the affinity of FMZ for the receptor, suggesting that decreased FMZ binding in the epileptic focus measured with PET is due to a decrease in the affinity of the tracer for the receptor.

Consistent with previous studies (30,31), we found no significant difference between the mean K_D of the epileptogenic neocortices and control tissue. Our study using group comparisons showed considerable interindividual variation of the cortex affinity and thus was insensitive to possible changes in the K_D parameter. Our paired comparison of spiking and nonspiking cortex from the same patients was more sensitive, however, than previous studies using nonspiking tissue from different subjects. In the intrasubject comparison, differences arising from the preparation methods, different anatomic locations, underlying mechanisms of epilepsy, age, duration of epilepsy, seizure frequency, and medication are minimized. This approach of detecting focal cortical binding abnormalities is also more comparable to the in vivo methods of analysis of FMZ binding where abnormal binding is based on the comparison of surrounding and contralateral homotopic cortical regions instead of using interindividual comparison.

As mentioned, the spiking cortex showed a higher receptor density in the cortical layers V–VI in all patients compared with nonspiking cortex. Cortical layer V contains neurons with appropriate membrane properties, intralaminar connections, neurotransmitter systems, and axonal outputs to generate highly synchronized activity (32–36). This layer initiates synchronized bursting when GABA-mediated inhibition is suppressed (37). In addition, a localized selective loss of GABAergic innervation in layer V of motor cortex in alumina gel-induced model of focal epilepsy was reported in monkeys, suggesting that this process may have a causal role in the development of seizure activity (38,39). Thus, the present finding of increased B_{max} in layers V–VI suggests there may be impaired GABAergic innervation (40) resulting in a compensatory increase of BZD-R in the human epileptogenic neocortex.

The finding of higher B_{max} values in epileptogenic cortex compared with nonspiking appears to be a paradoxical finding because in vivo FMZ binding studies show a decrease in the epileptic focus (41). One would expect that a higher B_{max} would result in higher FMZ binding in vivo; however, we have shown that there is a significant correlation between the B_{max} and K_D values, whereas no such correlation is found in nonspiking tissue. Furthermore, examination of the slope of the regression line reveals that for a onefold higher B_{max} value, the K_D is approximately twofold higher. In other words, higher B_{max} values in spiking tissue are associated with greater decreases in the affinity of FMZ for the receptor. Therefore, the observed decrease of in vivo FMZ binding may result from reduced affinity of FMZ for the receptor. This would suggest that the affinity of FMZ for the receptor, rather than the number of binding sites in the tissue, is the determining factor causing decreased FMZ binding in the epileptogenic cortex observed with PET in vivo.

In addition, our in vitro results are in contrast to PET findings of decreased in vivo B_{max} in epileptogenic regions (28,41). Several differences between the in vitro and in vivo approach of B_{max} and K_D estimation must be considered when comparing these findings. Using PET imaging, B_{max} and K_D values are estimated from Scatchard analysis using only two points. Because of the paucity of the data, the standard deviation of both parameters, especially that of K_D, increases. Large coefficients of variation for K_D were reported, indicating the limited reliability of estimation of K_D (42). Furthermore, based on some previous in vivo studies (41,43), it was assumed that K_D is a constant parameter in epilepsy, and the observed binding alteration is the consequence of the altered receptor density.

The correlation between the K_D and B_{max} of the epileptic cortex in our study indicates that these parameters are not independent. A similar correlation was previously found between in vivo measured B_{max} and K_D in normal cortex (43,44), but no in vitro correlation has been reported. Although the cause of this correlation in normal conditions is uncertain, in epileptic cortex the increased B_{max} can be considered as a result of a compensatory mechanism induced by decreased GABA-mediated inhibition (e.g., due to decreased affinity). The value of the regression coefficient for this correlation suggests that this compensation is disproportionate with the affinity decrease. Thus, it can be concluded from our in vitro findings that decreased receptor affinity is an alteration that can lead to reduced benzodiazepine receptor binding in vivo even when a compensatory B_{max} increase occurs.

The correlation between in vitro K_D of the spiking cortex and the degree of decreased in vivo FMZ binding of the corresponding spiking area compared to the contralateral homotopic region supports this assumption. Considering the multifactorial nature of epileptogenesis, several other, still unknown factors are likely to contribute to altered $GABA_A$-benzodiazepine receptor function (45). Furthermore, the positive correlation between the duration of the epilepsy and the KD values we observed suggests that repeated seizures can be associated with a progressive decrease of receptor affinity.

Our findings suggest that the observed changes in benzodiazepine receptor binding in epileptogenic neocortex cannot be explained simply by cell loss (46,47) or by other histopathological changes since alterations of binding parameters and receptor redistribution occurred with the same frequency in epileptic cortices with normal as well as with abnormal histology. Therefore, functional receptor changes can occur even without apparent morphological alteration of the cerebral cortex. This is supported by recent in vivo benzodiazepine receptor binding studies demonstrating the occasional reversibility of altered benzodiazepine receptor binding following either drug treatment (48) or epilepsy surgery (28).

$\alpha[^{11}C]$METHYL-L-TRYPTOPHAN (AMT) FOR MEASUREMENT OF SEROTONIN SYNTHESIS

Several lines of evidence implicate serotonergic mechanisms as playing a role in epileptogenesis. In the genetically epilepsy-prone rat (GEPR) model of generalized epilepsy, there is a decrease in brain concentration of serotonin (49) as well as decreased V_{max} for [H-3]serotonin uptake by synaptosomes and tryptophan hydroxylase activity (50). Pharmacologic treatments that facilitate serotonergic neurotransmission inhibit seizures in many animal models of epilepsy, including the GEPR rat, maximal electroshock model, pentylenetetrazol administration, kindling, and bicuculline microinjections in the area tempestas [reviewed by Statnick et al. (50)]. Conversely, the lowering of brain serotonin concentrations leads to an increase in seizure susceptibility in animal models of epilepsy (51,52) as well as in humans (53,54). Finally, in human brain tissue surgically removed for seizure control, levels of 5-HIAA (5-hydrox-yindole acetic acid, the breakdown product of serotonin) were found to be higher in actively spiking temporal cortex compared with normal controls (55,56). Increased 5HT immunoreactivity also has been reported in human epileptic brain tissue resected for the control of epilepsy (57).

AMT, which has been developed as a tracer for serotonin synthesis with PET in humans (58–60), is an analogue of tryptophan, the precursor for serotonin synthesis. This method is designed to measure serotonin synthesis in vivo since the intravenously injected ^{11}C-AMT is converted in the brain to $\alpha[^{11}C]$-methyl-serotonin, which is not a substrate for the enzyme monamine oxidase (61) and, therefore, accumulates in serotonergic terminals. We used AMT PET in patients with tuberous sclerosis complex (TSC) and medically intractable epilepsy (62). TSC is an autosomal dominant inherited disorder with a high spontaneous mutation rate, now known to result from mutations in at least two different genes, *TSC1* (63,64) and *TSC2* (65).

These genetic mutations result in tumorous growths in multiple organs, including the brain, skin, heart, and kidney (66,67). Intracranial lesions in TSC include cortical tubers (68–70), subependymal nodules, subependymal giant cell astrocytoma (71), and microscopic abnormalities such as microdysgenesis, heterotopic gray matter, and lamination defects (70,72). More than 80% of patients with TSC have seizures, and when these are uncontrolled, the prognosis is poor for normal cognitive function (66,73). Recent attempts at surgical removal of the epileptogenic tuber(s) met with some success (74–77), but the preoperative evaluation is generally invasive due to the frequent requirement of intracranial EEG monitoring with subdural electrodes. Scalp EEG lo-

calization may identify the lobe in which seizures are generated; however, this lobe may contain multiple tubers, only one of which may be responsible for the seizures. Anatomic neuroimaging with CT and MRI may demonstrate precisely the locations of tubers and calcifications (73,78–81) but does not differentiate between epileptogenic and nonepileptogenic lesions in the brain. Even currently available functional imaging studies are of limited use in patients with TSC. PET scanning with FDG shows decreased glucose metabolism corresponding to the locations of tubers and calcifications (82,83) but is not capable of distinguishing between epileptogenic and nonepileptogenic lesions unless a prolonged seizure fortuitously occurs during the tracer uptake period leading to focally increased glucose metabolism (ictal PET study) (84). Because of the short half-lives of PET isotopes, however, ictal PET studies are not practical. Although ictal studies using single-photon emission computed tomography (SPECT) have enjoyed more success in this regard, these are particularly difficult to accomplish in children with TSC, whose seizures are typically short lasting and are not ideal for ictal SPECT study.

Studies performed in our laboratory with AMT PET in patients with TSC and uncontrolled seizures have yielded exciting and promising results in allowing epileptogenic tubers [characterized by *high* (C-11)AMT accumulation] to be differentiated from nonepileptogenic ones [characterized by *low* (C-11)AMT accumulation] (Fig. 35.2) (62). We studied nine children with TSC and refractory epilepsy, all of whom underwent PET scans of glucose metabolism and AMT and EEG monitoring during both PET studies. Four of the eight children underwent video EEG monitoring of their seizures. Whereas all tubers showed decreased FDG uptake, five subjects showed one region of increased AMT uptake, three subjects showed two regions, and one subject showed three regions of increased AMT uptake compared with adjacent cortex. The magnitude of the regions of focal increase ranged from 5% to 111%, and the location of the increase was consistent with EEG ictal on-

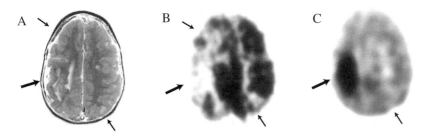

FIG. 35.2. MRI and PET scans in an 8-year-old girl with TSC and intractable epilepsy. **A:** MRI scan showing large tuber in the right central/parietal region (*bold arrow*) as well as other smaller lesions (*thin arrows*). **B:** The glucose metabolism PET scan shows cortical hypometabolism in the same regions as the lesions seen on MRI (*arrows*). **C:** AMT images display decreased tracer uptake in the location of small tubers compared to adjacent nonlesional cortex (*thin arrow*). The large right central tuber (*bold arrow*) shows a 110% increase in AMT uptake. Note that the left side of the image is the right side of the brain.

set localization in four of eight patients for whom ictal EEG data were available (two of the eight EEGs were nonlocalizing and nonlateralizing). In most subjects, the increase in AMT uptake was focal and nodular, located in the white matter underlying the tuber or located within the tuber itself. A second pattern that was seen consisted of a rim of increased [C-11]AMT uptake surrounding a tuber, and the increase was smaller in these cases.

The findings with AMT PET in patients with TSC and uncontrolled seizures strongly suggest that epileptogenic tubers (characterized by *high* AMT uptake) can be differentiated from nonepileptogenic ones (characterized by *low* ^{11}C-AMT uptake). Coregistration of the AMT PET images with MRI provides the necessary accurate spatial localization of the cortical lesions with high AMT uptake, which appears to correspond to EEG localization of seizure onset. For example, intracranial monitoring in the patient displayed in Fig. 35.2 showed excellent agreement between the region of high AMT uptake and seizure onset and propagation. Intracranial subdural grid electrode arrays were placed on posterior frontal, parietal, and temporal cortex for more precise localization of ictal onset prior to resective surgery. A volumetric MRI scan acquired with subdural electrodes in place was coregistered with the [C-11]AMT PET scan, and both MRI and PET scans underwent a

maximum intensity projection in three dimensions. The region of increased [C-11]AMT uptake was delineated and superimposed on the MRI showing the position of the subdural electrodes (Fig. 35.3). During the intracranial monitoring period, the patient had ten typical

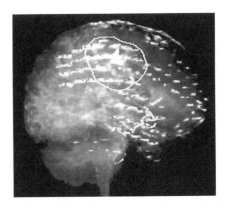

FIG. 35.3. MRI 3-D rendered image (patient shown in Fig. 35.2) using a maximum-intensity projection showing location of subdural grid electrode placement and delineation of region of increased AMT uptake. The position of the grid electrode array on top of the exposed cortical surface can be recognized because of the small distortions of the magnetic field in the vicinity of the metal electrodes. The *circular line* delineates the region of increased AMT uptake in the frontoparietal region. Ictal onset occurred at electrodes at the posterior border of the cortical region with increased AMT uptake and spread anteriorly around the border.

seizures, eight of which originated at electrodes at the posterior border of the [C-11]AMT PET abnormality, and the remaining two could not be localized. The eight seizures showed rapid spread to the anterior and inferior borders of the AMT PET abnormality. Although subependymal lesions were present in all nine children, none of these lesions could be visualized on the AMT PET scans, consistent with the notion that subependymal lesions are not epileptogenic. The data from human epileptic tissue are consistent with the findings of increased AMT uptake in epileptogenic tubers as well as AMT PET scans in non-TSC children with epilepsy (85), which showed that increased serotonin synthesis also correctly identifies epileptogenic cortex as indicated by ictal scalp EEG recordings.

SUMMARY

Our results and those of others demonstrate that the development of new PET probes with increasing sensitivity and specificity for epileptogenic brain regions is feasible. Further development of novel tracers guided by knowledge of the biochemical characteristics of epileptogenic cortex from basic studies is the logical next step in the application of neuroimaging to localize epileptogenic cortex. Furthermore, computational advances allowing coregistration of biochemical images with high-resolution MRI anatomic images, as well as electrophysiologic data sets, not only has practical value in guiding surgical resection of epileptogenic neocortex, but this approach contributes to further understanding of the biochemical mechanisms involved in the pathophysiology of neocortical epilepsy.

ACKNOWLEDGMENTS

This work was supported by funding from NIH grants NS-34488 (to H.T.C.) and NS-38324 (to D.C.C.). We are grateful to the faculty, students, and staff at the PET Center at Children's Hospital of Michigan for their collaboration and assistance in performing the studies described above. We further express our gratitude to Joel Ager, Ph.D., and James Janisse, M.A., from the Center for Health Care Effectiveness Research at Wayne State University for their collaboration in statistical analysis.

REFERENCES

1. Swartz BE, Halgren E, Delgado-Escueta AV, et al. Neuroimaging in patients with seizures of probable frontal lobe origin. *Epilepsia* 1989;30:547–558.
2. Swartz BE, Theodore WH, Sanabria E, et al. Positron emission and single photon emission computed tomographic studies in the frontal lobe with emphasis on the relationship to seizure foci. In: Chauvel P, Delgado-Escueta AV, Halgren E, Bancaud J, eds. *Frontal lobe seizures and epilepsies. Advances in neurology,* vol 57. New York: Raven Press, 1992;57:487–497.
3. Olson DM, Chugani HT, Shewmon DA, et al. Electrocorticographic confirmation of focal positron emission tomographic abnormalities in children with intractable epilepsy. *Epilepsia* 1990;31:731–739.
4. Engel J Jr. Functional explorations of the human epileptic brain and their therapeutic implications. *Electroencephalogr Clin Neurophysiol* 1990b;76:296–316.
5. Robitaille Y, Rasmussen T, Dubeau F, et al. Histopathology of nonneoplastic lesions in frontal lobe epilepsy: review of 180 cases with recent MRI and PET correlations. *Adv Neurol* 1992;57:499–513.
6. Langstrom B, Dannals RF, Stocklin G. Radiotracer production. In: Wagner HN, Szabo Z, Buchanan JW, eds. *Priniciples of nuclear medicine.* Philadelphia: WB Saunders, 1995;166–194.
7. Henry TR, Chugani HT, Abou-Khalil BW, et al. Positron emission tomography. In: Engel J Jr, ed. *Surgical treatment of the epilepsies,* 2nd ed. New York: Raven Press, 1993:211–243.
8. Engel J Jr, Henry TR, Risinger MW, et al. Presurgical evaluation for partial epilepsy: relative contributions of chronic depth electrode recordings versus FDG-PET and scalp-sphenoidal ictal EEG. *Neurology* 1990;40:1670–1677.
9. Engel J Jr. Functional explorations of the human epileptic brain and their therapeutic implications. *Electroencephalogr Clin Neurophysiol* 1990;76:296–316.
10. Theodore WH, Dorwart R, Holmes M, et al. Neuroimaging in refractory partial seizures: comparison of PET, CT, and MRI. *Neurology* 1986;36:750–759.
11. Henry TR, Engel J Jr, Sutherling WW, et al. Correlation of structural and functional imaging with electrographic localization and histopathology in refractory complex partial epilepsy. *Epilepsia* 1987;28:601.
12. Henry TR, Sutherling WW, Engel J Jr, et al. Interictal cerebral metabolism in partial epilepsies of neocortical origin. *Epilepsy Res* 1991;10:174–182.
13. Hosokawa S, Kato M, Otsuka M, et al. Positron emission tomography in epilepsy: correlative study. *Jpn J Psychiatry Neurol* 1989;43:349–353.
14. Latack JT, Abou-Khalil BW, Siegel GJ, et al. Patients with partial seizures: evaluation by MRI, CT, and PET imaging. *Radiology* 1986;159:159–163.
15. Sperling MR, Wilson G, Engel J Jr, et al. Magnetic resonance imaging in intractable partial epilepsy: correlative studies. *Ann Neurol* 1986;20:57–62.

16. Swartz BE, Halgren E, Delgado-Escueta AV, et al. Multidisciplinary analysis of patients with extratemporal complex partial seizures: I. Interest agreement. *Epilepsy Res* 1990;5:61–73.

17. Theodore WH, Holmes MD, Dorwart RH, et al. Complex partial seizures: cerebral structure and cerebral function. *Epilepsia* 1986d;27:576–582.

18. Swartz BE, Khonsari A, Brown C, et al. Improved sensitivity of [18]FDG-positron emission tomography scans in frontal and "frontal plus" epilepsy. *Epilepsia* 1995;36(4):388–395.

19. da Silva EA, Chugani DC, Muzik O, et al. Identification of frontal lobe epileptic foci in children using positron emission tomography. *Epilepsia* 1997;38:1198–1208.

20. Savic I, Ingvar M, Stone-Elander S. Comparison of [C-11]flumazenil and [F-18]FDG as PET markers of epileptic foci. *J Neurol Neurosurg Psychiatry* 1993;56:615–621.

21. Henry TR, Frey KA, Sackellares JC, et al. In vivo cerebral metabolism and central benzodiazepine-receptor binding in temporal lobe epilepsy. *Neurology* 1993;43:1998–2006.

22. Savic I, Thorell JO, Roland P. [11C]Flumazenil positron emission tomography visualizes frontal epileptogenic regions. *Epilepsia* 1995;36:1225–1232.

23. Muzik O, da Silva EA, Juhasz C, et al. Intracranial electrophysiological significance of flumazenil and glucose PET abnormalities in children with extratemporal lobe epilepsy. *Neurology* 2000;54:171–179.

24. Ryvlin P, Bouvard S, Le Bars D, et al. Clinical utility of flumazenil-PET versus [18F]fluorodeoxyglucose-PET and MRI in refractory partial epilepsy: a prospective study in 100 patients. *Brain* 1998;121:2067–2081.

25. Richardson MP, Koepp MJ, Brooks DJ, et al. Benzodiazepine receptors in focal epilepsy with cortical dysgenesis: an 11C-flumazenil PET study. *Ann Neurol* 1996;40:188–198.

26. Chugani HT, Shewmon DA, Khanna S, et al. Interictal and postictal focal hypermetabolism on positron emission tomography. *Pediatr Neurol* 1993;9:10–15.

27. Henry TR, Mazziotta JC, Engel J Jr, et al. Quantifying interictal metabolic activity in human temporal lobe epilepsy. *J Cereb Blood Flow Metab* 1990;10:748–757.

28. Savic I, Blomqvist G, Halldin C, et al. Regional increased in [11C]flumazenil binding after epilepsy surgery. *Acta Neurol Scand* 1998;97:279–286.

29. Nagy F, Chugani DC, Juhasz C, et al. Altered in vitro and in vivo flumazenil binding in human epileptogenic neocortex. *J Cerebral Blood Flow Metab* 1999;19:939–947.

30. Sherwin A, Matthew E, Blain M, et al. Benzodiazepine receptor binding is not altered in human epileptogenic cortical foci. *Neurology* 1986;36:1380–1382.

31. Olsen RW, Bureau M, Houser CR, et al. GABA/benzodiazepine receptors in human focal epilepsy. *Epilepsy Res Suppl* 1992;8:383–391.

32. Gutnick MJ, Connors BW, Prince DA. Mechanisms of neocortical epileptogenesis in vitro. *J Neurophysiol* 1982;48:1321–1335.

33. Connors BW. Initiation of synchronized neuronal bursting in neocortex. *Nature* 1984;310:685–687.

34. Connors BW. Neocortical anatomy and physiology. In: Engel J Jr, Pedley TA, eds. *Epilepsy.* Philadelphia: Lippincott–Raven, 1998:307–321.

35. White EL, Amitai Y, Gutnick MJ. A comparison of synapses onto the somata of intrinsically bursting and regular spiking neurons in layer V of rat SmI cortex. *Comp Neurol* 1994;342:1–14.

36. Castro-Alamancos MA, Connors BW. Cellular mechanisms of the augmenting response: short-term plasticity in a thalamocortical pathway. *J Neurosci* 1996;16:7742–7756.

37. Chagnac-Amitai Y, Connors BW. Horizontal spread of synchronized activity in neocortex and its control by GABA-mediated inhibition. *J Neurophysiol* 1989;61:747–758.

38. Ribak CE, Harris AB, Vaughn JE, et al. Inhibitory, GABAergic nerve terminals decrease at sites of focal epilepsy. *Science* 1979;205:211–214.

39. Houser CR, Harris AB, Vaughn JE. Time course of the reduction of GABA terminals in a model of focal epilepsy: a glutamic acid decarboxylase immunocytochemical study. *Brain Res* 1986;383:129–145.

40. Spreafico R, Battaglia G, Arcelli P, et al. Cortical dysplasia: an immunocytochemical study of three patients. *Neurology* 1998;50:27–36.

41. Savic I, Persson A, Roland P, et al. In vivo demonstration of reduced benzodiazepine receptor binding in human epileptic foci. *Lancet* 1988;2:863–866.

42. Abadie P, Baron JC, Bisserbe JC, et al. Central benzodiazepine receptors in human brain: estimation of regional B_{max} and K_D values with positron emission tomography. *Eur J Pharmacol* 1992;213:107–115.

43. Delforge J, Pappata S, Millet P, et al. Quantification of benzodiazepine receptors in human brain using PET, [11C]flumazenil, and a single-experiment protocol. *J Cereb Blood Flow Metab* 1995;15:284–300.

44. Millet P, Delforge J, Mauguiere F, et al. Parameter and index images of benzodiazepine receptor concentration in the brain. *J Nucl Med* 1995;36:1462–1471.

45. McDonald JW, Garofalo EA, Hood T, et al. Altered excitatory and inhibitory amino acid receptor binding in hippocampus of patients with temporal lobe epilepsy. *Ann Neurol* 1991;29:529–541.

46. Babb TL, Brown WJ, Pretorius J, et al. Temporal lobe volumetric cell densities in temporal lobe epilepsy. *Epilepsia* 1984;25:729–740.

47. Babb TL, Lieb JP, Brown WJ, et al. Distribution of pyramidal cell density and hyperexcitability in the epileptic human hippocampal formation. *Epilepsia* 1984;25:721–728.

48. Staedt J, Stoppe G, Kogler A, et al. Changes of central benzodiazepine receptor density in the course of anticonvulsant treatment in temporal lobe epilepsy. *Seizure* 1995;4:49–52.

49. Dailey JW, Reigel CE, Mishra PK, Jobe PC. Neurobiology of seizure predisposition in the genetically epilepsy-prone rat. *Epilepsy Res* 1989;3:317–320.

50. Statnick MA, Dailey JW, Jobe PC, et al. Abnormalities in brain serotonin concentration, high-affinity uptake, and tryptophan hydroxylase activity in severe-seizure genetically epilepsy-prone rats. *Epilepsia* 1996;37:311–321.

51. Wenger GR, Stitzel RE, Craig CR. The role of biogenic amines in the reserpine-induced alteration of minimal electroshock seizure thresholds in the mouse. *Neuropharmacol* 1973;12:693–703.

52. Lazarova M, Bendotti C, Samanin R. Studies on the role of serotonin in different regions of the rat central nervous system on pentylenetetrazol-induced seizures and

the effect of Di-n-propy-lacetate. *Arch Pharmacol* 1983;322:147–152.

53. Pallister PD. Aggravation of epilepsy by reserpine, associated with possible bleeding and clotting disturbances. *Rocky Mountain Medical Journal* 1982;56: 45–50.

54. Maynert E, Marczynski T, Browning R. The role of neurotransmitters in the epilepsies. *Adv Neurol* 1975;13: 79–147.

55. Louw D, Sutherland GB, Glavin GB, et al. A study of monoamine metabolism in human epilepsy. *Can J Neurol Sci* 1989;16:394–397.

56. Pintor M, Mefford IN, Hutter I, et al. The levels of biogenic amines, their metabolites and tyrosine hydroxylase in the human epileptic temporal cortex. *Synapse* 1990;5:152–156.

57. Trottier S, Evrard B, Vignal JP, et al. The serotonergic innervation of the cerebral cortex in man and its changes in focal cortical dysplasia. *Epilepsy Res* 1996;2 5:79–106.

58. Muzik O, Chugani DC, Chakraborty PK, et al. Analysis of [C-11]alpha-methyl-tryptophan kinetics for the estimation of serotonin synthesis rate in vivo. *J Cereb Blood Flow Metab* 1997;17:659–669.

59. Nishizawa S, Benkelfat C, Young SN, et al. Differences between males and females in rates of serotonin synthesis in human brain. *Proc Natl Acad Sci USA* 1997;94: 5308–5313.

60. Chugani DC, Muzik O, Chakraborty PK, et al. Human brain serotonin synthesis capacity measured in vivo with α[C-11]methyl-L-tryptophan. *Synapse* 1998;28: 33–43.

61. Missala K, Sourkes TL. Functional cerebral activity of an analogue of serotonin formed in situ. *Neurochem Int* 1988;12:209–214.

62. Chugani DC, Chugani HT, Muzik O, et al. Imaging epileptogenic tubers in children with tuberous sclerosis complex using α[11C]-methyl-L-tryptophan PET. *Ann Neurol* 1998;44:858–866.

63. Fryer AE, et al. Evidence that the gene for tuberous sclerosis is on chromosome 9. *Lancet* 1987;1:659–661.

64. van Slegtenhorst M, de Hoogt R, Hermans C, et al. Identification of the tuberous sclerosis gene TSC1 on chromosome 9q34. *Science* 1997;277:805–808.

65. Kandt RS, Haines JL, Smith M, et al. Linkage of an important gene locus for tuberous sclerosis to a chromosome 16 marker for polycystic kidney disease. *Nat Genet* 1992;2:37–41.

66. Gomez MR. Neurologic and psychiatric features. In: Gomez MR, ed. *Tuberous sclerosis,* 2nd ed. New York: Raven Press, 1988:21–36.

67. Roach ES, Smith M, Huttenlocher P, et al. Report of the diagnostic criteria committee of the National Tuberous Sclerosis Association. *J Child Neurol* 1992;7:221–224.

68. Ferrer I, Fabregues I, Coll J, et al. Tuberous sclerosis: a golgi study of cortical tuber. *Clin Neuropathol* 1984; 3:47–51.

69. Huttenlocher PR, Heydemann PT. Fine structure of cortical tubers in tuberous sclerosis: a golgi study. *Ann Neurol* 1984;16:595–602.

70. Machado-Salas JP. Abnormal dendritic patterns and aberrant spine development of Bourneville's disease—a golgi survey. *Clin Neuropathol* 1984;3:52–58.

71. Kingsley DPE, Kendal BE, Fritz CT. Tuberous sclerosis: a clinico-radiological evaluation of 110 cases with reference of atypical presentation. *Neuroradiology* 1986;28:38–46.

72. Boesel CP, Paulson GW, Kosnik EJ, et al. Brain hamartomas and tumors associated with tuberous sclerosis. *Neurosurgery* 1979;4:410–417.

73. Shepherd CW, Houser OW, Gomez MR. MR findings in tuberous sclerosis complex and correlation with seizure development and mental impairment. *Am J Neuroradiol* 1995;16:149–155.

74. Bye AM, Matheson JM, Tobias VH, et al. Selective epilepsy surgery in tuberous sclerosis. *Aust Paediatr J* 1989;25:243–245.

75. Andermann F, Palmini AL. Neuronal migration disorders, tuberous sclerosis, and Sturge–Weber syndrome. In: Lüders HO, ed. *Epilepsy surgery.* New York: Raven Press, 1992:203–211.

76. Duchowny M, Levin B, Jayakar P, et al. Temporal lobectomy in early childhood. *Epilepsia* 1992;33:298–303.

77. Bebin EM, Kelly PJ, Gomez MR. Surgical treatment for epilepsy in cerebral tuberous sclerosis. *Epilepsia* 1993;34:651–657.

78. Curatolo P, Cusmair R, Pruna D. Tuberous sclerosis: diagnostic and prognostic problems. *Pediatr Neuroscience* 1986;12:123–125.

79. Roach ES, Williams DP, Laster DW. Magnetic resonance imaging in tuberous sclerosis. *Arch Neurol* 1987; 44:301–304.

80. Nixon JR, Houser OW, Gomez MR, et al. Cerebral tuberous sclerosis: MR imaging. *Radiology* 1989;170: 869–873.

81. Cusmai R, Chiron C, Curatolo P, et al. Topographic comparative study of magnetic resonance imaging and electroencephalography in 34 children with tuberous sclerosis. *Epilepsia* 1990;31:747–755.

82. Szelies B, Herholz K, Heiss WD, et al. Hypometabolic cortical lesions in tuberous sclerosis with epilepsy: demonstration by positron emission tomography. *J Comput Assist Tomogr* 1983;7:946–953.

83. Rintahaka PJ, Chugani HT. Clinical role of positron emission tomography in children with tuberous sclerosis complex. *J Child Neurol* 1997;12:42–52.

84. Chugani HT, Rintahaka PJ, Shewmon DA. Ictal patterns of cerebral glucose utilization in children with epilepsy. *Epilepsia* 1994;35:813–822.

85. Chugani DC, da Silva EA, Muzik O, et al. Abnormal serotonin synthesis in epileptic foci of children: an in vivo study with alpha[C-11]methyl-tryptophan and positron emission tomography. *Epilepsia* 1997;38 (Suppl 3):45.

Neocortical Epilepsies.
Advances in Neurology, Vol. 84,
edited by P. D. Williamson, A. M. Siegel,
D. W. Roberts, V. M. Thadani, and M. S. Gazzaniga.
Lippincott Williams & Wilkins, Philadelphia © 2000.

36

Clinical Neuropsychology and Neocortical Epilepsies

M. Jones-Gotman

Departments of Neurology and Neurosurgery, Montreal Neurological Institute,
McGill University, Montreal, Quebec, Canada H3A 2B4

Neuropsychological evaluation is an integral part of the presurgical investigation of patients who are candidates for surgical treatment of epilepsy. It consists of a comprehensive assessment of cognitive functioning that includes intelligence, frontoexecutive skills, memory, attention, visuospatial abilities, and language. Some sensory functions and motor skills are also tested. Results from this thorough, usually standardized, assortment of measures provide a reliable way of characterizing and quantifying the nature and degree of cognitive dysfunction arising from epilepsy. The information gained from this evaluation is unique and cannot be gained or inferred from the other investigations, such as electroencephalography or neuroimaging, that are also carried out in these patients.

In temporal lobe epilepsy (TLE), the primary cognitive deficit is in learning and memory, owing primarily to the influence of the medial temporal lobe region in TLE. Because the vast majority of surgical candidates have TLE, information about those patients and about memory function is far more available than information about the rarer cases with neocortical epilepsies. This chapter focuses on what is known about the neuropsychology of those rarer cases, how they are investigated clinically, and what the results show in some such patients who have been investigated at the Montreal Neurological Institute (MNI).

The basic rationale underlying neuropsychological evaluations is to determine the dysfunctional hemisphere by comparing a patient's performance on verbal tasks with performance on visuospatial ones and, within the hemisphere, to determine the dysfunctional region by comparing performance on various kinds of tasks. These include memory tests, "frontal lobe tasks," and others expected to tap parietal or occipital functions, as will be discussed.

Lesions or foci in brain regions other than the temporal or frontal lobes are relatively rare. We went through our archives specifically for the Dartmouth symposium on neocortical epilepsies, seeking patients who had received neuropsychological assessments between 1970 and the present and who had a focal lesion or seizure onset other than in the medial temporal lobe. We excluded patients with a Full-Scale intelligence quotient (IQ) below 75, those younger than 15 years of age or older than 55, and subjects with a lesion or focus in more than one lobe. We found a small number of patients with focus confined to a parietal or occipital lobe, but there were 168 left temporal, 132 right temporal, 35 left frontal, and 44 right frontal lobe cases. Perhaps this is as good a testimony as any as to why in the epilepsy setting our efforts at test development have been in memory tests and frontal lobe tests far more than for parietal/occipital functions. The emphasis of this chapter is on the rarer lesions; therefore, we took a random sample of a small subset of the temporal lobe cases for the comparisons that were made specifically for this occasion.

FRONTAL LOBES

What functions are investigated in neuropsychological assessments? For frontal lobes, mental flexibility, planning, and fluency are all assessed. One of the best-known measures considered to be a test of frontal lobe function is the Wisconsin Card Sorting Test (WCST) (1,2). In 1997, Jelena Djordjevic, Ada Piazzini, and I compared performance on this task for 50 patients with unilateral resection from a frontal lobe (25 left, 25 right), randomly selected from our archives between 1971 and 1994, and 40 randomly selected patients with unilateral resection from a temporal lobe (20 left, 20 right) (3). We found that the left frontal lobe group achieved significantly fewer categories than did the right frontal or left temporal lobe groups, but they did not differ from the right temporal lobe group. The same pattern was observed for error scores, total errors, and perseverative and unique errors. Further inspection of the WCST scores (number of categories achieved) as they related to site of lesion within the frontal lobes showed no consistent relationship between performance and the subregion of lesion within the frontal lobe. Although these data are from patients who have undergone operation, the same pattern is observed in unoperated cases: The number of categories achieved and the errors differ significantly in patients with a left frontal lobe focus compared with other patient groups.

To be noted in these results is that the right frontal lobe group did not differ at all from the left temporal lobe group on the WCST. A different result is seen when one looks at figural fluency. We use the Design Fluency Test to measure fluency in the nonverbal mode (4,5). The task requirements are that the patient must create original abstract designs that do not represent anything and cannot be named, and they must draw as many different designs as they can in 5 minutes. On average, normal subjects produce about 16 acceptable drawings.

Patients with right frontal lobe or right central lesions are impaired on this task, producing on average five or six acceptable designs; patients with left frontal lesions or left or right temporal lobe lesions are not impaired (4,5). There were no groups in this study (4) with parietal or occipital lesions, although the earlier study (5) did include a few parietal cases, and those patients also performed normally on this task. The performance of patients with damage in the right frontal lobe is characterized in some cases by a steady production of drawings, which, however, are all the same or highly similar; in other cases, the patient makes few drawings and claims that there is nothing else to draw. Comparing an individual patient's performance on paired verbal and visuoperceptual tasks that are as similar as possible except for the actual material (e.g., words versus designs) of each task aids in teasing out subtle deficits. This is especially useful in preoperative evaluations, when determination of a focus is most important. In this case, comparing verbal to figural fluency within an individual patient can be instructive. In terms of group data, a specific deficit in verbal fluency is not observed for any group in unoperated patients, but postoperatively patients with surgical excision from the left frontal lobe show a loss in word fluency; their performance after surgery becomes significantly impaired. This is not true of other lesion groups.

Another measure used to evaluate frontal lobe function is the Stroop test (6–8), which requires mental flexibility in its "interference condition." In that condition, patients are shown color names printed in a color other than the one named; they must name the color of the ink and inhibit the more common response to read the words. Planning abilities are tested with the so-called tower tests—Tower of Hanoi, Tower of London, Tower of Toronto (8,9)—and the well-known Trail-Making Test (10). These tasks allow one to explore further, or to clarify, a subject's suspected frontal lobe deficit.

Motor tasks are used to evaluate frontal lobe function as well. These include finger-tapping tests, sequential tapping, strength tasks using hand or pinch dynamometer, and manual dexterity tasks as measured by the Purdue or Grooved Pegboard tests (11,12). Large differences between the hands in performance on such tests suggest dysfunction in the contralateral motor cortex, although in our sample, we did not find significant group differences either before or after surgery on a hand dynamometer task. We are currently collecting data measuring pinch strength instead of handgrip strength because the pinch strength measure is believed to be more sensitive. Again, in individual cases, a pattern of unilateral weakness or lack of dexterity on more than one of these tasks adds strength to the findings and allows one to make a diagnosis.

TEMPORAL NEOCORTEX

One of the most important cognitive functions to be assessed, other than memory, is word-retrieval skills (e.g., 13–19). Word-finding difficulties are among the first complaints from patients with a lesion or focus in the dominant hemisphere, and the importance of confrontation naming measures in documenting postsurgical decline is well established (4,20,21). Using the Boston Naming Test, we demonstrated a difference between left and right temporal lobe focus in unoperated patients. Of interest to us in Quebec, where a large proportion of our patients are francophone, is that we found a difference between anglophone and francophone healthy subjects on the task: the mean score of francophone subjects was about three points lower than that of the anglophone subjects (22). The left temporal lobe deficit was, of course, present in both language groups when patients were compared with the appropriate control group.

In the nondominant temporal lobe, impairments in visuospatial and visuoperceptual functioning are investigated. These are more difficult to document (13,14,20,21) than are the naming deficits seen from the dominant

hemisphere, except in the less frequent cases of patients with severe deficits. This difficulty in demonstrating subtle perceptual inefficiencies may simply reflect inadequacies in the traditional instruments used to assess these functions (13).

In a study carried out at the MNI, in collaboration with C. Guerreiro (23), we studied 62 patients who were divided into groups according to MRI scan measurements of medial temporal lobe regions. The groups were patients with normal volumes, amygdala atrophy only, hippocampal atrophy only (one group with unilateral hippocampal atrophy, one with bilateral), or amygdala plus hippocampal atrophy. For memory studies, we did an additional, separate grouping, blind to the MRI groupings: Based on the pattern of results from the memory tests, patients were assigned to one of the following four memory-function categories: unimpaired, unilateral left or unilateral right dysfunction, or bilateral dysfunction.

The IQ results were analyzed with a one-way analysis of variance (ANOVA) that showed a significant difference among the groups ($F = 4.68, p = 0.002$). Inspection of the means showed that the two groups without hippocampal atrophy had higher IQ ratings than did the three groups with hippocampal involvement. Post hoc comparisons showed that this difference was significant for the group with atrophy in both the amygdala and the hippocampus; that group differed from the normal values group and from the amygdala-only group. This finding of higher IQ in patients with normal volumes or atrophy confined to the amygdala suggests that long-term damage in the hippocampus contributes to ongoing learning deficits.

The groups also differed on the memory measure, as shown by a chi-square test ($p = 0.03$). This difference reflected a more pronounced memory impairment in patients whose atrophy included hippocampus than in patients with amygdala atrophy alone or in patients with normal volumes. These results strongly suggest that amygdala damage alone will not produce memory deficits.

PARIETAL LOBES

The traditional tests of parietal lobe function in patients with stroke, tumor, or other large lesions are well known. Demonstration of parietal lobe dysfunction in patients with epilepsy arising from a parietal lobe focus is more difficult, and the frank impairments seen after extensive lesions are not seen or are attenuated. A poor or distorted copy of the complex Rey–Osterrieth figure (24,25) points to interference in parietal lobe function, and our data with a small number of subjects suggest that this is true only of patients with a right parietal focus. In contrast, our results with the same sample of patients show the least efficient reading in the small group of patients with a left parietal focus.

Somatosensory tests are also used to evaluate the parietal region (9,13,26). Our results from a systematic two-point discrimination task show raised thresholds contralateral to the focus in the right parietal group compared with the left. As with many other tasks, the difference is more pronounced after surgery.

OCCIPITAL LOBES

In a search through almost 30 years of records, only five cases of focal occipital lobe damage were found, all of which were right-sided. Had the criteria been less stringent, more cases probably would have been selected, but still this small number points out the rarity of such cases. Among the tests chosen for analysis, no clear findings emerged for the occipital cases, although the group means for hand strength were low for both hands. Tasks aimed specifically at visual perception were not analyzed.

OVERVIEW

The ability to localize dysfunction based on neuropsychological performance is dependent on the sensitivity and specificity of the measures used. Important factors to consider in interpreting neuropsychological findings include overall level of cognitive perfor-

mance, age of seizure onset, and chronological age at the time of testing (e.g., 20). It should also be emphasized that no interpretations should be based on performance on a single test; rather, one should analyze the *pattern of results* on a battery of carefully selected tests (9,13). This procedure allows convergent lines of evidence to support a conclusion of dysfunction; an overreliance on single test measures can be misleading.

Finer analyses of the dysfunctions associated with focal epilepsy are beginning to emerge. Dissection of impairments through the judicious use of tests that tap specific aspects of different functions allows neuropsychologists to offer a more informed diagnosis and to offer better advice to patients regarding details of their cognitive difficulties.

Postsurgical changes in cognitive functioning are dependent partly on the presurgical abilities of the patient. In the case of memory, for example, the patients who are most likely to show postoperative memory decrements are those with good memory preoperatively or with normal hippocampal volumes according to measurements made of medial structures on MRI scans (27,28). This is especially noticeable if the resection is made from the dominant temporal lobe. Nevertheless, many of the deficits discussed in this chapter are more pronounced in operated patients, and some of the deficits are observed clearly only after surgical lesions and are not seen reliably with the seizure focus alone.

Quality-of-life issues are a growing area of concern in the context of epilepsy surgery (29,30). Whereas methods of investigating quality of life have been developed for other diseases, issues specific to epilepsy have been addressed far more recently. This topic is beyond the scope of the present chapter.

INTRACAROTID AMOBARBITAL PROCEDURE

Most neuropsychological assessments also include determination of cerebral dominance for language. This is typically achieved using the intracarotid amobarbital procedure (IAP), which was introduced originally at the MNI in 1955 by Juhn Wada (31). The IAP is a method of temporary hemianaesthesia of the brain that Wada had developed earlier in Japan (32). The technique involves injection of a barbiturate into each hemisphere in turn, anaesthetizing it briefly, during which time the awake hemisphere can be tested for its capacity for language and memory. In the original application, the test was used for preoperative determination of which hemisphere is dominant for speech. The memory application, initiated by Milner and associates (33), was an extension of the procedure designed to estimate the functionality of the medial temporal lobe structures of each hemisphere. Because this application of the IAP is not meant to test neocortex, it will not be discussed further in this chapter.

The IAP is a stressful, invasive procedure, and some low-functioning or highly emotional patients may be unable to cooperate sufficiently to undergo it. The amobarbital effect is short; thus, there is only a brief period during which to assess the patient. The assessment can be complicated by transient aphasia, mental confusion, agitation, transient visual-field defects, and (rarely) seizures or medication effects. Cross-flow into the contralateral hemisphere occurs in about 30% of cases (34), but this is unrelated to slow waves contralateral to injection (35) or to reduced metabolism contralateral to injection (measured as hypoperfusion via single photon emission tomography, or SPECT) (36). These findings make the significance of angiographic cross-filling uncertain.

Most centers, including the MNI, consider the IAP's role in determining cerebral dominance for language to be critical in left-handed patients and in those whose pattern on cognitive tests is discordant with the expected laterality of seizure focus. At the MNI and in some other centers, patients with atypical cerebral dominance according to the IAP undergo an additional positron emission tomography (PET) cognitive activation study for language. These experimental studies are promising but will not supplant the IAP in the near future because at present only one discrete aspect of language can be tested in a single PET study, leaving questions about other aspects of language unanswered (37).

Interpretation of results that suggest bilateral representation of language is the most controversial aspect of the speech IAP (38), and at the same time those results are particularly important for decisions about the extent of surgical excision from a potentially dominant or codominant hemisphere. Cooperative PET and IAP studies carried out in the same patients should lead to a clearer understanding of the nature and extent of bilateral representation of speech functions.

ACKNOWLEDGMENTS

This work was supported in part by grant MT-10314 from the Medical Research Council of Canada. I thank Dr. A. Olivier for the continuing opportunity to study his patients and Mr. Bernhard Baier for extraction of data from the neuropsychology archives. I also thank staff and fellows of the MNI neuropsychology unit for carrying out the many evaluations represented in this data bank.

REFERENCES

1. Grant DA, Berg GA. A behavioral analysis of degree of reinforcement and ease of shifting to new responses in a Weigl-type card-sorting problem. *Journal of Experimental Psychology* 1948;38:404–411.
2. Milner B. Some effects of frontal lobectomy in man. In: Warren JM, Akert K, eds. *The frontal granular cortex and behavior.* New York: McGraw-Hill, 1964:313–334.
3. Djordjevic J, Piazzini A, Jones-Gotman M. Two scoring systems for the Wisconsin Card Sorting Test: same or different measures? *Epilepsia* 1997;38(Suppl 8):163.
4. Jones-Gotman M. Localization of lesions by psychological testing. *Epilepsia* 1991;32(Suppl 5):41–52.
5. Jones-Gotman M, Milner B. Design fluency: the invention of nonsense drawings after focal cortical lesions. *Neuropsychologia* 1977;15(1):653–674.
6. Stroop JR. Studies of interference in serial verbal reactions. *Journal of Experimental Psychology* 1935;18:643–662.
7. Perret E. The left frontal lobe of man and the suppression of habitual responses in verbal categorical behaviour. *Neuropsychologia* 1974;12:323–330.
8. Spreen O, Strauss E. *A compendium of neuropsychological tests,* 2nd ed. New York: Oxford University Press, 1998.
9. Lezak MD. *Neuropsychological assessment,* 3rd ed. New York: Oxford University Press, 1995.
10. Reitan RM. Trail making test results for normal and

brain-damaged children. *Perceptual and Motor Skills* 1971;33:575–581.

11. Bornstein RA. Normative data on intermanual differences on three tests of motor performance. *Journal of Clinical and Experimental Neuropsychology* 1985;8:12–20.

12. Tiffin J, Asher EJ. The Purdue pegboard: norms and studies of reliability and validity. *Journal of Applied Psychology* 1948;32:234–247.

13. Jones-Gotman M, Smith ML, Zatorre RJ. Neuropsychological testing for localizing and lateralizing the epileptogenic region. In: Engel J Jr, ed. *Surgical treatment of the epilepsies*, 2nd ed. New York: Raven Press, 1993;245–261.

14. Jones-Gotman M. Psychological evaluation: testing hippocampal function. In: Engel J Jr, ed. *Surgical treatment of the epilepsies*, 2nd ed. New York: Raven Press, 1993;203–211.

15. Smith ML. Memory disorders associated with temporal-lobe lesions. In: Boller F, Grafman J, eds. *Handbook of neuropsychology*, vol 3. New York: Elsevier, 1989: 91–106.

16. Rausch R, Babb TL. Hippocampal neuron loss and memory scores before and after temporal lobe surgery for epilepsy. *Archives of Neurology* 1993;50:812–817.

17. Hermann BP, Seidenberg M, Schoenfeld J, et al. Neuropsychological characteristics of the syndrome of mesial temporal lobe epilepsy. *Archives of Neurology* 1997;54: 369–376.

18. Sass KJ, Sass A, Westerveld M, et al. Specificity in the correlation of verbal memory and hippocampal neuron loss: dissociation of memory, language, and verbal intellectual ability. *Journal of Clinical and Experimental Neuropsychology* 1992;14:662–672.

19. Mayeux R, Brandt J, Rosen J, et al. Interictal memory and language impairment in temporal lobe epilepsy. *Neurology* 1980;30:120–125.

20. Trenerry MR. Neuropsychologic assessment in surgical treatment of epilepsy. *Mayo Clinic Proceedings* 1996; 71:1196–1200.

21. Hermann BP, Seidenberg M, Dohan FC, et al. Reports by patients and their families of memory change after left anterior temporal lobectomy: relationship to degree of hippocampal sclerosis. *Neurosurgery* 1995;36: 39–45.

22. Hermann BP, Wyler AR, Somes G, et al. Pathological status of the mesial temporal lobe predicts memory outcome from left anterior temporal lobectomy. *Neurosurgery* 1992;31:652–657.

23. Majdan A, Sziklas V, Jones-Gotman M. Performance of healthy francophone and anglophone subjects and patients with resection from the temporal lobe on matched

tests of verbal and visuoperceptual learning. *Journal of International Neuropsychological Society* 1996;2:37.

24. Guerreiro C, Cendes F, Li L, et al. Clinical patterns of patients with temporal lobe epilepsy and pure amygdalar atrophy. *Epilepsia* 1999;40:453–461.

25. Rey A. L'examen psychologique dans les cas d'encephalopathie tramatique. *Archives of Psychology* 1942; 28:112.

26. Osterrieth P. Le test de copie d'une figure complexe. *Archives of Psychology* 1944;30:206–356.

27. Corkin S, Milner B, Rasmussen T. Somatosensory thresholds: contrasting effects of post-central gyrus and posterior parietal-lobe excisions. *Archives of Neurology* 1970;22:41–58.

28. Trenerry M, Jack C, Ivnik R, et al. MRI hippocampal volumes and memory function before and after temporal lobectomy. *Neurology* 1993;43:1800–1805.

29. Vickery B, Hays R, Graber J, et al. A health-related quality of life instrument for patients evaluated for epilepsy surgery. *Med Care* 1992;30:299–319.

30. Perrine K, Hermann BP, Vichrey BG, et al. The relationship of neuropsychological functioning to quality of life in epilepsy. *Archives of Neurology* 1995;52:997–1003.

31. Wada J. Youthful season revisited. *Brain and Cognition* 1997;33(1):7–10.

32. Wada J, Rasmussen T. Intracarotid injection of sodium Amytal for the lateralization of cerebral speech dominance: experimental and clinical observations. *Journal of Neurosurgery* 1960;17:226–282.

33. Milner B, Branch C, Rasmussen T. Study of short-term memory after intracarotid injection of sodium Amytal. *Transactions of the American Neurological Society* 1962;87:224–226.

34. Silfvenius H, Fagerlund J, Saisa M, et al. Carotid angiography in conjunction with amytal testing of epilepsy patients. *Brain and Cognition* 1997;33(1):33–49.

35. Gotman J, Bouwer M, Jones-Gotman M. Intracranial EEG study of brain structures affected by internal carotid injection of amobarbital. *Neurology* 1992;42:2136–2143.

36. McMacklin D, Dubeau F, Jones-Gotman M, et al. Assessment of the functional effect of the intracarotid sodium amobarbital procedure using co-registered MRI/HMPAO-SPECT and SEEG. *Brain and Cognition* 1997;33:50–70.

37. Jones-Gotman M, Smith ML, Wieser H-G. Intraarterial amobarbital procedures. In: Engel J Jr, Pedley T, eds. *Epilepsy: a comprehensive textbook*, vol 2. New York: Raven Press 1998;1767–1775.

38. Risse G, Gates J, Fangman M. A reconsideration of bilateral language representation based on the intracarotid amobarbital procedure. *Brain and Cognition* 1997;33: 118–132.

Neocortical Epilepsies.
Advances in Neurology, Vol. 84,
edited by P. D. Williamson, A. M. Siegel,
D. W. Roberts, V. M. Thadani, and M. S. Gazzaniga.
Lippincott Williams & Wilkins, Philadelphia © 2000.

37

Cerebral Lesions, Psychoses, and Epilepsy: Disease Versus Illness

David C. Taylor

Neurosciences Unit, Institute of Child Health and Great Ormond Street Hospital,
The Wolfson Centre, Mecklenburgh Square, London, WC1N 2AP, UK

The idea that epilepsy is a cause of madness is as old as history.

If it is true, then the precise conditions for such a relationship are of practical and theoretic interest. The practical interest is in the prevention of psychosis when treating persons with epilepsy. The theoretic interest is in the genesis and mechanisms of the psychoses in general. Confusion and dispute persist despite some research, partly because both *epilepsy* and *psychosis* are weak categories (1). They are too large, imprecise, and diverse. There is no certainty as to which is a subcategory of the other or whether both are simply aspects of cerebral disease. The apparent priority in "the psychoses of epilepsy" depends on the point of reference.

A study might be made of epilepsy among people diagnosed as psychotic or of psychosis arising in people with epilepsy. Researchers have had a variety of perspectives and purposes (2–6). Robust data are rare or are not gathered in useful quantities. The duration and the natural history of the various psychoses vary considerably. The aggregation of cases for analyses must be considered carefully when mechanisms are being sought rather than a series of patients being monitored. The idea that the mechanism of autism could not be connected with that of schizophrenia may be the basis for neglecting autism as a psychosis of epilepsy by epileptologists (*but* see 7–11). To be interesting, psychosis rates would have to be raised in pesons with epilepsy (and vice versa). It would be more interesting if the association was specific, not just an effect of "brain damage."

My perspective is *developmental* (12–17). Precisely, it is that the late consequence of an untoward event in the brain can be understood only in the context of (a) the nature and precise location of the event (lesions are not all the same); (b) the patient's age at the time of the event (between the fetus and late adult life); (c) contingent and intermediate events (the patient's biography); (d) the conditions at the time of the inquiry (the ambient state); (e) the genetic potential (for mental disorder); and (f) the area of interest (cognition, growth, state, mental states). Events producing what are later regarded as "the pathological basis" of epilepsy, such as neuronal migration defects, tumors, scars, or anoxic damage, will themselves have had different times of origin in ontogeny. They will have biased subsequent development in different ways. Their eventual impact in the area of interest (here it is psychosis) will be influenced by intermediate experiences and by others operating around the time of the onset of the psychosis. These include the reorganization of the brain reactive to, or compensatory to, the initial event, and that which is simply a part of normal development such as puberty. Consequently, brain events as causes, epilepsies as intermediate expressions, and psychoses as "outcomes" will be extremely complex relationships. Thus, a given genetic event leading to a tuber in tuberous sclerosis (TS) may relate to a variety of psychoses: autism, manic–depressive illness, schizophrenia, or confusional psychosis, depending on the preceding conditions of (a) to (e) (above). In what way can the TS be said to have *caused* these different outcomes?

The two principal sorts of chronic psychoses relate to (a) activity level and mood (affective) and (b) thought and speech (schizophrenic/autistic). Even so, they are not entirely separable (hyperkinetic autistic children, schizoaffective adults). The phenomenology of the psychoses of epilepsy is seen to vary with age and the developmental level, as does the semiology of the seizures, because the subject will have arrived at different levels of cerebral organization, life experiences, and age-related life concerns. Similar basic mechanisms thus may be found to underlie "psychoses" that are seen phenomenologically, and even biologically in some ways, to be different. It is a recurrent truth in medicine that the late consequences of an event can appear in a different guise from the original expression of it. Early encephalitis and later Parkinsonism, staphylococcal infection, chorea, mitral stenosis, syphilitic rash, and a presenile dementing illness proved to be causally connected. The modern biological, more developmental, approach to schizophrenia seems to acknowledge this logic, although it ignores the relevance of epilepsy in schizophrenia almost entirely (18–20).

My other perspective is from the philosophy of science, which recognizes the profound differences between the sorts of categories used in medicine; a calcifying haemangioma, mania, and a harsh upbringing are different *sorts* of categories. Only the first is a *thing*. In philosophy, it is said to have "substance," which allows it to be discussed with continual reference to its structure. The second is evident to behold only as it occurs and relies subsequently on description to be communicated to others. It can be agreed on by reference to formulae such as those of the *Diagnostic and Statistical Manual of Mental Disorders* (DSM) (21) or International Classification of Diseases (ICD), but description becomes constrained by them. The third depends on evocation by inquiry and empathic understanding of the unfolding account (which might be a lie but could be corroborated). Neuropsychiatric research depends on finding the relationships between such categories. Structure (what I call *disease*) is likely to be the most reliable. It is what is most satisfying to most doctors.

PSYCHOSES OF EPILEPSY

This chapter is not a general review. It is an account of various personal studies of psychoses related to epilepsy. The purpose of the studies has been to try to contribute to the understanding of the nature of the psychoses. The psychoses of epilepsy are of clinical importance in themselves. The larger ambition was to make discoveries that went beyond that data and contributed to the understanding of all psychotic processes. The studies all concern patients who have been treated for epilepsy by surgery. This group of patients provided what was, 30 years ago, a unique opportunity to know about the pathological basis of epilepsy. This, in turn, afforded the possibility of determining whether causal connections exist between the pathological changes in the brain and the psychoses.

The *null position* is that there is no connection between epilepsy, cerebral lesions, and psychosis. If there is no such connection, the psychoses of epilepsy simply would fail as a model for the study of psychosis. All the risk would be taken up by the genes, or by social process, or factors that remain unknown. Other sorts of study will be quoted here only if they relate to themes of these studies. To a limited extent, the opportunity these studies once afforded might seem to have been superseded by modern scanning. Even so, it would still be worth giving what is already known more thoughtful consideration because we are so far from understanding these processes.

Schizophrenia-like Psychoses

My first research on the topic was the Gowers Memorial Prize Essay for 1967 (22). The essay was a correlation analysis that was made possible only by the then recent acquisition by London University of the Atlas computer. One hundred patients who had undergone surgery and 100 variables were entered. The correlation analysis, which was massive for its time, allowed the meaning of the broad psychiatric categorizations used *(normal, neurosis, psychopathy,* and *psychosis)* to be made plain in a way that previously would not have been possible. It showed what was consistently said about the "psychotic" group. The items to which these terms related in a meaningful way were evident in the correlation matrix. Sixteen of the 100 patients in the study were categorized as "psychotic" before surgery. Eight subjects had "schizophreniform" psychoses; two were children with autistic spectrum disorders; one had a manic episode awaiting surgery; one had a schizoaffective disorder; and four had depressive psychoses. All these sorts of psychoses have been since studied independently. The variety of the psychoses included in the study weakened possible correlations for schizophrenia-like psychosis. It also made such suggestions that emerged from the analysis more persuasive. Almost all the correlations of the mental states were with items of social process. *Psychosis* was the only category to correlate with *pathology in the resected lobe.* Less mesial temporal sclerosis (MTS) and more focal lesions than expected were found, reminiscent of the concurrently published findings of Malamud (23) showing an association between schizophrenic states and limbic system tumors. *Age at onset* appeared as a correlate for *psychopathy* (young at onset) and *psychosis* (older at onset).

It formed the key lecture of my first American lecture tour, in 1969, to say that people

with TLE who developed schizophrenic symptoms were predictable from a prior knowledge of various risk characteristics. Something was wrong with the way their brain was working. What had gone wrong had happened a long time before it became evident that things were wrong (neurosyphilis again). The lecture was received politely in the department of psychiatry at a great university. The chairman praised the presentation, the method, and the English in which it was spoken in his words of thanks. In private, however, he counseled me that I was not talking about *psychiatry*. The psychoses, he explained patiently, were functional disorders that were defined as being inexplicable in structural terms. Imperfections in the brain would be *neurology*. This was the peak time for psychoanalytic domination of American psychiatry. Faced by such established beliefs, and by persisting in having the prize essay published as it was actually written, I waited until 1972 for it to appear in print. The paper also contained 16 detailed biographies illustrating the basis of diagnosis and illuminating the cases. These were regarded as irrelevant by most medical journal editors.

A relatively increased risk of schizophrenia-like psychosis for female subjects was evident in the material but not strong enough to be evident in the correlation analysis. It had been observed by others (24,25) who had no "ax to grind" and did not notice it. It is, interestingly, also evident in the recent paper by Mellers et al. (26), who did not notice it either.

In 1971, I applied the developmental approach to the data of Slater et al. (2) as well as that of (16) Falconer and Flor-Henry (27). The article showed that national statistics supported the finding of an excess of female patients (relative to the sex ratio in epilepsy) hospitalized with psychoses of epilepsy. The Slater et al. series (2) and Flor-Henry's (27) figures also showed a relative excess of female subjects. These series also supported the later than usual age of onset of epilepsy in patients developing schizophrenia-like psychosis. MTS would be less likely to be seen in epilepsies starting in later childhood and adolescence if prolonged febrile convulsions were part of its cause because age of onset was deemed as that at the first-ever seizure. In Slater et al.'s (2) series, the peak quinquennium of onset of established epilepsy was 10 to 14 for girls but 15 to 19 for boys. The peak age of onset of psychosis was also earlier in females. If only those epilepsies with onset before the age of 20 years are considered, 2 of 24 male patients, but 12 of 30 female subjects, had their onset of psychosis before the age of 20 years, suggesting that the onset of psychosis was linked to a developmental process. In general, female subjects are ahead of male subjects in all aspects of development. Slater et al.'s notion of some significant interval between the onset of the epilepsy and of the psychosis proved to be artefactual. Their material showed that exactly the same number of people became psychotic in every decade that passed after the onset of epilepsy. Besides, the psychosis follows the epilepsy by definition, and so there is certain to be a figure that describes the mean interval, however pointless it is to know it unless it is fairly constant.

From the point of view of the outcome of epilepsy surgery, the issues of age and interval are important. Fortunately, the emergence of schizophrenia is rare in surgical series. Manchanda et al. (28) saw 4.3% in a series of 300 patients seen for possible epilepsy surgery. Schizophrenic symptoms generally emerge early. Surgical teams have been reluctant to operate on patients displaying such symptoms. Monitoring the Irish series of more than 100 cases since 1994 revealed no patient offered for surgery with florid schizophrenic symptoms and only two in whom there was a perceptible risk that schizophrenia might supervene (Taylor and Moran, unpublished data). The trend is toward earlier surgery, however, and it becomes inevitable that patients at risk for later onset of schizophrenia will undergo surgery. Then it will appear as though there has been a causal connection between the surgery and the psychotic outcome.

From the point of view of the origin and nature of the schizophrenic process, the highly variable interval suggests that many factors will contribute to the effect. It appears that some patients' susceptibility around the time of the onset of epilepsy is such that the two processes are more or less synchronous. In others, it appears that a further process of cerebral dilapidation with age or the effects of seizures or medications is required before the psychotic process is revealed. In practical terms, operating despite schizophrenic symptoms or in the light of a high risk of their later occurrence is acceptable, provided the situation is made clear (29); that is, it will be for the comfort factor of not having seizures (22,30).

In 1975, patients from the Falconer series with at least 3 years' follow-up numbered 255. It was possible by then to set up a deliberate contrast between all 47 patients with "alien tissue" (AT) in the temporal lobe and 41 consecutive patients with MTS (13). The contrast was between psychosis rates and the distribution of psychotic patients by sex, by side, and by handedness, between those two groups of patients. The null position was that there was no, a priori, reason to believe that they may be different. Eleven of the 47 AT patients were psychotic as compared with 2 of the MTS. group. Psychotic patients also were preponderant in the left-operated, female, left-handed, later onset, patients. The bulk of these patients suffered from schizophrenia-like psychosis. An important "side issue" is that the excess of left-handedness cannot be explained in terms of "pathological left-handedness." First, because the excess is located only in the AT group and, second, because the left-handed group underwent operation for lesions on the left and right sides equally. The excess of left-handed persons seems to be the result of a developmental deviation consequent to the presence of a cerebral lesion early in development, usually prior to birth. It is a marker that cerebral organization is unusual. An excess of left-handedness was found among schizophrenics by Lishman and McMeekan (31). This 1975 study showed that various small-scale studies of epilepsy and schizophrenia will suggest various associations, depending on the age, sex, and handedness of the samples. Studies that exclude any of these groups in the belief that it provides for purity of effect are in danger of being biased against the usual trend in such cases.

At a meeting in Boston in 1976, I pressed the argument further (14). First, I drew attention to the fact that I would not be referring (as I am not now) to brief psychotic episodes or postictal states but only to psychoses that endured and were seen in clear consciousness. The inclusion of patients with only these brief states will cloud the issue of causal specificity hopelessly and will say nothing about the mechanism of schizophrenia.

Second, I drew attention to the fact that psychiatry, at the time of emergent classification, originally classified epilepsy as a major *functional* psychosis because there was no *particular* cerebral lesion accepted as its cause. Whereas the concept of there being other functional psychoses had survived from that time, epilepsy had come to be seen as a phenomenon resulting from a variety of causes. Could there equally be a "schizophrenic phenomenon" that could be promoted by a variety of causal agents? If so, then there could be variety even among those that were associated with temporal lobe epilepsy (TLE). Third, there was good reason, on the face of it, to compare the general phenomenology of the experience of a psychomotor seizure to the content of a psychosis. The first-rank symptoms of schizophrenia of Schneider compared closely to the "mental symptoms" of TLE described by Gastaut (32). The French had called the more exotic of them *micropsychoses*. There was no evidence, however, from a detailed study of aura experiences in this group of patients, later published in full (33), that the rich, exotic, experiential auras were associated with schizophrenia.

In view of the inaccessibilty of the original publication, I quote from the end of the paper, pages 35–36:

> One of the mysteries of schizophrenia, and the real implication of the problem of "interval" between epilepsy onset and psychosis onset,

has been why the schizophrenia waits before declaring itself. Here I turn to aphasiology for evidence and help. Jason Brown (34,35) has suggested that the developmental sequence in organizing the neural base of language is one that extends into middle life. It consists of a progressive condensation or contraction into highly specialized (and highly vulnerable) language areas. Supposing that there were, in the developing brain, a lesion that provoked epilepsy but which was not gross enough to produce a major reorganization of the developmental strategy in the brain. Such a lesion would not, in youth, necessarily produce serious consequences while the language system was extensively deployed through the hemisphere, though it may create some diffusion of language organization. As the normal contraction and condensation of language proceeds, however, the disruption created by the lesion may increase quite markedly and suddenly. If the disorder produced is to be described as schizophrenia then it will be both subtle and to some extent flexible. It has some of the characteristics of a semantic paraphasia. Interestingly, semantic paraphasias are associated with bilateral temporal and mild generalized cerebral disorder, as indeed were the epilepsies which Slater et al. and Flor-Henry described as those most likely to show schizophrenic breakdown. The other important component of psychosis is what aphasiologists call "denial" and what psychiatrists regard as a "failure of insight." The error is essentially uncorrectable because that is the nature of the error....Looking at the brain through the window provided by the surgery of temporal lobe epilepsy...I see a whole group of language/ thought disorders starting from Infantile Autism and extending into the late paraphrenias.

The metaphor I have used since, is that the resident librarian in the newly opened library (of the brain that will be schizophrenic) is an efficient eccentric whose memory allows the recovery of volumes on request despite an unusual filing system. Later, a more conventional person takes over the library and finds serious difficulties whenever he or she attempts conventional search.

In pursuing the issue of unusual brain organization further, a study was made of the responses of 31 patients who had undergone surgery to the Eysenck Personality Questionnaire. Left-operated male patients showed less extraversion than did right-operated male subjects, and left-operated female subjects had the highest Lie scores (36). The lie scale was used so heavily used that it strongly suggested a loss of contact with reality. These patients were the group of women who would be susceptible to developing schizophrenia. They were also much older as a group than any other sex-by-side group. A detailed and complex analysis was made of changes in Verbal and Performance IQ scores after surgery. This same group of female patients with AT lesions operated on the left proved to show anomalous changes in IQ scores unlike those seen in any other grouping (37). In a lecture to the American Epilepsy Society, I illustrated the effect of Falconer's decision not to operate on any more patients with schizophrenia. It happened that he personally did no more operations that involved removing AT lesions from the left temporal lobe of a female patient.

The paradigm case of schizophrenia following epilepsy was outlined by Falconer (16), his case 1; surgery was done on this patient in February 1951. The case is described also in Falconer et al. (38) and as case 7 of Cavanagh (39) inter alia. The importance of the case is the detail of the information and the length and accuracy of the follow-up. The child had many advantages of birth and upbringing and received the best available medical care throughout her life.

The 1953 paper reports that this child was of normal birth and early development and walked and started a few words at the age of 12 months. By 14 months, however, she became fretful, irritable, and oppositional. She would stamp and scream for no apparent reason. At the age of 2 years, epileptic attacks were typified by behavioral arrest and a blank stare. The right arm might extend, and she would appear to be plucking at an object. Coarse nystagmoid movements and head drops would follow; the whole attack lasted up to 3 minutes and was followed by confusion. From that time, she did not regress or progress in her development. Electroencephalogphy (EEG) was obtainable in deep sleep and revealed relative flattening over the left temporal and occipital areas. Irregular spike and wave was seen over both hemispheres. Skull radiographs and ventriculography showed a mass lesion of the temporal lobe 5.5 × 2.2 cm with calcification. Neurosurgical intervention was decided on after much consideration. Cavanagh's paper describes the lesion best. Professor Michael Farrell recently looked at the papers and confirmed that the description would not be changed in modern terminology. In the specimen, the tumor occupied the posterior third of the left temporal pole. "...the most striking features of which were large numbers of calcareous granules and numerous cystic spaces. The tumor tissue was composed of an intimate mixture of astrocytes of relatively normal but hyperplastic type and oligodendroglia."

The initial response to surgery was excellent, although she had an extensive hemianopia. Within 8 months, her behavior and speech had improved, and she was seizure free. By age 5, she was seen as having made considerable progress. Subsequently, although seizure free, she was prone to tiresome and oppositional behaviours. There was a period of school refusal shortly after starting school at age 6, and throughout her education, teachers found her difficult. Her intellectual functioning was, however, below that expected in the type of schools she attended. She was tried in several private secondary schools, but her results were generally disappointing. She was strongly left-handed, as were other members of her family. She spent a period of time working in another country in a simple occupation but that was not satisfactory.

By the age of 19, it was clear that she had a mental illness, but it was less clear what this illness was. Much had been attributed to interpersonal problems in the family, but it became gradually clearer that she had paranoid ideas. She fixed on the idea that she had an intravaginal tampon. Gradually, there appeared auditory but also visual hallucinations. She believed that radar was spying on her and that she had appeared on her own television set.

She was agitated, insomniac, and showed incongruous affect. At other times, her preserved warm affect made her psychiatrists doubt whether this was "real" schizophrenia. Despite the continuing absence of seizures, she was treated with antiepileptic drugs as well as antipsychotics and electroconvulsive therapy (ECT). She spent increasing lengths of time in sheltered situations or in mental hospitals. Her last measured IQ was P77 and V85. Her left-handedness might have been familial, and her speech, in her right brain as there was no initial loss, but rather a gain in speech following surgery.

Schizophrenia is a hazard waiting to be uncovered by events. For some patients, TLE and its antecedents are among the events. Some of the relevant elements are accessible from analysis of the relatively few cases that provide worthwhile information and that are available for study worldwide. The null positions are that having an unusually made brain does no harm, does not affect behavior, or is a positive thing. Of course, for much of the subject's life that may have been true. There is another problem: The psychoses are mainly episodic or chronically recurrent, which makes it more difficult to see them as brain dysfunctions. Much of psychiatric practice does not take the qualities of the brain into consideration seriously because of the obvious interposition of the person and of the events of the person's biography. It was the nature of the person with which the psychiatry of my American chairman was concerned. We are mostly inclined to judge human behavior in moral terms. That is to say, we are not, instinctively, inclined to see it as an aberration of brain functioning. On the other hand, there is a general credence given to the notion that there is some association between cerebral malfunction and behavioral problems. Syphilis, acquired immunodeficiency syndrome (AIDS), and rabies serve as reminders. All the research referred to in the preceding sections will go for nothing unless it can be shown not only that there is some general increase of risk but also there are specific associations between cerebral lesions and particular psychiatric states. The following stand in the way of the endeavor:

1. The general weakness of research strategies, for example, ignorance of relevant but unmeasured elements
2. Weakness in our understanding of development and the import of time and of aging
3. Psychiatric nomenclature, that is, its weak categories and definitions
4. Environmental, situational, interpersonal, or intrapsychic elements of great effect
5. Interactions between items 1 through 4 that add to the improbability of finding coherent associations between the brain lesion and the behavior

This means that we should be obliged to try to make sense of each case as far as we can and each research result insofar as possible.

Asperger's Syndrome

At the time when Falconer's early cases were being studied, nothing was known of the syndrome of autistic psychopathy, described by Asperger (40). His work owes its recognition in the West to Lorna Wing (41). The deficits of persons with this personality construction are similar to many of those described in the older vocabulary of "epileptic personality," and they will be recognized by epileptologists. They imply (42), first, severe impairment of reciprocal social interaction; second, some all-absorbing narrow interest that tends to be foisted onto others; third, problems of speech and language, including some possible delay of their development, and rather pedantic speech forms with odd prosody; fourth, nonverbal communication problems, including limited use of gesture, gauche body language, and inappropriate, stiff, facial expression. Szatmari et al. (43) gave particular attention to the aloneness and problems of making friends and the inability to read the meaning of the facial expressions and emotions of others. It is a disorder of empathy. In the study by Falconer et al. (44), patients 13 and 23 seem to meet the criteria from among the first 31 operated cases that I have rereviewed.

Case 13 was given up for adoption. He appeared to be blind and was treated as such, although he later proved not to be blind. Seizures began at the age of 3 years. He also had outbursts of rage and overactivity interspersed with quiet periods. His development was delayed, and his early life was punctuated by admissions to various facilities for persons with epilepsy. He underwent operation at the age of 13 with findings of MTS in the left temporal lobe. He became seizure free, improved cognitively, and developed good musical skills. He was regarded as unusually "blunt" and to have fixed and determined ideas. Although he continued to do well in adult life, he remained "odd." He never read a frivolous book, only those on world affairs, which he took seriously. He did not smile at people, which, he explained, was not in his nature. He continued his academic studies in another country.

Case 23 underwent right temporal lobectomy at age 36 with findings of MTS. At the age of 19 months, he suffered a prolonged febrile convulsion. A sense of not daring to move for a few moments soon supervened. Noticeable complex partial seizures (CPS) followed at the age of 7 years. He was of superior intelligence and did well at school. His passion was arithmetic, and he would use difficult mental mathematics to drive away his seizures. He was not fully relieved of seizures as occasional nocturnal grand mal occurred. He suffered depressive feelings both before and after surgery. He wrote to me, in response to my inquiry, 22 years after his operation. His letter was couched in rather convoluted business language that separated him as its subject. He was engaged in precise mathematical work as his profession and in precise activities by way of recreation. The letter contained the details of the mathematics in which he was engaged in generous quantity.

Both these operations would have to be counted as a success because they altered the biographies of these two men in positive directions. Contemporary cases, seen in Ireland, are of more intensely affected persons who remain invalids because of their mental condition, which tends to produce a period of deterioration around puberty. Children with these traits also vary considerably in their general level of functioning depending on their intelligence and the usefulness of whatever comes to absorb their interest.

Affective Disorders

Falconer and colleagues were working alongside psychiatrists who were treating people with epilepsy. The endeavor was relatively new and untried. Looking again at the first group of 31 cases they reported (44), the prevalence of depression and suicide is striking. The reason is plainly that those most likely to be put forward at that time were the most desperate. Let me set the scene for those who might not otherwise understand the scale and frequency of the psychopathology to which we refer.

The *first* case is given above.

The *second* was a woman who had a single convulsion in infancy and established TLE from the age of 15 years. At the age of 20, she had developed paranoid schizophrenia. She was 43 at the time of her left temporal lobectomy. She did not recover consciousness after the operation.

The *third* patient first had a right and then a left lobectomy and died in status epilepticus 6 months after the second operation.

The *fourth* patient was described before operation as rigid, demanding, self-pitying, querulous, hypochondriacal, and depressive. He had lived at an epilepsy colony. Left temporal lobectomy was a successful intervention.

The *fifth* patient was a 9-year-old girl who had been sexually abused (called "seduced" in the notes) while at an epilepsy colony. She had been sent there for her flagrantly sexualized behavioral problem (Cavanagh case 8). She was aggressive, violent, willful, and manipulative. This kind of behavior is seen in our studies at Great Ormond Street and also in Dublin in girls with mass lesions of the right temporal lobe starting to have epilepsy around the middle of their first decade. She became seizure free but experienced many psychological problems. She also suffered a severe postnatal depression some 20 years later.

The *sixth* patient was a 45-year-old man whose first seizure was a febrile convulsion with chicken pox in 1910. He had also lived in an epilepsy colony for several years and had been unemployed most of his life. He was described, before operation, as "colorless, with slow deliberate speech, suspicious, and moody." His seizures gradually abated after right temporal lobectomy, which revealed MTS. His depression was treated after operation with ECT on more than one occasion. He later gained paid employment and died of cancer of the lung 12 years after the operation.

The *seventh* patient suffered posttraumatic epilepsy from the age of 18 years until his operation at the age of 45. He had been "psychotically depressed" in bouts for the previous 8 years. After right lobectomy, seizures were reported as rare. They were, anyway, probably hysterical as was the disorder that confined him much of the time to a wheelchair. He had recurrent bouts of depression, treated with ECT until his death from a cerebrovascular accident (CVA) 16 years later.

The *eighth* patient suffered a right-sided transient paresis on the right following his first febrile seizure at the age of 2 years. His subjective auras were distressing abdominal pain, tenesmus, and the passage of flatus. By the time of his admission for operation at the age of 23, he was a deteriorated, drunken man with gross social incapacity and flagrant sexual behavior. Right lobectomy revealed MTS, and the seizures stopped, but he died of alcoholism in a rooming house for derelicts 2 years later.

The *ninth* patient was a businessman who had developed seizures at age 21. They interfered with his work and were an embarrassment. Two years later, a small neuroglial lesion was removed from the left temporal lobe (Cavanagh case 6) (39). I last saw him 20

years after the operation. He had an occasional ecstatic aura when exercising that may coincide with making an unusual error in his game of squash. He was a successful businessman who was happily married with a family.

The *tenth* patient started CPS in his forties, characterized by smell and reminiscence of the content of a war incident. This seems like the release of a posttraumatic stress disorder. He would verbalize the incident in his attacks. Left temporal lobectomy revealed no lesion (missed cortical dysplasia?). Seizures occurred sporadically over the next 20 years, but 3 years after his operation, he became subject to bouts of low mood.

This is enough to establish that a tradition of detailed biographic and psychiatric inquiry was established stemming from the sort of work done at the country's principal postgraduate psychiatric hospital and its conjoined Institute of Psychiatry. This element of preoperative workup became standard for every patient as a psychiatrist was allocated to the team from the earliest days. The postoperative inquiries came from Falconer's annual recall for interview and assessment at 10 years. To this endeavour was added the work of a series of psychiatric research assistants. Thus, it arose that patients would be followed up for 20 years or longer, exceeding by far the years over which patients had suffered epilepsy before operation. To say, as the neuropathologist Bruton said, that the incidence of depression rose from 0.4% to 10% is simply an error (45). It is one of several rather serious errors in such a prestigious book (46). Postoperative depression is a serious issue. Probably it is best predicted from the family and preoperative history and the nature of the patient's predicament. To the predicament and the genetic potential is added the cerebral and psychological trauma of surgery, and to that is added the burden of success or of failure. Postoperative suicide is a serious issue. It is probably best predicted from the preoperative mental state and the history of previous suicide attempts. All successful suicides will be postoperative but not necessarily will have surgery as the cause but only, necessarily, be located in that period of time (47).

In 1989, I reviewed some of the literature on epilepsy and affective disorder and reconsidered some of the lessons of Falconer's series (13). Cases were added of current youths with epilepsy who were part of my current practice. A particular concern was to illustrate the value of studying the much rarer phenomenon of hypomania when looking for brain/behavioral relationships. The reason was because hypomania is far less likely to be reactive or situational than depression. That can readily fade into sadness and situational distress and will run at some 20% of the population who might be "cases" on any given day.

Flor-Henry's original study (27) included cases from Falconer's series as well as Slater's. He found, in these seriously and chronically sick people, a trend toward right-sided foci among those with affective disorders, which contrasted with an opposite trend in schizophrenia. These trends have not been found consistently, although the basis for diagnosis has been extremely inconsistent and the timing of events is rarely given. The value of more consistent findings would be that they might suggest something about the cerebral mechanism involved. The most consistent finding of all has been the association of organic mania to right hemisphere damage. There is also a substantial body of evidence in psychology that suggests that the right brain plays a major role in the recognition and management of affective stimuli. A seminal case was first given before an audience at a meeting in Waterville, Maine, about 25 years ago:

One of the items of interest was that his "obscure" illness led him to be seen by Dr. Sargant, the country's leading general psychiatrist, who immediately referred him to Professor Denis Hill. Actually, the problem was evident in the raindrop calcification at the tip of the right temporal pole seen in the straight radiograph of the skull. He was 19 by the time the lobectomy was done that revealed the haemangioma. All was well until he became delirious with measles and mumps together at the age of 5 years. Initially, his results at school were consistent with his IQ (preoperatively, V144; P128); after the age of 11, they deteriorated away from group and family expectations. Around this time, his episodic disturbing "dreams," reminiscences, and déjà vu began, together with low moods. He thought much about suicide and first attempted it at the age of 12 with a massive dose of aspirin after a disappointing examination result. At 14, he suffered adenoviral encephalitis and lost 3 months from school. He was mercilessly bullied by boys and felt despised by masters. He left school as soon as possible and was unable to proceed to university. Grand mal started at 16, with further changes of mood, which began to include swings in which he would work furiously, experience elation, and change jobs. He was neat, overly friendly, and garrulous. Then he would crash to depression and sleep 18 of 24 hours. He made further overdose attempts but changed his mind. After his operation, his fits stopped, but his mood swings continued. One evening, he spoke to his psychiatrist on the telephone to tell him he was well. Around midnight, he spoke to his father. He requested a call from his landlady for 6.20 a.m. so he could go to church with friends. When she called, he was dead. He had consumed a massive quantity of a drug that he had secreted in the garden over a period of time.

This is an example of the impulsive suicide of the young. There is no family history of affective disorder. The prenatally acquired lesion expressed itself perhaps through some facilitation of two separate bouts of viral encephalitis, through biasing his IQ scores, though the "dream" sequence, through rich subjective CPS, and via the grand mals. Should we doubt that it also affected his mood state? The seizures and subclinical attacks reduced his efficiency and created a negative social evaluation, all of which led him into a totally different part of the social system than he might otherwise have occupied.

Over the years, since I reported this case, similar scenarios have been seen. The case is important because it is a bridge between the more adult and the childhood form of the psychiatric presentation of this type of lesion. A similar female teenager was referred to me by Dr. Rasmussen. In our study at Great Ormond Street, we have seen a number of children presenting at around 5 to 9 years of age with mass lesions and marked oppositional behaviour. In girls, this is often colored with sexually explicit and rude behavior.

Suicide

The study (47) was designed to inquire further into the nature of suicides prompted by the five per mean 5 years of follow-up reported by Taylor and Falconer (48). When the series was at 296, there were 193 patients who had more than 5 years of follow-up. Thirty-seven had died, four of the late results of their original small tumor, seven of other natural causes, eight during epileptic seizures, three in accidents, six in unclear circumstances that could have been suicides, and nine by unequivocal suicide. Eight of 11 deaths in the first 2 years of follow-up were by suicide (5) or in unclear circumstances (3). The suicides and unclear deaths aged around twenty years died by impulsive acts. The next group of them was aged between 30 and 40 (a decade younger than the peak decade in the general population). There was a high loading of the usual suicide risk factors, such as isolation, bereavement, divorced or single status, physical illness, and aging. Even from the small sample briefly described already, it can be seen that this population was one at exceptional risk, up to 50 times expectation. Half the patients who died by suicide had had no fits since their operation. On the other hand, there was no other period of risk anywhere near as high as that in the first 2 postoperative years. It is possible that some patients see surgery as the last defense against a wretched life, and when it seems to have failed to modify their plight, they kill themselves. This highlights the fact that it is their plight, rather than their epilepsy, that is at issue. My most recent experience of suicide postoperatively confirmed for this me. Suicide is intensely

multifactorial and has "accidental" factors added from outside the individual's control, such as the chance of rescue from otherwise certain death. That makes it unlikely that there will prove to be brain–behavior correlations.

Autistic Syndromes

Epileptology has been dominated by an adult perspective. The neocortical epilepsies have grown in prominence from the possibilities offered by surgical treatment. Surgical treatment, too, has been dominated by an adult perspective. Yet the inexorable direction of surgical treatment is toward shortening the interval between onset of epilepsy and investigation and between investigation and surgery. Given the age-related incidence of epilepsy, this will lead to an increase in the treatment of children by surgery, which, in turn, focuses attention on the surgical treatment of developmental regression occurring at the onset of epilepsy in early childhood. The possibilities were recently reviewed (49). Developmental regression is obvious enough and worrying enough to deserve attention without too close analysis of the nature of that process; however, it is where recent advances in the surgery of epilepsy meet the older issue of childhood autism and the autistic spectrum of disorders.

The possibility exists that where the epilepsies associated with autistic regression have a lesional basis, their study might throw light on a mechanism of autism. The problem is to make assessments of the nature of the regression that are as accurate and elegant as the rest of the work. Autistic regression is a severe and intractable disorder. Although it sometimes improves over time, it is less likely to do so when associated with mental retardation. There are close parallels with the situation in the early years of temporal lobe surgery in adults. The closest attention must be given to the whole state of being of these children and their families. Falconer operated on two children with autism, both of whom died within a few years of the operation unrelieved of any symptoms.

Autistic syndromes are rarely included in reviews of the psychoses of epilepsy. Yet the incidence of epilepsy in autism makes it by far the most common association between epilepsy and psychosis. About 40% of people with autism have seizures at some time, with half of them starting before the age of 3 years. This close association between epilepsy and autism was first observed by Schain and Yannet (50). The epilepsy might start before language develops, or language may regress at the onset of epilepsy. Autism in that case might be a form of Landau–Kleffner syndrome (epileptic aphasia). Some children react with increased activity, becoming distractible, inappropriate, and frantic. Others move into a world of their own, showing features of disorders in the autistic spectrum (51). Infantile spasms are a minority form of the epilepsies that lead into autistic regression, but all such seizures are of remarkably early onset. In the study by Wong (11), 80% had onset before 12 months of age.

In the process of being considered for surgical treatment, extensive data are accumulated regarding the locality, nature, and lateralization of the lesion as well as the neurologic and psychiatric diagnoses. These data have been studied in the program of epilepsy surgery at Great Ormond Street. One hundred operations were performed from 1991 to 1997, and more than 400 children referred for consideration of surgical treatment have been reviewed or are still under review. The program does not solicit or reject subjects with mental retardation (learning difficulties), language disorder, neurologic signs, or behavioral problems. All potential candidates for surgery are seen by a neuropsychiatrist. The clinical interview is to ascertain the nature and severity of psychiatric disorder in the child and family and classify them where they are namable. A DSM-IV diagnosis was made for all the children seen by the neuropsychiatrist except those who showed no symptoms and those so retarded (but not autistic) that no useful statement could be made. The hemisphere affected (side) refers to the balance of MRI and EEG and clinical evidence in those who are unoperated (left, right, uncertain) or the side of the operation or proposed operation. *Mass lesions* refer to all lesions, whether imaged on MRI or revealed on pathological examination, that show aggregations of abnormal cells replacing normal structures, such as dysembryoplastic neuroepithelial tumours (DNETs), tubers, astrocytomas, cortical dysplasia or other mass structures. Age at onset of epilepsy is taken as the time of the first seizure ever. The diagnosis of mental retardation given here was made on clinical grounds.

Ninety-eight patients were seen by the neuropsychiatrist between 1993 and 1996. There were 37 mass lesions (20 right, 17 left), and 35 of the children (36%) were retarded. Eight children had Asperger's syndrome (DSM-IV 299.8). Three were boys; six had abnormalities in the right brain. Two of the eight had mass lesions with an onset of epilepsy at 60 months. One of the eight was mentally retarded. There were 11 children in the group with autistic syndromes. Nine were boys. Ten of the 11 were affected in the right brain, and 10 of the 11 showed some kind of mass lesion (six DNETs), of which nine were in the right temporal lobe. Nine of the 11 were retarded. The age at onset of epilepsy for those mass lesions was 9 months.

This study suggested that those with autistic spectrum disorders (other than Asperger's syndrome) had different associations from those with other psychiatric diagnoses. More boys than girls were affected, there were more right- than left-sided lesions, the lesions were more likely to be mass lesions of prenatal origins, and onset of epilepsy was particularly early.

The excess of right-sided lesions is compatible with many neuropsychological reports, summarized and developed by Shields et al. (52), suggesting that early onset right cerebral dysfunction produces deficits that, in some respects, resemble autistic spectrum disorders. Bolton and Griffiths (53), in a study of 18 patients with TS, that the closest association between TS and autism was where there was a tuber in a temporal lobe. They found no bias as to side, and gender was not reported. Our study confirms the association between mass lesions of the temporal lobes and autistic features in a sample in whom early onset epilepsy is an important intervening variable. Given these conditions, mental retardation is likely to coexist with autism, as it does generally.

A cluster of factors were associated with autism in our series: right temporal lesions of prenatal origin, male sex, and seizure onset in the first year of life. The causal relationship between these elements is unknown, and a further genetic factor may be required to produce an autistic outcome. Children with Asperger's syndrome were considered separately. The factors associated with that syndrome were different by sex, by side, by nature of lesion, by IQ, and by a different preponderance as to the right side; however, numbers of cases in the psychiatric groups are small. The general importance of epilepsy and EEG abnormalities in pervasive development disorders (PDD) was clarified in the study by Tuchman and Rapin (54). A third of their sample of nearly 600 children with PDD or autistic spectrum disorders had suffered regression. Although only 11% had suffered seizures, 8% of the remainder had epileptiform EEGs. In the context of this study, early onset of epilepsy almost demands a cerebral lesion of prenatal origin.

From a practical, clinical standpoint, it is clear that a subgroup of children with early onset epilepsy and mass lesions of the neocortex will be at high risk of autistic and global regression. Surgical treatment can be offered as a matter of urgency. Initial appraisal suggests that usually some of the intensity is removed from unwanted behaviors. The outcome of such treatment must await a significant period of follow-up. There remains the haunting memory of Falconer's case 1.

Envoi

Over the last 30 years, the study of the psychoses of epilepsy has been confined largely to case reports and analyses of particular groups, such as those arising in particular series. There has been little hypothesis-generated research to test the validity of claims that certain cascade sequences and aggregations of risk factors are overrepresented to the point that they might suggest a causal mechanism. Because there are relatively few cases being studied, each study might contain considerable biases arising from selection processes, some of which might not be realized by the study authors. Progress might improve if cases were explored in detail, in depth, and over time. By operating on young people with neocortical epilepsy, the possibility exists that more of the serious mental disorders will arise postoperatively rather than preoperatively. This effect will not be caused by surgery, but it will provide for the possibility of predicting (from the presence of certain elements) who is at risk. Alternatively, good, original data will allow following back to uncover what the factors of risk to the various psychoses might be. Work in hand at several centers throughout the world will enable this sort of audit to be fruitful.

In my model (1), three major components must be considered if a sickness is to be understood. The sickness in question here is a complex conjoining of two illnesses, arising in a given sequence, arising in turn from a range of possible tissue changes, arising in turn from a whole range of potential causes. Starting from the concept the *neocortical epilepsies* (at least *some* limitations are imposed), we are unlikely to arrive at much understanding. Most advances in medicine have come from microbiology. They have come from using the medical model, which is to reduce a problem gradually to the finest possible level of analysis. Over the next 30 years, I hope we will begin to treat each of the lesions arising in the brain as an individual disease whose natural history needs to be known. This cannot be achieved by the "lumping" that is needed to achieve the case numbers that editors and scientists seem to consider needed to produce a publishable paper. To some extent, TS has led the way, although it is a multisystem disease, largely because it is relatively common. Psychotic states and epilepsies are at a level removed from the disease to which they draw attention. We are distracted by habit from the fact that they are intangible ephemera. They are just messages from a brain made distraught by its lesion. Somehow, we have the trick of mind that still argues that, because there is not always a lesion, the messages are the real thing. What is real is that in such a case we do not yet know what the disease is. So we pretend it is the illness. That was the history of schizophrenia, too. Having invented the construct, we are faced with the problem of how to solve its causation or understand its mechanism in a way that applies to the whole construct. It seems likely that there are lesions of a sort that, when placed in such a place at a particular time, make certain people more likely than others to suffer epilepsy or become psychotic at a future time. It is just a matter of filling in the gaps.

I just cannot get over the feeling that we did not listen to what we were told by Falconer's case 1.

REFERENCES

1. Taylor D. The components of sickness. In: Ounsted C, Apley J, eds. *One child.* London: SIMP Heinemann, 1982.
2. Slater E, Beard A, Glithero E. The schizophrenia-like psychoses of epilepsy. *Br J Psychiatry* 1963;109:95–150.
3. Kim W. Psychiatric aspects of epileptic children and adolescents. *J Am Acad Child Adolesc Psychiatry* 1992;30:252–265.
4. Mace C, Trimble M. Psychosis following temporal lobe surgery: a report of six cases. *J Neurol Neurosurg Psychiatry* 1991;54:639–644.
5. Mace C. Epilepsy and schizophrenia. *Br J Psychiatry* 1993;163:439–455.
6. Bruton C, Stevens J, Frith C. Epilepsy, psychosis, and schizophrenia: clinical and neurological correlations. *Neurology* 1994;44:34–42.
7. Rutter M. Autistic children: infancy to adulthood. *Seminars in Psychiatry* 1970;2:435–450.
8. Volkmar F, Douglas N. Seizure disorders in Autism. *J Am Acad Child Adolesc Psychiatry* 1990;29:127–129.
9. Gillberg C, Coleman M. *The biology of the autistic syndromes,* 2nd ed. Oxford: MacKeith Press, 1992.
10. Deonna T, Ziegler A-L, Mourra-Serra J, et al. Autistic regression in relation to limbic pathology: report of two cases. *Dev Med Child Neurol* 1993;35:158–176.
11. Wong V. Epilepsy in children with autistic spectrum disorder. *J Child Neurol* 1993;8:317–322.
12. Taylor D. Ontogenesis of epileptic psychoses: a reanalysis. *Psychol Med* 1971;1:247–253.
13. Taylor DC. Affective disorder in epilepsies: a neuropsychiatric review. *Behav Neurol* 1989;2:49–68.
14. Taylor D. Epileptic experience, schizophrenia, and the temporal lobe. *McLean Hospital Journal Special Issue* 1977;June:22–39.
15. Taylor DC. Factors influencing the occurrence of schizophrenia-like psychosis in patients with temporal lobe epilepsy. *Psychol Med* 1975;5:249–254.
16. Falconer M. Reversibility by temporal lobe resection of the behavioural abnormalities of temporal lobe epilepsy. *N Engl J Med* 1973;289:451–455.
17. Rourke B. The syndrome of non-verbal learning disabilities: developmental manifestations in neurological disease, disorder, and dysfunction. *Clinical Neuropsychologist* 1988;2:293–330.
18. Buckley P, Moore C, Long H, et al. ¹H-Magnetic resonance spectroscopy of the left temporal and frontal lobes in schizophrenia: clinical, neurodevelopmental, and cognitive correlates. *Biol Psychiatry* 1994;36:792–800.
19. Castle D, Abel K, Takei N, et al. Gender differences in schizophrenia: hormonal effect or sub-types? *Schizophr Bull* 1995;21:1–12.
20. Trojanowski J, Arnold S. In pursuit of the molecular neuropathology of schizophrenia. *Arch Gen Psychiatry* 1995;52:274–276.
21. American Psychiatric Association. *Diagnostic and statistical manual of mental disorders,* 4th ed, 1994.
22. Taylor DC. Mental state and temporal lobe epilepsy: a correlative account of 100 patients treated surgically. *Epilepsia* 1972;13:727–765.
23. Malamud N. The epileptic focus in temporal lobe epilepsy from a pathological standpoint. *Arch Neurol* 1967;14:113–123.
24. Rodin E, De Jong R, Waggoner R, et al. Relationship between certain forms of psychomotor epilepsy and schizophrenia. *Arch Neurol Psychiatry* 1957;77:449–463.
25. Glaser G. The problem of psychosis in psychomotor temporal lobe epilepsies. *Epilepsia* 1964;5:271–278.
26. Mellers J, Adachi N, Takei N, et al. SPET of verbal fluency in schizophrenia and epilepsy. *Br J Psychiatry* 1998;173:69–74.
27. Flor-Henry P. Psychosis and temporal lobe epilepsy: a controlled investigation. *Epilepsia* 1969;10:363–395.
28. Manchanda R, Schaefer B, McLachlan R, et al. Psychiatric disorders in candidates for surgery for epilepsy. *J Neurology Neurosurg Psychiatry* 1996;61:82–89.
29. Taylor DC, Neville BGR, Cross JH. New measures of outcome needed for the surgical treatment of epilepsy. *Epilepsia* 1997;38:625–630.
30. Reutens DC, Savard G, Andermann F, et al. Results of surgical treatment in temporal lobe epilepsy with chronic psychosis. *Brain* 1997;120:1929–1936.
31. Lishman A, McMeekan E. Hand preference patterns in psychiatric patients. *Br J Psychiatry* 1976;129:148–166.
32. Gastaut H. So-called "psychomotor" or temporal lobe epilepsy. *Epilepsia* 1953;2:59–96.
33. Taylor D, Lochery M. Temporal lobe epilepsy: origin and significance of simple and complex auras. *J Neurol Neurosurg Psychiatry* 1987;50:673–681.
34. Brown J. The neural organization of language: aphasia and neuropsychiatry. In: Reiser M, Arieti S, eds. *American handbook of psychiatry,* vol 4. New York: Basic Books, 1975.
35. Brown J, Jaffe J. Hypothesis on cerebral dominance. *Neuropsychologia* 1975;13:107–110.

36. Taylor D, Marsh S. The influence of sex and side of operation on personality questionnaire responses after temporal lobectomy. In: Gruzelier J, Flor-Henry P, eds. *Hemisphere asymmetries of function in psychopathology.* Amsterdam: Elsevier, 1979.

37. Taylor D. Developmental stratagems organising intellectual skills: evidence from studies of temporal lobectomy for epilepsy. In: Knights R, Bakker D, eds. *The neuropsychology of learning disorders: theoretical approaches.* Baltimore: University Park Press, 1976.

38. Falconer M, Pond D. Temporal lobe epilepsy with personality and behaviour disorders caused by an unusual calcifying lesion. *J Neurol Neurosurg Psychiatry* 1953; 16:234–244.

39. Cavanagh J. On certain small tumours in the temporal lobe. *Brain* 1958;81:389–405.

40. Asperger H. Die autistischen Psychopathen im Kindesalter. *Archiv für Psychiatrie und Nervenkranken* 1944; 117:76–136.

41. Wing L. Asperger's syndrome: a clinical account. *Psychol Med* 1981;11:115–129.

42. Gillberg C. *Clinical child neuropsychiatry.* Cambridge: Cambridge University Press, 1995.

43. Szatmari P, Brenmer R, Nagy J. Asperger's syndrome: a review of the clinical features. *Can J Psychiatry* 1989; 22:554–556.

44. Falconer M, Hill D, Meyer A, et al. Treatment of temporal lobe epilepsy by temporal lobectomy. *Lancet* 1955;1:827–835.

45. Bruton C. *The neuropathology of temporal lobe epilepsy.* Oxford: Oxford University Press, 1988.

46. Taylor D. Review of Bruton 1988. *Psychol Med* 1989;19:525–526.

47. Taylor D, Marsh S. Implications of long term follow-up in epilepsy: with a note on the causes of death. In: Penry J, ed. *Epilepsy: the eighth international symposium.* New York: Raven Press, 1977.

48. Taylor D, Falconer M. Clinical, socio-economic, and psychological changes after temporal lobectomy for epilepsy. *Br J Psychiatry* 1968;114:1247–1261.

49. Engel J Jr, Cascino G, Shields D. Surgically remediable syndromes. In: Engel J Jr, Pedley T, eds. *Epilepsy: a comprehensive textbook.* Philadelphia: Lippincott–Raven, 1997.

50. Schain R, Yannet H. Infantile autism: an analysis of 50 cases and a consideration of certain relevant neuropsychological concepts. *J Pediatr* 1960;57:560–567.

51. Wing L. The autistic spectrum. *Lancet* 1997;2: 1761–1766.

52. Shields J, Varley R, Broks P, et al. Hemispheric functioning developmental language disorders and high-level autism. *Dev Med Child Neurol* 1996;38:473–486.

53. Bolton P, Griffiths P. Association of tuberous sclerosis of temporal lobes with autism and atypical autism. *Lancet* 1997;349:392–395.

54. Tuchman R, Rapin I. Regression in pervasive developmental disorders: seizures and epileptiform electroencephalogram correlates. *Pediatrics* 1997;99:560–566.

Neocortical Epilepsies.
Advances in Neurology, Vol. 84,
edited by P. D. Williamson, A. M. Siegel,
D. W. Roberts, V. M. Thadani, and M. S. Gazzaniga.
Lippincott Williams & Wilkins, Philadelphia © 2000.

38

Cortical Dysplasias and Epilepsy: A Review of the Architectonic, Clinical, and Seizure Patterns

Frederick Andermann

*Departments of Neurology and Neurosurgery, Montreal Neurological Institute,
McGill University, Montreal, Quebec, Canada H3A 2B4*

Abnormalities of cortical structure and organization have been described since the early days of neuropathology. These descriptions usually were based on brains studied at autopsy, and the clinical background and history were often sketchy. The relationship to epilepsy, in particular to intractable epilepsy, could not be easily or well determined under these circumstances.

The tradition of surgical treatment for intractable epilepsy at the Montreal Neurological Hospital goes back more than 60 years. The resections were carried out by gyral emptying, and the tissue obtained was not ideal for pathological analysis. In the United Kingdom, Murray Falconer, a New Zealander, developed surgical treatment at the Kings-Maudsley, a tradition that has been continued until now. He used a different technique. The epileptogenic tissue, electrically defined, was resected en bloc and studied by the pathologists Clive Bruton and Nicholas Corsellis, who realized that some of the tissue obtained showed abnormal organization. These early patients were described by the neuropsychiatrist David Taylor in a paper entitled "Focal Dysplasia of the Cerebral Cortex in Epilepsy." I quote from the original description:

An unusual microscopic abnormality has been identified in the lobectomy specimens removed surgically from the brains of ten epileptic patients. The abnormality could seldom be identified by palpation or by the naked eye. Histologically, it consisted of congregations of large bizarre neurons which were littered through all of the first cortical layer. In most but not in all cases, grotesque cells, probably of glial origin were also present in the depth of the affected cortex and in the subjacent white matter. This kind of abnormality appears to be a malformation. The picture is reminiscent of tuberous sclerosis but too many distinguishing features both in the clinical and in the pathological aspects make this diagnosis untenable. The cases are therefore looked on provisionally, since all but one are still alive, as comprising a distinct form of cortical dysplasia in which localized exotic populations of nerve cells underlie the electrical and clinical manifestations of certain focal forms of epilepsy.

This definition has withstood the test of time and quite remarkably was made before modern imaging was available (1). The description of the findings is hard to improve, and the most common form of cortical dysplasia is now described as the *Taylor type*.

A number of years ago, a young man with megalencephaly who had focal seizures involving the arm and leg on one side only was referred to us. During most of these attacks, he remained conscious but occasionally would fall; he had a mild hemiparesis. He had an extremely unusual ongoing or continuous focal epileptic abnormality over the contralateral central area consisting of moderate- to high-voltage sharp waves at six to eight cycles per second. Dr. Rasmussen operated and found that the epileptogenic abnormality arose in the greatly enlarged precentral and postcentral gyri. Because the patient's hemiparesis was mild, he carried out only a resection anterior and posterior to this epileptogenic area, and this had little effect on the seizures. Years later, a magnetic resonance scan was carried out and clearly showed the enlarged gyri. There was also lesser contralateral enlargement of the precentral and postcentral gyri without, however, any epileptogenic abnormality arising in these. This patient showed the unusual ongoing epileptic electroencephalographic (EEG) abnormalities associated with dysplasia, which were much later identified and studied by Palmini and colleagues (2). This was the first patient in whom we suspected that a dysplastic abnormality was the cause of the epilepsy.

The computed tomography (CT) scan enabled recognition of some of the more gross structural developmental abnormalities, but it was the advent of magnetic resonance imaging (MRI) that led to recognition of many more dysplastic lesions during life. An example of this distinction is provided by a young man with focal seizures involving the foot and leg, which caused frequent falls, made it impossible for him to attend school, and led to progressive weakness of the leg. Numerous high-quality CT scans could not demonstrate an abnormality, but the first MRI showed a focal lesion of the foot area (Fig. 38.1), which turned out to be a benign glial tumor with dysplastic changes surrounding it, of a type later described by Prayson and Estes (3). The resection shown in the figure led to considerable improvement and cessation of the attacks involving the lower extremity. He now requires a light plastic brace and has had no increase in leg weakness. He continues to have seizures that now involve the upper extremity, but in these attacks, he does not fall. This patient illustrates that residual dysplastic tissue may be present and still lead to recurrent seizures.

Cortical dysplasia may be associated with overlying skin changes, such as the ectodermal dysplasia shown in the patient illustrated in Fig. 38.2. Underneath, there was obvious thickening of gray matter and calcification, a rather unusual finding in dysplasia. The resection led to complete cessation of seizures and eventually gradual reduction and finally

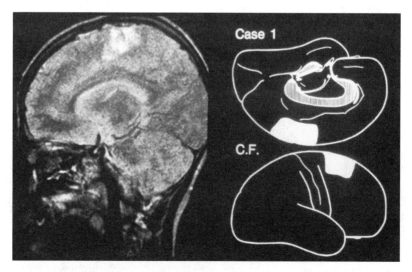

FIG. 38.1. Sagittal MRI showing a benign glial tumor surrounded by cortical dysplasia in the foot area. This lesion was not visible on several high-quality CT scans. Resection of the lesion led to considerable improvement but not to any additional deficit in the foot.

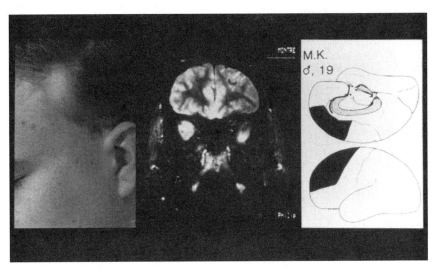

FIG. 38.2. An area of frontal ectodermal dysplasia overlying a dysplastic lesion. The MRI shows thickening of the gray matter and calcification seen as a void signal in this coronal scan. Pathological diagnosis was cortical dysplasia of Taylor type. Resection of the lesion led to cessation of attacks.

cessation of the medication by his neurologist. He had a recurrence, with a single seizure 2 years later. The medication was restarted in low doses, and some days later, he was found dead in bed, presumably as a result of a second, more severe seizure.

Other skin lesions associated with cortical dysplasias are multiple hemangiomata and, in particular, linear nevus sebaceous as illustrated in Fig. 38.3. This is not infrequently as-

sociated with hemimegalencephaly, as is achromic nevus of Ito. The skin lesions are usually over the head and neck but may involve other parts of the body; the underlying dysplastic abnormalities are usually ipsilateral but on occasion are contralateral to the cutaneous abnormality. The changes of dysplasia, however, are not always visible on imaging and may produce epilepsia partialis continua even in the absence of recognizable

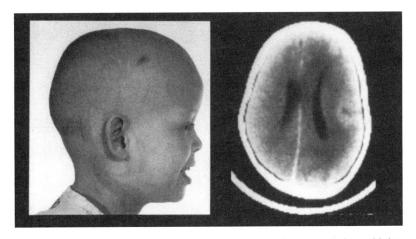

FIG. 38.3. Linear nevus sebaceous of Jadassohn on the neck of this young boy with intractable partial epilepsy. Hemimegalencephaly was present on the side of the skin lesion.

MRI changes (4). These changes may be bilateral, although the severity of the epilepsy is not always the same on both sides. This issue requires further investigation. In one of our patients, the contralateral dysplastic abnormality was recognized only at post mortem, although during life seizures had been originating only on one side.

A major challenge has been the search for increasingly subtle dysplastic abnormalities underlying intractable partial epilepsy. A recent important development was the introduction of surface coil MRI studies in which three-dimensional (3-D) acquisition with appropriately placed surface coils is carried out, leading to an increased signal-to-noise ratio and improved contrast between gray and white matter. This enabled Dr. Barkovich and his group to recognize dysplastic lesions not otherwise seen with high-quality MRI (5).

At the Montreal Neurological Institute, Dr. Alexandre Bastos developed curvilinear reformatting based on a high-quality 3D MR acquisition. Symmetric curved slices are obtained from a previously determined brain surface and can be rendered in 3-D. The advantages of this technique are reduced partial volume effect, symmetric visualization of the cortical structures, and preservation of surface landmarks (Fig. 38.4). The yield from this imaging technique is greater than can be obtained by studying orthogonal slices in which oblique cuts or slices along the long axis of a gyrus may create the false impression of gray matter thickening (6) (Fig. 38.5). In a number of patients, small dysplastic lesions could be demonstrated only by this technique. Their resection led to an excellent result (Figs. 38.6 through 38.8).

The prospect for improved MRI in epilepsy also includes the utilization of morphometry as carried out at the National Hospital for Neurology and Neurosurgery and by the Montreal Neurological Hospital (7,8). One can measure the volumes of gray and white matter of a lobe and compare the gyral patterns of the two hemispheres. These approaches are time consuming and as yet do not have the practical significance of some of the other imaging methods.

Functional MRI as well as diffusion and perfusion studies also may be expected to provide as yet unsuspected information. Eventually, one hopes to be able to visualize regional cerebral abnormalities caused by channel disorders.

Electrocorticography has shown an unusual pattern of virtually continuous but at times intermittent rhythmic epileptogenic discharge arising from dysplastic tissue (Fig. 38.9). This

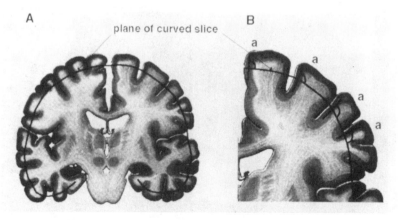

FIG. 38.4. The technique of curvilinear construction. The plane of the curved slice is illustrated in **A** and **B**. The computer program allows the creation of parallel slices at 1 or 2 mm increasing depth.

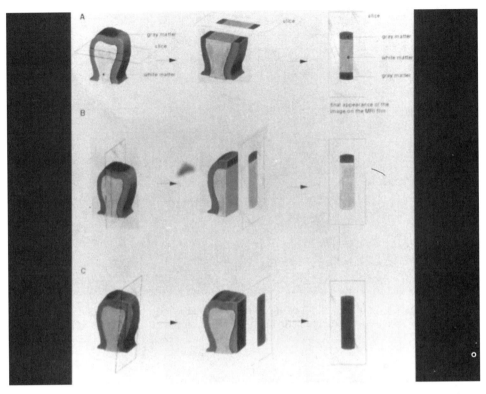

FIG. 38.5. Artifactual cortical thickening resulting from orthogonal slices can be identified. Areas of cortical thickening or gray–white matter blurring indicating dysplasia may be recognized.

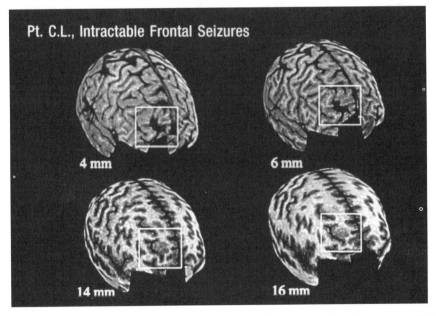

FIG. 38.6. A patient with intractable frontal seizures. Curvilinear reconstruction at increasing depths enables visualization of the dysplastic lesion, which was successfully resected.

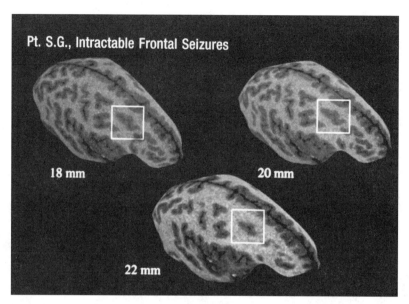

FIG. 38.7. A patient with intractable focal seizures. An area of cortical dysplasia corresponding to the clinical and electrographic changes can be seen. The lesion was resected, and this led to a good result.

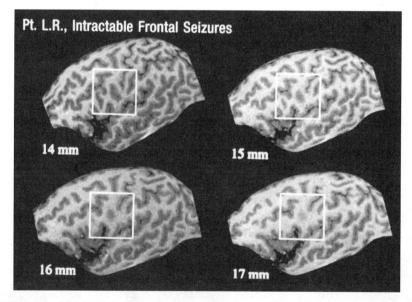

FIG. 38.8. A patient with intractable frontal seizures. Curvilinear reconstruction shows an area of blurred gray–white matter interface corresponding to the dysplastic abnormality resected at surgery. The patient's seizures ceased.

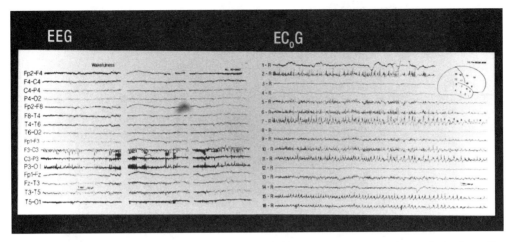

FIG. 38.9. An EEG from a patient with cortical dysplasia shows abundant, almost rhythmic, epileptogenic abnormality from areas overlying the dysplastic tissue. Virtually continuous epileptogenic interictal abnormality is found in the corticogram of a patient with cortical dysplasia of Taylor type.

was described by Palmini and colleagues; this abnormality was not found in patients who had seizures associated with tumors (2). Whether other lesions also can produce this kind of abnormality remains as yet uncertain. The EEG also shows abnormalities of a similar pattern, although these are less well defined compared with these seen at corticography (9). Thus, it has become clear that this type of electrographic abnormality originates in dysplastic tissue itself, which distinguishes these abnormalities from classic glial tumors. The recognition of abnormalities of this type has considerable practical significance because it has been shown by Palmini et al. that not only maximal resection of the visible lesion but additional resection of the area generating this type of continuous epileptiform discharge is required to obtain a good result (2).

These imaging and electrographic findings illustrate that a wide spectrum of dysplastic lesions exists, ranging from small areas that can be completely resected with complete cessation of seizures, to more widespread abnormalities that cannot be seen by current imaging studies, ranging all the way to the diffuse hemispheral dysplastic abnormalities recognized by Chugani (10)

and also by our own group. These abnormalities involving an entire hemisphere are not necessarily associated with enlargement of the hemisphere.

Functional imaging has been helpful in some patients. It may show abnormalities that are not revealed by MRI, as illustrated by a girl with intractable occipital seizures, leading eventually to loss of the visual hemifield, and whose MRIs were consistently normal. An interictal single-photon emission computed tomography (SPECT) scan showed evidence for hypoperfusion in the parietal occipital region, and the dysplastic nature of the abnormality was confirmed by pathological examination of the surgical specimen. The interictal scans, however, are of limited value as a rule, even in patients with dysplasia whose ictal scans provide more useful information. Reduced FDG uptake may be shown in positron emission tomography (PET) studies. This is illustrated in a young girl with a small cingulate, presumably dysplastic, lesion that led to more widespread frontal hypometabolism (Fig. 38.10).

Ligands such as alpha-methyl-tryptophan may show increased uptake in dysplastic tissue as it does in tuberous sclerosis (Fig. 38.11). Whether this is related to increased epileptic activity or to properties of the le-

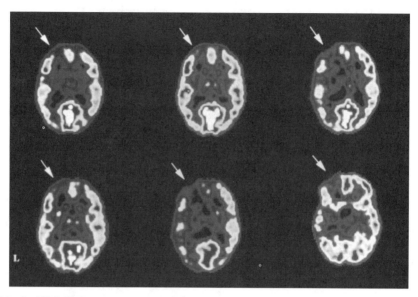

FIG. 38.10. An FDG PET scan of a young girl who has a small cingulate lesion. The scan shows more widespread frontal hypometabolism.

sion itself is not yet clear. Additional ligand studies using methionine, a marker of protein synthesis, may provide valuable information as well.

In our center, magnetic resonance spectroscopy (MRS) carried out by Li et al. demonstrated maximal reduction of *N*-acetyl-aspartate in the lesional area with lesser reduction in the perilesional area of interest and minimal changes far from the lesion (11).

Attempts have been made to grade the severity of dysplastic lesions. The least abnormality consists of vertical and horizontal dyslamination translating a disorder of migration.

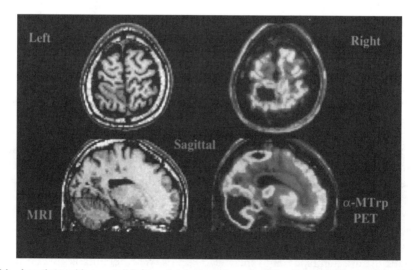

FIG. 38.11. A patient with a small left parietal area of cortical dysplasia (**left panels**). Alphamethyl-triptophan PET study (**right panels**) shows increased uptake of the ligand in the area of the lesion.

Abnormal neurons resulting from cortical malpositioning are most likely premature. In these lesions, features of both migrational and maturational abnormality are present. Finally, differentiation abnormalities also may be present, leading to the occurrence of balloon cells. These are primitive elements not fully differentiated between glial and neuronal cell lines. The presence of balloon cells has been linked to the occurrence of the most severe epileptic abnormalities.

As in other aspects of epilepsy, no classification is likely to satisfy all workers in the field; however, the classification established by Barkovich and colleagues is workable and provides a useful framework on which to build (12).

In summary, dysplastic cortical abnormalities are characterized by thickening of the gray matter and poor distinction between gray and white matter. Small dysplastic abnormalities are frequently situated at this interface, in the bottom of sulci but occasionally in the crowns of gyri, and they may have variable extension.

Subcortical heterotopia usually is associated with some cortical abnormality as well. Their resection may be limited by the involvement of essential somatomotor, sensory, or language areas. This is illustrated by the MRI of a young woman whose heterotopia could not be resected because this would have led to unacceptable deficit (Fig. 38.12). Fortunately, her seizures were of less than maximal severity; she derived some benefit, although by no means full seizure control, from pharmacologic treatment.

Periventricular nodular heterotopia are more common than suspected and may also be associated with intractable epilepsy. In some of the patients there are more obvious additional lesions overlying the periventricular nodules (Dubeau et al., personal communication) whereas in others microdysgenesis overlying the periventricular nodules has been described (Meencke et al., personal communication). It is now clear that the epileptogenic abnormalities may occur at a distance from the periventricular nodules which tend to predominate over the posterior wall of the ventricular system (Fig. 38.13). Several centers have carried out temporal resections, sometimes without being aware of the presence of these nodules. The results have been unsatisfactory in the majority (13) and there is still considerable debate as to whether the lesions themselves are epilepto-

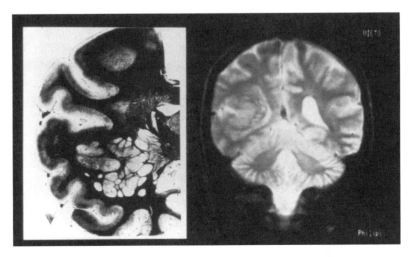

FIG. 38.12. Large subcortical heterotopia and epilepsy. **Left:** Pathological findings. **Right:** A virtually identical finding on MRI. The lesion could not be excised because to do so would have led to unacceptable deficit. The seizures are imperfectly controlled by antiepileptic medication.

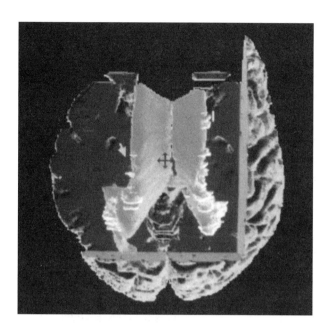

FIG. 38.13. Reconstruction of the ventricles in a patient with periventricular nodular heterotopia. The lesions predominate over the posterior aspect of the lateral ventricles and at times are found in the temporal horns as well.

genic or whether it is the dysplastic overlying cortex which is responsible for the epileptic discharge. These patients now require invasive recording for clarification of the origin of the epileptic discharge. Whether dual pathology, that is additional sclerosis of mesial temporal structures, is present in these patients, is not entirely clear.

Contiguous periventricular nodules are often a manifestation of a sex-linked dominant disorder. The first family, with the malformation in female members spanning four generations, was described by Huttenlocher et al. (14). No living males were born to these women (Fig. 38.14), but they had an increased number of abortions. The abnormality seems to be lethal in male children, although sporadic affected males with this defect have been described. The genetic basis of this abnormality, a gene on xq28, was identified by Eksioglu et al. working in Walsh's laboratory (15).

Band heterotopia or the double-cortex syndrome was identified during life by Livingston and Aicardi (16). Our own earliest description was inadequate because the quality of the imaging did not permit recognition of the characteristic malformation of a band of white matter underlying the cortex, with a band of gray matter below (17). There is great variation in the degree of cortical abnormality associated with this subcortical migration defect. There is also considerable variation in the thickness and extent of the band (18). Most of the patients are female. Affected women may transmit the abnormality to daughters, whereas the sons may have lissencephaly (19). The underlying genetic abnormality, a gene on xq22, putatively involved in signaling, also was identified by Ross et al. (20) and by Des Portes et al. (21). Although the structural abnormalities are much rarer in male subjects, it has now been described in 18 sporadic male epileptic patients with a considerable range in the severity of the epilepsy and of the associated cognitive abnormality (D'Agostino, unpublished) (Figs. 38.15 and 38.16). It has become clear that the band is not necessarily symmetric, and in one of our patients, it was much thicker in one hemisphere compared with the other. Focal or rather pseudofocal epileptic abnormalities may be encountered. Resection of more or less extended areas in seven patients with such EEG findings was usually unhelpful. Extensive cortical transection in a patient with pseudofocal abnormalities carried out by

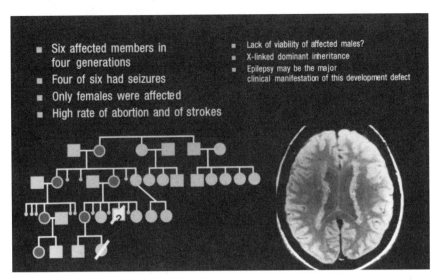

FIG. 38.14. Pedigree of the family described by Huttenlocher et al. Periventricular contiguous nodular heterotopia was found in female members of four generations, suggesting that the malformation was inherited as a sex-linked dominant. There were no affected males in this pedigree; thus, the malformation may be lethal for male children. (From Huttenlocher PR, Taravath S, Mojtahedi S. Periventricular heterotopia and epilepsy. *Neurology* 1994;44:51–55, with permission.)

Morrell and Whisler also did not result in useful outcome (Bernasconi et al., unpublished).

Generalized pachygyria may present with severe and uncontrollable epileptic seizures. In one of our patients with this malformation and secondary generalized epilepsy, a callosal section led to only limited improvement in the attacks (Fig. 38.17).

Micropolygyria is a disorder of cortical organization that occurs later in pregnancy com-

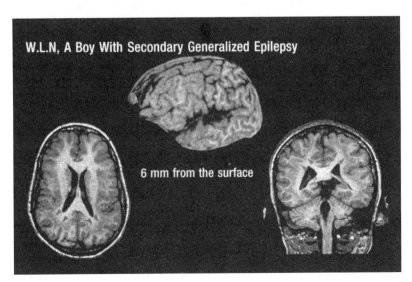

FIG. 38.15. Coronal and axial MRI and curvilinear reconstruction in a boy with band heterotopia. The band is separated from the cortex by a thin layer of white matter, best seen in the coronal plane and behind the central sulcus. The curvilinear reconstruction is at 6 mm from the surface. The findings also suggest a degree of anterior pachygyria.

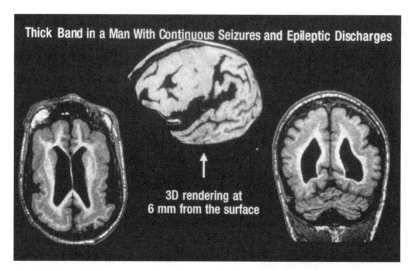

FIG. 38.16. A thick band of linear subcortical heterotopia in a man with quadriplegia, continuous seizures, and epileptic discharges. The band is much thicker compared with that in Fig. 38.15, illustrating the range of anatomic abnormalities correlating with the severity of clinical changes.

pared with the dysplastic lesions described in the preceding. Whether it can develop postnatally is still open to discussion. These lesions also have been recognized during life with the help of modern imaging. In bilateral perisylvian micropolygyria, the wide area of micropolygyria found on CT (Fig. 38.18) was first interpreted to represent pachygyria, and only later was the nature of the abnormality correctly identified. The polymicrogyria is best demonstrated by curvilinear reconstruction (Fig. 38.19). The seizures are usually secondary generalized, but in some patients consistently focal abnormalities may be found in addition, often originating in mesial temporal areas. The clinical abnormality consists of an at times striking pseudobulbar palsy with complete anarthria but an ability to pronounce

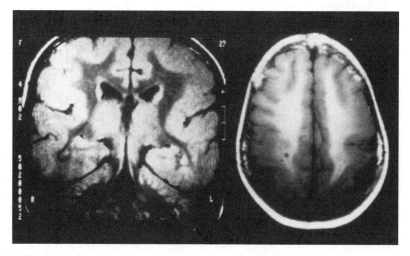

FIG. 38.17. MRI of a patient with generalized pachygyria and generalized epileptic abnormalities. A callosotomy led to no significant improvement in the seizures.

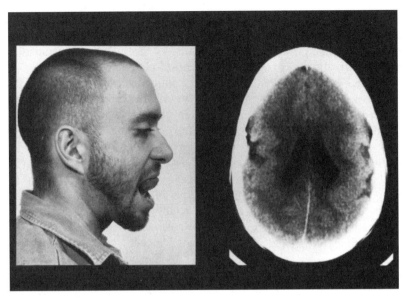

FIG. 38.18. A patient with bilateral perisylvian polymicrogyria shown during a maximal attempt at protruding his tongue. CT scan showing a thick band of gray matter over the lateral aspect of the hemisphere. This was first interpreted as pachygyria and later shown to represent polymicrogyria.

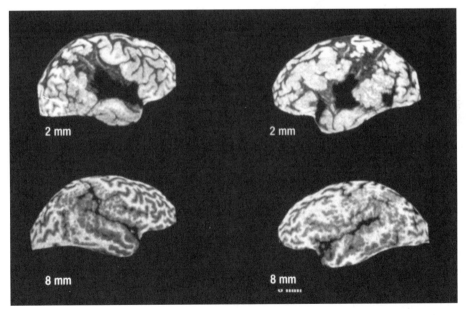

FIG. 38.19. The polymicrogyria is best demonstrated by curvilinear reconstruction with cuts at different depths. In this patient, the lesions are almost symmetric.

vowels. The patients may not be able to protrude the tongue and usually cannot move it
sideways. In other patients, presumably more
in those whose abnormalities are not exactly
homologous, the speech abnormality may be
much milder or not at all noticeable. A mild
hemiparesis with difficulty in rapid alternating
movements of the fingers and in toe tapping
may be present, and this may be unilateral or
bilateral. More recently, patients with neurologic abnormalities of this type but without
seizures have been described, and emphasis
has been placed on early recognition (22). In
about 10% of patients, there is associated
arthrogryposis multiplex congenita, possibly
resulting from an inflammatory process. This,
however, is still conjectural.

Polymicrogyria also may be inherited as a
sex-linked dominant trait, but perhaps other
modes of inheritance may occur as well (23)
(Fig. 38.20). It is likely that the early patients
with pseudobulbar palsy described by
Worster-Drought may have had this malformation of cortical organization as well (24).

Bilateral micropolygyria may occur over
occipital regions bilaterally, which may be related to a watershed vascular abnormality.
These patients often have a generalized
epileptic disorder. Bilateral frontal micropolygyria has been described, and these patients present with developmental delay, but
their epileptic problems are often not as severe.

Hypothalamic hamartoma has been a long-
standing clinical puzzle. Early laughing attacks often are followed by considerable behavioral abnormalities and the development
of a secondary generalized epileptic process,
which occurs late in the first decade, and
there is deterioration in cognitive function
with striking and intractable aggression, hy-
peractivity, and poor judgment. These abnormalities have been attributed to more widespread hemispheral changes, but resection of
focal areas, showing at times interictal or ictal
epileptogenic discharges, invariably led to
failure (25). That epileptogenic abnormalities
can arise in the hamartoma itself was shown

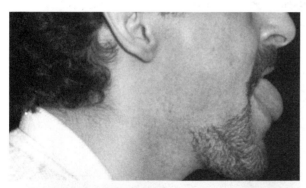

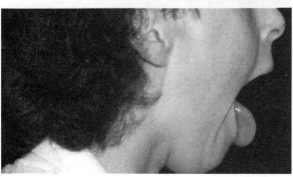

FIG. 38.20. A brother and sister with
bilateral perisylvian polymicrogyria
and severe dysarthria. Here they are
attempting to protrude the tongue.

by Munari and colleagues (26). Surgical resection may lead to cessation of seizures or to considerable improvement. A series of thirteen patients from four centers are currently being reported by Palmini et al. (unpublished). Radiosurgery also has been used by Kuzniecky and colleagues with good results (27). Further confirmation that the hamartoma is in fact responsible for abnormality was demonstrated by Tasch and colleagues, who showed reduced N-acetylaspartate in the hypothalamic lesion (28).

Not all patients with hypothalamic hamartoma, however, have severe epileptic or behavioral abnormalities. Both Berkovic and our group recently studied patients with small hypothalamic lesions (+5 mm in diameter) who merely had an urge to laugh; they had no more overt clinical manifestations (Fig. 38.21) (29).

Studies of neurotransmitter function in dysplastic tissue, based on histochemical analysis, were performed in several patients by Spreafico and colleagues (30). These investigators convincingly showed an increase in excitatory, glutaminergic function coupled with a decrease in GABAergic inhibitory activity.

SUMMARY

Since the nineteenth century, various abnormalities of cortical development resulting from migration defect, disorders of maturation, and disorders of cortical organization were described in brains at autopsy. Cortical dysplasia then was recognized in tissue resected during surgical treatment of patients with intractable epilepsy, but this finding remained largely unappreciated until the development of modern imaging. CT allowed glimpses of the more obvious malformations, but it was the advent of MRI that enabled the recognition and classification of the different types of lesions.

In the Taylor type of cortical dysplasia, it became clear that there was a wide range in the severity and, above all, in the extent of the abnormality. The lesions range from small ar-

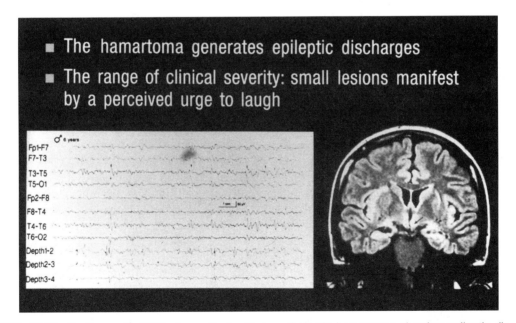

FIG. 38.21. (Left panel): EEG of a patient with hypothalamic hamartoma showing epileptic discharge arising in the lesion (**right panel**). A 5-mm hypothalamic hamartoma in a different patient leading to seizures with retained consciousness and a desire to laugh. She has normal behavior and intelligence.

eas, often difficult to identify, to extensive lesions surrounded by a halo or penumbra of presumably less severe, but still clinically significant, structural abnormality. Functional imaging (SPECT, PET, and MRS) have provided additional insights and led to strategies for surgical treatment. Even lesions involving the central strip may at times be successfully resected, but in such patients much depends on the preoperative neurologic status. Recognition of the fact that dysplastic lesions are in themselves epileptogenic has been another milestone in our understanding of these abnormalities.

Subcortical heterotopias, in particular periventricular nodular heterotopias, have been recognized as causing intractable epilepsy in some but not in all patients. Surgical approaches to these lesions are now being planned. The hereditary nature of the lesions in some patients has explained the familial occurrence of epilepsy in a number of instances.

Generalized epileptic abnormalities and generalized disorders of migration and maturation have been described as band heterotopia or the double-cortex syndrome. Here, too, sex-linked dominant inheritance may occur, and progress has been made in our understanding of the mechanisms of these genetically determined lesions. Focal resection in patients with band heterotopia, however, has been of little value in the small number of patients in whom it has been carried out.

Cortical malformations due to disorganization, occurring later in intrauterine life, are represented by micropolygyria. These lesions are often bilateral and perisylvian, but at times they are unilateral and in some patients may be occipital or frontal. Several syndromes have emerged, the most common being the one characterized by severe pseudobulbar palsy and mild pyramidal deficit (31). In some patients with such cortical abnormalities, particularly those with micropolygyria, the epilepsy may not be intractable, and full control may be obtained by medical treatment (32).

Interesting and important clinical features of patients with bilateral perisylvian polymicrogyria were described by Guerrini et al. (33) and Caraballo et al. (34). In some patients who develop a secondary generalized electrographic abnormality and drop attacks early in the first decade, there is eventual improvement and cessation of the epileptic abnormality toward the end of the first decade or somewhat later. These investigators stressed that callosotomy should be considered with caution in patients with micropolygyria and this electroclinical pattern.

Hypothalamic hamartomata and the associated epileptic syndrome have been better understood in recent years. Despite the risks of surgery, resection of the lesion offers hope of improvement in seizure control and of the often extremely severe behavioral abnormalities. On the other hand, patients with small lesions leading only to a "need to laugh" without more overt epileptic or behavioral manifestations are now being recognized.

Finally, initial investigations have begun to uncover the transmitter abnormalities in patients with cortical dysplasia. An increase in excitatory glutaminergic activity and a decrease in inhibitory gabaergic activity have been identified in tissue from patients treated surgically for their intractable epilepsy (30).

Recognition of the cortical dysplasias has turned over a new leaf in our understanding of intractable epilepsy in many patients. This is best illustrated by a patient with focal seizures investigated by Dr. Rasmussen 25 years ago. No cause for this patient's problem could be identified, and Dr. Rasmussen suggested to the family that they might want to return in 25 years when advances in investigation could provide a clearer explanation of their son's epilepsy. This family literally accepted this advice, and when they returned, as suggested, 25 years later, the MRI showed a typical example of transmantle dysplasia (35) (Fig. 38.22). In this man, rather exceptionally, the epileptic abnormality was not sufficient to justify surgical intervention, and his seizures, although not of maximal severity, have continued.

Recognition of more subtle structural abnormalities, clarification of the significance of microdysgenesis, and the search for rational

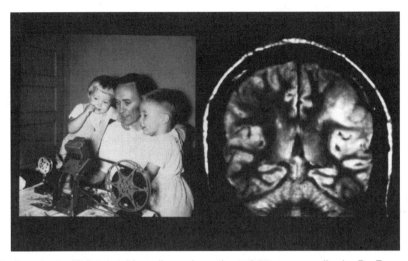

FIG. 38.22. A patient with intractable epilepsy investigated 25 years earlier by Dr. Rasmussen. The cause of the epilepsy could not be identified. The family was advised to return later, hoping for advances in investigation. MR now demonstrated transmantle dysplasia (**right panel**). The patient's seizures continue but are not sufficiently severe to justify an attempt at resecting the lesion.

therapy based on better understanding of the transmitter abnormalities are challenges for the present. Prevention of dysplastic abnormalities remains a challenge for the future and will depend on further progress in neuroscience.

REFERENCES

1. Taylor DC, Falconer MA, Bruton CJ, et al. Focal dysplasia of the cerebral cortex in epilepsy. *J Neurol Neurosur Psychiatry* 1971;34:369–387.
2. Palmini A, Gambardella A, Andermann F, et al. Intrinsic epileptogenicity of human dysplastic cortex as suggested by corticography and surgical results. *Ann Neurol* 1995;37:476–487.
3. Prayson RA, Estes ML, Morris HHD. Coexistence of neoplasia and cortical dysplasia in patients presenting with seizures. *Epilepsia* 1993;34:609–615.
4. Desbiens R, Berkovic SF, Dubeau F, et al. Life threatening focal status epilepticus due to occult cortical dysplasia. *Arch Neurol* 1993;50:695–700.
5. Barkovich AJ, Rowley HA, Andermann F. MR in partial epilepsy: value of high-resolution volumetric techniques. *Am J Neuroradiol* 1995;16:339–343.
6. Bastos AC, Comeau RM, Andermann F, et al. Diagnosis of subtle focal dysplastic lesions: curvilinear reformatting from three dimensional magnetic resonance imaging. *Ann Neurol* 1999;46:88–94.
7. Sisodiya SM, Free SL, Stevens JM, et al. Widespread cerebral structural changes in patients with cortical dysgenesis and epilepsy. *Brain* 1995;118:1039–1050.
8. Lee JW, Andermann F, Dubeau F, et al. Morphometric analysis of the temporal lobe in temporal lobe epilepsy. *Epilepsia* 1998;39:727–736.
9. Gambardella A, Palmini A, Andermann F, et al. Usefulness of focal rhythmic discharges on scalp EEG of patients with focal cortical dysplasia and intractable epilepsy. *Electroencephalogr Clin Neurophysiol* 1996; 98:243–249.
10. Chugani HT. PET in preoperative evaluation of intractable epilepsy. *Pediatr Neurol* 1993;9:411–413.
11. Li LM, Cendes F, Bastos AC, et al. Neuronal metabolic dysfunction in patients with cortical developmental malformations: a proton magnetic resonance spectroscopic imaging study. *Neurology* 1998;50:755–759.
12. Barkovich AJ, Kuzniecky RI, Dobyns WB, et al. A classification scheme for malformations of cortical development [Review]. *Neuropediatrics* 1996;27:59–63.
13. Li LM, Dubeau F, Andermann F, et al. Periventricular nodular heterotopia and intractable temporal lobe epilepsy: poor outcome after temporal lobe resection. *Ann Neurol* 1997;41:662–668.
14. Huttenlocher PR, Taravath S, Mojtahedi S. Periventricular heterotopia and epilepsy. *Neurology* 1994;44: 51–55.
15. Eksioglu YZ, Scheffer IE, Cardenas P, et al. Periventricular heterotopia: an x-linked dominant epilepsy locus causing aberrant cerebral cortical development. *Neuron* 1996;16:77–87.
16. Livingston JH, Aicardi J. Unusual MRI appearance of diffuse subcortical heterotopia or "double cortex" in two children. *J Neurol Neurosurg Psychiatry* 1990;53: 617–620.
17. Marchal G, Andermann F, Tampieri D, et al. Generalized cortical dysplasia manifested by diffusely thick cerebral cortex. *Arch Neurol* 1989;46:430–434.
18. Barkovich AJ, Guerrini R, Battaglia G, et al. Band heterotopia: correlation of outcome with magnetic resonance imaging parameters. *Ann Neurol* 1994;36: 609–617.

19. Pinard JM, Motte J, Chiron C, et al. Subcortical laminar heterotopia and lissencephaly in two families: a single x-linked dominant gene. *J Neurol Neurosurg Psychiatry* 1994;57:914–920.

20. Ross ME, Allen KM, Srivastava AK, et al. Linkage and physical mapping of x-linked lissencephaly/SBH (XLIS): a gene causing neuronal migration defects in human brain. *Hum Mol Genet* 1997;6:555–562.

21. Des Portes V, Pinard JM, Billuart P, et al. A novel CNS gene required for neuronal migration and involved in x-linked subcortical laminar heterotopia and lissencephaly syndrome. *Cell* 1998;92:51–56.

22. Miller SP, Shevell M, Rosenblatt B, et al. Congenital bilateral perisylvian polymicrogyria presenting as congenital hemiplegia. *Neurology* 1998;50:1866–1869.

23. Guerreiro ML, Andermann E, Guerrini R, et al. Familial perisylvian polymicrogyria: a new familial syndrome of cortical maldevelopment. *Annals of Neurology* 2000 (in press).

24. Worster-Drought C. Suprabulbar paresis: congenital suprabulbal paresis and its differential diagnosis, with special reference to acquired suprabulbar paresis. *Dev Med Child Neurol* 1974(Suppl 30);30:1–33.

25. Cascino GD, Andermann F, Berkovic SF, et al. Gelastic seizures and hypothalamic hamartoma: evaluation of patients undergoing chronic intracranial EEG monitoring and outcome of surgical treatment. *Neurology* 1993; 43:747–750.

26. Munari C, Tassi L, Berta E, et al. Case of a child with gelastic seizures and hypothalamic hamartoma [Letter, Comment]. *Epilepsia* 1997;38:1364–1365.

27. Kuzniecky R, Guthrie B, Mountz J, et al. Intrinsic epileptogenesis of hypothalamic hamartomas in gelastic epilepsy. *Ann Neuro* 1997;42:60–67.

28. Tasch E, Cendes F, Li LM, et al. Hypothalamic hamartomas and gelastic epilepsy—a spectroscopic study. *Neurology* 1998;51:1046–1050.

29. Sturm JW, Andermann F, Berkovic SF. "Pressure to laugh": an unusual epileptic symptom associated with small hypothalamic hamartomas. *Neurology* 2000; 971–973.

30. Spreafico R, Battaglia G, Arcelli P, et al. Cortical dysplasia: an immunocytochemical study of three patients. *Neurology* 1998;50:27–36.

31. Kuzniecky R, Andermann F, Guerrini R. Congenital bilateral perisylvian syndrome: study of 31 patients. The CBPS Multicenter Collaborative Study. *Lancet* 1993; 341:608–612.

32. Ambrosetto G. Treatable partial epilepsy and unilateral opercular neuronal migration disorder. *Epilepsia* 1993;34:604–608.

33. Guerrini R, Genton P, Bureau M, et al. Multilobar polymicrogyria, intractable drop attack seizures, and sleep-related electrical status epilepticus. *Neurology* 1998;51:504–512.

34. Caraballo R, Cerosimo R, Fejerman N. A particular type of epilepsy in children with congenital hemiparesis associated with unilateral polymicrogyria. *Epilepsia* 1999;40:865–871.

35. Barkovich AJ, Kuzniecky RI, Bollen AW, et al. Focal transmantle dysplasia: a specific malformation of cortical development. *Neurology* 1997;49:1148–1152.

Neocortical Epilepsies.
Advances in Neurology, Vol. 84,
edited by P. D. Williamson, A. M. Siegel,
D. W. Roberts, V. M. Thadani, and M. S. Gazzaniga.
Lippincott Williams & Wilkins, Philadelphia © 2000.

39

Cortical Dysplasia: Developmental Effects

Gregory L. Holmes and *Nicolas Chevassus au Louis

*Department of Neurology, Harvard Medical School, Division of Clinical Neurophysiology
and Epilepsy, Children's Hospital, Boston, Massachusetts 021125; *Laboratoire de Epilepsie
et Ischémie Cérébrale, Institut National de la Santé de la Recherche Medical, Paris, France*

Brain development is a dynamic process of choreographed cellular interactions that often involve dramatic reorganization and cell migration during specific time periods. Cerebral cortical development consists of waves of neuronal division and migration with subsequent formation of neuronal circuits. Certain neurons will travel remarkably long distances from their site or origin to their ultimate destination. Following migration, neuron growth continues with increasing dendritic and axonal arborization. The growth and increased differentiation of selected populations of neurons are balanced by the elimination of cells through programmed cell death.

Brain development may be profoundly disturbed by internal and external factors such as gene defects, metabolic disturbances, prenatal or perinatal cerebral infarction, hypoxia, ischemia, trauma, irradiation, or drugs. The consequences of brain injury are highly dependent on the timing and location of the injury (1). A brain insult during the proliferation phase will result in a deficit of cortical neurons, whereas an injury during migration will result in the aberrant positioning of neurons.

Not surprisingly, the structural consequences of disturbances of brain development are quite varied, consisting of such disorders as diffuse pachygyria, lissencephaly, subcortical laminar heterotopia, polymicrogyria, and four-layered microgyria (2–5). The nosology of cerebral malformations are evolving with the increasing improvements in neuroimaging. Some investigators used a traditional classification of cerebral malformations that consists of four main groups: (a) agyria/pachygyria-lissencephaly; (b) microgyria-polymicrogyria; (c) dysplastic cortical architecture; and (d) heterotopias (6). Others have based classification of these malformations on the timing of the developmental process, encompassing terms such as *neuronal migration deficits* (5–8), *cerebral dysgenesis* (9,10), or *synaptic dysgenesis* (11). In this chapter, cerebral dysgenesis and dysplasia are used to refer to any type of abnormality of cortical architecture resulting from disturbances of cellular proliferation, migration, terminal differentiation, programmed cell death, synapse elimination, and cortical remodeling.

On a cellular level, human dysplastic tissue is associated with significant malformations, including microgyria, cytomegaly with associated cytoskeletal abnormalities, displaced pyramidal neurons in layer I and the white matter, inverted pyramidal neurons, loss of columnar architecture, excessive basal dendritic branching, and pyramidal cells with bifurcated and trifurcated apical dendrites (12–14). Cerebral dysgenesis is an important cause of functional impairment, including epilepsy and developmental delay in both children and adults (9,15–17). Many cortical malformations result in severe seizure disorders, which may be refractory to antiepileptic drug (AED) therapy (5).

Because of the refractory nature of epilepsy in children with cerebral dysgenesis, there has

497

been an increased interest in treating intractable epilepsy in selected patients with resection of the dysplasia (7). A surgical strategy raises important questions. Is the epileptogenic region totally confined to the dysplastic lesion? To answer this question, it is necessary to ask first whether the dysplastic lesion is epileptogenic and, second, whether the altered excitability associated with the dysplasia extends beyond the dysplastic lesion. A second major question to be answered regards the long-term effects of cortical dysplasia on brain development.

IS THE EPILEPTOGENIC REGION CONFINED TO THE DYSPLASTIC LESION?

Clinical Studies

Few studies have carefully examined the altered physiology occurring in human dysplastic tissue. In a study of dysplastic tissue obtained from three patients undergoing surgical resection for intractable epilepsy, Mattia et al. (18) found seizure-like discharges when the tissue was exposed to 4-aminopyridine (4AP). In neocortical tissue from control patients epileptiform activity was not produced by similar concentrations of 4AP.

In attempts to understand the pathophysiologic basis for epilepsy in cortical dysplasia, tissue from patients with cortical dysplasia has been subjected to a number of immunohistologic evaluations. Babb and colleagues (19,20) demonstrated alterations in glutamate receptor subunit proteins in tissue from patients with cortical dysplasias. The N-methyl-D-aspartate (NMDA) receptor has two families of subunit proteins: NMDAR1 and NMDAR2. The NMDAR1 gene generates eight alternate splice variants; the NMDAR2 gene has four gene products generating NR2A-NR2D subunits. Dysplastic tissue was intensely stained for NMDAR2A/B, whereas nondysplastic tissue was not immunoreactive to NMDAR2A/B. A number of antibodies selective to NMDAR1 splice variants were labeled dysplastic but not nondysplastic tissue. The findings suggested that hyperexcitability seen in cortical dysplasia may result from the presence of NMDAR2 subunits and selectively expressed NMDAR1 splice variants in dysplastic neurons. In addition, specimens from patients with intractable epilepsy have shown decreases in parvalbumin, calbindin D-28 k, and somatostatin immunoreactive cells, implying a reduction in inhibition (21,22). Spreafico et al. (23) reported a decrease of GABAergic interneurons as well as abnormal baskets of parvalbumin-positive terminals around excitatory neurons, also indicating that the microdysgenetic lesion may have impaired inhibition.

Animal Studies

Investigators evaluating cerebral excitability in animal models of cortical dysplasia found evidence for both augmented excitability as well as impaired inhibition. As will be discussed, both factors may play a role in altered seizure susceptibility in cortical dysplasias.

Augmentation of Excitation

To mimic the dysplastic lesion occurring in humans, investigators have taken advantage of the freeze lesion model (24–29). In this model, a freeze lesion is applied through the intact skull in newborn rats, resulting in a focal region of cortical microdysgenesis that resembles human four-layered microgyria (27,28). The microdysgenesis is a discrete lesion, surrounded by normal appearing cortex (Fig. 39.1). The microdysgenesis is easily produced, it is uniform from animal to animal, and it is associated with minimal morbidity and mortality. It is a useful animal model in which to investigate the structural and functional migration disorders occurring during early brain development (26,30); however, it should be noted that the rats do not develop spontaneous seizures. There are now a number of studies using in vitro intracellular recordings from animals with neonatal freeze lesions demonstrating that the region around the microdysgenetic lesion is hyperexcitable.

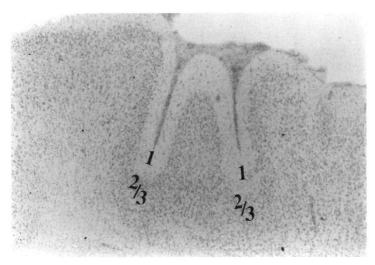

FIG. 39.1. Examples of microgyria in rats with a freeze lesion. Note the abnormal cortical lamination pattern (numbers refer to cortical layers, calibration bar = 50 μm).

Jacobs et al. (31) found a focal region of hyperexcitability around the margin of microdysgenesis, with field potentials evoked by electric stimulation, demonstrating prolonged, multiphasic, and variable latencies. The hyperexcitability appeared within 12 days and persisted until adulthood. Intracellular recordings demonstrated that the neurons generated orthodromic bursts of spikes during the field potential events. The epileptiform activity could be generated only in a cortical zone extending a few millimeters from the microgyrus but *not* within the microgyrus itself. In recordings from the anatomically intact layer V, animals with freeze lesions had higher peak amplitudes of inhibitory postsynaptic currents (IPSCs) than controls. In addition, when NMDA and non-NMDA excitatory receptors were blocked in the tissue, the percent decrease in spontaneous IPSCs was significantly greater for cells near the freeze lesion than controls. It was suggested that this finding reflected an increased activation of interneurons (which innervate GABAergic cells) or an enhancement of GABA function through axonal sprouting, or both, in animals with freeze lesions.

Supporting evidence for an increase in excitability around the dysplasia came from Luh-mann and Raabe (2), who found that in control animals orthodromically evoked synaptic activation was spatially restricted to a narrow cortical column about 1 mm in diameter in normal control animals, whereas, in rats with cortical dysplasia, the same electric stimuli elicited a long-lasting epileptiform response that propagated in horizontal directions over distances of at least 3 to 4 mm, well beyond the margins of the microdysgenetic lesion. Spontaneous epileptiform activity also could be observed only in cortical slices with migrational abnormalities, indicating that structural or functional modifications induced a long-term hyperexcitability within the cortical network. The authors found that epileptiform responses were not significantly affected by APV (DL-2-amino-5-phosphonovaleric acid), an NMDA blocker, but were blocked by (+/−)-alpha-amino-3-hydroxy-5-methlisoxazole-4-propionic acid (AMPA) antagonist 6-nitro-7-sulphamoyl-benzo(f)quinoxaline-2,3-dione (NBQX), which suggests that the expression and propagation of epileptiform activity in dysplastic cortex depends predominately on the activation of AMPA receptors.

A factor contributing to the hyperexcitability of surrounding tissue could be the excess of excitatory glutamatergic projections that has been described in the area bordering the microgyrus (24). These fibers are thalamic afferent fibers that were rerouted as a result of the absence of their normal target (i.e., the layer 4 neurons) in the microgyric area (32,33). Figure 39.2 presents in schematic form the pathological process occurring with the freeze lesion. As demonstrated in the figure, because of the final location of the rerouted thalamocortical fibers, the margins of the microdysgenetic lesion are the most excitable. As a further indication of the adverse effects of cortical dysplasias on neighboring tissue, Prince et al. (34) found that the microgyrus itself was not necessary for generating epileptiform events. When a transcortical cut was made separating the microgyrus from the surrounding cortex, epileptiform activity still could be evoked from the adjacent cortex. The authors also found that immunocytochemical staining for a 68-kDa neurofilament protein was enhanced in the area around the microgyrus, further suggesting that the injury induced synaptic reorganization.

In addition to electrophysiologic studies demonstrating abnormal physiologic responses extending beyond the margins of the microdysgenetic region (2,34), far-reaching changes in excitatory neurotransmitter receptor also have been described in animals with freeze lesions. At age 3 months, rats with freeze lesions induced on day 1 were evaluated for binding of NMDA, AMPA, kainate, $GABA_A$, and $GABA_B$ using radioactive binding techniques by Zilles and colleagues (35). In the cortical dysplasia, binding to NMDA, AMPA, and kainate receptors was significantly increased. Of significant interest was the finding that the whole hemisphere containing the microgyria was shown to exhibit increased glutamate binding.

Impairment of GABAergic Inhibition

In addition to enhanced excitability, some studies implicated alterations in inhibition (36,37). Luhmann et al. (36) found that excitatory postsynaptic potentials of regular spiking cells in microgyric cortex were characterized by their long-duration, multiphasic components, burst discharge, and sensitivity to the NMDA-receptor–mediated late component of depolarization, demonstrating an enhanced NMDA response. In addition, polysynaptic IPSPs mediated by $GABA_A$ and $GABA_B$ receptors were either absent or reduced in peak conductance in the microdysgenetic lesion. Because monosynaptic IPSPs recorded in the presence of glutamate receptor blockers were similar in animals with freeze lesions and controls, it was suggested that GABAergic neurons in microgyric cortex had a weaker excitatory input. The authors suggested that the epileptiform activity elicited by microdysgenesis is caused by an increase in NMDA-receptor–mediated excitation in pyramidal neurons and a concurrent decrease of glutamatergic input onto in-

FIG. 39.2. Pathogenesis of experimental cortical microgyria. At P0, a cold lesion induces focal necrosis of the cortical plate *(CP)* postmitotic neurons *(hatched symbols)*. Radial glial fibers are damaged, but their cell bodies, which lie in the ventricular zone *(VZ)* are unaffected. Thalamic afferents are waiting in the subplate *(SP)*. At P5, the glial reaction *(stars in P0)* has cleared damaged cells. Radial glial fibers have regenerated and allowed the migration of external layer neurons. These neurons will form the four-layered cortex, which contains a molecular layer 1, two external cortical layers, and a deep layer that is in continuity with layer 6b. Thalamic fibers that invade the microgyria fail to find their appropriate target (i.e., layer 4 neurons) and are rerouted in the borders of the microgyrus. In adults, the four-layered microgyric cortex is conserved and is associated with the conservation of some immature features, such as conservation of Cajal–Retzius *(CR)* neurons and radial glial fibers. The normally transient subpial Cajal–Retzius neurons exert an important synaptic control on the terminal bouquet of neocortical dendrites. *WM,* white matter. [Based on the work of Dvorák and Feit (26), Rosen et al. (25,65), Prince et al. (34,66), and Supèr et al. (68).]

hibitory interneurons, resulting in decreased inhibition.

As described, Zilles et al. (35) found widespread increases in binding to NMDA, AMPA, and kainate receptors in the hemi-

sphere ipsilateral to the hemisphere with the dysplasia. In addition, the authors also found extensive decreases in binding to $GABA_A$ and $GABA_B$ receptors. These findings suggest that the microgyrus is associated with distur-

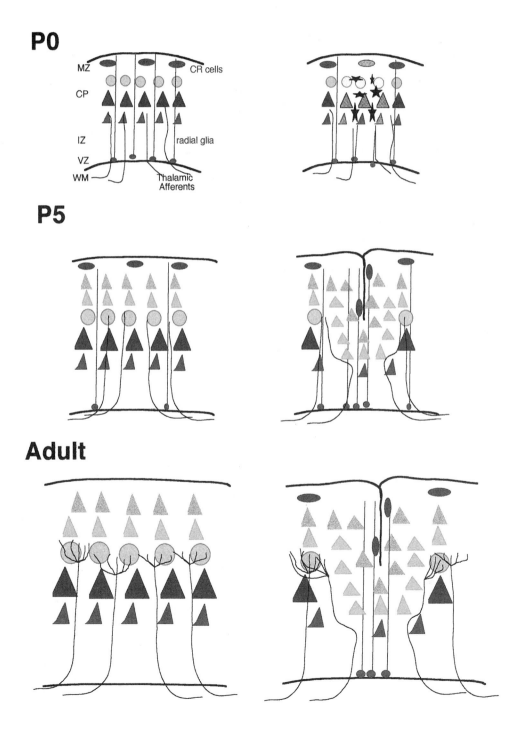

bances of the excitation to inhibition balance that are far reaching.

A number of authors reported a decrease in parvalbumin, a calcium-binding protein that is colocalized in GABAergic cells, in the microdysgenetic lesion in animal models, as in humans (31,37). Whereas GABA markers are decreased within the microgyrus itself, this does not necessarily indicate that decreased inhibition is responsible for the increased excitability associated with these lesions. As described, the electrophysiologic studies have demonstrated that inhibition is present, and perhaps even enhanced, in the microdysgenetic lesion and surrounding tissue.

CONCLUSIONS

Together, these results suggest a profound reorganization of the cortical network bordering the malformed region involving rerouting of excitatory afferent fibers, which causes the hyperexcitability of the microgryrus. The mechanisms involved in these changes are likely to resemble those described in posttraumatic adult epilepsy (38), that is, sprouting of lesioned axons, rerouting of afferent fibers, and a change in local circuits (39). These changes in local circuits could involve both enhanced excitation as well as impaired inhibition. These aberrant networks appear to set up a pathological process that involves neurons at sites quite distant from the cortical dysplasia.

WHAT ARE THE LONG-TERM CONSEQUENCES OF DYSGENETIC REGIONS?

There is increasing evidence from both clinical and animal studies that dysplasia may have widespread effects on brain excitability, extending beyond the actual region of dysplasia. As will be seen, these alterations in brain excitability raise concern over the effectiveness of surgical intervention in patients with cortical dysplasias.

Clinical Studies

The coexistence of dysplasia with mesial temporal sclerosis has been noted by numerous authors (10,40–44). Cendes et al. (40) used magnetic resonance imaging (MRI) volumetric studies to assess hippocampal size. Abnormal hippocampal volumes were present in some patients with both temporal and extratemporal lesions. Dual pathology was considerably more common in patients with dysplasia (25%), porencephalic cysts (31%), and gliosis (23.5%) than in those with tumors (2%) and vascular malformation (9%). Patients with a history of febrile seizures had a higher incidence of hippocampal atrophy than did those without such a history. No relationship was found between the location of the dysplasia and hippocampal pathology.

Other investigators also noted the propensity of cortical dysplasia to result in dual pathology. Levesque et al. (41) reviewed both hippocampal and extrahippocampal pathology in 178 patients who underwent en bloc temporal lobectomy for intractable epilepsy. Hippocampal cell loss was far more serious in patients with heterotopias than in patients with tumors as dual pathology. In a series of 100 patients with hippocampal sclerosis defined by MRI, 15 patients had cortical dysplasia (10).

It is not clear why there is such a high incidence of dual pathology in patients with cortical dysplasia versus tumors. It is possible that there is a common pathogenetic process that leads to both the dysplasia and hippocampal sclerosis. Another possibility is that recurrent seizures arising from the dysplasias lead to the changes in the hippocampal formation (17). For example, dyplasias may predispose the child to febrile seizures (40).

These studies raise concerns about whether patients with cerebral cortical dysplasia will remain at risk for seizures following the focal resection because pathological changes can occur in cortical areas outside the dysplasia. Not all studies, however, demonstrated a clear increase in hippocampal pathology in patients with cortical dysplasia. In a pathological study of temporal lobes from 28 children undergoing surgery for severe epilepsy, Mathern et al. (45) found that although these children had decreased numbers of granule cells, there was minimal Ammon's horn neuronal loss and mossy fiber sprouting. These findings suggested to the authors that repeated, non-hippocampal seizures did not lead to the development of hippocampal sclerosis.

Animal Studies

To address the question of whether cerebral dysgenesis can cause alterations in brain development and cerebral excitability in regions distant from the dysgenetic region, we used the freeze model to examine hippocampal function. To determine whether this limited area of microdysgenesis resulted in changes in hippocampal excitability, we evaluated kindling in prepubescent rats, assessed early gene activation following kainic acid, and measured mossy fiber distribution in the hippocampus in rats that received either one or three freeze lesions on the first day of life (46).

Rats receiving freeze lesions did not differ behaviorally from littermate controls in an obvious manner. Spontaneous seizures were not observed. When these rats were killed as adults, clearly defined, four-layered cerebral microdysgenetic lesions were detected (Fig. 39.1). No cell loss was seen in the hippocampus by using routine histologic staining; however, when Timm staining was used, we found that the rats with freeze lesions had a modest increase in sprouting of dentate granule cell axons (mossy fibers) in the CA3 region compared with controls. Figure 39.3 shows a normal example of Timm staining, and Fig. 39.4 shows mossy fiber sprouting in a rat with a freeze lesion. A comparison of CA3 sprouting in a control and in a rat with a freeze lesion is provided in Fig. 39.5. Note the increased sprouting in the rat with the freeze lesion. Quantification of the mossy fiber sprouting using computer density measurements confirmed that there were significant differences in the amount of Timm staining in the controls and animals subjected to a freeze lesion.

Mossy fiber sprouting in the CA3 intrapyramidal region has been demonstrated to display a considerable degree of plasticity under a variety of experimental conditions, including malnutrition (47), hyperthyroidism (48), perinatal alcohol exposure (49), CA3 lesions (50), prenatal exposure to methylazoxymethanol

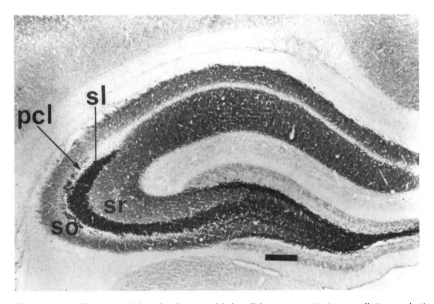

FIG. 39.3. Example of Timm staining (*pcl*, pyramidal cell layer; *sr*, stratum radiatum; *sl*, stratum lucidum; *so*, stratum oriens) (calibration bar = 100 μm). The Timm stain specifically colors zinc in the mossy fiber axons and boutons of the dentate granule cells. Note the heavy staining in the hilus and CA3 region.

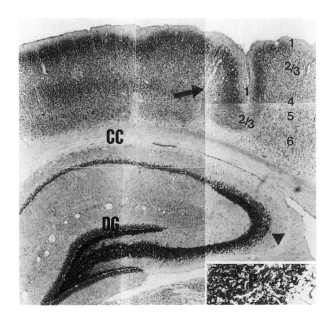

FIG. 39.4. Example of Timm stained section from rat with a single freeze lesion. Note the microgyria *(arrow)* with abnormal cortical lamination pattern. CA3 region is demonstrated by *arrowhead* and insert. *CC,* corpus callosum; *DG,* dentate granule cell layer; *P,* pyramidal cell layer.

(51), following status epilepticus induced with kainic acid (KA) (48,52,53), amygdala kindling (53–55), or following recurrent seizures during early brain development (56,57). It is unclear whether the sprouting we observed is secondary to the heightened excitability around the freeze lesion.

To assess whether freeze lesion-induced microgyri are more susceptible to seizure activation, we induced seizures by systemic injection of KA. The pattern of neuronal activation following KA-induced seizures was evaluated using *c-fos* immunostaining. Fos is a protein produced by a member of the family of immediate–early genes. It is sparsely expressed at baseline. A rapid transient induction of Fos, however, may follow excitatory neuronal activation, as in seizures (58). KA seizures were induced in rats with freeze lesions at postnatal (P) day 10, 20, or 30.

We found that microdysgenesis resulted in greater intensity of *c-fos* staining ipsilateral to the lesion in P30 rats. This asymmetry in *c-fos* was not seen in P10 or P20 rats, suggesting that the effect of the microdysgenesis on the hippocampus requires a mature innervation of hippocampal pathways, is a time-dependent

process, or both (Fig. 39.6). Because the cortical microdysgenesis did not involve the hippocampus, the asymmetry of *c-fos* staining indicated that the effects of microdysgenesis were related to ipsilateral connections between the microdysgenesis and hippocampus. Despite the preferential activation of early genes ipsilateral to the microdysgenesis, KA did not cause increase staining in the microdysgenetic lesion itself. The microdysgenesis did not appear to play a role in the generation of the seizures.

The reason for the altered *c-fos* activation and sprouting in the animals with the microdysgenesis is not clear, but it may relate to the altered excitability that occurs within the microdysgenetic lesion as well as extending beyond the immediate region of the lesion. We found no significant differences in afterdischarge threshold or kindling rate in rats with freeze lesions and controls, however.

It is possible that both the CA3 sprouting and *c-fos* activation are secondary to enhanced excitability, which, through activity-dependent mechanisms, alters hippocampal excitability. There are extensive efferents into the entorhinal cortex, which subsequently innervate hip-

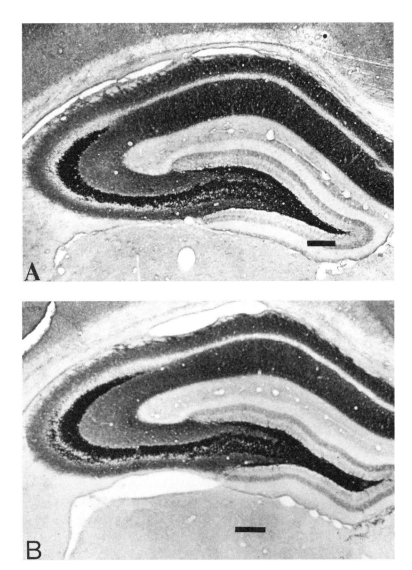

FIG. 39.5. Examples of Timm stained section from a control rat **(A)** and rat with a single freeze lesion **(B)**.

pocampal structures through the perforant pathway. Because synaptic activity appears to be an important factor in the development of both the excitatory and inhibitory neurotransmitter receptors (59,60), it is conceivable that a hyperexcitable cortical lesion over an extended period could alter hippocampal physiology and connectivity. For example, it is known that CA3 sprouting can be induced by kindling (53–55). Increased cortical excitability could have other effects, such as increasing dentate granule cell neurogenesis (61) or modulating development of hippocampal interneurons (62). For example, Marty and Onténiente (62) found that the levels of expression of somatostatin and calretinin in maturing hippocampal interneurons was dependent on the endogenous balance of excitatory and inhibitory activity.

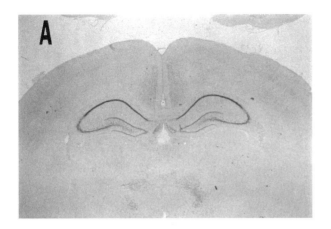

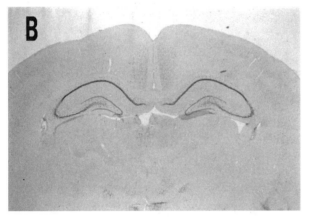

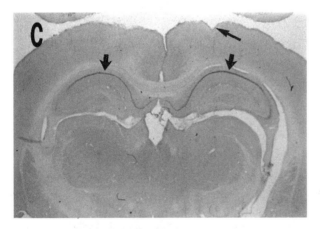

FIG. 39.6. *c-fos* staining in P10 **(A)**, P20 **(B)**, and P30 **(C)** rats that received a freeze lesion on P0. No differences were noted between the controls (not shown) and rats with the freeze lesions at P10 or P20. In P30 rats there was an asymmetry in *c-fos* staining, with greater staining in CA1 *(short arrow)* on the side of microdysgenesis *(long arrow)*.

SUMMARY

Taken together, these results demonstrate that the effects of cortical dysplasia may extend beyond the margins of the dysplasia. Electrophysiologic studies demonstrated that the region of hyperexcitability is not confined to the dysplasia, and studies of glutamate and GABA binding have found abnormalities throughout the entire hemisphere of adult rats with freeze lesions. Cortical dysplasia in animals leads to changes in neuronal activation of principal cells of the hippocampus during seizures and causes sprouting of dentate granule cell axons in CA3. Whereas the relevance of rodent data to the human condition is questionable, a number of human studies showed a high incidence of hippocampal pathology in patients with cortical dysplasia. Whereas the success rate for surgery in patients with cortical dysplasias who have medically intractable seizures is high, the animal and human studies presented here may help to explain why some patients continue to have seizures despite removal of the cortical lesion.

ACKNOWLEDGMENTS

This research was supported by the Emily P. Rogers Research Fund, Institut National de la Santé de la Recherche Medical, American Epilepsy Society, and grants to G.L.H. from the NINDS (NS27984) and Fogarty Foundation.

REFERENCES

1. Palmini A, Andermann F, De Grissac H, et al. Stages and patterns of centrifugal arrest of diffuse neuronal migration disorders. *Dev Med Child Neurol* 1993;35: 331–339.
2. Luhmann HJ, Raabe K. Characterization of neuronal migration disorders in neocortical structures. I. Expression of epileptiform activity in an animal model. *Epilepsy Res* 1996;26:67–74.
3. Marín-Padilla M. Prenatal and early postnatal ontogenesis of the human motor cortex: a golgi study. I. The sequential development of the cortical layers. *Brain Res* 1970;23:167–183.
4. Meencke H-J, Janz D. Neuropathological findings in primary generalized epilepsy: a study of eight cases. *Epilepsia* 1984;25:8–21.
5. Palmini A, Andermann F, Olivier A, et al. Focal neuronal migration disorders and intractable partial epilepsy: a study of 30 patients. *Ann Neurol* 1991;30: 741–749.
6. Rorke LB. A perspective: the role of disordered genetic control of neurogenesis in the pathogenesis of migration disorders. *J Neuropathol Exp Neurol* 1994;53:105–117.
7. Palmini A, Andermann F, Olivier A, et al. Focal neuronal migration disorders and intractable partial epilepsy: results of surgical treatment. *Ann Neurol* 1991;30:750–757.
8. Barth PG. Disorders of neuronal migration. *Can J Neurol Sci* 1987;14:1–16.
9. Raymond AA, Fish DR, Sisodiya SM, et al. Abnormalities of gyration, heterotopias, tuberous sclerosis, focal cortical dysplasia, microdysgenesis, dysembryoplastic neuroepithelial tumour, and dysgenesis of the archicortex in epilepsy: clinical, EEG, and neuroimaging features in 100 adult patients. *Brain* 1995;629–660.
10. Raymond AA, Fish DR, Stevens JM, et al. Association of hippocampal sclerosis with cortical dysgenesis in patients with epilepsy. *Neurology* 1994;44:1841–1845.
11. Becker LE. Synaptic dysgenesis. *Can J Neurol Sci* 1991;18:170–180.
12. Belichenko P, Sourander P, Dahlström A. Morphological aberrations in therapy-resistant partial epilepsy (TRPE): confocal laser scanning and 3D reconstructions of Lucifer Yellow injected atypical pyramidal neurons in epileptic human cortex. *Mol Neurobiol* 1994;9: 245–252.
13. Palmini A, Andermann E, Andermann F. Prenatal events and genetic factors in epileptic patients with neuronal migration disorders. *Epilepsia* 1994;35:965–973.
14. Mischel PS, Vinters HV. Neuropatholog of developmental disorders associated with epilepsy. In: Engel J Jr, Pedley TA, eds. *Epilepsy: a comprehensive textbook.* Philadelphia: Lippincott–Raven, 1997:119–132.
15. Hardiman O, Burke T, Phillips J, et al. Microdysgenesis in resected temporal neocortex: incidence and clinical significance in focal epilepsy. *Neurology* 1988;38: 1041–1047.
16. Holmes GL. Epilepsy and other seizure disorders. In: Berg B, ed. *Principles of pediatric neurology.* New York: McGraw-Hill, 1997:223–284.
17. Ho SS, Kuzniecky RI, Gilliam F, et al. Congenital porencephaly and hippocampal sclerosis: clinical features and epileptiform spectrum. *Neurology* 1997;49: 1382–1388.
18. Mattia D, Olivier A, Avoli M. Seizure-like discharges recorded in human dysplastic neocortex maintained in vitro. *Neurology* 1995;45:1391–1395.
19. Ying Z, Babb TL, Comair YG, et al. Increased expression of NMDAR2 proteins and differential expression of NMDAR1 splice variants in dysplastic neurons of human epileptic neocortex. *J Neuropathol Exp Neurol* 1998;57:47–62.
20. Babb TL, Ying Z, Hadam J, et al. Glutamate receptor mechanisms in human epileptic dysplastic cortex. *Epilepsy Res* 1998;32:24–33.
21. Ferrer I, Olivier B, Russi A, et al. Parvalbumin and calbinden-D28k immunocytochemistry in human nocortical epileptic foci. *J Neurol Sci* 1994;123:18–25.
22. Ferrer I, Pineda M, Tallada M, et al. Abnormal local-circuit neurons in epilepsia partialis continua associated with focal cortical dsyplasia. *Acta Neuropathol* 1998; 83:647–652.
23. Spreafico R, Battaglia G, Arcelli P, et al. Cortical dysplasia: an immunocytochemical study of three patients. *Neurology* 1998;50:27–36.
24. Humphreys P, Rosen GD, Press DM, et al. Freezing lesions of the developing rat brain: a model for cerebrocortical microgyria. *J Neuropathol Exp Neurol* 1991;50: 145–160.
25. Rosen GD, Press DM, Sherman GF, et al. The development of induced cerebrocortical microgyria in the rat. *J Neuropathol Exp Neurol* 1992;51:601–611.
26. Dvorák K, Feit J. Migration of neuroblasts through partial necrosis of the cerebral cortex in newborn rats—contributions to the problems of morphological development and developmental period of cerebral microgyria. *Acta Neuropathol (Berl)* 1977;38:203–212.
27. Rosen GD, Sigel EA, Sherman GF, et al. The neuropro-

tective effects of MK-801 on the production of microgyria by freezing injury to the newborn rat neocortex. *Neuroscience* 1995;69:107–114.

28. Rosen GD, Sherman GF, Galaburda AM. Birthdates of neurons in induced microgyria. *Brain Res* 1996;727: 71–78.

29. Rosen GD, Waters NS, Galaburda AM, et al. Behavioral consequences of neonatal injury of the neocortex. *Brain Res* 1995;681:177–189.

30. Dvorak K, Feit J, Jurankova Z. Experimentally induced focal microgyria and status verrucosis deformis in rats—pathogenesis and interrelation: histological and autoradiographical study. *Acta Neuropathol* 1978;44: 121–129.

31. Jacobs KM, Gutnick MJ, Prince DA. Hyperexcitability in a model of cortical maldevelopment. *Cereb Cortex* 1996;6:511–523.

32. Rosen GD, Galaburda AM. Thalamocortical and corticothalamic conectivity in induced neocortical microgyria. *Soc Neurosci Abst* 1998;224:12.

33. Jacobs KM, Mogenson M, Warren L, et al. Experimental microgyri disrupt the cytochrome oxydase identified barrel formation in rat somatosensory cortex. *Soc Neurosci Abst* 1997;317:5.

34. Prince DA, Jacobs KM, Salin PA, et al. Chronic focal neocortical epileptogenesis: does disinhibition play a role? *Can J Physiol Pharmacol* 1996;75:500–507.

35. Zilles K, Qû M, Schleicher A, et al. Characterization of neuronal migration disorders in neocortical structures: quantitative receptor autoradiography of ionotropic glutamate, GABA$_A$ and GABA$_B$ receptors. *Eur J Neurosci* 1998;10:3095–3106.

36. Luhmann HJ, Karpuk N, Qû M, et al. Characterization of neuronal migration disorders in neocortical structures. II. Intracellular in vitro recordings. *J Neurophysiol* 1998;80:92–102.

37. Hablitz JJ, DeFazio T. Excitability changes in freeze-induced neocortical microgyria. *Epilepsy Res* 1998;32: 75–82.

38. Salin P, Tseng G-F, Hoffman S, et al. Axonal sprouting in layer V pyramidal neurons of chronically injured cerebral cortex. *J Neurosci* 1998;15:8234–8245.

39. Marín-Padilla M. Developmental neuropathology and impact of perinatal brain damage. I. Hemorrhagic lesions of neocortex. *J Neuropathol Exp Neurol* 1996;55: 758–773.

40. Cendes F, Cook MJ, Watson C, et al. Frequency and characteristics of dual pathology in patients with lesional epilepsy. *Neurology* 1995;45:2058–2064.

41. Levesque MF, Nakasato N, Vinters HV, et al. Surgical treatment of limbic epilepsy associated with extrahippocampal lesions: the problem of dual pathology. *J Neurosurg* 1991;75:364–370.

42. Prayson RA, Reith JD, Najm IM. Mesial temporal sclerosis: a clinicopathologic study of 27 patients, including 5 with coexistent cortical dysplasia. *Arch Pathol Lab Med* 1996;120:532–536.

43. Jay V, Becker LE, Otsubo H, et al. Pathology of temporal lobectomy for refractory seizures in children. *J Neurosurg* 1993;79:53–61.

44. Prayson RA, Estes ML. Cortical dysplasia: a histopathologic study of 52 cases of partial lobectomy in patients with epilepsy. *Hum Pathol* 1995;26: 493–500.

45. Mathern GW, Babb TL, Mischel PS, et al. Childhood generalized and mesial temporal epilepsies demonstrate different amounts and patterns of hippocampal neuron loss and mossy fibre synaptic reorganization. *Brain* 1996;119:965–987.

46. Holmes GL, Sarkisian M, Ben-Ari L, et al. Consequences of cortical dysplasia during development in rats. *Epilepsia* 1999 (in press).

47. Hartmann D, Frotscher M, Sievers J. Development of granule cells, and afferent and efferent connections of the dentate gyrus after experimentally induced reorganization of the supra- and infrapyramidal blades. *J Neurosci Res* 1994;35:419–427.

48. Represa A, Tremblay E, Ben-Ari Y. Aberrant growth of mossy fibers and enhanced kainic acid binding sites induced in rats by early hyperthyroidism. *Brain Res* 1987; 423:325–328.

49. West JR. Long-term effects of developmental exposure to alcohol. *Neurotox* 1986;7:245–256.

50. Laurberg S, Zimmer J. Lesion-induced rerouting of hippocampal mossy fibers in developing but not in adult rats. *J Comp Neurol* 1980;190:627–650.

51. Cheema SS, Lauder JM. Infrapyramidal mossy fibers in the hippocampus of methylazoxymethanol acetate-induced microcephalic rats. *Dev Brain Res* 1983;9: 411–415.

52. Represa A, Tremblay E, Ben-Ari Y. Kainate binding sites in the hippocampal mossy fibers: localization and plasticity. *Neuroscience* 1987;20:739–748.

53. Represa A, Jorquera I, Le Gal La Salle G, et al. Epilepsy induced collateral sprouting of hippocampal mossy fibers: does it induce the development of ectopic synapses with granule cell dendrites? *Hippocampus* 1993;3:257–268.

54. Van der Zee CEEM, Rashid K, Le K, et al. Intraventricular administration of antibodies to nerve growth factor retards kindling and blocks mossy fiber sprouting in adult rats. *J Neurosci* 1995;15:5316–5323.

55. Represa A, Ben-Ari Y. Kindling is associated with the formation of novel mossy fiber synapses in the CA3 region. *Exp Brain Res* 1992;92:69–78.

56. Holmes GL, Gaiarsa J-L, Chevassus-Au-Louis N, et al. Consequences of neonatal seizures in the rat: morphological and behavioral effects. *Ann Neurol* 1998;44:845–857.

57. Holmes GL, Sarkisian M, Ben-Ari Y, et al. Mossy fiber sprouting following recurrent seizures during early development in rats. *J Comp Neurol* 1999;404:537–553.

58. Morgan JI, Cohen DR, Hempstead JL, et al. Mapping patterns of c-fos expression in the central nervous system after seizure. *Science* 1997;237:192–197.

59. Stelzer A, Slater NT, ten Bruggencate G. Activation of NMDA receptors blocks GABAergic inhibition in an in vitro model of epilepsy. *Nature* 1987;326:698–701.

60. Ben-Ari Y, Gho M. Long-lasting modification of the synaptic properties of rat CA3 hippocampal neurones induced by kainic acid. *J Physiol* 1988;404:365–384.

61. Parent JM, Yu TW, Leibowitz RT, et al. Dentate granule cell neurogenesis is increased by seizures and contributes to aberrant network plasticity in the adult hippocampus. *J Neurosci* 1997;17:3727–3738.

62. Marty S, Onténiente B. The expression pattern of somatostatin and calretinin by postnatal hippocampal interneurons is regulated by activity-dependent and -independent determinants. *Neuroscience* 1997;80:79–88.

63. Supèr H, Pérez Sust P, Soriano E. Survival of Cajal–Retzius cells after cortical lesions in newborn mice: a possible role for Cajal–Retzius cells in brain repair. *Dev Brain Res* 1997;98:9–14.

64. Marín-Padilla M. Cajal–Retzius cells and the development of the neocortex. *Trends Neurosci* 1998;21:64–71.

65. Rosen GD, Sherman GF, Galaburda AM. Radial glia in the neocortex of adult rats: effects of neonatal brain injury. *Dev Brain Res* 1994;82:127–135.

66. Prince DA, Jacobs K. Inhibitory function in two models of chronic epileptogenesis. *Epilepsy Res* 1998;32:83–92.

Neocortical Epilepsies.
Advances in Neurology, Vol. 84,
edited by P. D. Williamson, A. M. Siegel,
D. W. Roberts, V. M. Thadani, and M. S. Gazzaniga.
Lippincott Williams & Wilkins, Philadelphia © 2000.

40

Evaluation and Surgical Treatment of Localization-related Epilepsy in Infants

Michael Duchowny

Neuroscience Program, Miami Children's Hospital, Miami, Florida 33155

Intractable localization-related seizures and infantile spasms are common in early life and often are associated with dignostic uncertainty and treatment dilemmas (1). Seizure frequencies can be extremely high, bordering on status epilepticus, and medications often prove ineffective. Furthermore, seizure onset in infancy carries a poor prognosis with respect to seizure control and psychosocial status (2,3).

The use of neocortical resection for medically resistant seizures in early life was virtually unknown 10 years ago. With several notable exceptions, such as hemispherectomy in select circumstances (e.g., Sturge–Weber syndrome), debilitating seizures in infants were treated by continued medical manipulation in the face of dwindling evidence that further intervention was likely to be successful. In selected circumstances, surgical therapy now offers an opportunity to reverse the epileptic encephalopathy and facilitate developmental progress (4).

CLINICAL MANIFESTATIONS OF LOCALIZATION-RELATED SEIZURES IN EARLY POSTNATAL LIFE

Symptomatic

Partial seizures with onset in infancy are frequently symptomatic of underlying structural brain damage. More than half of the patients with partial epilepsy reported by Dravet et al. (5), two thirds of those reported by Duchowny (6) and Nordli et al. (7), and three fourths of patients described by Ohmori et al. (8) had evidence of structural lesions and underlying encephalopathy. Whereas lesions may occur throughout the cerebral cortex, frontal and temporal lobe involvement is particularly common.

Altered behavioral responsiveness and motor convulsions characterize most seizures. Altered responsiveness is accompanied by decreased motor activity and probable but undefined alterations in awareness without grossly observable automatisms (9). These "hypomotor" events are more likely to arise from temporal or temporoparietal sites. In contrast, motor convulsive activity consisting of tonic, atonic, or clonic movement show a greater predilection for frontal, frontocentral, or frontoparietal regions (9).

Tonic seizures present as stiffening and extension of the extremities and are frequently bilateral and asymmetric. The coordinated bilateral movement synchrony of older patients is often absent in the infant. Head and eye version is common but can shift laterality, rendering it unreliable as a lateralizing sign (6).

Clonic extremity movements are more often unilateral, whereas facial or eyelid clonus is more typically bilateral. Single or repetitive myoclonic jerks may precede or follow other motor convulsive patterns (10). Seizure duration of less than 5 minutes is the rule.

Automatisms are a less common seizure manifestation and tend to be relatively simple, in keeping with the overall immaturity of the cerebral cortex (7,11). Oromotor and gross gestural movement characterize most behaviors. Gestures more often precede convulsions, whereas oromotor manifestations are more likely to follow them (12). Autonomic changes including pallor, flushing, mydriasis, apnea, and tachycardia are commonly observed (13).

A firm diagnosis of localization-related related epilepsy is difficult and not always possible in some infants, prompting many investigators to question the reliability of the International League Against Epilepsy (ILAE) classification in this population (7). Typical features of partial epilepsy in older subjects are often lacking, and the presenting symptoms in infancy may be extremely subtle, such as hypomotor or autonomic changes. In some cases, it may be difficult to decide accurately whether seizures are generalized or localized. Even video/EEG monitoring may be confusing in the infant but remains the single most valuable technique for diagnosing localization-related epilepsy in early postnatal life.

Benign Partial Epilepsy in Infancy

Watanabe and collaborators first described a population of infants with localization-related seizures and benign course (14,15). Typically, affected patients are neurologically normal, and the interictal electroencephalogram (EEG) has a normal background and absence of electrographic seizure activity. Seizures are easily controlled by first-line antiepileptic drugs (AEDs). Seizures last less than 5 minutes, and seizure onset often localizes to the temporal lobe.

The semiology of seizures in benign partial epilepsy in infancy is indistinguishable from symptomatic localization-related seizures. Behavioral arrest, motor convulsions, automatisms, and autonomic manifestations are typical. A subgroup of infants with benign partial epilepsy evolving to epilepsy with secondarily generalized seizures also has been reported (16). Affected patients more often demonstrate seizure origin in central cortical regions, suggesting primary involvement of sensorimotor cortex, but pure focal clonic seizures have not been reported. Ictal EEG reveals secondary bilateral synchrony.

Infantile Spasms

Excisional surgery is a novel approach to treat patients with West syndrome. Infantile spasms are now regarded as a cortically modulated disorder related to the presence of a circumscribed lesion rather than a generalized epileptic disturbance. Excision of the localized epileptogenic region is therefore possible once it can be adequately defined. Surgical methodology offers hope for affected patients who otherwise have a poor prognosis for seizure control and high morbidity and mortality (17).

Surgical candidacy is most suitable in West syndrome patients with localizing signs. While evidence of localized structural damage on MR imaging simplifies the preoperative evaluation, patients with normal or nonspecific imaging findings may still exhibit asymmetric spasms and lateralized hypsarrhythmia (18–20). Asynchrony of the hypsarrhythmia may reflect agenesis of the corpus callosum (21). Even hemihypsarrhythmia may occur in the absence of unilateral imaging findings (22). As many as two thirds of patients demonstrate evidence of focality in at least one preoperative modality (23). Asymmetric spasms tend to be more frequent than symmetric ones (19,22).

A more specific relationship between infantile spasms and partial epilepsy is observed in some patients. Partial seizures may evolve into infantile spasms (13) or appear concurrently (24). The occurrence of focal electrographic discharges before the hypsarrhythmic burst suggests a facilitatory role of partial seizure activity in some patients (25). Despite correlation with focal pathology, focal features do not correlate with age of onset or outcome (22).

Focal cortical lesions associated with infantile spasms are commonly located in the central and posterior hemisphere regions rather than in the anterior cerebral cortex (26). Occipital lesions produce the earliest onset of spasms, whereas frontal lesions are rare and associated with later spasm onset (27). Frontal lesions are also less likely to produce focal EEG changes, including spikes and attenuated background. This anteroposterior gradient based on age correlates closely with the normal sequence of brain maturation (28).

Special Syndromes

A high proportion of infants with medically resistant partial epilepsy are born with clinical syndromes that present with a constellation of known signs and symptoms. Their recognition plays a critical role in candidate selection because the prognoses of many syndromes are generally well known. Although syndromic patients can exhibit marked individual differences, the overall predictive power of the diagnosis promotes more diligent efforts to control seizures and prepare families for eventual surgical referral.

Neurocutaneous disorders are particularly overrepresented at centers performing epilepsy surgery in early postnatal life. Aside from the more well-known disorders, such as tuberous sclerosis complex and Sturge–Weber syndrome, a large number of lesser-known conditions produce localization-related seizures. These include syndromes such as hypomelanosis of Ito, linear nevus sebaceous syndrome, incontinentia pigmenti, and neurocutaneous melanosis. Patients with these disorders are highly susceptible to medically resistant seizures and catastrophic presentations in the first year of life.

CANDIDATE SELECTION AND PREOPERATIVE EVALUTION

Medical Intractability in Infancy

Pediatric epileptologists caring for infants with medically refractory epilepsy recognize the inadequacy of adult criteria for establishing intractability. Seizure frequency in infants can be extreme, with multiple daily or even hourly recurrences. Although many infants already are developmentally delayed as a result of underlying brain damage, the combination of high seizure frequency and adverse drug effects may lead to further retardation of development and may lead to a loss of developmental milestones.

The high seizure frequencies of many infants permits more rapid determination of AED efficacy. Thus, although drug failure typically takes several years to detect in older patients, determinations in infants may require only weeks or months. When drug resistance is established in the setting of deteriorating development, especially in patients with special syndromes, earlier rather than later surgical intervention is easily justified.

Interestingly, many of the reasons for reconsidering surgical referral in older subjects are not an issue with regard to infants. Medication noncompliance is virtually nonexistent, and psychogenic seizures do not contribute to diagnostic uncertainty. Severe mental retardation is not a surgical contraindication because future potential cannot be objectively defined. Lastly, family dysfunction is less an issue, as the social dynamics of parent–infant interactions are relatively focussed.

EEG Evaluation

Infants and young children display rapidly changing EEG features reflecting dynamic postnatal processes, including maturation of myelination, synaptic connectivity, and neuronal dropout. The relatively immature neonatal cortex cannot support sustained or widespread hypersynchronized cortical discharges, even in the presence of diffuse pathological changes. As a consequence, EEG localization of clinical seizures in early life may be difficult. Clinical seizure patterns may be temporally and spatially dissociated from electrographic seizure patterns. With advancing chronologic age, the EEG and clinical semiology of partial seizures become more robust and seizures propagate more rapidly (10).

Ictal EEG patterns in infants are often regional rather than localized and display a wide variety of artifacts that obscure EEG interpretation. There is generally good correlation of ictal and interictal data, but fewer than half of interictal spiking is detected at the scalp (29). Infants are also susceptible to bilaterally synchronous and multifocal discharges. When EEG localization is not possible, regionalization may allow the planning of further invasive studies. Magnetic resonance imaging (MRI) and functional imaging may be used to confirm equivocal electrophysiologic findings.

The task of defining consistent focality is particularly challenging when focal epileptiform activity propagates rapidly. Not uncommonly, focal epileptiform patterns are identified interictally prior to the phase of generalization (21). The appearance of generalized epileptiform patterns is restricted to a finite window of time and is thus a phase in a developmental continuum. Focality also may be defined by alterations of EEG background, such as polymorphic slowing or attenuation of fast frequencies. In some cases, focal, intermittent fast activity provides the only clue to primarily localized epileptogenic dysfunction (30).

Neuroimaging

For the detection of most pediatric lesions, MRI is superior to computed tomographic (CT) scanning and is the imaging modality of choice for evaluating young pediatric epilepsy surgery candidates. The high specificity and sensitivity of MRI facilitate accurate definition of the pathologic substrates of many developmental disorders, including cortical dysplastic lesions, migrational disturbances, and developmental tumors (i.e., dysembryoplastic neuroepithelial tumors, gangliogliomas, and others). The high brain water content in the first 6 months of life may compromise gray–white differentiation on MRI and render interpretation more difficult. For this reason, CT may be preferable. MRI can identify a pathologic substrate in more than 80% of children with intractable partial epilepsy (31). Of 98 children and adolescents with partial epilepsy undergoing CT and MRI investigations, 30 had negative CT, and MRI showed lesions that were responsible for their epilepsy (32).

In addition, MRI studies also can document a high incidence of hippocampal sclerosis (HS) in childhood, and hippocampal volume loss can be documented (33). In 53 children with temporal lobe epilepsy (TLE) undergoing detailed MRI investigations, 30 showed either HS or regions of abnormal hippocampal signal in the absence of a mass lesion (34). HS has been documented in infants with medically resistant seizures. A developmentally delayed infant with a normal baseline MRI reportedly developed unilaterally increased signal in the hippocampus within 24 hours of an episode of status epilepticus (35).

Neuroimaging of pediatric epilepsy surgery candidates generally involves the use of techniques to maximize yield similar to adult imaging paradigms. T1-weighted data are optimally acquired in an oblique coronal orientation, orthogonal to the long axis of the hippocampi (36). Sequencing includes thin (1–1.5 mm) images without gaps, especially through the hippocampal regions. Further sequences such as fluid attenuated inversion recovery (FLAIR) may help to demonstrate subtle abnormalities. We routinely perform MRI at our institution after video/EEG monitoring for more detailed examination of the candidate seizure region.

Functional Imaging

Functional imaging of the epileptogenic region may help to define the seizure focus, especially when other modalities yield equivocal or divergent findings. Several techniques are presently available.

Positron Emission Tomography

Positron emission tomography (PET) uses radioactive tracers with short half-lives linked to cerebral blood flow. [18]Fluorodeoxyglucose (FDG) is a marker of the interictal focus, correlating with the epileptogenic region, usually the temporal lobe, in about 80% of adult cases (37). Ictal capture is unlikely and should not be induced by convulsant agents because of the technical limitations of the scanning process.

The requirement for sedation and higher proportion of extratemporal seizures limits the clinical utility of PET in children. Newer isotopes bound to receptor-specific compounds such as ^{11}C-flumazenil bind directly to the benzodiazepine receptor and hold promise for enhanced localization (38).

Single-Photon Emission Computed Tomography

Imaging with single-photon emission computed tomography (SPECT) uses isotopes such as HMPAO for qualitative measures of regional cerebral perfusion (rCP). Early studies were performed in the interictal state, but ictal injections are acknowledged to yield more accurate localization of the epileptogenic region (39). The high yield of ictal SPECT has supplanted PET in the functional evaluation of pediatric epilepsy surgery candidates (40).

Proton Magnetic Resonance Spectroscopy

Magnetic resonance spectroscopy (MRS) studies in epilepsy utilize *N*-acetyl aspartate (NAA), creatine, and phosphocreatine-containing compounds; several lines of evidence indicate that NAA is primarily intraneuronal and an indicator of neuronal well-being (41). ^{1}H-MRS can be added to routine imaging and provides important lateralizing information, especially in TLE (42). Recent MRS studies documented deranged neuronal function in dysplastic lesions and revealed correction of

metabolic derangement at mirror temporal foci after successful surgery (43).

Functional Mapping

The high incidence of neocortical epilepsy in children mandates careful assessment of cortical function. The standard adult paradigm whereby baseline stimulation is increased in 0.5- to-1.0 mA steps until an afterdischarge, functional response, or 15-mA ceiling is obtained is rarely successful in younger patients (44,45). Electric responsiveness increases in direct proportion to age, whereas the threshold for functional responsiveness decreases until adolescence (45).

Cortical responses are more reliably elicited in children by increasing both stimulus intensity and stimulus duration in a stepwise fashion (45). In comparison to the adult paradigm, only dual stimulation successfully evokes both afterdischarges and functional responses in patients 4 years of age and younger (45).

Sensorimotor Mapping

Dual-stimulation mapping of sensorimotor responses in pediatric epilepsy surgery candidates reveals that anatomic representation of cortical function is similar to that in the adult. Despite the overall similarities, however, elicited responses display several important maturational features (46). Children under the age of 4 years show predominantly tonic rather than clonic movements, and movement of the tongue is unusual. Before the age of 6 years, hand but not individual finger movement occurs in response to stimulation. As a rule, tonic finger movement appears earlier than clonic finger movement, a developmental sequence mirroring the ontogenetic expression of motor seizure patterns in childhood (11,47).

In children younger than 2 years of age, facial motor responses are often bilateral (46), resembling a grimace and lasting several seconds. Bilateral facial movement cannot be elicited in older children, suggesting that bilateral facial innervation is a transient postnatal pattern that predates axonal or synaptic elimination (48,49). With maturation, ipsilateral lower facial innervation is gradually lost. The observed bilateral facial movement is also consistent with facial sparing in congenital but not acquired hemiplegia (50).

Cortical mapping in patients with aberrant cortical development reveals unexpected anomalies of the motor homunculus (46). A hand region lying superior to the primary shoulder region and a double shoulder region above and below hand and finger cortex have been observed in selected patients. Aberrant cortical motor organization is more common when there is dysplastic tissue (51). Experimental studies in the primate brain indicate that prenatal lesions are capable of inducing anomalous cortical sulci and functional reorganization at remote cortical sites in both cerebral hemispheres (52–54).

Language Mapping

Whereas postnatal lesions of the dominant hemisphere in early childhood lead to significant reorganization of language cortex, there is little information about language representation in children with partial seizures and anomalous cortical development. Clarification of this problem has obvious implications for surgical evaluation of children with these lesions and seizures originating within or adjacent to language cortex (54).

A recent investigation of electric stimulation of language cortex in 34 predominantly pediatric patients with implanted subdural grid electrodes identified 28 with MRI or histologic evidence of developmental pathology (55). Patients with developmental lesions had language cortex in frontal and temporal sites, anatomically similar to the adult. The "adult" representation has been documented in an epilepsy patient as young as 4 years and has been encountered in a 2-year-old child undergoing mapping prior to tumoral surgery. The actual amount of square surface area of cortex devoted to language (based on the number of subdural electrodes with language representation) is also similar to the adult (56,57), suggesting that language sites are committed in early life and conserved anatomically over the lifespan.

OUTCOME

Localization-related Seizures

Historically, large resections have been the surgical treatment of choice for medically resistant partial seizures. Popular since the start of the second half of this century, hemispherectomy has been used to prevent death in status epilepticus and progressive neurologic decline as a consequence of repeated seizures and cumulative medication toxicity. The effectiveness of hemispherectomy for seizure control is well documented, and the temporary decline in the number of hemispherectomies worldwide resulted from danger inherent in superficial hemosiderosis of the ventricular wall and the development of progressive and occasionally fatal obstructive hydrocephalus.

Advances in the selection and preoperative evaluation of young epilepsy surgery patients now make it possible to identify patients with circumscribed seizure foci in the absence of any lateralized neurologic deficits (e.g., hemiparesis, homonomous hemianopia). Although hemispherectomy is a consideration for such cases, more precise delineation of the primary epileptogenic zone permits more selective resection with potential sparing of critical cortex. Whereas it may be argued that neural plasticity is fully operative in early life, there is evidence that cortical functions are not spared equally and that long-term recovery may be incomplete.

Significant reversal of catastrophic localization-related seizures in infants by neocortical resection was first reported in five patients younger than 1 year (4). Three became seizure free, and two improved significantly. This preliminary experience demonstrated that, in selected patients, hemispherectomy may not be necessary for complete seizure control.

Further confirmation of favorable seizure outcome using procedures tailored to the neurologic and seizure presentation appeared in two larger series. Wyllie (58) described 12 infants undergoing neocortical resection or hemispherectomy. Ten patients had abnormalities on MRI, and the two infants with negative studies had regions of cortical dysplasia localized by interictal SPECT. At mean 32-month follow-up, six were seizure free, three had rare seizures, and two had worthwhile improvement. There was catchup development following surgery, with parents reporting rapid acquisition of new skills after surgery.

In another series, 16 of 26 infants became seizure free, and four additional patients had a greater than 90% reduction in seizure occurrence (59). No significant differences were noted between patients undergoing hemispherectomy/multilobar resection versus patients undergoing lobar resection or between temporal versus extratemporal resection. Seizure outcome was also independent of the amount of neocortex removed from nonlesional patients. Only the presence of a discrete lesion correlated with a favorable outcome.

Infantile Spasms

A report by Shewmon et al. (60) revealed a high rate of immediate cessation of infantile spasms in infants actively exhibiting spasms at the time of resection. Of 28 cases, 26 (93%) exhibited immediate cessation of their spasms, only three of whom showed later relapse. The long-term prognosis was somewhat less optimistic: Only 11 patients were seizure free, five of whom were still taking medication. Considering the prognosis for patients with infantile spasms, the degree of seizure control in this population represents a significant improvement over medical therapy.

Improvement in adaptive function has been noted in patients undergoing surgery for infantile spasms (61). Adaptive levels for communication, daily living, and socialization skills improved after surgery for infantile spasms. The degree of improvement is as good or superior to children treated with adrenocorticotrophic hormone or sodium valproate. Children undergoing surgery earlier had the best developmental outcomes.

MORBIDITY AND MORTALITY

Young patients undergoing large procedures such as hemispherectomy and multilobar resection, demonstrate the expected deficits when eloquent cortical regions are excised. Hemiparesis and homonymous visual field defects are present after motor strip and posterior cortical ablation, although either may be spared with more limited resections. In most instances, similar disturbances are present preoperatively and are not made appreciably worse.

Postoperative complications are similar to those of older patients and include wound infection and subdural hematoma; however, postoperative mortality may be higher in young patients. One patient reported by Wyllie et al. (58) died of unexplained causes several hours after frontal lobectomy, and a 10-month-old infant reported by Duchowny et al. (59) died 3 weeks after functional hemispherectomy from sepsis and dehydration. A third patient died of acute hydrocephalus 4 months after functional hemispherectomy (59). This patient presented to a local hospital in a distant city with signs of intracranial pressure but was discharged without neurodiagnostic studies or treatment.

Including the absence of mortality in the three patients reported by Duchowny et al. (4), the three reported deaths occurred in a surgical cohort of 46 patients, yielding an estimated mortality of 7%. Although this figure appears to be considerably greater than the mortality rates for older children and adults, it is probably in part attributable to overall mortality associated with large resections.

CONCLUSION

The expression of epilepsy in early life constitutes a wide spectrum that includes benign partial and generalized disturbances as well as medically refractory disorders. A subset of infants with localization-related seizures may experience a particularly catastrophic course characterized by unresponsiveness to drug treatment and deterioration in developmental milestones. Postictal hemiparesis and convulsive apnea are characteristic symptoms in this age group. Infants suffering from West syndrome also may have an underlying localized cortical disturbance. Long-term outlook is generally disappointing, with prognosis for seizure persistence and mental handicap even poorer than for infantile spasms. Surgery in the setting of catastrophic deterioration is therefore an important and justifiable treatment option.

A high proportion of infants with catastrophic localization-related seizures have underlying disorders of cortical development. Cortical malformations may be localized or part of a more fully developed syndrome (e.g., hemimegalencephaly) in patients with linear nevus sebaceous syndrome. The neocortex is often involved, and neocortical seizures are therefore prevalent. Developmental lesions in medically uncontrolled infants are more often multilobar and associated with extremely high seizure frequencies.

As in older patients, the preoperative evaluation for neocortical resection in infancy depends on high-resolution MRI in conjunction with functional imaging and EEG localization. As a result of widespread lesional involvement, severe epileptogencity, and aberrant propagation patterns, however, resections in infants tend to be large multilobar excisions or hemispherectomies.

Despite these challenges, it is possible to achieve high rates of seizure freedom after surgery in infants for localization-related epilepsy. Seizure control in patients with infantile spasms is also favorable (60). Seizure freedom results in gratifying arrest of the preoperative clinical deterioration; long-term seizure outcome and psychological status remain unknown.

REFERENCES

1. Shields WD, Peacock WJ, Roper SN. Surgery for epilepsy: special pediatric considerations. *Neurosurg Clin N Am* 1993;4:301–10.
2. Chevrie JJ, Aicardi J. Convulsive disorders in the first year of life: neurological and mental outcome and mortality. *Epilepsia* 1978;19:67–74.
3. Chevrie JJ, Aicardi J. Convulsive disorders in the first year of life: persistence of epileptic seizures. *Epilepsia* 1979;20:643–649.
4. Duchowny MS, Resnick TJ, Alvarez LA, et al. Focal resection for malignant partial seizures in infancy. *Neurology* 1990;40:980–984.
5. Dravet C, Catani C, Bureau M, et al. Partial epilepsies in infancy: a study of 40 cases. *Epilepsia* 1989;30:807–812.
6. Duchowny MS. Complex partial seizures of infancy. *Arch Neurol* 1987;44:911.
7. Nordli DRJ, Bazil CW, Scheuer ML, et al. Recognition and classification of seizures in infants. *Epilepsia* 1997;38:553–560.
8. Ohmori I, Ohtsuka Y, Oka E, et al. Electroclinical study of localization-related epilepsies in early infancy. *Pediatr Neurol* 1997;16:131–136.
9. Acharya JN, Wyllie E, Lüders HO, et al. Seizure symptomatology in infants with localization-related epilepsy. *Neurology* 1997;48:189–196.
10. Duchowny M. The syndrome of partial seizures in infancy. *J Child Neurol* 1992;7:66–69.
11. Jayakar P, Duchowny MS. Complex partial seizures of temporal lobe origin in early childhood. In: Duchowny MS, Resnick TJ, Alvarez LA, eds. *Pediatric epilepsy surgery*. New York: Demos, 1990:41–46.
12. Yamamoto N, Watanabe K, Negoro T, et al. Complex partial seizures in children: ictal manifestations and their relation to clinical course. *Neurology* 1987;37:1379–1382.
13. Luna D, Dulac O, Plouin P. Ictal characteristics of cryptogenic partial epilepsies in infancy. *Epilepsia* 1989;30:833–838.
14. Watanabe K, Yamamoto N, Negoro T. Benign complex partial epilepsies in infancy. *Pediatr Neurol* 1987;3:208–211.
15. Watanabe K, Yamamoto N, Negoro T, et al. Benign infantile epilepsy with complex partial seizures. *J Clin Neurophysiol* 1990;7:409–416.
16. Watanabe K, Negoro T, Aso K. Benign partial epilepsy with secondarily generalized seizures in infancy. *Epilepsia* 1993;34:635–638.
17. Jeavons PM, Bower BD, Dimitrakoudi M. Long-term prognosis of 150 cases of "West syndrome." *Epilepsia* 1973;14:153–164.
18. Donat JF, Wright FS. Simultaneous infantile spasms and partial seizures. *J Child Neurol* 1991;6:246–250.
19. Donat JF, Lo WD. Asymmetric hypsarrhythmia and infantile spasms in West syndrome. *J Child Neurol* 1994;9:290–296.
20. Drury I, Beydoun A, Garofalo EA, et al. Asymmetric hypsarrhythmia: clinical electroencephalographic and radiological findings. *Epilepsia* 1995;36:41–47.
21. Gaily EK, Shewmon DA, Chugani HT, et al. Asymmetric and asynchronous infantile spasms. *Epilepsia* 1995;36:873–882.
22. Kramer U, Sue WC, Mikati MA. Hypsarrhythmia: frequency of variant patterns and correlation with etiology and outcome. *Neurology* 1997;48:197–203.
23. Kramer U, Sue WC, Mikati MA. Focal features in West syndrome indicating candidacy for surgery. *Pediatr Neurol* 1997;16:213–217.
24. Donat JF, Wright FS. Unusual variants of infantile spasms. *J Child Neurol* 1991;6:313–318.

25. Carrazana EJ, Lombroso CT, Mikati M, et al. Facilitation of infantile spasms by partial seizures. *Epilepsia* 1993;34:97–109.
26. Chugani HT. Functional brain imaging in pediatrics. *Pediatr Clin North Am* 1992;39:777–799.
27. Koo B, Hwang P. Localization of focal cortical lesions influences age of onset of infantile spasms. *Epilepsia* 1996;37:1068–1071.
28. Chugani HT, Hovda DA, Villablanca JR, et al. Metabolic maturation of the brain: a study of local cerebral glucose utilization in the developing cat. *J Cereb Blood Flow Metab* 1991;11:35–47.
29. Jayakar P, Duchowny M, Resnick TJ, et al. Localization of seizure foci: pitfalls and caveats. *J Clin Neurophysiol* 1991;8:414–431.
30. Shewmon A. Electroencephalography as a localizing tool. *Neurosurg Clin N Am* 1995;6:481–490.
31. Kuzniecky R, Murro A, King D, et al. Magnetic resonance imaging in childhood intractable partial epilepsies: pathologic correlations. *Neurology* 1993;43:681–687.
32. Resta M, Dicuonzo PF, Spagnolo P, et al. Imaging studies in partial epilepsy in children and adolescents. *Epilepsia* 1994;35:1187–1193.
33. Kuks JB, Cook MJ, Fish DR, et al. Hippocampal sclerosis in epilepsy and childhood febrile seizures. *Lancet* 1993;342:1391–1394.
34. Grattan-Smith JD, Harvey AS, Desmond PM, et al. Hippocampal sclerosis in children with intractable temporal lobe epilepsy: detection with MR imaging. *AJR Am J Roentgenol* 1993;161:1045–1048.
35. Nohria V, Lee N, Tien RD, et al. Magnetic resonance imaging evidence of hippocampal sclerosis in progression: a case report. *Epilepsia* 1994;35:1332–1336.
36. Duncan JS. Imaging and epilepsy. *Brain* 1997;120:339–377.
37. Engel J Jr. PET scanning in partial epilepsy. *Can J Neurol Sci* 1991;18:588–592.
38. Savic I, Thorell JO, Roland P. [11C]flumazenil positron emission tomography visualizes frontal epileptogenic regions. *Epilepsia* 1995;36:1225–1232.
39. Duncan R, Patterson J, Roberts R, et al. Ictal/postictal SPECT in the pre-surgical localisation of complex partial seizures. *J Neurol Neurosurg Psychiatry* 1993;56:141–148.
40. Harvey AS, Bowe JM, Hopkins IJ, et al. Ictal 99mTc-HMPAO single photon emission computed tomography in children with temporal lobe epilepsy. *Epilepsia* 1993;34:869–877.
41. Connelly A, Jackson GD, Duncan JS, et al. Magnetic resonance spectroscopy in temporal lobe epilepsy. *Neurology* 1994;44:1411–1417.
42. Gadian DG, Connelly A, Duncan JS, et al. 1H magnetic resonance spectroscopy in the investigation of intractable epilepsy. *Acta Neurol Scand* 1994;152(Suppl):116–121.
43. Cendes F, Andermann F, Dubeau F, et al. Normalization of neuronal metabolic dysfunction after surgery for temporal lobe epilepsy: evidence from proton MR spectroscopic imaging. *Neurology* 1997;49:1525–1533.
44. Alvarez LA, Jayakar P. Cortical stimulation with subdural electrodes: special considerations in infancy and childhood. *J Epilepsy* 1990;3(Suppl):125–130.
45. Jayakar P, Alvarez LA, Duchowny MS, et al. A safe and effective paradigm to functionally map the cortex in childhood. *J Clin Neurophysiol* 1992;9:288–293.
46. Duchowny M, Jayakar P. Functional cortical mapping in children. *Adv Neurol* 1993;63:149–154.
47. Brockhaus A, Elger CE. Complex partial seizures of temporal lobe origin in children of different age groups. *Epilepsia* 1995;36:1173–1181.
48. Innocenti GM, Caminitti R. Postnatal shaping of callosal connections from sensory areas. *Brain Res* 1980;38:381–394.
49. Rakic P, Bourgeois JP, Eckenhoff MF, et al. Concurrent overproduction of synapses in diverse regions of the primate cerebral cortex. *Science* 1986;232:231–232.
50. Lenn NJ, Freinkel AJ. Facial sparing as a feature of prenatal-onset hemiparesis. *Pediatr Neurol* 1989;5:291–295.
51. Maegaki Y, Yamamoto T, Takeshita K. Plasticity of central motor and sensory pathways in a case of unilateral extensive cortical dysplasia: investigation of magnetic resonance imaging, transcranial magnetic stimulation, and short-latency somatosensory evoked potentials. *Neurology* 1995;45:2255–2261.
52. Goldman PS. Neuronal plasticity in primate telencephalon: anomalous projections induced by prenatal removal of frontal cortex. *Science* 1978;202:767–768.
53. Goldman PS, Galkin TW. Prenatal removal of frontal association cortex in the fetal rhesus monkey: anatomical and functional consequences in postnatal life. *Brain Res* 1978;152:451–485.
54. Berger MS, Kincaid J, Ojemann GA, et al. Brain mapping techniques to maximize resection, safety, and seizure control in children with brain tumors. *Neurosurgery* 1989;25:786–792.
55. Duchowny M, Jayakar P, Harvey AS, et al. Language cortex representation: effects of developmental versus acquired pathology. *Ann Neurol* 1996;40:31–38.
56. DeVos KJ, Wyllie E, Geckler C, et al. Language dominance in patients with early childhood tumors near left hemisphere language areas. *Neurology* 1995;45:349–356.
57. Lesser RP, Lüders HO, Dinner DS. The location of speech and writing functions in the frontal language area: results of extraoperative cortical stimulation. *Brain* 1985;107:275–291.
58. Wyllie E. Surgery for catastrophic localization-related epilepsy in infants. *Epilepsia* 1996;37:S22–S25.
59. Duchowny M, Jayakar P, Resnick T, et al. Epilepsy surgery in the first three years of life. *Epilepsia* 1998;39:737–743.
60. Shewmon DA, Shields WD, Sankar R, et al. Follow-up on infants with surgery for catastrophic epilepsy. In: Tuxhorn I, Holthausen H, Boenigk H, eds. *Pediatric epilepsy syndromes and their surgical treatment.* London: John Libbey, 1997:513–25.
61. Asarnow RF, LoPresti C, Guthrie D, et al. Developmental outcomes in children receiving resection surgery for medically intractable spasms. *Dev Med Child Neurol* 1997;39:430–440.

Neocortical Epilepsies.
Advances in Neurology, Vol. 84,
edited by P. D. Williamson, A. M. Siegel,
D. W. Roberts, V. M. Thadani, and M. S. Gazzaniga.
Lippincott Williams & Wilkins, Philadelphia © 2000.

41

Outcome After Neocortical Resections in Pediatric Patients with Intractable Epilepsy

Elaine Wyllie

*Department of Neurology, Pediatric Epilepsy Program,
The Cleveland Clinic Foundation, Cleveland, Ohio 44195*

Few seizure outcome data are available from neocortical resections in pediatric patients. A recent series (1) illustrated some of the issues involved in the strategy for these procedures. This series included 136 pediatric patients who had epilepsy surgery at the Cleveland Clinic Foundation (CCF) during a 5.5-year period from January 1990 through June 1996 (1). The procedure was neocortical resection for 31% of children (3 months to 12 years of age) and 39% of adolescents (13 to 20 years of age).

In the CCF series (1), 22 (46%) of the 48 extratemporal resections were frontal; the remainder were parietal, occipital, perirolandic, or multilobar (frontal and temporal, temporal and occipital, or temporo–parieto–occipital). Magnetic resonance imaging (MRI) revealed the focal epileptogenic lesion (tumor, dysplasia, vascular malformation, or encephalomalacia) in 41 cases (85%). An additional four patients had focal cortical dysplasia that was diagnosed histopathologically but not seen on preoperative MRI. Therefore, 45 (94%) of the 48 extratemporal or multilobar resection patients had lesional epilepsy, and the remaining three patients had unknown etiology with normal MRI and nonspecific histopathology. The most common etiologies were focal cortical dysplasia (46% of patients) and low-grade tumor (39% of patients). Overall, MRI revealed the focal abnormality in 91% of the lesional

cases and clearly played a critical role in the selection of surgical candidates.

One to 7.5 (mean, 3.6) years after surgery, seizure-free outcome was the result for 54% of patients (58% of children and 52% of adolescents) (1). This was significantly less frequent than for patients who had temporal resection (78% were seizure free); however, differences in seizure outcome based on surgery type diminished when results were analyzed by etiology. Among patients with low-grade tumor, postoperative freedom from seizures was achieved for similar percentages of patients who had temporal (86%) versus extratemporal or multilobar (75%) resection. Results also tracked etiology instead of surgery type in the setting of cortical dysplasia (56% of patients were seizure free after temporal resection, 50% of patients were seizure free after extratemporal or multilobar resection). Dysplasia was significantly more frequent among patients who required extratemporal or multilobar resection (46%) than among those who required temporal resection (12%), perhaps contributing to the lower frequency of seizure-free outcome after extratemporal and multilobar procedures. The difference in outcome between patients with cortical dysplasia versus low-grade tumor was significant for the group as a whole. Other diverse series (2–5) have reported variable results after surgery for focal cortical dysplasia.

In addition to the patients with seizure-free outcome, another nine patients (19%) in the CCF series (1) had rare seizures after extratemporal or multilobar resection. Although complete freedom from seizures is the definition of acceptable outcome after epilepsy surgery in adults (6), the analysis may be different for some children. The goals for epilepsy surgery in adults are usually driving, employment, and independence, whereas the goals for surgery in children are often relief from catastrophic epilepsy, resumption of developmental progression, and improvement in behavior. For children with a high preoperative seizure burden, postoperative reduction to either rare or no seizures may represent a crucial improvement.

In contrast to the CCF results (1), Fish and colleagues (7) reported good outcome with rare or no postoperative seizures for only 27% of 45 children and adolescents (excluding tumor cases) who had frontal lobe resection at the Montreal Neurologic Institute during the pre-MRI era between 1940 and 1980. The more favorable results from the CCF series (1) may be due to the high percentage of patients with a focal epileptogenic lesion seen on preoperative MRI. Others also noted that the presence of a focal lesion on preoperative MRI is the key to a better prognosis for extratemporal resection. In a predominantly adult series, Zentner and colleagues (8) reported results almost identical to those from the CCF series (1), with freedom from seizures after extratemporal resection for 54% of 56 patients. In both series, almost all the patients had a focal lesion on histopathology, almost all of the lesions were identified on preoperative MRI, and a higher percentage of lesional than nonlesional patients were seizure free. The striking similarity in the results from these two contemporary series appears to reflect the positive impact of modern MRI on the selection of candidates for extratemporal or multilobar resection.

Clinical presentations may differ between pediatric and adult candidates for neocortical resection, but age-related differences in seizure manifestations do not appear to affect outcome. The most striking example is that of infantile spasms and hypsarrhythmia resulting from a focal epileptogenic lesion, usually cortical dysplasia (9–11). Even though these infants lack a key feature that is usually considered critical to the identification of surgical candidacy, that is, partial seizures with localized electroencephalographic (EEG) onset, their chance for good postoperative seizure outcome does not appear to be diminished. Chugani and colleagues (10) reported seizure-free outcome after cortical resection or hemispherectomy for 65% of 23 infants who presented with this seizure type. In these cases, positron emission tomography (PET) and MRI played especially critical roles in identifying the zone of cortical abnormality.

Similar to results from Chugani and colleagues (10), the CCF series (1) also noted that young age does not preclude favorable outcome after epilepsy surgery. The percentages of patients with postoperative freedom from seizures were similar in infancy, childhood, and adolescence. Duchowny and colleagues (12) also reported favorable results after epilepsy surgery early in life. These results suggest that epilepsy surgery should be considered at whatever age patients present with severe focal epilepsy.

In the CCF series (1), the most common complication of epilepsy surgery was wound infection, seen in four (2.9%) of the 136 study patients. Chronic implantation of subdural electrodes, performed in three of these four infected patients, appeared to be a factor. During recent years, as MRI has become more sensitive for identification of epileptotogenic lesions, the use of subdural electrodes has decreased at the CCF. Some investigators (5) believe that evaluation with subdural electrodes may be important for best outcome in the setting of focal cortical dysplasia, whereas others (1) believe that the use of subdural electrodes should be reserved for special cases requiring detailed localization of eloquent cortex in relation to a nearby epileptogenic zone.

Other complications of epilepsy surgery, including neocortical resection, are hemorrhage, infarction, new neurologic deficits, or perioperative death. During the 5.5-year study period of the CCF series (1), two of 149 (1.3%) died perioperatively. Other pediatric series (4,13) also included a small number of deaths. These cases emphasize that epilepsy surgery should be reserved for patients with severe, intractable epilepsy and poor quality of life. The risk may be increased in infancy. The surgical mortality at any age must be balanced against the mortality of uncontrolled seizures treated medically, however, which was estimated by Nashef and colleagues (14) to be 1:295 per year for children and adolescents. The surgical risk may be reduced by a dedicated team of pediatric neurosurgeons, anesthesiologists, and intensivists.

CONCLUSION

In summary, neocortical resections are frequently the procedures that come under consideration for pediatric patients with severe intractable epilepsy because of the relatively high incidence of developmental pathology in this age group. The chance for freedom from seizures after these procedures appears lower than for patients who have mesial temporal resection, but recent series have reported favorable outcome for most patients who had a focal epileptogenic lesion identified by MRI. Outcomes including rare or no postoperative seizures are especially gratifying in this group of patients who typically present with a high preoperative seizure burden. The potential risk:benefit ratio for surgery must be weighed carefully for each child in light of many complex age-related issues, and complicated cases warrant referral to specialized pediatric centers.

REFERENCES

1. Wyllie E, Comair YG, Kotagal P, et al. Seizure outcome after epilepsy surgery in children and adolescents. *Ann Neurol* 1998;44:740–748.
2. Palmini A, Andermann F, Olivier A, et al. Focal neuronal migration disorders and intractable partial epilepsy: results of surgical treatment. *Ann Neurol* 1991;30:750–757.
3. Hirabayashi S, Binnie CD, Janota I, et al. Surgical treatment of epilepsy due to cortical dysplasia: clinical and EEG findings. *J Neurol Neurosurg Psychiatry* 1993;56:765–770.
4. Vining EPG, Freeman JM, Pillas DJ, et al. Why would you remove half a brain? The outcome of 58 children after hemispherectomy—the Johns Hopkins experience: 1968–1996. *Pediatrics* 1997;100:163–171.
5. Mihara T, Matsuda K, Tottori T, et al. Focal cortical dysplasia and epilepsy surgery. *No To Hattatsu* 1997;29:134–144.
6. Sperling MR, Saykin AJ, Roberts FD, et al. Occupational outcome after temporal lobectomy for refractory epilepsy. *Neurology* 1995;45:970–977.
7. Fish DR, Smith SJ, Quesney LF, et al. Surgical treatment of children with medically intractable frontal or temporal lobe epilepsy: results and highlights of 40 years' experience. *Epilepsia* 1993;34:244–247.
8. Zentner J, Hufnagel A, Ostertun B, et al. Surgical treatment of extratemporal epilepsy: clinical, radiologic, and histopathologic findings in 60 patients. *Epilepsia* 1996;37:1072–1080.
9. Chugani HT, Shields WD, Shewmon DA, et al. Infantile spasms: I. PET identifies focal cortical dysplasia in cryptogenic cases for surgical treatment. *Ann Neurol* 1990;27:406–413.
10. Chugani HT, Shewmon DA, Shields WD, et al. Surgery for intractable infantile spasms: neuroimaging perspectives. *Epilepsia* 1993;34:764–771.
11. Wyllie E, Comair YG, Kotagal P, et al. Epilepsy surgery in infants. *Epilepsia* 1996;37:625–637.
12. Duchowny MS, Resnick TJ, Alvarez LA, et al. Focal resection for malignant partial seizures in children. *Neurology* 1990;40:980–984.
13. Chugani HT, Shewmon DA, Peacock WJ, et al. Surgical treatment of intractable neonatal-onset seizures: the role of positron emission tomography. *Neurology* 1988;38:1178–1188.
14. Nashef L, Fish DR, Garner S, et al. Sudden death in epilepsy: a study of incidence in a young cohort with epilepsy and learning difficulty. *Epilepsia* 1995;36:1187–1193.

Neocortical Epilepsies.
Advances in Neurology, Vol. 84,
edited by P. D. Williamson, A. M. Siegel,
D. W. Roberts, V. M. Thadani, and M. S. Gazzaniga.
Lippincott Williams & Wilkins, Philadelphia © 2000.

42

Antiepileptic Drugs in the Treatment of Neocortical Epilepsies

Jacqueline French, Peter Crino, and *Roger J. Porter

Epilepsy Center, Hospital of the University of Pennsylvania, Philadelphia, Pennsylvania 19104;
*Wyeth-Ayerst Research, Philadelphia, Pennsylvania 19101-8299

This chapter reviews differentiation of the medical therapy of the neocortical epilepsies from other syndromes, with emphasis on the potential difference between the treatment of mesial temporal epilepsies and the neocortical epilepsies. The treatise will be divided into three sections. First, we consider the differences between these two syndromes at a fundamental pharmacologic and neurophysiologic level. We then turn to current therapy to see whether any of the current drugs are particularly favored in the effort to treat neocortical epilepsies. Finally, we consider the role of new drugs in the treatment of this syndrome.

PHARMACOLOGIC FUNDAMENTALS

Seizures in patients with neocortical epilepsy are often particularly difficult to control by using conventional antiepileptic drugs (AEDs). Many patients with epilepsy resistant to medications require surgery to resect an epileptogenic focus. A frequent pathological finding in patients with medically intractable epilepsy is a region of disrupted cerebral cortical cytoarchitecture, which may result from low-grade tumor, for example, ganglioglioma, glial scar, encephalomalacia or, commonly, focal cortical dysplasia (FCD) (1–3). FCD may be identified in any cortical region although temporal and frontal neocortex are common locations. FCD may be isolated lesions, or it may exist as multiple foci throughout the brain. FCD, regions surrounding low-grade neoplasms, and encephalomalacic cortex are highly epileptogenic as determined by intraoperative electrocorticography (4,5), which reveals repetitive bursts of rhythmic spikes. Like other epileptogenic foci, FCD exhibits hypometabolism on positron emission tomography (PET) scans (6). Many tumors, vascular malformations, or larger dysplastic foci such as polymicrogyria or pachygyria can be identified by MRI (7), but microscopic tumors, scars, or FCD may be difficult to detect (8,9). FCD is often identified histologically in resected cortex from patients without radiographically detectable lesions.

Epileptogenesis in FCD and Neocortical Epilepsy

It is likely that the neuropharmacologic profiles of neurons within neocortical foci may render these regions resistant to the effects of most AEDs. The cellular substrates for epileptogenesis in neocortical foci are distinct from those in hippocampal or mesial temporal lobe seizures. Indeed, the high prevalance of lesions, for example, tumors or FCD, in neocortical epilepsy versus seizures of hippocampal onset suggests important pathogenic differences. Direct comparisons between the electric features of neocortical and hippocampal seizures in human may be helpful in distinguishing the effects of distinct AEDs in these epilepsies.

Alterations in both laminar cytoarchitecture and cellular morphology in a variety of brain lesions—including tumors, vascular malformations, focal cortical dysplasia, encephalomalacia secondary to ischemic stroke or trauma, and gliosis—likely serve as important contributors to epileptogenesis. For example, direct electrophysiologic recordings from FCD slice specimens have revealed either repetitive, seizure-like discharges or isolated negative-going field potentials following treatment with 4-aminopyridine (5,10). Whereas little is understood about the electrophysiologic properties of neocortical heterotopia, recent evidence suggests that heterotopic neurons in hippocampal sector CA1 may provide an electric bridge between the hippocampal formation and temporal neocortex (11). Electrical field potentials in human neocortical temporal lobe tissue resected for treatment of pharmacoresistant epilepsy exhibited spontaneous population spikes (12). In patients with ganglioglioma, stimulation of entorhinal cortex evoked an abnormal response of greater complexity and shorter latency in the ipsilateral hippocampus (13) than in control hippocampus.

Altered expression of select genes and their encoded proteins, for example, neurotransmitter receptor complexes, may be the key factors in seizure initiation and propagation. The molecular neuropharmacologic features of dysplastic neurons may provide etiologic clues to their aberrant migration as well as potential epileptogenic mechanisms. The current view regarding epileptogenesis in FCD is that there is an imbalance in excitatory and inhibitory control of neural firing. Thus, there is either too much excitatory or too little inhibitory synaptic activity. Specifically, one proposed hypothesis for the epileptogenic properties of neocortical foci is diminished inhibitory tone resulting either from reduced GABAergic neurons or $GABA_{A/B}$ receptor-mediated neurotransmission. Epileptogenic FCD exhibits reduced binding of ^{123}I-iomezanil or ^{11}C-flumazenil to the benzodiazepine binding sites (14). Previous evidence suggested that there are too few GABAergic neurons within FCD or in neocortex adjacent to neocortical lesions. A decrease in the number of inhibitory neurons within dysplastic cortex may contribute to the epileptogenicity of these regions (15). It is not known whether reductions in the number of GABAergic neurons result from selective cell death, failed expression of genes that regulate glutamic acid decarboxylase (GAD) synthesis, or migratory failure of GABAergic neurons. Indeed, heterotopic neurons in subcortical white matter express the calcium-binding proteins calbindin and parvalbumin, which are typically enriched in inhibitory neurons (15). Thus, heterotopic neurons might reflect a subpopulation of GABAergic cells that fail to reach the cortical mantle during corticogenesis. As such, they fail to make appropriate inhibitory synaptic connections with neurons within dysplastic or surrounding normal cortex, and this results in excessive excitation and seizure propagation.

Alterations in the relative abundances of excitatory amino acid neurotransmitter receptor mRNAs and proteins may have functional consequences relating to the firing properties of dysplastic neurons and other lesions in neocortical epilepsy. Increased glutamate-mediated synaptic activity may enhance excitation in these regions. For example, in rodents with FCD resulting from methoxyazoxymethanol treatment, reductions in NMDA 1 and increases in GluR2 mRNA were identified (16). In single microdissected dysplastic neurons, reductions in GluR1 and NMDA2A and increases in GluR4 and R6 and NMDA 2B and 2C subunit mRNAs have been demonstrated (17). Recent immunohistochemical analyses of human epilepsy tissue demonstrated increased NR 1, 2A, and 2B receptor subunit immunoreactivity in dysplastic neurons (18). Other studies, however, failed to identify consistent differences in GABAergic or glutamatergic markers in FCD (19). Increased NR2A/B and GluR2/3 receptors in dysplastic neurons suggests that seizures emanating from these lesions may result from enhanced excitatory synaptic transmission. Altered abundances of GAD, GABA, GABAergic, and glutamatergic receptor subunits also have been reported in regions surrounding dysembryoblastic neuroepithelial tumors (DNTs), gangliogliomas, and tubers (19). Several lines of evidence have suggested that decreases in postsynaptic inhibition may have a role in epileptogenesis in cortical structures. Human neocortical neurons recorded intracellularly under normal conditions generate stimulus-induced and spontaneous potentials that are mediated by the activation of postsynaptic $GABA_A$ and $GABA_B$ receptor subtypes. Pharmacologic blockade of the $GABA_A$ receptor makes epileptiform bursts appear in response to extracellular focal stimuli, thus indicating that inhibition mediated through the activation of the $GABA_A$ receptor exerts an important role in controlling neuronal excitability in the human neocortex (20). A more complex interaction between $GABA_A$ and $GABA_B$ receptor subunits may contribute to epileptogenesis. For example, postsynaptic blockade of $GABA_B$ receptors induces an amplification of epileptiform activity in neocortical slices disinhibited by $GABA_A$ receptor antagonists. Additional blockade of presynaptic $GABA_B$ receptors reduces the inhibitory autofeedback control of GABA release, leading to a displacement of competitive antagonists from the postsynaptic $GABA_A$ receptor and hence to suppression of epileptiform activity induced by $GABA_A$ receptor antagonists (21).

The well-documented efficacy of benzodiazepines and barbiturates on seizure control, especially in status epilepticus, argues that regulation of GABAergic tone in seizure foci is essential for seizure control. In light of these data, it is not surprising that several newer AEDs, including vigabatrin, tiagabine, and gabapentin, which act specifically to facilitate GABA-mediated synaptic activity, are proving effective in select groups of patients. Assessment of these agents for specific use in neocortical epilepsy is warranted.

Animal Models

A few animal models of FCD have been evaluated that may aid in understanding the pathogenesis of neocortical epilepsy (22).

These include direct trauma (needlestick or cortical freeze lesion) to the cortical plate, fetal ionizing radiation (23), administration of alcohol or methylmercury to fetal rats, and several spontaneous and transgenic mouse mutant strains. Most of the animal systems cause focal or diffuse disruption of cortical cytoarchitecture and underscore the hypothesis that disruption of cell morphology and lamination are major factors in epileptogenesis. In experimental models of FCD, the expression of epileptiform activity in affected cortex likely results from an imbalance between excitatory and inhibitory synaptic transmission as reported in human specimens. An increase in NMDA-receptor–mediated excitation in pyramidal neurons and a concurrent decrease of glutamatergic input onto inhibitory interneurons yield a functional diminution of inhibitory tone (24). Exposure of fetal rats to external gamma irradiation produces diffuse cortical dysplasia and neuronal heterotopia. Electroencephalographic studies in these animals revealed an increased propensity for electrographic seizures and in vitro neocortical slices containing dysplastic cortex demonstrate enhanced excitability when $GABA_A$ receptor–mediated inhibition is blocked with bicuculline. In contrast, newborn rats receiving a focal freeze lesion to the cerebral cortex were investigated anatomically and in vitro electrophysiologically after survival times of up to 5 months (25). Loss of normal cortical lamination (focal microgyrus) and presence of ectopic cell clusters in layer I and in the white matter (heterotopia) are observed in these animals. Prominent hyperexcitability of the disorganized neocortical network is detected, and electric stimulation of slice afferents elicits epileptiform responses that propagated over greater than 4 mm in the horizontal direction. Epileptiform responses are blocked by 2,3-dihydroxy-6-nitro-7-sulfamoyl-benz(F)-quinoxaline (NBQX), indicating that AMPA receptors play a prominent role in the generation and propagation of this pathophysiologic activity. These researchers suggested that excessive excitation rather than disinhibition induces epileptogenesis. A contrasting view was proposed by other investigators using the freeze microgyrus system (26). They demonstrate that sprouting of axonal arborizations of pyramidal cells onto interneurons, upregulation of GABAergic neurons, and perhaps sprouting of inhibitory axons that make increased numbers of contacts onto pyramidal cells all may contribute to increased, rather than diminished, inhibitory drive. Their results do not support the disinhibitory hypothesis of chronic epileptogenesis. Further investigation of the respective roles of excitatory and inhibitory synaptic transmission in neocortical epilepsy, especially in the setting of neocortical lesions, will provide answers to these dilemmas.

Several lines of evidence underscore a possible role of voltage-gated Na^+ channels (NaCH) in epilepsy (27). Altered expression of NaCh mRNAs was identified in kainate(KA)-treated rats with seizures. These investigators postulated that the KA-induced upregulation in NaCh mRNAs likely induced an increase in hippocampal neuronal excitability and a propensity for seizures. Further studies of Na^+ and K^+ channel expression in human neocortical foci remain a necessity. Clearly, because AEDs, including carbamezapine, phenytoin, and lamotrigine, work as Na^+ channel blockers, alterations in Na^+ channel kinetics, number, or functional composition may impact on the effects of these AEDs in neocortical epilepsy.

ROLE OF CURRENT MEDICATIONS

Phenobarbital, phenytoin, carbamazepine, and valproate have been the mainstay of the treatment of neocortical epilepsies since each of these drugs was marketed. In addition, the use of these medications for neocortical epilepsies has remained, in the eyes of most clinicians, undifferentiated from the treatment of partial epilepsies in general. The reason for this undifferentiated approach has been the paucity of data suggesting that some of these medications are better for the control of seizures arising from the mesial temporal region and that others are better for attacks arising from the neocortex.

In many ways, our inability to differentiate is surprising. We are able to differentiate the effects of several other antiepileptic drugs, both in relation to seizure types and to the various epilepsies; we can partition drugs among the syndromes. Ethosuximide is effective against absence epilepsy and is limited in its scope. Valproate is not only effective against absence epilepsy but is highly effective in certain myoclonic syndromes, where phenytoin is useless at best. Even the special case of infantile spasms has its own peculiar pattern of drug responsiveness. These syndromes are pathophysiologically distinct, and, as we might expect, the various medications partition differentially among them. Remarkable then, if one then considers the neuroanatomic, neurophysiologic, and clinical dissimilarities between neocortical and mesial temporal epilepsies, is the failure to see prominent partition of the various medications between these two syndromes.

What are the data on the difference in the effectiveness of the various older medications on neocortical and mesial temporal seizures? The data are exceedingly limited; they come from two disparate sources and yield differing opinions.

The most generally applicable data come from the first Veterans Administration (VA) study (28) of the comparison of carbamazepine, phenobarbital, phenytoin, and primidone in the treatment of partial seizures. In an interesting comparative analysis of the patients who had either extratemporal or temporal seizures, Mattson (29) was able to find 63 patients with extratemporal seizures and 66 with temporal lobe onset. Seizures were controlled in 55% of the temporal but only 30% of the extratemporal group. Although the difference in response to medical therapy (using one of the four aforementioned drugs) could not be statistically analyzed because of the small sample size, one interesting observation stood out: The use of either phenobarbital or primidone was associated with complete seizure control in six of the eight extratemporal patients even though the overall control in the partial seizure patients with these two medications was only 32%. Despite these observations, the author noted that convincing data are not available to make a selection between drugs used for temporal and extratemporal seizure control (29).

The second line of data on the potential differentiation of commonly used antiepileptic drugs in neocortical epilepsies comes from a much more highly selected group of patients whose seizures arise from the frontal lobe. The syndrome of autosomal dominant nocturnal frontal lobe epilepsy is known in the English literature as *ADNFLE*. This syndrome is characterized by clusters of brief nocturnal motor seizures with hyperkinetic and tonic characteristics. An aura may be present, and some authors note that consciousness may not be lost during some attacks (30). The seizures typically start in childhood and persist into adulthood.

The reason that neocortical frontal lobe epilepsy is of particular interest is that carbamazepine appears, anecdotally to be sure, to be particularly effective against such seizures—more so than some other drugs. During the study by Scheffer et al. (30), 38 patients with the disorder were on medical therapy for seizure control. Of these, 15 were taking carbamazepine, and 12 were well controlled. When carbamazepine was withdrawn in adulthood, seizures were likely to recur. These researchers noted that phenytoin was also effective in some older patients but that valproate was "generally not effective." When patients were switched from valproate to carbamazepine, "a dramatic improvement in seizure control was seen" (30).

This differentiation was further documented in one patient by Thomas et al. (31), who studied five affected patients in one family and directly compared the effectiveness of valproate and carbamazepine. At the doses used, carbamazepine is much more effective than valproate in this syndrome.

Additional data come from the study of Oldani et al. (32), who studied 38 patients with ADNFLE and treated 15 of these for 6 months. Eleven patients experienced a good response; of these, eight were treated with carbamazepine, two with clonazepam, and one with lamotrigine. Finally, in an earlier study, Fusco et al. (33) studied eight patients and noted that one patient had experienced a good response on phenytoin.

Clearly, from these data, it is impossible to make a definitive judgment, especially for an individual patient, on the merits of selecting various classic medications for the treatment of neocortical epilepsy. No controlled studies are available to assist us in this effort. Whether one is intrigued by the data on phenobarbital from the VA study or whether one is impressed by the anecdotal data from the studies of ADNFLE, firm conclusions are simply not possible.

NEWER ANTIEPILEPTIC DRUGS

As is the case for the standard antiepileptic drugs, little data are available about the differential effects of the newer antiepileptic drugs on neocortical epilepsy versus mesial temporal lobe epilepsy. Yet there may be better reasons for investigating the newer agents in this regard. The standard AEDs, discussed in the previous section, share similar mechanisms of action, such as sodium channel blockade, which are for the most part, not receptor specific. In addition, older drugs tend to have multiple, less well-defined mechanisms. In comparison, newer antiepileptic drugs tend to have more selective, receptor-based mechanisms of action. Table 42.1 subdivides newer and established AEDs by mechanism of action. As discussed earlier in this chapter, we are learning an increasing

TABLE 42.1. *Mechanisms of some new and old antiepileptic drugs*

Sodium channel blockade	Receptor-specific mechanism	Multiple mechanisms
Phenytoin	*Vigabatrin* (GABA)	*Topiramate*
Carbamazepine	*Tiagabine* (GABA)	*Felbamate*
Lamotrigine	*Gabapentin* (GABA-related)	*?Valproic acid*
	Phenobarbital	

Newer drugs are in italics.

amount about the changes in receptors in cortex that contains specific pathology, such as cortical dysplasia. It is also possible that different lobes of the brain have different connections, which utilize specific neurotransmitters to a greater or lesser extent, or have a greater or lesser density of certain receptors. It stands to reason that neocortical epilepsy, with its more varied pathological substrate and potentially more varied underlying pathophysiology, would require an expanded pharmacopoeia for effective treatment. It is in this patient population, if anywhere, that we might expect to identify subgroups of patients who demonstrate a selective mechanism-based drug response.

Although these concepts are intellectually appealing, there has been no convincing evidence to date that supports the effectiveness of a given AED for such a subpopulation. In part, this lack of evidence may stem from the difficulty of obtaining such information. There are no good animal models for selective drug testing. Specifically, no models of frontal versus temporal versus occipital epilepsy are available for AED screening. Also, there is no good comparison model of neocortical versus mesial temporal disease. Most information about the effectiveness of new AEDs derives from placebo-controlled, adjunctive trials. Little or no attempt has been made to subdivide populations in these trials to determine whether some groups might have greater benefit than others. Such an attempt would in any case be fraught with peril. How would subgroups be chosen? By underlying pathology? More often than not, this is unknown. By lobe of seizure onset (e.g., frontal versus temporal versus parietal)? Again, this is frequently unknown, as focal electroencephalographic spikes can be notoriously misleading, and patients with well-defined foci frequently undergo epilepsy surgery rather than entering investigational drug trials. Even if a subgroup could be accurately identified, it might be too small to provide meaningful data, as it was in the VA cooperative study discussed previously. Nonetheless, efforts are under way to better characterize clinical trial populations to "tease out" characteristics of drug-sensitive patients.

Randomized controlled trials have not provided information about which of the newer antiepileptic drugs may be beneficial in neocortical epilepsies. The scant existing data was derived from observational studies. Again, there are great potential biases in studies such as these, but they may provide some preliminary pilot data. One small study (34) evaluated 105 children aged 5 months to 22 years, treated with either vigabatrin or lamotrigine. Of these, 47 were believed to have localization-related epilepsy. Five of eleven children with frontal lobe epilepsy responded to lamotrigine, whereas only one of nine children with temporal lobe epilepsy responded. Children with localization-related seizures treated with vigabatrin had a better response overall, which was independent of localization in this small sample. Another, larger observational study was performed in 566 refractory epilepsy patients receiving lamotrigine. Children and adults were included. Patients with partial seizures that secondarily generalized did better that those with complex partial seizures. Studies indicated that patients with pure mesial temporal lobe epilepsy often have complex partial seizures only (35). Therefore, this differential effect may indicate better effectiveness for neocortical epilepsy.

CONCLUSION

There is a large clinical gap between our understanding on a basic level of substrate and pharmacology of neocortical epilepsy and our ability to use this information clinically to choose a treatment for a given patient. Much more information is needed. It is hoped that the emergence of new antiepileptic drugs, with specific mechanisms will stimulate research that will close this gap.

ACKNOWLEDGMENTS

We acknowledge the efforts of Susan Rymer, Toni Roulston, and Kathleen Treen in the preparation of this manuscript. Without their help, it could not have been accomplished.

REFERENCES

1. Taylor DC, Falconer M, Bruton MJ. Focal dysplasias of the cerebral cortex in epilepsy. *J Neurol Neurosurg Psychiatry* 1971;34:369–387.
2. Barth PG. Disorders of neuronal migration. *Can J Neurosci* 1987;14:1–16.
3. Wolf HK, Muller MB, Spanle M, et al. Ganglioglioma: a detailed histopathological and immunohistochemical analysis of 61 cases. *Acta Neuropathol* 1994;88:166–173.
4. Palmini A, Gambardella A, Andermann F, et al. Intrinsic epileptogenicity of human dysplastic cortex as suggested by corticography and surgical results. *Ann Neurol* 1995;37:476–487.
5. Preul MC, Leblanc R, Cendes F, et al. Function and organization in dysgenic cortex. Case report. *J Neurosurg* 1997;87:113–121.
6. Henry TR, Sutherland NW, Engel J Jr, et al. Interictal cerebral metabolism in partial epilepsies of neocortical origin. *Epilepsy Res* 1991;10:174–182.
7. Kuzniecky R, Morawetz R, Faught E, et al. Frontal and central lobe focal dysplasia: clinical, EEG, and imaging features. *Dev Med Child Neurol* 1995;37:159–166.
8. Hardimann O, Burke T, Phillips J, et al. Microdysgenesis in resected temporal neocortex: incidence and clinical significance in focal epilepsy. *Neurology* 1998;38:1041–1047.
9. Rojiani AM, Emery JA, Anderson KJ, et al. Distribution of heterotopic neurons in normal hemispheric white matter: a morphometric analysis. *J Neuropathol Exp Neurol* 1996;55:178–183.
10. Mattia D, Olivier A, Avoli M. Seizure-like discharges recorded in human dysplastic neocortex maintained in vitro. *Neurology* 1995;45:1391–1395.
11. Chavassus-Au-Louis N, Congar P, Represa A, et al. Neuronal migration disorders: heterotopic neocortical neurons in CA1 provide a ridge between the hippocampus and the neocortex. *Proc Natl Acad Sci USA* 1998;95:10263–10268.
12. Luhmann HJ, Raabe K, Qû M, et al. Characterization of neuronal migration disorders in neocortical structures: extracellular in vitro recordings. *Eur J Neurosci* 1998;10:3085–3094.
13. Rutecki PA, Grossman RG, Armstrong D, et al. Electrophysiological connections between the hippocampus and entorhinal cortex in patients with complex partial seizures. *J Neurosurg* 1989;70:667–675.
14. Richardson MP, Koepp MJ, Brooks DJ, et al. 11C-flumazenil PET in neocortical epilepsy. *Neurology* 1998;51:485–492.
15. Spreafico R, Battaglia G, Arcelli P, et al. Cortical dysplasia: an immunocytochemical study of three patients. *Neurology* 1998;50:27–36.
16. Rafiki A, Chevassus-Au-Louis N, Ben-Ari Y, et al. Glutamate receptors in dysplasic cortex: an in situ hybridization and immunohistochemistry study in rats with prenatal treatment with methylazoxymethanol. *Brain Res* 1998;782:142–152.
17. Crino PB, French J, Dichter M, et al. Gene expression analysis of single neurons in focal cortical dysplasia. American Epilepsy Society Abstract, 1999.
18. Ying Z, Babb TL, Comair YG, et al. Induced expression of NMDAR2 proteins and differential expression of NMDAR1 splice variants in dysplastic neurons of human epileptic neocortex. *J Neuropathol Exp Neurol* 1998;57:47–62.
19. Wolf HK. Glioneuronal malformative lesions and dysembryoblastic neuroepithelial tumors in patients with chronic pharmacoresistant epilepsies. *J Neuropathol Exp Neurol* 1995;54:245–254.
20. Avoli M, Hwa G, Louvel J, et al. Functional and pharmacological properties of GABA-mediated inhibition in the human neocortex. *Can J Physiol Pharmacol* 1997;75:526–534.
21. Sutor B, Luhmann HJ. Involvement of GABA(B) receptors in convulsant-induced epileptiform activity in rat neocortex in vitro. *Eur J Neurosci* 1998;10:3417–3427.
22. Chavassus-Au-Louis N, Baraban SC, Gaiarsa JL, et al. Cortical malformations and epilepsy: new insights from animal models. *Epilepsia* 1999;40:811–821.
23. Roper SN, King MA, Abraham LA, et al. Disinhibited in vitro neocortical slices containing experimentally induced cortical dysplasia demonstrate hyperexcitability. *Epilepsy Res* 1997;26:443–449.
24. Luhmann HJ, Karpuk N, Qû M, et al. Characterization of neuronal migration disorders in neocortical structures. II. Intracellular in vitro recordings. *J Neurophysiol* 1998;80:92–102.
25. Luhmann HJ, Raabe K. Characterization of neuronal migration disorders in neocortical structures. I. Expression of epileptiform activity in an animal model. *Epilepsy Res* 1996;26:67–74.
26. Prince DA, Jacobs KM, Salin PA, et al. Chronic focal neocortical epileptogenesis: does disinhibition play a role? *Can J Physiol Pharmacol* 1997;75:500–507.
27. Bartolomei F, Gastaldi M, Massacrier A, et al. Changes in the mRNAs encoding subtypes I, II, and III sodium channel alpha subunits following kainate-induced seizures in rat brain. *J Neurocytol* 1997;26:667–678.
28. Mattson RH, et al. Comparison of carbamazepine, phenobarbital, phenytoin, and primidone in partial and secondarily generalized tonic–clonic seizures. *N Engl J Med* 1985;313:145–151.
29. Mattson RH. Drug treatment of partial epilepsy. *Adv Neurol* 1992;57:643–650.
30. Scheffer IE, Bhatia KP, Lopes-Cendes I, et al. Autosomal dominant nocturnal frontal lobe epilepsy: a distinctive clinical disorder. *Brain* 1995;118:61–73.
31. Thomas P, Picard F, Hirsch E, et al. Epilepsie frontale nocturne autosomique dominante. *Rev Neurol* 1998;154:228–235.
32. Oldani A, Zucconi M, Asselta R, et al. Autosomal dominant nocturnal frontal lobe epilepsy: a video-polysomnographic and genetic appraisal of 40 patients and delineation of the epileptic syndrome. *Brain* 1998;121:205–223.
33. Fusco L, Iani C, Faedda MT, et al. Mesial frontal lobe epilepsy: a clinical entity not sufficiently described. *J Epilepsy* 1990;3:23–135.
34. Belanger S, Coulombe G, Carmant L. Role of vigabatrin and lamotrigine in the treatment of childhood epileptic syndromes. *Epilepsia* 1998;39:878–883.
35. French JA, Williamson PD, Thadani VM, et al. Characteristics of medial temporal lobe epilepsy. I. Results of history and physical examination. *Ann Neurol* 1993;34:774–780.

Neocortical Epilepsies.
Advances in Neurology, Vol. 84,
edited by P. D. Williamson, A. M. Siegel,
D. W. Roberts, V. M. Thadani, and M. S. Gazzaniga.
Lippincott Williams & Wilkins, Philadelphia © 2000.

43

Surgery of Parietal and Occipital Lobe Epilepsy

André Olivier and Warren Boling, Jr.

Montreal Neurological Institute, McGill University, Montreal, Quebec, Canada H3A 2B4

The approach taken in this chapter considers both the parietal and occipital lobes together because of their close anatomic and functional relationships. The same reasoning could be applied for the central area. It is indeed impossible to discuss surgery of the parietal lobe without consideration of the central area and particularly of the postcentral gyrus.

Many obstacles are encountered in obtaining excellent surgical results in parietal lobe epilepsy. These include difficulty in interpreting the semiology, the lack of a visible lesion on imaging, the presence of highly eloquent areas in the vicinity of the resection zones, and the intricacies of the surgical anatomy including its vascular components.

Modern anatomicofunctional imaging has revolutionized the field of epilepsy surgery by revealing more discrete lesions responsible for the epilepsy and by providing the surgeon with tools to reach these lesions with precision and safety. This approach combines frameless stereotaxy with preoperative and perioperative functional mapping of sensory, motor, and speech functions (1–4).

Few series have been published on the surgical treatment of parietal and occipital epilepsy and even fewer on the modern surgical and technical aspects (5–17). After a brief historical overview, a summary of the surgical anatomy of the parietal and occipital lobes is presented. The clinical manifestations of parietal and occipital epilepsy, which are so cru-cial in establishing the hypothesis of the site of seizure onset, are presented from a practical surgical perspective. The technical aspects and various modalities of resections pertaining also are addressed. The core of the presentation consists of an analysis of several representative cases with emphasis on the operative approaches, findings, and results.

HISTORICAL PERSPECTIVE

Horsley, considered the father of epilepsy surgery, maintained that there was no separation of sensory and motor function between the precentral and postcentral gyrus, although he did state that in the postcentral gyrus, "probably provision for sensorial coordination is greater" (18). In 1909, Cushing presented two patients with epilepsy and sensory auras in the right hand (19). He was able to awaken the patients after the dura was exposed and stimulate the central area. He concluded that stimulation of the postcentral gyrus gave definite sensory impressions not elicited from the precentral gyrus and that motor responses resulted only from precentral stimulation. This description of the sensory somatotopical organization of the postcentral gyrus supplemented with brain maps represents a significant historical landmark in the surgery of parietal lobe epilepsy.

Foerster in 1926 reported an astonishing series of patients with traumatic epilepsy treated surgically, which included seven occipital, seven parietal, and 11 postcentral cases (20). He also provided a detailed map of cortical stimulation results including sensory and motor responses from the central area. In 1930, Foerster and Penfield presented their results in the surgical treatment of traumatic epilepsy and the role of brain injury as an etiologic factor (21,22). They emphasized the importance of diagnostic imaging with pneumoencephalography and seizure semiology for localizing the cortical scar. They also stressed the importance of performing the operation under local anesthesia to allow the cortical surface to be mapped by electric stimulation and to excise the scar completely.

The epilepsy surgical series at the Montreal Neurological Institute (MNI) began in 1929 (23). When Penfield and associates classified patients by regions, they found that surgery in the parietal lobe produced the least favorable outcome (24,25). Rasmussen reported the MNI experience up to 1980 for surgery of parietal, central, and occipital epilepsy (10); 203 patients had nontumoral epileptogenic lesions, and 56% became seizure free or had a marked reduction of seizure tendency following surgery. Three hundred forty-seven patients presented with a tumor and a prime complaint of focal epilepsy (26). The lesions were located in the central area in 65, parietal in 45, and occipital in 2. The removal of meningiomas, benign gliomas, and vascular malformations resulted in excellent results on the seizure tendency with 81%, 70%, and 67%, respectively, arrest or marked reduction in seizure frequency for each of these conditions. The worst seizure outcome was in malignant gliomas, with only 43% of the patients obtaining a significant effect.

Salanova et al. in 1992 reported on 42 patients with nontumoral occipital lobe epilepsy who underwent surgery at the MNI prior to 1991 (11). Of these, 67% became seizure free or had a significant reduction in seizure frequency. In 1995, Salanova et al. reported a series of 82 patients with nontumoral parietal lobe epilepsy who underwent surgery at the MNI between 1929 and 1988 (12). A significant benefit was achieved in 65% of these pa-

tients. Thirty-four patients with tumoral parietal lobe epilepsy from the MNI also were reviewed by Salanova et al. (13). All these patients had slow growing tumors confined to the parietal lobe. After a mean follow-up of 12.3 years, 75% were seizure free or had rare seizures.

Williamson et al. described 16 patients with occipital epilepsy and surgery in the occipital lobe (17). All these patients had a lesion; 14 became seizure free. The same year, Williamson et al. reported 10 patients with parietal epilepsy and surgery in the parietal lobe (16). Resection of a lesion found in all the patients resulted in 100% freedom from seizures. Cascino et al. evaluated ten patients with a parietal lesion and intractable epilepsy (7). Diverse pathology types were included, and lesionectomy resulted in seizure freedom in nine.

Blume et al. reported 19 patients with and without lesions who underwent surgery in the occipital lobe for intractable epilepsy (6). Thirty-two percent became seizure free and an additional 42% achieved seizure reductions greater than 50%.

SURGICAL ANATOMY OF PARIETAL LOBE

The boundaries of the parietal lobe, as described by neuroanatomists, here had little revision since Turner proposed the central sulcus as the line of separation between the frontal and parietal lobes (28–33). On the lateral convexity, the anterior boundary corresponds to the central sulcus and on the mesial surface either to a vertical line drawn from the termination of the central sulcus down to the cingulate sulcus (31,34) or to the marginal branch of the cingulate sulcus (33,35) (Fig. 43.1). The posterior boundary on the mesial surface is the parietooccipital sulcus and, on the lateral convexity, an arbitrary line drawn from the parietooccipital sulcus superomedially to the preoccipital notch inferiorly. On the lateral convexity, the limits of the parietal lobe are ill defined because it blends without clear demarcation with the temporal and oc-

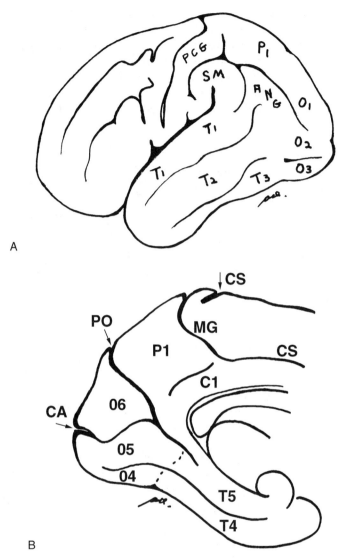

FIG. 43.1. **A:** Anatomy of parietooccipital area (lateral surface). The superior temporal gyrus bifurcates to form the posterior limb of the supramarginal gyrus *(SM)* and the anterior limb of the angular gyrus *(ANG)*. P1, the superior parietal lobule, is continuous with 01 the superior occipital gyrus. T2 and the angular gyrus merge into 02. T3 is continuous with 03. Taken together, the supramarginal gyrus and angular gyrus form the inferior parietal lobule. They are separated from P1 by the intraparietal sulcus. *PCG,* postcentral gyrus; *T2,* 2nd temporal gyrus; *P1,* superior parietal lobule; *T3,* 3rd temporal gyrus; *SM,* supramarginal gyrus; *01,* 1st occipital gyrus; *Ang,* angular gyrus; *02,* 2nd occipital gyrus; *T1,* 1st temporal gyrus; *03,* 3rd occipital gyrus. **B:** Anatomy of parietooccpital area (mesial surface). T5 (parahippocampal gyrus) is split posteriorly by the anterior limb of the calcarine fissure to become superiorly the isthmus of the cingulate gyrus (C1) and inferiorly the lingual gyrus. *06,* the cuneus, and *05,* the lingual gyrus, are separated by the posterior limb of the calcarine fissure *(CA)*. *PO,* parietooccipital fissure; *04,* lateral occipital gyrus; *CA,* calcarine fissure; *05,* lingual gyrus; *CS,* central sulcus; *06,* cuneus; *MG,* marginal ramus of CS; *CS,* callosomarginal (cingulate) sulcus; *T5,* parahippocampal gyrus; *C1,* cingulate gyrus.

cipital lobes (Fig. 43.1A). The anterior–inferior boundary of the parietal lobe corresponds to the sylvian fissure and more posteriorly to an arbitrary line drawn from the sylvian fissure to the preoccipital notch. The inferior boundary of the parietal lobe on the mesial surface is the subparietal sulcus, a discontinuous sulcus that separates the precuneus from the cingulate gyrus (Fig. 43.1B).

The parietal lobe contains five anatomically distinct gyral regions. Although presenting numerous variations from one person to the other, the intraparietal sulcus is the key structure for identifying each region on the convexity of the parietal lobe. Named the *intraparietal sulcus* by Turner, it forms a "T" lying on its side, with the vertical part forming the postcentral sulcus and the horizontal arm dividing the parietal lobe into superior and inferior lobules (28) (Fig. 43.1A). The horizontal limb then continues into the occipital lobe as the superior occipital sulcus. The superior parietal lobule (P1) includes all the area found on the convexity above the intraparietal sulcus and is bound by the postcentral sulcus anteriorly and the occipital lobe posteriorly (Fig. 43.1A). The convolution of the superior parietal lobule extends onto the mesial surface of the brain as the precuneus. The boundaries of the precuneus are anteriorly, the marginal branch of the cingulate sulcus, inferiorly the subparietal sulcus, and posteriorly the parietooccipital sulcus (Fig. 43.1B).

The supramarginal and angular gyri together constitute the inferior parietal lobule (P2). The supramarginal gyrus caps the posterior termination of the sylvian fissure and is the gyrus just posterior to the lower postcentral gyrus with which it is continuous. The angular gyrus is posterior to the supramarginal gyrus and caps the posterior termination of the superior temporal sulcus (Fig. 43.1A). Considerable variation may be found in the classic pattern of the inferior parietal lobule just described.

The postcentral gyrus is one of two vertical convolutions in the central area, functionally part of the central area but anatomically part of the parietal lobe. It is bound anteriorly by the central sulcus and posteriorly by the postcentral sulcus. It takes a sinusoidal shape following the curves of the central sulcus (Fig. 43.1A).

SURGICAL ANATOMY OF OCCIPITAL LOBE

The occipital lobe encompasses all of the structures posterior to the parietooccipital sulcus medially and to a line drawn from the parietooccipital sulcus to the preoccipital notch over the convexity. The most characteristic topographic feature of the occipital lobe is the calcarine fissure. It is confined to the mesial surface and continuous with the parietooccipital sulcus (Fig. 43.1B). An anterior limb of the calcarine fissure divides the parahippocampal gyrus into the isthmus of cingulate gyrus and the lingual gyrus, and a posterior limb separates the occipital lobe into the cuneus (O6) above and the lingual gyrus (O5) below. The calcarine fissure bulges into the occipital horn to form the calcar avis; O5 extends anteriorly to merge with the parahippocampal gyrus; and O4 corresponds to the occipital portion of the occipitotemporal or fusiform gyrus. The gyral pattern over the convexity of the occipital lobe is variable, but generally it can be divided into three separate convolutions: the superior, middle, and inferior occipital gyri (O1, O2, and O3) (Fig. 43.1A).

Gyral Continuum

The simplest and most surgically meaningful approach to the gyral anatomy of the parietal and occipital lobes is that taken by the French anatomists of the nineteenth century (33,36,37). The value of this approach is also emphasized by Yasargil (32). The convolutions of the brain can be viewed as continuous ribbons of cortex folded into predictable patterns. By adhering to the nomenclature of the early anatomists, this concept is even more easily understood (Fig. 43.1A). Thus, the inferior extent of the postcentral gyrus is continuous through a gyral bridge with the supramarginal gyrus of P2, which in turn passes directly into the angular gyrus, which then leads into O2. The postcentral gyrus also forms a continuous ribbon at its superior extent, where P1 takes root and extends posteriorly to blend directly into O1. Just as the intraparietal sulcus divides P1 from P2, it divides O1 from O2 as the superior occipital sulcus (Fig. 43.1A). The postcentral gyrus also forms a continuous gyral connection with the precentral gyrus, inferiorly through the subcentral gyrus and superiorly through the paracentral lobule. Likewise, on the mesial surface, the precuneus is continuous with the cingulate gyrus through gyral bridges creating a discontinuous subparietal sulcus (Fig. 43.1B).

At the junction of the temporal lobe with the parietal lobe, T1 and T2 gyri contribute to the formation of P2. The T1 gyrus splits posteriorly to form the posterior limb of the supramarginal gyrus and the anterior limb of the angular gyrus. The T2 gyrus also extends posteriorly to become the posterior part of the angular gyrus and the O2 portion of the occipital lobe. The T3 gyrus extends posteriorly to become the O3 gyrus, without contributing to the parietal lobe proper (Fig. 43.1A).

Functional Anatomy of the Parietooccipital Region

The fiber connections of the parietal lobe were summarized by Crosby et al. (38). The postcentral gyrus functions as the primary somatic sensory area. Its connections can be grouped into three major components: association and commissural fibers, sensory radiations, and efferent connections to the motor system. Intercortical and association fibers interconnect regions of the frontal and parietal lobes with the postcentral gyrus. The superior longitudinal association bundle connects the somatic sensory area with the frontal cortex and visual association cortex. Temporal opercular fibers pass to the lower somatic sensory area, and the upper sensory area receives fibers from the cingulum. The corpus callosum carries fibers interconnecting the

two sensory areas as well as connections to other regions in the contralateral hemisphere. The thalamic sensory radiations are predominantly composed of reciprocal connections with the nucleus ventralis posterior of the thalamus through the posterior limb of the internal capsule. The postcentral gyrus also has fibers affecting the motor system through extrapyramidal pathways to the basal ganglia, brainstem, spinal cord, and cerebellum. Additionally, fibers pass through the pyramidal system to the motor areas of the spinal cord and brainstem.

The precuneus and superior parietal lobules function as sensory association areas and are composed of reciprocal connections with the pulvinar and the lateral thalamic nuclei. Corticotegmental fibers from this parietal area have been traced to the midbrain tegmentum. Association fibers connect this same area with the cingulate gyrus, the occipital region, the superior temporal gyrus, and postcentral gyrus in the ipsilateral hemisphere as well as the homologous areas in the opposite hemisphere through commissural fibers. The angular and supramarginal gyri are associative areas absent in subprimate animals. The angular gyrus is connected by association fibers with several cortical areas, in particular, the occipital and adjacent parietal association areas. The supramarginal gyrus is richly connected as well with association fibers, linking it with the auditory, visual, and sensory association areas. Fibers from the long association pathways of the inferior occipitofrontal and the inferior longitudinal fasciculi also are associated with the supramarginal gyrus, providing additional connections with the occipital, temporal, frontal, and parietal areas.

The largest input to the primary visual cortex is through the geniculocalcarine fibers from the lateral geniculate nucleus. These fibers run in the sublenticular and postlenticular segment of the internal capsule. Fibers from the superior retinal fields pass almost directly posterior to the superior lip of the calcarine fissure. Fibers from the inferior retinal fields loop into the temporal lobe, with the most peripheral visual representation more anterior and the macular fibers mostly by-passing the temporal lobe.

The secondary visual areas of the occipital lobe are connected to the primary visual cortex in the same and opposite hemispheres. They also are interconnected through the long association bundles with prefrontal, sensory, motor, auditory, insular, and temporal areas. The superior longitudinal and inferior frontooccipital bundles connect the occipital and frontal lobes. Corticotectal or corticotegmental fibers relay impulses for eye movements.

Seizure Patterns and Clinical Manifestations

The ictal manifestations of occipital and parietal lobe epilepsy often arise from structures distant to the seizure focus (14). The aura may arise from the lobe of seizure origin but the early ictal semiology often is determined by the pathways of seizure spread. The scalp electroencephalogram (EEG) in both parietal and occipital epilepsies typically shows extension to surrounding structures and is often unreliable for localization. In parietal lobe epilepsy, the most commonly reported aura is somatosensory resulting from involvement of or spread to the central area (12,16,39,40). In addition, the presence of a somatosensory aura is highly correlated with a seizure origin in the parietal lobe (40).

Early ictal phenomena in parietal lobe epilepsy can manifest themselves with either a convulsive or nonconvulsive pattern. The nonconvulsive manifestations are characterized by manual or oral automatisms suggestive of temporal lobe seizures and result from ictal spread to the temporolimbic structures. Convulsive phenomena can take the form of focal motor clonic activity from involvement of the central area or asymmetric tonic posturing from the supplementary motor area (SMA) (16,41). Ajmone-Marsan and Goldhammer found that an early ictal pattern of unilateral clonic convulsions of the limbs and face was a reliable lateralizing sign and that tonic adversive turning of head and eyes and tonic extension of an arm

was not (42). The location of the epileptic focus can determine the pattern of seizure spread. Salanova et al. found that ictal spread to the SMA with tonic posturing arose most commonly from an electric focus in the superior parietal lobule, and patients with automatisms usually have an epileptogenic zone involving the inferior parietal lobule (12).

Visual auras are the hallmark of occipital lobe epilepsy, being present in most patients in recent series (5,6,11,17,43). Most commonly, the aura consists of elementary visual hallucinations described as lights or geometric shapes, that may have color and may be moving or flashing. Spread to the temporolimbic structures may give rise to complex hallucinations and epigastric or cephalic sensations (9,17,44). Visual phenomena arising from the occipital lobe typically appear contralateral to the seizure origin (45). In patients with a visual-field defect, the visual hallucination may appear within the blind field (45).

The ictal manifestations of occipital lobe epilepsy are variable and are determined by the pathway of seizure spread. As is the case for parietal lobe epilepsy, automatisms are especially common and result from spread to the temporolimbic structures (5,11,15,17,44, 46). Seizure spread also may result in tonic posturing or clonic motor activity (43). Contralateral head and eye deviation was found to be a useful lateralizing sign by Salanova et al. (11). Williamson et al. found that 44% of patients with occipital lobe epilepsy had two or more different seizure types (17).

In occipital lobe epilepsy, scalp EEG is unlikely to localize the epileptic focus. Salanova et al. found 18% of patients had interictal epileptiform discharges restricted to the occipital lobe and that ictal onsets were confined to the occipital lobe in 17% of patients (11). The interictal activity and ictal onset often were widespread and usually involved the temporooccipital region. Williamson et al. found the most common localization of interictal paroxysmal activity to be temporal (17). Therefore, surface EEG is often not localizing, and intracranial recording is frequently required (47). In patients with automatisms or focal motor manifestations, it is important not to miss a visual aura or a visual-field deficit. Any of these findings may be indicative of occipital lobe seizure origin.

Brain Imaging

Because of difficulty in recognizing the seizure origin, neuroimaging techniques, especially MRI, have become particularly useful for identifying potentially epileptogenic lesions. Even in the face of noncongruent EEG findings, the presence of a potentially epileptogenic lesion in a patient being evaluated for surgery must be hypothesized to be the seizure origin (7,16,48).

INVESTIGATIVE OPTIONS

Stereoelectroencephalography

Scalp EEG is often not sufficient for the evaluation of epilepsy arising in the parietal and occipital regions. Because these areas give rise to diverse types of seizure semiologies and the risk of deficit from surgery, especially visual-field deficits from occipital

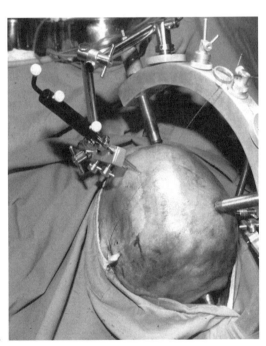
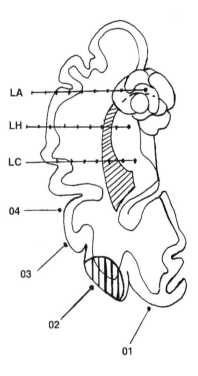

A   B

FIG. 43.2. A: Placement of intracranial surface and depth electrodes is now routinely done by a computer-guided, frameless stereotactic approach using preoperative imaging. The compact stereotactic apparatus and optical pointer (*) are shown. (*) Traxtal: SNN (ISG, Mississauga, Ontario, Canada). **B:** Intracranial recording can be used to solve a problem of localization within one hemisphere in the presence of conflicting findings. The task was to establish the primary focus in a patient presenting with epileptic discharges predominant in the temporal lobe and a clear occipital lesion. Electrodes are inserted in the amygdala, hippocampus, and parahippocampus within the temporal lobe and over the occipital cortex and lesion. The primary focus turned out to be in the occipital area. *LA*, left amygdala; *01*, occipital pole behind the lesion; *LH*, left hippocampus; *02*, over the lesion; *LC*, left parahippocampus; *03*, occipital cortex in front of the lesion; *04*, occpitotemporal area.

resections, intracranial monitoring is commonly required to confirm the suspected site of seizure onset. At the MNI, intracranial electrodes are placed using MRI-guided frameless stereotaxy and a computer program that allows a potential trajectory to be displayed when the pointer is placed on the scalp (1–4). A specially designed device (wander) guides the multicontact depth electrode along a selected trajectory as it is inserted to a target point (Fig. 43.2). Epidural cortical electrodes can be placed precisely to overlie a gyrus of interest identified on the three-dimensional (3-D) surface reconstruction or an abnormal area seen on the two-dimensional (2-D) MRI (Fig. 43.3). Because many of these surface electrodes can be easily and precisely inserted over the cerebral cortex, chronic electrocorticography (ECoG) can be carried out through multiple small twist drill holes, thus avoiding craniotomy for placement of subdural grids. The intracranial surface (cortical) and depth (subcortical) electrodes provide a better appraisal of the 3-D features of the epileptic process and of the seizure spread. Depth and epidural

(epicortical) electrodes are held in place by a hollow bone peg.

Preoperative Mapping

Preoperative brain mapping has now become an integral part of the surgical planning for all procedures in the frontal, central, and parietal areas. It consists essentially of integrating the topographic data provided by 2-D and 3-D MRI and the functional information provided by functional MRI and positron emission tomography (PET) scanning. Display of the vascular anatomy is also provided by a double dose of gadolinium (Gadopentate Dimeglumine, Berlex, Canada) used as an angiogram.

At the MNI, PET scan activation is used routinely to map the sensorimotor areas (Fig. 43.4A,B) and the speech centers (Figs. 43.5.B, 43.6A, 43.6B). The anatomofunctional brain reconstruction then is combined to the technique of frameless stereotaxy. This approach is a great help to the surgeon in planning placement of intracranial electrodes and in performing craniotomies, cortical stimulations, and resections (3).

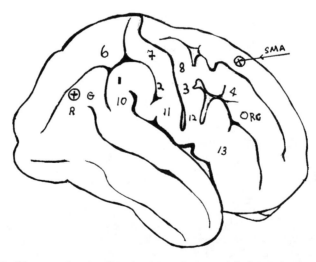

FIG. 43.3. Case J.L. Diagram showing the placement intracranial electrodes inserted over predetermined sites with the frameless stereotactic technique. The purpose of the study was to clarify a problem of seizure onset over the parieto–centro–frontal area SMA: depth electrode directed at the supplementary motor area. ⊕ depth electrode going through the parietal lobe. Predominant interictal and ictal epileptic activity was recorded at electrodes 11 and 12 over the lower central area. *RC,* right cingulate; *R,* referral electrode; *G,* ground electrode.

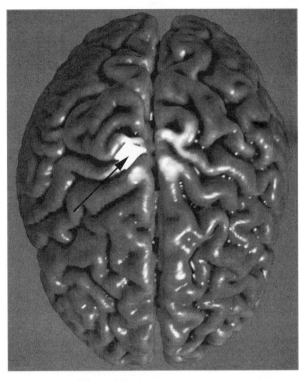

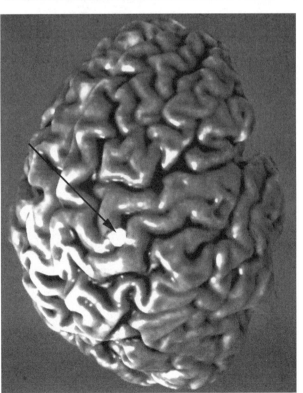

FIG. 43.4. A: 3-D MRI reconstruction with H2O15 PET showing area of hand–motor activation *(arrow)*. Immediately behind is the central sulcus. Posterior and parallel to the central sulcus is the postcentral gyrus. This combination of topographic and functional data forms the basis for preoperative mapping. **B:** 3-D MRI reconstruction showing position of PET foot sensory activation at the upper limit of the postcentral gyrus *(arrow)*. See the difference in configuration (better seen on the opposite side) between the upper central sulcus and the marginal sulcus posterior to it. Notice also configuration of the intraparietal sulcus. *Continued on next page.*

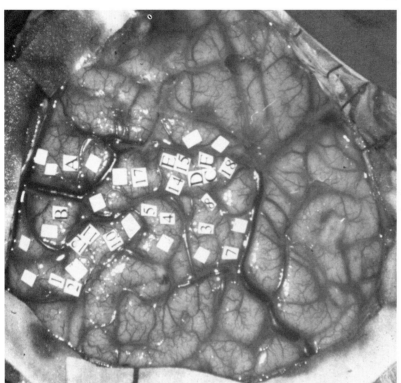

D

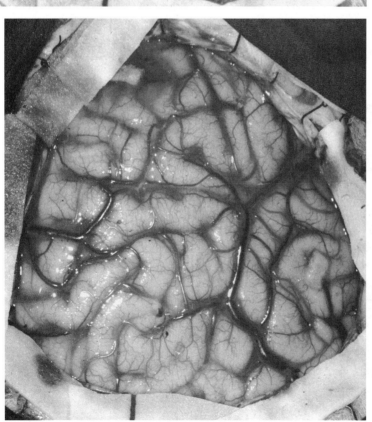

C

FIG. 43.4. *Continued.* **C:** Central area. The parietofrontal area is exposed. Notice the paucity of clear topographic landmarks to recognize the structures of the central area, that is, the central sulcus and the precentral and postcentral gyri. **D:** Central area. Extensive sensory and motor stimulation of the central area has been performed providing excellent localization. The boundary between the parietal and frontal lobe (central sulcus) is well established. *1.* 1.5V stimulation elicited little finger sensation on the left; *2.* numbness in the left little finger; *3.* 2V sensation left lateral tongue; *4.* sensation in left upper lip; *7.* sensation in right side of tongue; *10.* sensation tip of left thumb; *11.* sensation in index finger and corner of mouth; *12.* sensation in index finger; *13.* tingling in middle and ring fingers; 2.5-V stimulation-induced transient twitching in left hand; 3.5-V stimulation started focal motor contractions of right hand; *18.* 3.0-V stimulation sensation felt on side of mouth and unable to talk briefly.

542

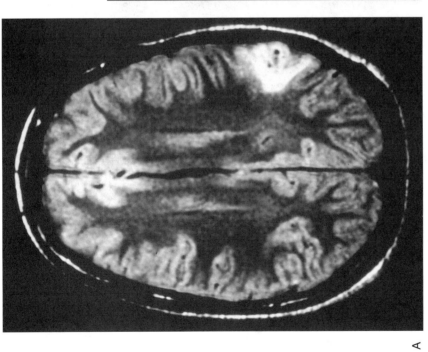

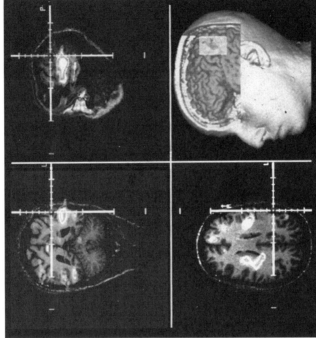

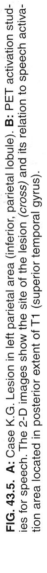

FIG. 43.5. A: Case K.G. Lesion in left parietal area (inferior, parietal lobule). **B:** PET activation studies for speech. The 2-D images show the site of the lesion (*cross*) and its relation to speech activation area located in posterior extent of T1 (superior temporal gyrus).

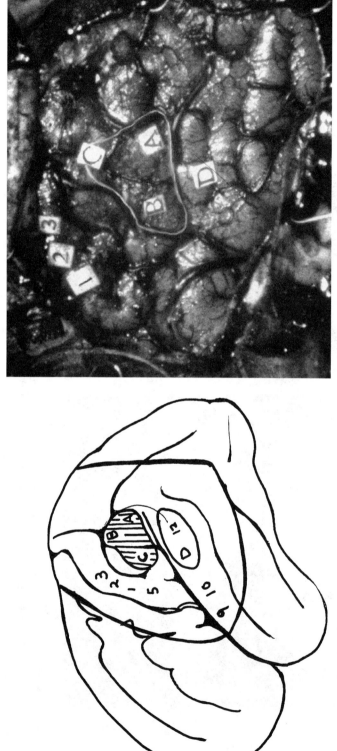

FIG. 43.6. A: Operative diagram showing physiologic data and epileptic activity in relation to lesion. *1.* 4.5-V stimulation. Patient felt tingling over upper lips and tip of tongue; *2.* Same as #1; *3.* stimulation at 5.5 V; patient felt sensation in tongue, side of mouth, and lip; *5,9,10.* sites of ECoG recording; *12.* speech interference with stimulation at 4.0V; *A,B,C.* spiking activity over the lesion; *D.* speech interference upon stimulation at 4.0V and the site of PET activation for language task. **B:** Operative photograph; refer to Fig. 43.15A for orientation. Lesion is not visible on the surface, and its boundaries have been delineated with the stereotactic pointer and encircled with a thread. Epileptiform activity (A,B,C) is over the lesion. D is the site of speech in reference (compare with Fig. 43.14B).

SURGICAL TECHNIQUES

Principle of Image-guided Craniotomy for Epilepsy

At the MNI since 1992, virtually all procedures for surgical treatment of epilepsy are performed with image guidance systems, also called *frameless stereotaxy* or *neuronavigation* (1–4). The patient undergoes a preoperative MRI, which is used for 3-D reconstruction of the head and brain. When a reopening is contemplated, a double-dose gadolinium scan is used to display the large surface veins to preserve them during the dural opening. A series of common natural anatomic landmarks then are coregistered between the patient's head and its 3-D reconstruction. This crucial step of the procedure is called *registration*. From then on, the stereotactic pointer can be used to optimize the scalp flap and center the craniotomy in relationship with underlying cerebral structures. The technique is particularly useful when combined with preoperative mapping. It is now a routine approach at the MNI to carry out somatosensory activation of the foot, hand, tongue, or lips to locate over the scalp, dura, and brain, the actual position of the postcentral gyrus. The location of speech centers also can be indicated (Fig. 43.5B) (3,49).

Choice of Anesthesia

Local or General

In our experience, "local anesthesia" is in fact a combination of local and neuroleptanalgesia (50,51). Local anesthesia has advantages and inconveniences. Its main disadvantages are the limitation in head fixation, the need for constant supervision by a trained anesthetic team, and the time involved. It can be done only in intelligent and well-motivated patients. These restrictions aside, local anesthesia and neuroleptanalgesia remain most useful techniques to approach an epileptic focus located in a crucial functional zone. ECoG and cortical stimulation can be carried out with greater facility, and verbal, motor, or memory testing can be performed at any time during the procedure. It is definitely safer for dominant hemisphere procedures because it allows for speech mapping. When preoperative EEG and imaging studies indicate that the epileptogenic zone is in a noncrucial area, general anesthesia can be used satisfactorily. It is faster, easier, and more comfortable for the patient, the anesthetist, and the surgeon. Head positioning and immobilization under general anesthesia are essential for procedures such as callosotomy or amygdalohippocampectomy. It is difficult to obtain selective and adequate motor response with the patient under general anesthesia, and it is impossible to map speech centers; however, general anesthsia using nitrous oxide supplemented with fentanyl and droperidol is still compatible with adequate recording (50,51). Since the advent of image guidance, we have been able to routinely combine head clamp fixation to local and neuroleptanalgesia (Fig. 43.7A). Once the brain is exposed, a meticulous study of the surface topography is always carried out, whether the patient is asleep or not. Correlations between surface topography and 3D-MRI mapping are particularly useful with the patient under general anesthesia.

Scalp Incisions and Craniotomies

When the head registration has already been done, the scalp incisions are fashioned using the stereotactic pointer. For parietal exposures, an inverted U-shaped incision is used with the horizontal limb on the midline. The anterior limb extends anterior to the precentral gyrus and the posterior one to the level of the parietooccipital sulcus. The craniotomy is done by making three burr holes between 5 to 10 mm from the midline and joining them with the Gigli saw. Gadolinium venography is particularly useful for locating the superior sagittal sinus with precision. If more mesial exposure is needed, further craniectomy along the midline is achieved with rongeurs or power tools. Two additional burr holes are made just below the level of the sylvian fis-

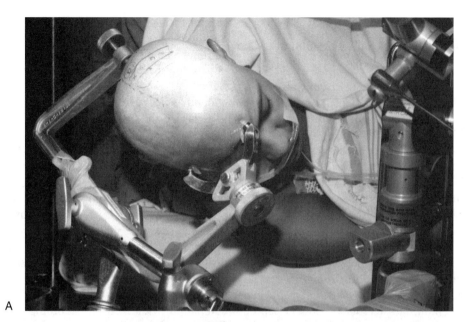

A

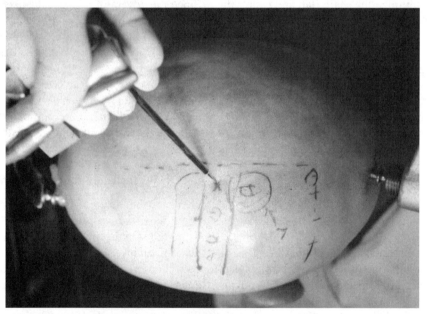

B

FIG. 43.7. A: Case A.H. Operative setup under local anesthesia and neurolepanalgesia using a neu-ronavigation system (viewing wand). Position of midline (superior sagittal sinus) is indicated by *dot-ted line.* Local anesthesia is used at the pin sites. **B:** Case A.H. Stereotactic wand pointing to the foot sensory activation area as projected over the scalp. Note the location of the lesion behind and rep-resented by a *circle.* The actual position of the midline is indicated by the *dotted line.* The stereotac-tic pointer helps to optimize the scalp incision and size of craniotomy in relation to lesion and mid-line. *PCG* represents the position of the postcentral gyrus.

sure. The dura is retracted mesially toward the midline.

For occipital exposures, a curvilinear incision is used with the mesial limb on the midline reaching down to the external occipital protuberance. The lateral limb detaches itself from the midline in front of the parietooccipital fissure and goes in the direction of the ear. The craniotomy is also made with 3 burr holes lateral to the midline and extends into the lower burr holes. The anterior superior one is placed in front of the parietooccipital sulcus and the anterior inferior one in front of the temporooccipital notch. The dura is opened laterally and retracted over the midline.

Electroencephalography

The first condition for an adequate ECoG is sufficient brain exposure. The suspected areas should be readily recognizable and reachable. A total of 16 electrodes are usually used. Their tip is made of a carbon ball supported by a flexible wire. They can be used to record from the cortical surface and from structures deep within a cavity, which is particularly useful in postresection ECoG. The electrodes can be arranged in any montage in a bipolar or monopolar fashion. Typically, with a large parietal exposure, four parallel rows of four electrodes are disposed to cover the exposed cortex. Flexible subdural electrodes are used to record from the mesial surface of the parietal lobe, the undersurface of the temporal and occipital lobes, or from cortex covered by dura. EcoG provides both diagnostic and prognostic information by further delineating the active zone prior to resection and by indicating the areas of residual discharges after cortical removal. It is particularly useful in dealing with cortical dysplasias (52–54). ECoG is an integral part of cortical mapping by stimulation and serves to detect poststimulation afterdischarges. Areas of epileptic activity are indicated with letter tags placed on the cortical surface (Figs. 43.6 and 43.8).

Perioperative Cortical Mapping

The identification of the sensorimotor strip, especially of the postcentral gyrus, is an essential step in many cortical resections. It is best determined by electric stimulation under local anesthesia, carried out with a constant current generator starting at 0.5 V with increments of 0.5 V. Most responses are obtained around 3 V. The postcentral gyrus is best identified by obtaining sensory responses from the tongue area, which corresponds to the lower part of the postcentral gyrus, above the sylvian fissure and behind the central sulcus (Fig. 43.4C,D). The idea is to concentrate on sensory responses over the postcentral gyrus rather than repeated motor stimulations over the precentral gyrus, which are usually obtained at higher threshold and have a greater propensity to cause seizures. Only a few motor responses are needed to confirm the position of the precentral gyrus, which is often not necessary. Based on these responses, the central, precentral, and postcentral sulci are identified. Stimulation also is used to identify speech areas. Positive responses to stimulation are indicated with numbers, sites of epileptic activity with letters, and negative responses with blanks (Fig. 43.9). If a seizure is induced by stimulation, it is quickly stopped by the intravenous injection of a fast-acting barbiturate, such as Brietal (Methohexital Sodium, Eli Lilly, Canada, Inc.). When about to stimulate in the central area, the surgeon must ensure that the anesthetist is aware of the situation and ready for an impending clinical seizure. All measures should be taken to avoid a major convulsive seizure and its hazardous consequences, such as the patient falling off the operating room table, brain contusions, and hemorrhages.

Technique of Endopial Resection

This is a modification of the basic "subpial technique," in which a series of small holes are made with the sharp tips of a bipolar forceps. Each of these small holes is opened further and enlarged with the ultrasonic dissector (CUSA [Valley Lab, Boulder, CO, U.S.A.]) set at low parameters of vibration and suction (0.12% and 12%). The holes then are interconnected subpially by fragmenting and aspirating the

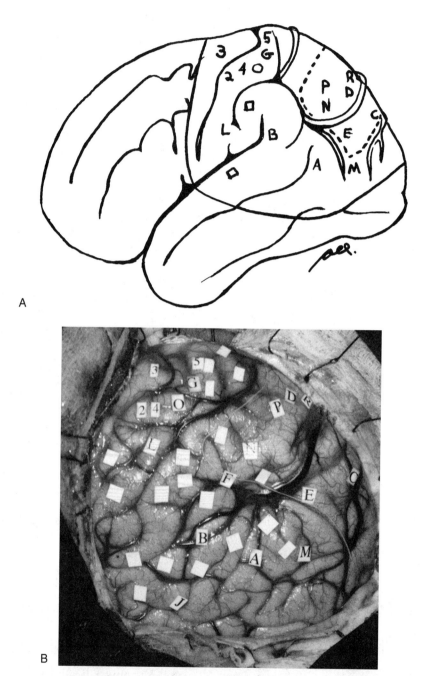

FIG. 43.8. A: Case L.M. Lateral surface diagram showing physiological responses and extent of resection *(dotted line)*. *2,* 2.5-V sensation in the right hand, index and middle fingers; *3,* 2.5-V flexion of the elbow; *4,* 3-V sensation in index finger; *R,* Electrographic seizure; *5,* 3-V sensation in right arm; *E,* electrographic seizure; blanks, negative stimulations; *N,R,D,P,C,* principal sites of epileptic activity. **B:** Case L.M. Actual operating room photograph. Notice the presence of a large vein overlying the lesion and draining region of inferior parietal lobule (see Fig. 43.8A for orientation).

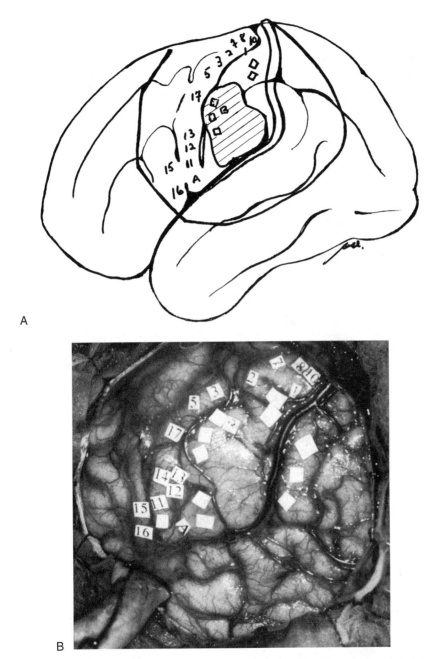

FIG. 43.9. A: Case P.Y. Operative diagram for orientation showing site of lesion *(slash bars)* sites of epileptic activity (A and B) and physiological responses to stimulation. *3,* stimulation at 2.2 V produced contraction at corner of mouth; *8,* 3.0-V stimulation: patient felt sensation in 4th finger, clonic contraction of fingers; *11,* stimulation at 4.0 V produced arrest of counting; stimulation at 3.0 V produced tongue contraction; *15,* stimulation at 3.0 V produced arrest of counting; *16,* arrest of counting, could not find his words; contraction of mouth and tongue; *A,B,* site of epileptiform activity. **B:** Case P.Y. Actual operative photograph. Note configuration of large ascending parietal vein draining from region of sylvian fissure (refer to Fig. 43.9A for orientation).

cortex and white matter and leaving in place the pia and bypassing arteries and veins. Once this is accomplished, a thorough coagulation is performed along the line of resection, and the pia and vessels are divided. This technique is used to go around the incision line in en bloc resections. When an en bloc resection is performed, that is, when arteries and veins are divided, the full consequence of their obliteration must be assessed beforehand to avoid any undue ischemia or swelling.

Multicompartment Endopial Technique

This is a modification of the "subpial technique" used when no vessels are sacrificed. A

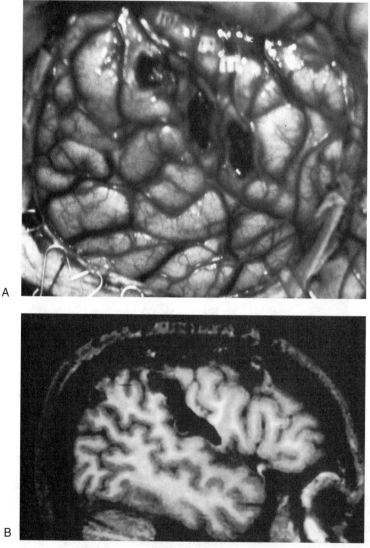

FIG. 43.10. A: Case J.L. Operative photograph showing the actual resection. This is an example of the endopial cortical resection technique performed through multiple separate compartments leaving all bypassing arteries and veins intact. **B:** Case J.L. Postoperatove MRI showing the full extent of the endopial cortical resection, which involves the lower postcentral gyrus and most of the supramarginal gyrus. Compare with Figs. 43.5A,B and 43.6A. The true extent of the resection is seen.

series of pial openings is made between by-passing arteries or veins, taking care to leave these vessels undisturbed (Fig. 43.10A). The various cavities are interconnected by using a subpial circumvascular approach. The end result is best seen not at the time of surgery (Fig. 43.10A) but on the postoperative MRI (Fig. 43.10B). The technique is particularly useful in resection of the lower central area, such as the lower postcentral gyrus and opercular resection, and resection in the region of the inferior parietal lobule (Fig. 43.10A,B). The actual tissue removal is also performed by using the ultrasound dissector set at low parameters of vibration and suction.

Technical Pitfalls in Parietal and Occipital Resections

The complications in parietal and occipital lobe epilepsy surgery can be avoided only if the main pitfalls are constantly kept in mind. First, one must consider and avoid direct injury to the major venous trunks, that is, the superior longitudinal and transverse sinuses. No large ascending central or parietal veins should be divided or large arterial trunk interrupted. When large vessels are present in the resection field, the technique of "multicompartment endopial emptying" must be used.

Other major pitfalls are inadequate identification of the precentral primary motor and the postcentral primary sensory areas. Of capital importance also is the recognition of speech centers in the dominant hemisphere, identified by preoperative or peroperative mapping and stimulation (Figs. 43.5 and 43.6).

Visual Loss Following Occipital Surgery

Most cases of occipital lobe epilepsy arise from the mesial surface of the occipital lobe, that is, the calcarine region, and the vast majority of patients are treated by an occipital lobectomy that involves the primary visual cortex; therefore, a contralateral homonymous hemianopsia is expected. When the deficit and its impact are discussed in detail with the patient, the hemianopsia should be considered an unavoidable side effect rather than a complication. Of crucial importance is the fact that occipital lesions are often bilateral and that a visual-field deficit may exist on the side of the contemplated occipital resection, which could give rise to blindness. The surgeon must be absolutely aware of the preoperative status of the visual fields and of the eventual impact of additional deficits. Finally, the anterior extent of the occipital resection on the dominant hemisphere should not be inadvertently extended in the angular gyrus, which is best avoided by preoperative speech mapping and peroperative neuronavigation (Figs. 43.5 and 43.6).

ILLUSTRATIVE CASES

Parietal Lobe Epilepsy

Case J.L.

J.L. was 17 years old at the time of surgery. He was a right-handed boy with intractable epilepsy of unknown etiology for the preceding 7 years. Initially, his seizures were heralded by an aura of the hand becoming "as big as the hospital." The sensation of macropsia ended soon after seizure onset, and at his presentation to the MNI, he described an aura of numbness in the whole left hand with a sharp demarcation of paraesthesia at the wrist without a march. The seizures were predominately nocturnal, and the pattern consisted of abruptly sitting up, eye blinking, and tonic extension of the left arm. The frequency was almost daily. Surface EEG showed right centroparietal interictal spiking. The MRI revealed no lesion. Ictal single-photon emission computed tomography (SPECT) demonstrated hyperperfusion in the right lower central area.

Because of the initial aura of macropsia and the curious somatosensory sensation involving the whole hand without a march of symptoms, it was postulated the seizure origin was either in the primary somatosensory cortex of the postcentral gyrus or posterior to it. In an attempt to localize the seizure origin better, stereo electroencephalography (SEEG) was performed (Fig. 43.3). Two multicontact depth electrodes were inserted frontally and targeted to the SMA and the anterior cingulate. One multicontact depth electrode was inserted through the inferior parietal lobule and targeted to the mesial parietal cortex. A series of epidural cortical electrodes were placed over the central and pericentral area. The seizure origin was localized to the right lower central area (Fig. 43.3). To obtain greater precision in mapping the central area, the patient had a PET activation study of hand motor function. At surgery with the patient under local anesthesia, a right frontotemporoparietal craniotomy was performed using MRI-guided frameless stereotaxy. The sylvian fissure, central region, and parietal lobe were well exposed. ECoG demonstrated a clear focus of spike activity at the lower postcentral and supramarginal gyrus (Fig. 43.11A,B). Cortical stimulation mapped the tongue and hand somatosensory areas, and stimulation of the supramarginal gyrus elicited a hand paraesthesia similar to his usual aura. The patient had a seizure on the table at the conclusion of the stimulation, which was quickly aborted with intravenous Brietal. He subsequently underwent removal of the lower central area, up to the hand region, and resection of the supramarginal gyrus by the technique of subpial microdissection, leaving intact all the pial vessels passing through the central area (Fig. 43.10). Pathology of the specimen revealed neuronal heterotopia. After surgery, the patient has remained seizure free with a follow-up now of 1 year and without a deficit.

This case illustrates the typical somatosensory aura and seizure spread of parietal lobe epilepsy. Intracranial recording was able to improve localization of the seizure focus from scalp EEG. ECoG provided additional information for identifying the involved gyri. Patient J.L. also demonstrates that the lower postcentral gyrus can be removed safely for a distance of up to 3 cm from the sylvian fissure as long as the bypassing vessels are left intact. More superior resections carry the risk of hand sensory and motor deficits. A safe re-moval can be accomplished in all parts of the parietal lobe in the nondominant hemisphere behind the postcentral sulcus. In the dominant hemisphere, resections above the intraparietal sulcus will avoid the eloquent regions of P2.

Case A.H.

A.H. was a 19-year-old woman at the time of surgery. She initially had febrile convulsions at 14 months of age but was well controlled with anticonvulsants for 3 years. Her medication was tapered off at 4 years of age, and for 9 years she remained asymptomatic. At 13 years of age, her seizures recurred with a generalized convulsion; however, her predominant seizure pattern became an elevation and tonic–clonic contractions of the right upper limb with rotation of the head toward the right side. This was followed by a slow fall to the ground. She had no warning. Despite multiple drug regimens, her seizure frequency remained one per month. EEG telemetry revealed a frequent paroxysmal disturbance of cerebral activity recorded from the midline central and parietal regions. Her neurologic examination was normal, and her initial MRI scans, performed prior to her presentation to the MNI, did not reveal a focal abnormality; however, fine-cut MRI with curvilinear reformatting performed at the MNI revealed a 1-cm area of thickened cortex in the left mesial precuneus with a close relationship to the paracentral lobule (Fig. 43.12A).

To determine the relationship of the lesion to foot function, a PET activation study was performed (Fig. 43.12B) and revealed foot sensory function to be located in the gyrus anterior to the lesion. At surgery, a left parietocentral craniotomy was performed with the patient under local anesthesia (Fig. 43.7A) The position and extent of the craniotomy in relation to the lesion and foot area were established with the frameless stereotactic technique. Surface ECoG showed polymorphic slow-wave activity over the lesion and a depth electrode inserted to the lesion revealed sharper activity. After Brietal injection, low-

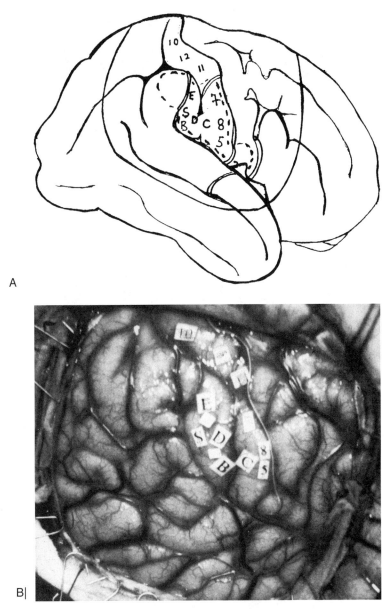

A

B|

FIG. 43.11. A: Case J.L. Operative diagram showing the results of brain mapping, including sites of epileptic activity, and stimulation data. Stimulation at letter *S* produced the patient's typical convulsive seizure. Dotted line shows extent of resection which includes the lower postcentral gyrus and most of the supramarginal gyrus. *5,* Simulation with 2.5 V elicited sensation in the middle of the tongue; *7,* numbness of tongue felt more posteriorly; *8,* numbness felt on tip of tongue; *10,* stimulation with 3.0 V elicited sensation in little finger; *11,* sensation again felt in little finger; *12,* sensation felt in middle finger; *B,C,D,E,* maximum spike activity and continuous delta activity. **B:** Case J.L. Operative photograph (see Fig. 43.5A for orientation). The *white thread* corresponds to the central sulcus. Note the configuration of the supramarginal gyrus (B, D, S, and E are over its anterior limb).

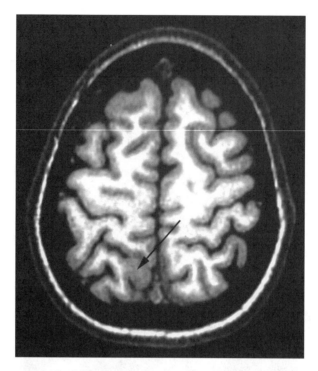

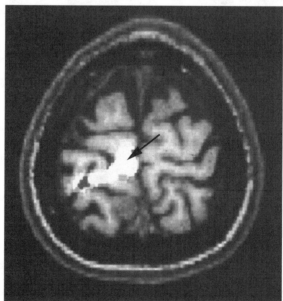

FIG. 43.12. A: Case A.H. Transverse preoperative MRI showing lesion in parasagittal parietocentral area (left side). Whether the lesion is actually in the postcentral gyrus or in P1 (superior parietal lobule) is difficult to ascertain. Compare with Fig. 43.7B. **B:** Case A.H. Transverse PET showing zone of foot sensory activation with postcentral gyrus well in front of the lesion. Compare with Fig. 43.7A.

amplitude spikes were recorded from the lesion. Stimulation of the postcentral gyrus at 1 and 1.5 V mapped thumb, finger, and foot areas (Fig. 43.13A). A response of tingling in the foot obtained from postcentral gyrus stimulation corresponded to the site of PET activation. MRI-guided frameless stereotaxy was used to locate the lesion and define its margins (Fig. 43.13A,B). All the apparent gray–brown lesion was selectively removed, preserving the functioning cortex in the postcentral gyrus and the adjacent draining veins (Fig. 43.14A,B). Histologic analysis showed cortical dysplasia with disorganization of cortical layering and abundant heterotopic neurons in the white matter. The patient made a quick recovery from surgery and had no deficits; however, she had a seizure 35 days after surgery similar to her habitual seizures. The postoperative MRI suggested some residual dysplasia in the surgical cavity. She continued to have seizures at the same frequency as before surgery, except for a 4-month period when she was seizure free. Additionally, the seizure pattern changed with a bilateral myoclonic jerking of the upper extremities replacing the lateralized tonic clonic movement she had before surgery.

This patient continued to have seizures, most likely because a remnant of cortical dysplasia was not resected. Either the lesion was subtotally removed, or a dysplasia was present adjacent to the recognized lesion but was too subtle to be detected with available imaging modalities. Cortical dysplasia may not have sharply demarcated borders, and the lesion may be larger than what can be identified with even the most sophisticated imaging. The striking epileptogenicity of dysplasia is evident by this patient's persistent seizures despite a removal of all the grossly apparent lesion (Fig. 43.14).

At the MNI, neuronavigation using MRI-guided frameless stereotaxy has become an indispensable part of all intracranial procedures for epilepsy. Using the Viewing Wand system (ISG Canada), 300 patients who had craniotomy for intractable epilepsy were reported (8). The incorporation of frameless stereotaxy into the surgical protocol improved the patient's management in a number of ways. In presurgical planning, the scalp incision, craniotomy flap, and angle of approach can be optimized by identifying the underlying brain structures before an incision is made. More selective approaches can be facilitated by precise placement of the scalp incision and the craniotomy over a lesion or localized area planned for resection (Fig. 43.12). Topographic localization of important blood vessels, sinuses, and gyri can be improved with image guidance. Intracranially, the central sulcus can be identified to facilitate cortical stimulation. The sites of ECoG recording can be identified on the cortical surface and displayed on a large screen for the benefit of the electroencephalographers or others in the gallery. Also, the sites of stimulation responses and epileptic activity are now registered with labels placed over the 3-D reconstruction of the brain and archived for storage.

Case D.A.

Patient D.A. was a 19-year-old right-handed man at the time of surgery. His seizures began at the age of 9 years and were intractable to medication. His mother's pregnancy was normal, but at delivery there was an episode of hypoxia, and a left hemiparesis became apparent when he started to walk at the age of 1 year. The predominant seizure pattern was an unpleasant but difficult to describe sensation in the upper left arm, which traveled to the hand, usually followed by tonic stiffening and elevation of the left arm. These attacks occurred several times each day. About once per month, he had attacks beginning with a stare, arrest of activity, and leftward deviation of the head and eyes. One third of his attacks were preceded by a sensation of fear. Neurologic examination revealed no useful movements of the hand on the left, but his arm strength was better than antigravity. There was a left-sided hemisensory disturbance to pinprick, position sense, and vibration.

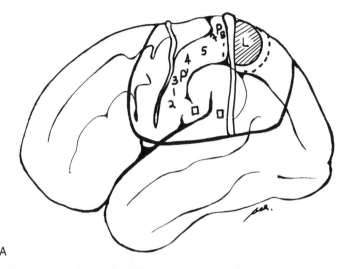

A

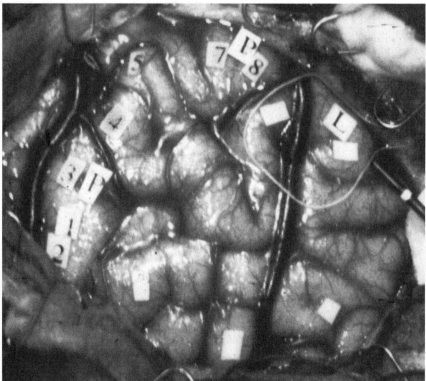

B

FIG. 43.13 A: Case A.H. Brain map showing physiologic responses to stimulation, correlation with PET scan, and the location of lesion. *L,* lesion; *P,* site of sensory foot activation with PET; *1,* stimulation with 1.0 V elicited tingling in right thumb; *2,* tingling again felt in right thumb; *3,* a sensation of finger flexion felt in the right hand; *P1,* negative response. **B:** Case A.H. Exposed cortex at surgery. A recording electrode is inserted into the lesion *(L)*. Note the presence of large ascending vein draining the inferior parietal lobule and running over the lesion (see Fig. 43.9A for orientation).

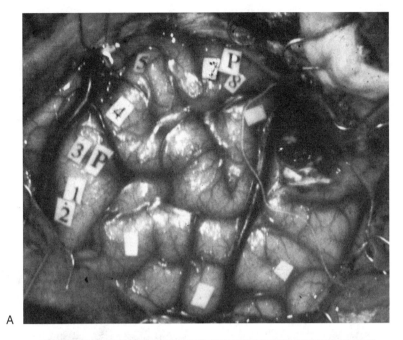

A

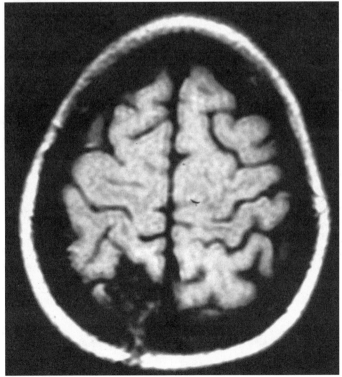

B

FIG. 43.14. A: Case A.H. Operative photograph showing the actual resection. The large central ascending vein has been left intact. The resection is extended anterior to it by the subpial approach. **B:** Case A.H. Transverse postoperative MRI showing the extent of removal, including the lesion. Compare with preoperative MRI on Fig. 43.7A.

A neuropsychological evaluation demonstrated deficits pointing primarily to the frontal and central areas. Scalp EEG showed interictal sharp and slow-wave activity from the right centroparietal region. Ictal discharges were recorded from the right centroparietal area as well. The MRI demonstrated a large cerebrospinal fluid (CSF)-filled cavity in the right frontocentrotemporal area. The posterior and superior margins showed scarring, atrophy, and gliosis. Intracarotid amobarbitol testing revealed left-sided speech representation.

A right frontoparietal craniotomy was performed with the patient under general anesthesia and exposed a large frontocentroparietal cyst (Fig. 43.15). ECoG found rhythmic spiking above and behind the cyst. Cortical stimulation produced strong flexion of the left wrist and elbow with elevation of the shoulder reminiscent of a seizure (point 2). A resection of the parietal lobe and central area was performed and included the areas of maximal ECoG spiking, preserving the cingulate gyrus (Fig. 43.15A). Pathology showed neuronal loss and gliosis. Eighteen months after surgery, D.A. had one nocturnal tonic seizure related to medication taper, and he had no further deficit other than his congenital hemiparesis.

This case demonstrates the approach to epilepsy resulting from a large cyst. The seizure origin was localized to a region around the cyst by the semiology and electrical findings. The resection was tailored to the area of seizure onset without removing the cyst. Identifying the site of seizure onset on the periphery of a large cyst is akin to locating a cabin around the shore of a lake. The less the actual cyst is disturbed, the better.

Case P.Y.

P.Y. was a 36-year-old left-handed man at the time of surgery. He had seizure onset at the age of 5 years. A computed tomography (CT) scan was performed when he was 25 years of age and showed a hypodense lesion in the frontoparietal area. His seizures were heralded by a tingling sensation on the right side of the face and mouth, which progressed to a shooting paraesthetic sensation in the right arm and movement of the tongue. There was no loss of consciousness, but he was unable to speak. Rarely, the attacks progressed to a generalized convulsion. The seizure frequency was one to two per day and intractable to medication. The neurologic examination was normal. Scalp EEG revealed left frontotemporal epileptiform activity. The MRI performed at 36 years of age demonstrated a hypointense lesion involving the lower precentral and postcentral gyri consistent with a glioma and unchanged in size from the previous CT scan.

A left fronto–temporo–parietal craniotomy was performed with the patient under local anesthesia. This revealed a fullness and whitish discoloration of the central area (Fig. 43.9A). ECoG showed spiking activity above and in front of the lesion. Cortical stimulation mapped sensory and motor responses anterior and above the lesion. Stimulation anterior to the motor responses produced speech arrest (Fig. 43.9). A soft, grayish lesion with ill-defined borders was removed. It measured 3 cm in the vertical direction and was centered primarily in the postcentral gyrus (Fig. 43.16). Pathology revealed an oligodendroglioma, and there was no resulting deficit. Six months after surgery, his seizures recurred with a brief generalized convulsion, and he continued to have smaller attacks with a shocklike sensation through his body and automatic movements of his tongue without a loss of consciousness. At 5 years of follow-up, the seizure frequency was markedly reduced from before surgery, with the seizures occurring in clusters one day each month. A CT scan showed a complete resection of the tumor.

Case K.G.

Patient K.G. was a 26-year-old right-handed woman at the time of surgery in 1995. Her seizures began at the age of 8 years and were intractable to anticonvulsant medication. She had different seizure types. One started

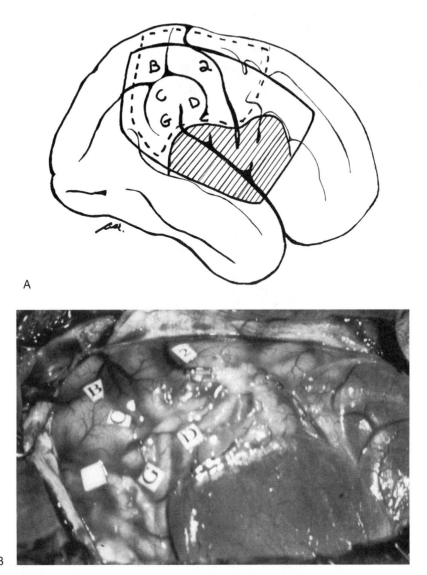

FIG. 43.15. A: Case D.A. Operative diagram showing physiologic responses, site of epileptic activity, and the actual lesion (cyst) indicated by *bars*. The extent of removal is indicated by the dotted line. *B,C,* rhythmic sharp wave activity; *2,* 4.0V stimulation elicited wrist and elbow flexion and shoulder elevation reminiscent of a typical seizure. **B:** Case D.A. Operative photograph. Notice the thin cortex at the upper limit of the cyst (refer to Fig. 43.11A for orientation).

with tingling in the right arm, most prominent in the hand, which sometimes affected her ability to speak and also often proceeded to a painful sensation around the elbow. Another seizure type began with a visual hallucination of a scene containing people she could not quite identify but gave her a feeling of dread. Either of these attacks could proceed to a loss of contact and lip smacking. The seizure frequency was several times per week. A CT scan obtained soon after seizure onset suggested the presence in the parietal lobe of a vascular lesion not seen on angiography. She underwent a craniotomy and exploration of

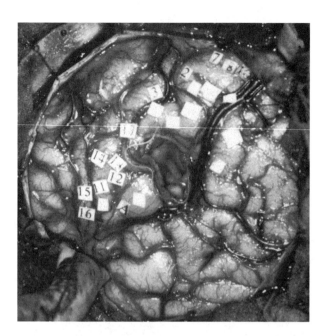

FIG. 43.16. Case P.Y. The tumor has been resected.

the lesion, but it was not resected because it was considered too close to the speech area and was not apparent on the surface. Intracarotid amobarbitol evaluation showed left-hemisphere language dominance. Scalp EEG demonstrated interictal epileptiform activity over the centrotemporal and centroparietal areas. The MRI performed in 1995 revealed an area of cortical thickening and high signal in the left supramarginal gyrus consistent with dysplasia (Fig. 43.5A).

Preoperative mapping and planning included MRI reconstruction and PET activation of somatosensory and speech function. The lesion was found to be located above the speech activation (Fig. 43.5B). A left centroparietal craniotomy was performed with the patient under local anesthesia. Using the MRI-guided frameless stereotaxy and 3-D surface reconstruction, the sulcal and gyral anatomies were identified and the dysplastic lesion localized on the cortex. The arachnoid over the lesion appeared indurated. ECoG demonstrated spiking over the lesion and cortical stimulation elicited lower lip and tongue tingling anterior to the lesion (Fig. 43.6). There was no speech arrest with stimulation in the lesion. A grossly com-

plete resection was made of the gray—brown soft lesion. Speech function was tested continuously during the resection. Severe speech interference by stimulation was found at the site of speech activation with PET (Fig. 43.6). Pathology revealed the lesion to be a ganglioglioma. After surgery, she had no language deficits and was seizure free until four partial complex seizures occurred 8 months postoperatively. She continued to have an occasional aura of numbness in the right hand and had three more partial complex seizures 2 years after surgery.

The marked epileptogenicity of gangliogliomas probably results from elements of dysplasia commonly in close relationship with the tumor (55). Patient K.G. had a good result in reduction of her seizure frequency, but her persistent seizure tendency may result from residual rests of dysplasia not seen on MRI.

Case L.M.

L.M. was 39 years of age in 1999. She was right-handed, and her seizure onset was at the age of 5 years. She demonstrated three seizure types. The first was a drop attack with an occasional aura of numbness in the right foot, sometimes preceded by an epigastric rising sensation. Another type was a scream followed by loss of consciousness and fall. Additionally, she had generalized convulsions. Her seizure frequency was 20 each month. Her neurologic examination showed a mild right hemiparesis, extinction, decreased pinprick and light touch sensation on the right, and her visual fields were normal. Scalp EEG demonstrated left central parietal epileptic discharge. CT scan performed in 1983 showed a hyperdense area in the left posterior parietal region.

L.M. underwent her first surgery in 1984. A left temporal parietal occipital craniotomy performed with local anesthesia exposed a lesion in the superior parietal lobule. ECoG demonstrated a wide field of abnormal electric activity (Fig. 43.8). The intraparietal sulcus was identified, and cortical stimulation in the superior and inferior parietal lobule was negative for speech arrest. A subtotal resection of the lesion was performed measuring 4.5 × 5 cm (Fig. 43.17A). Pathology showed astroglial changes and ectopic neurons in the white matter compatible with hamartoma (Fig. 43.17B). She developed no additional deficits. After surgery, her seizure frequency decreased by 50%, and the seizures were much less severe. Her seizure pattern changed to a slow fall as a result of leg weakness and jerking of the right arm without loss of consciousness. When an MRI study was done, it showed a large area of residual dysplasia extending from the occipital horn and atrium to the superior parietal lobule. In 1988, she underwent a reopening of the left craniotomy under general anesthesia and had further removal of the lesion. The resection was halted, however, after only a subtotal resection because a large cortical draining vein was thought to have been disrupted. She again had no further deficit after surgery.

L.M. had a marked reduction in her seizure frequency after surgery with the introduction of a new medication. The improvement, however, was transient, and by 1997 she had several attacks each month and two or three each month in which she would fall violently. In preparation for additional surgery, she had a PET activation study for language and intracarotid amobarbitol testing, which demonstrated left-hemisphere speech dominance and activation outside the lesion.

In 1999, she underwent reopening of the left parietal craniotomy. By using a double-dose gadolinium scan, the MRI-guided frameless stereotactic approach allowed identification of the large draining veins prior to dural opening. The dura was open parallel to the draining veins and over the resection cavity, affording a good view of the residual lesion. The lesion margins were identified with the navigation system, and the regions of language PET activation were identified on the patient's cortex, allowing a safe and gross total resection of the lesion with no additional deficit after surgery.

Functional neuroimaging is an integral part of the peroperative planning for surgery near the central and language areas. By coregistering the PET or fMRI data with the patient's anatomic MRI, the functional imaging for a desired task can be incorporated in the neuronavigation system. The 3-D surface reconstruction demonstrates the gyral and sulcal pattern better than direct visualization of the cortical surface and allows for the integration of information important for a successful surgery. The location of a lesion, the seizure origin, and any functionally important areas to be avoided can all be viewed on the 2-D and 3-D images for surgical planning. For surgery in the central or language areas, PET or fMRI can guide the cortical stimulation directly to the activation site, making stimulation more efficient and less likely to induce a seizure. For surgery outside the language or central areas, functional imaging confirms the location of important areas without having to expose them to perform cortical stimulation. The craniotomy is therefore smaller and centered only on the planned resection.

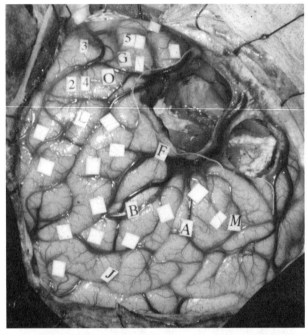

A

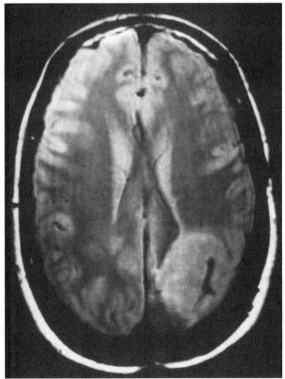

B

FIG. 43.17. **A:** Case L. M. Operative photograph. Cortical resection through the superior parietal lobule. The large vein draining the inferior parietal lobule has been left undisturbed. **B:** Case L.M. Large hamartomatous lesion extending from the ventricle to the cortical surface incompletely resected at time of initial surgery. Note the enlarged intraparietal sulcus.

Occipital Lobe Epilepsy

Case B.B.

Patient B.B. was an 11-year-old right-handed girl at the time of surgery. She had a congenital left hemiparesis, and her seizure onset was at 6 years of age. Her seizure pattern was characterized by a visual hallucination of various colored patterns followed by deviation of the head and eyes to the left and oral automatisms, which occurred three to five times per week. Another, rarer seizure pattern consisted of the same visual hallucination followed by shaking of the left arm and rigid extension of the remaining extremities. Scalp EEG consistently demonstrated active epileptiform activity in the right occipital region. Visual-field examination did not show a deficit. A CT scan revealed a porencephalic area and cortical atrophy in the superior parietal parasagital zone. Intracarotid amobarbital testing confirmed no speech representation in the right hemisphere.

A right parietal occipital craniotomy was performed with the patient under general anesthesia (Fig. 43.18). ECoG showed high voltage spiking activity posterior to the lesion on the convexity of the occipital lobe (Figs. 43.18 and 43.19A). An occipital lobectomy was performed, and postresection ECoG demonstrated residual spiking at the resection margin, which was removed until no residual spiking remained (Figs. 43.18 and 43.19). Pathology demonstrated focal neuronal loss and gliosis, and she developed an expected hemianopsia. She was seizure free until 6-1/2 years after surgery, when she had three convulsive episodes without a visual warning; these were different from her habitual seizures, and she had one more attack 9 years after.

This case demonstrates the characteristic seizure pattern of occipital lobe epilepsy and the usefulness of ECoG in delineating the seizure focus.

Case T.

Patient T. was an 11-year-old, right-handed boy with a 7-year history of intractable epilepsy at the time of surgery. He described no aura. His seizure pattern consisted of an initial staring, eye and head deviation to the left, followed by complex automatisms of the right hand with repetitive tapping on the right thigh. These occurred several times per day. The physical examination revealed a decreased ability to perform rapid movements of the left hand, left inferior quadrantanopsia, and optokinetic nystagmus, suggesting a right

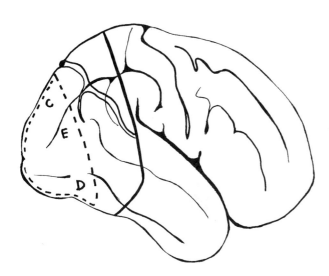

FIG. 43.18. Case B.B. Diagram showing the extent of right craniotomy, the ECoG data, and the extent of resection *(dotted line)*.

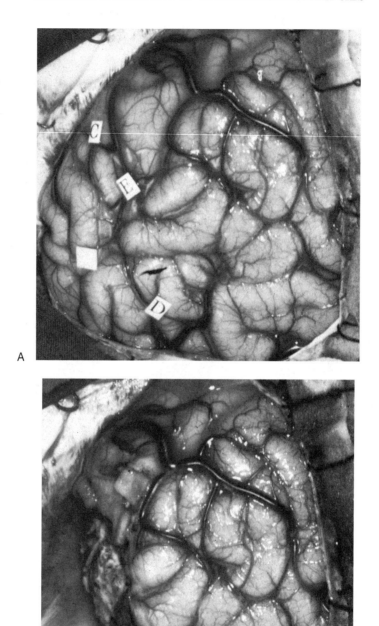

FIG. 43.19. A: Case B.B. Photograph of exposed cortex and sites of epileptic activity. *C,D,E,* sites of high voltage repetitive spike activity. **B:** Case B.B. Operative photograph showing the actual resection (refer to Fig. 43.19A for orientation).

parietal defect. Surface EEG showed diffuse interictal spiking over the right frontocentral, right occipital, right temporal, and right parietooccipital areas. Ictal onset was right parietooccipital. MRI demonstrated a right occipital cortical abnormality and dilated right atrium as well as a left parietooccipital hemosiderin deposit. Ictal SPECT showed an area of hyperperfusion in the right temporal lobe.

With congruence of the scalp EEG, physical examination and the dominant lesion on the MRI, the patient proceeded to surgery for a right occipital lobectomy and resection of the right occipital cortical abnormality (Figs. 43.20). Preresection ECoG showed spiking over the right occipital lobe, and a postresection ECoG demonstrated residual spiking, which led to additional posterior parietal re-

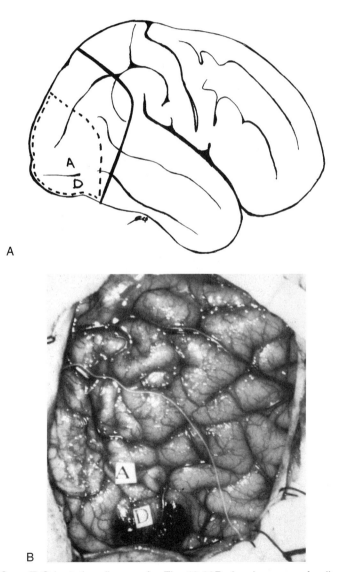

A

B

FIG. 43.20. A: Case T. Orientation diagram for Fig. 43.20B showing zone of epileptic activity *(A and B)* and occipital resection (dotted line). **B:** Case T. Note the area of occipital polymicrogyria, more conspicuous behind letter A. The *black area* at the bottom of the picture is a small operative contusion.

section (Fig. 43.20B). Pathology of the specimen showed polymicrogyria, focal cortical dysplasia, and white matter neuronal heterotopias. The patient has now been seizure free for 7 years after surgery.

This case illustrates the importance of the physical examination, EEG, and MRI in identifying the seizure origin. Reliance on the ictal SPECT would have been misguided because it demonstrated only seizure spread. The newer technologies used to evaluate epilepsy, such as FDG-PET, SPECT, and magnetic resonance spectroscopy can be helpful in some cases, but they can also compound the ambiguity if too much weight is placed on them.

Case J.G.

J.G. was a right-handed 39-year-old man at the time of surgery. His seizures began at the age of 8 years, and his seizure pattern was predominantly of a partial complex type. Most of the seizures began with an aura of a visual sensation described as a blurring in the right upper quadrant. In a minority of attacks, the aura was a feeling of fear or an ascending epigastric sensation. The seizures then proceeded to a loss of contact, staring, and dystonic posturing of the right hand. During a seizure, he might grasp at objects with either hand or walk around the room. Once a month, he had a generalized convulsion, and the partial complex seizures occurred twice a week. All the seizure patterns were uncontrolled by medication. Scalp EEG recorded many seizures showing onsets in the inferomesial temporal, lateral temporal, posterior temporal, occipital, and parietooccipital areas. Neuropsychological testing was consistent with lateral cortical dysfunction in the left hemisphere as well as less severe dysfunction of left mesial temporal structures. He did not have a visual-field defect, and the remainder of the neurologic examination did not detect any deficits. The initial MRI study demonstrated mild cortical atrophy of the left temporal pole without hippocampal atrophy. With additional fine-cut MRI studies and curvilin-

ear reconstruction, several small subependymal nodules were discovered in the lateral wall of the occipital horn consistent with hertertopias (Fig. 43.21A).

Although the occipital lesion was small, its location was consistent with the seizure generator on the scalp EEG. The resection of a deep-seated occipital lesion would carry an almost certain risk of some visual deficit. Therefore, to confirm the lesion as the site of seizure onset and to rule out other potential sites of onset, SEEG was performed (Fig. 43.22C). Four multicontact depth electrodes were inserted in the left hemisphere, one directed at the amygdala, one at the posterior hippocampal area, one in the subependymal nodule. Another depth electrode was inserted; targeted to the mesial structures between the lesion and the posterior hippocampus. Intracranial recording demonstrated the seizures arising from the region of the nodule. The patient proceeded to surgery, and a left occipital craniotomy was performed (Fig. 43.22A,B). A transcortical microsurgical approach was made to the occipital horn using MRI-guided frameless stereotaxy (Fig. 43.22C). The ependymal brownish lesion was well identified, and a selective resection of the nodule was accomplished. After surgery, visual-field testing revealed an incomplete right lower homonymous field defect. At 1-year follow-up, the patient has been seizure free except for a single nocturnal generalized convulsion.

This case illustrates the effectiveness of selectively removing small areas of dysplasia proven to be the site of seizure origin. It also illustrates clearly the potential for subependymal lesions to be the cause and origin of seizures. This causal relationship could be demonstrated only with the intracranial recording technique (i.e., SEEG) (Figs. 43.3, 43.4, and 43.22C).

Case H.

Patient H. was a 29-year-old right-handed man at the time of surgery. His seizure onset was at 5 years of age with no known etiology. Most of his seizures began with an aura of colored spots in the right upper quadrant of the vi-

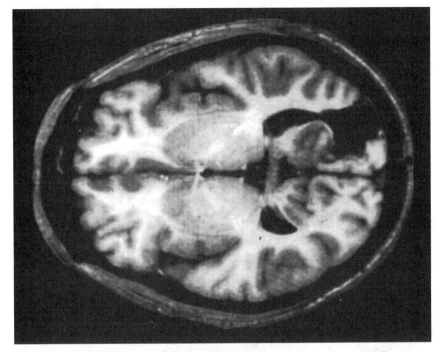

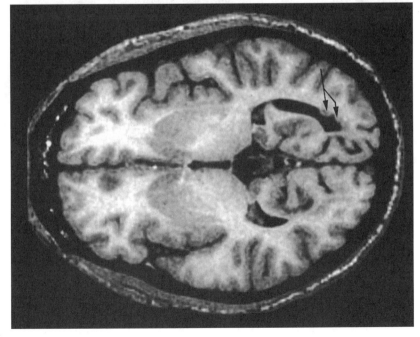

FIG. 43.21. A: Case J.G. Left paraventricular (subependymal) occipital heterotopias indicated by double arrow. **B:** Case J.G. Postoperative MRI showing removal of lesion. Compare with A.

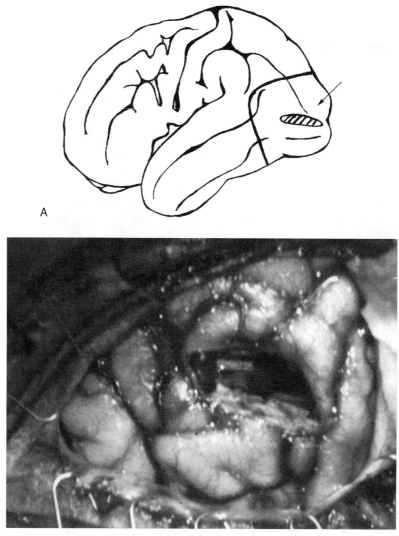

FIG. 43.22. A: Case J.G. Operative diagram for orientation. Site of cortical incision shown *(lines and arrow)*. **B:** Case J.G. Operative photograph showing actual cortical incision (see A).

sual field. He also experienced auras of déjà vu with an accompanying sense of euphoria. He then had one of three different seizure patterns: a generalized convulsion, an isolated visual aura or an aura of déjà vu and euphoria followed by loss of contact and automatic behavior. Scalp EEG showed interictal spiking in the left posterior temporal occipital and left occipital areas. MRI revealed neocortical atrophy of the left temporal lobe and gliosis of the left hippocampus. Intracranial recording then was performed with depth electrodes on the left tar- geted to the supracalcarine and infracalcarine parts of the occipital lobe, the amygdala, the anterior hippocampus, and the posterior parahippocampus. The seizure origin was localized to the left occipital lobe. The patient was counseled on the inevitable right hemifield visual defect that would result from surgery. At surgery, a preresection ECoG revealed diffuse left posterior parietal and occipital spiking, and a left occipital lobectomy was performed. He has been seizure free for 3 years since the surgery.

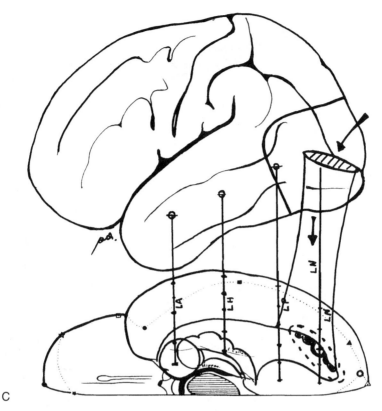

C

FIG. 43.22. *Continued.* **C:** Composite diagram showing placement of electrodes for intracranial recording. Also shows transcortical resection of ventricular nodule. Electrode A is in the amygdala LH in body of hippocampus, LP in posterior temporal area LN is inserted through the paraventricular heterotopic nodule.

Postoperatively, patient H.'s case was complicated by depression and anxiety over the resulting visual-field defect. The patient had been examined by an ophthalmologist before surgery, and, thinking the surgery was for a temporal lobe focus, the ophthalmologist informed the patient that a visual-field defect was not expected. The patient chose to accept the ophthalmologist's assessment of risk to the visual field over the surgeon's. The patient's grief over the visual-field deficit was present for many months, but other adjustment problems related to his new seizure-free life also became apparent. He longed for the euphoric auras, which had given him frequent highs.

Our experience has been that patients are not concerned by a visual-field defect resulting from surgery in the occipital lobe if they can anticipate a significant reduction in their seizure frequency. It must be stressed to the patient repeatedly and documented that they may end up with persistence of seizures and a visual-field defect. They must be counseled on this eventuality. Patient H. is unusual in his unacceptance of the deficit, especially after an excellent seizure outcome, mostly attributable to poor communication.

Multilobar Epilepsy

Case T.C.

At the time of surgery, T.C. was a 5-year-old girl with intractable epilepsy since the age of 2 days. The initial seizures consisted of stiffening and flickering of the eyelids. At the time of surgery, the seizures were manifested by turning the head to the left, flickering the eyelids, and stiffening the left arm and leg. She had many seizures every day, occasionally up to 40, and her left side would become weaker after a flurry of attacks. The more severe attacks would precipitate a fall. Her neurologic examination was remarkable for a left hemianopsia, a paucity of movements, and some neglect of the left side of the body. She also walked with a circumduction of the left leg. The MRI showed macrogyria of the posterior aspect of the temporal, parietal, and occipital lobes (Fig. 43.23). The white matter in these regions had an abnormally low signal intensity, and there was a loss of cortical/medullary differentiation. Scalp EEG demonstrated a severe epileptic abnormality with an abnormal background involving all the right hemisphere (Fig. 43.24).

A widespread abnormality existed in the right hemisphere; however, the seizure onset seen on the EEG correlated with the most severe structural abnormality identified on the MRI. Therefore, a resection of the structurally abnormal region was proposed in an effort to lower the seizure tendency. The patient underwent a temporo–parieto–occipital craniotomy under general anesthesia. The boundaries of the lesion identified on MRI were outlined on the surface of the brain using the MRI-guided frameless stereotaxy (Fig. 43.24A). Preresection ECoG demonstrated active diffuse interictal discharges over the right temporo–parieto–occipital region (Fig. 43.24). Two electrographic seizures were recorded, with the maximum over the temporal and occipital lobes below the level of the sylvian fissure. The central area was mapped by cortical stimulation. (Responses at 4.0 V: points A, C, and D flexion of all left fingers and point E flexion of 4th and 5th fingers on the left.) A large resection was subsequently performed, which encompassed the right temporal, occipital, and posterior parietal lobes in addition to a corticectomy of the lower postcentral gyrus (Fig. 43.24A). The resection included most of the visible lesion on MRI in addition to the cortex exhibiting the maximal epileptic activity on ECoG. Pathology examination demonstrated abnormal large and binucleate neurons

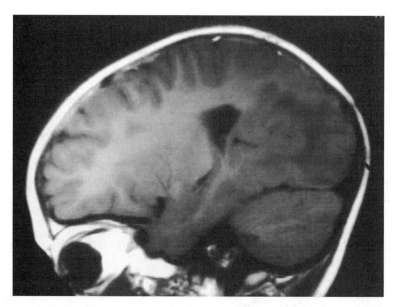

FIG. 43.23. Case T.C. Preoperative MRI showing extensive area of dysplasia and hypomyelination in occipito–parieto–temporal area.

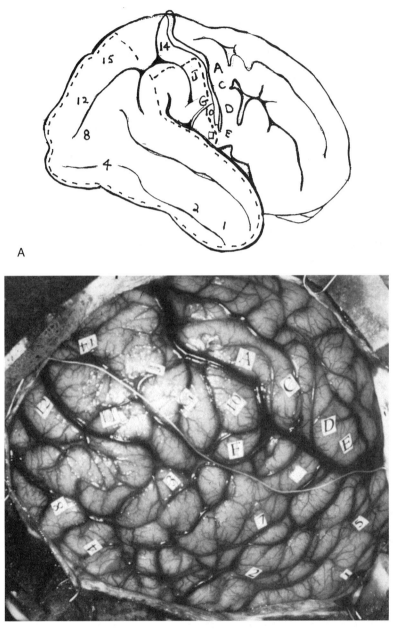

FIG. 43.24. A: Case T.C. Operating room diagram showing physiologic responses, sites of epileptic activity, and extent of resection *(dotted line).* The resection comprises the occipital lobe, the temporal lobe, and part of the parietal lobe. *A,* 4.0-V stimulation produced flexion of fingers on the left; *C,* left-hand contraction and flexion of fingers; *D,* flexion of all fingers on the left; *E,* flexion of 4th and 5th fingers on the left; *1,2,4,8,10,12,14,15,16,* diffuse interictal spike activity and several electrographic seizures recorded. **B:** Case T. Operating room photograph showing physiologic responses, sites of epileptic activity, and extent of removal *(dotted line)* (see A for orientation). *4,5,7,* ECoG recording sites. A diffuse epileptogenic abnormality was recorded with several electrographic seizures over the lesion and the central area. *F,* stimulation at 4.0 V produced a slight movement of the left hand.

throughout the cortical layer and a paucity of myelin in the white matter. After surgery, she was seizure free for 3 months. Some seizures recurred, but she has maintained a 90% improvement in seizure frequency for over 3 years and no longer has severe attacks with falls.

This case illustrates several of the difficulties in dealing with widespread multilobar cortical dysplasia. Incomplete removal does not stop the seizure tendency; however, a subtotal removal of a large area of cortical dysplasia can be beneficial in cases where the area of maximal interictal epileptogenic focus has been identified and resected. Finally, this patient demonstrates that dysplasia may possibly involve an entire hemisphere even though gross imaging changes may be quite localized.

The importance of dysplasia as the etiology of intractable epilepsy is seen in patients J.L., A.H., L.M., T., J.G., and T.C. The dysplastic cortex is intrinsically epileptogenic as opposed to other recognized etiologies of seizure, such as tumor or scar that produce their effect by irritating surrounding cortex (54). The recognition of cortical dysplasia in the evaluation of a patient for epilepsy surgery is critical because good seizure control is incumbent on as complete a resection as possible of the dysplasia (52,43,56,57). Also, the prospect for good seizure control from surgery is much lower if a lesion is not detected (58,59). The most commonly missed lesions are small areas of dysplasia that may require more sophisticated techniques such as curvilinear reconstruction to detect them (27,56).

At surgery, dysplasia may be impossible to detect on the cortical surface, even if readily seen on MRI. Indeed, abnormalities that can be identified on the cortical surface have margins that are usually not discernible at surgery. Therefore, to locate small lesions and identify the boundaries of larger ones, MRI-guided frameless stereotaxy and 3-D surface reconstruction have become essential at the MNI for the treatment of these abnormalities (2). The stereotaxic pointer can be used to outline the margins of the dysplasia on the surface of the scalp to tailor the scalp incision and the craniotomy. When the surface of the brain is exposed, the dysplasia can be localized with the stereotaxic pointer to guide placement of the ECoG and plan the resection. Because these lesions are better seen on MRI than at surgery, identification of the margins using frameless stereotaxy is essential to be confident of an adequate removal.

SURGICAL RESULTS

Table 43.1 shows the total number of patients in the authors' series who have undergone a procedure involving the parietal and occipital lobes. Cases of the central area that have had removal of the lower post central gyrus also are included. Multilobar cases are those where various extents of parietooccipital resections have been performed. Results on the seizure tendency will be presented for the strictly parietal or occipital cases. There were 39 patients in the parietal group, for a total of 59 procedures, and 30 patients in the occipital group, for a total of 39 procedures. The various etiologies found in these two groups are listed in Table 43.2 and Table 43.3.

Table 43.4 shows the classification of the results used in the authors' series and the results for the parietal group. Class I is the seizure-free category, which may comprise patients who have residual subjective auras. Class II is made up of patients who have had a reduction of more than 90% in the frequency of their seizures. Class III represents the group of patients with a seizure frequency decrease between 60% and 90%. Finally,

TABLE 43.1. *Surgery involving parietal and occipital lobes*[a]

Procedure	No. of procedures	(No. of patients)
Parietal	59	(39)
Occipital	39	(30)
Central	59	
Multilobar	24	
Total	181	

[a]A. Olivier's series.

TABLE 43.2. *Parietal lobe pathology (39 patients)*

Type of pathology	Percent of patients
Benign tumors	34
Gliosis	26
Dysplasias	24
Cavernous hemangiomas	8
Cysts	8
Arteriovenous malformation	3
Scars	3
Vascular lesions	3

TABLE 43.3. *Occipital lobe pathology (30 patients)*

Type of pathology	Percent of patients
Benign tumors	33
Gliosis	27
Dysplasias	17
Arteriovenous malformation	13
Cysts	13
Cavernous hemangiomas	10
Infarct microscopic	7
Encephalic	7
Sturge–Weber	3

TABLE 43.4. *Parietal resections surgical outcome (39 patients)*

Class	Outcome	Percent of patients
I	Seizure free	52
II	>90% Reduction	30
III	60%–90% Reduction	11
IV	<60% Reduction	7

TABLE 43.5. *Occipital resections surgical outcome (30 patients)*

Class	Outcome	Percent of patients
I	Seizure free	71
II	>90% reduction	18
III	60%–90% reduction	7
IV	<60% reduction	4

TABLE 43.6. *Complications of parietal lobe resections*

Complication	No. of patients
Hematomas	3
Osteomyelitis	1
Empyema	2
Quadranopsia	2
Hemianopsia	1
Hemiparesis	2

group IV is the "failure" group, with a seizure reduction of less than 60%.

In the parietal group (Table 43.4), 52% became seizure free, 30% had a reduction of more than 90%, and 11% had a reduction of 60% to 90%. Failure to alter the seizure tendency in a significant way occurred in 7% of the patients.

Table 43.5 shows the results for the 30 patients in the occipital group. Seventy-one percent became seizure free, and 18% obtained a reduction of more than 90%. Seven percent were in the 60% to 90% category and 4% in the failure group.

Complications

Complications in this series were few and are listed in Table 43.6. *Hematomas* refer to subdural or epidural hematomas. There were no mortality or severe neurological deficits.

CONCLUSION

Parietal and occipital lobe epilepsy may be difficult to localize by seizure semiology because distant structures are often involved early; however, the presence of a somatosensory aura strongly implicates the parietal lobe, and seizures heralded by elementary visual hallucinations are convincing for occipital lobe onset. The surface EEG also may not be localizing because it often shows the initial ictal and interictal activity distant from the seizure origin in both parietal and occipital epilepsy. SEEG (intracranial recording) is often necessary to validate clinical and EEG impressions.

A lesion discovered in a patient being evaluated for epilepsy surgery must be suspected to be the site of seizure origin even if it is incongruous with the surface EEG. Increasingly, dysplasia is being recognized as the etiology of intractable neocortical epilepsy, and a diligent search using MRI and other neuroimaging modalities may be required to discover it. The prognosis for a good seizure outcome is greatly improved if a lesion is detected and removed as completely as possible.

At the MNI, MRI-guided frameless stereotaxy is an integral part of surgical planning. The 3-D surface reconstruction of the brain shows the gyral and sulcal anatomy better than the view of the exposed cortical surface. Frameless stereotaxy used in conjunction with preoperative mapping can be used for tailoring the craniotomy flap, localizing regions of functional activation, and identifying a lesion. It is essential for the resection of dysplasia because the boundaries of a lesion seen on the MRI may not be evident on the exposed cortex.

The advent of modern computer-guided surgery has provided the surgeon with means to avoid many of the technical pitfalls involving the parietooccipital area as well as a tool to delineate and resect epileptogenic lesions with increased safety to obtain better seizure control.

REFERENCES

1. Olivier A, Germano I, Cukiert A, et al. Frameless stereotaxy for surgery of the epilepsies: preliminary experience [Technical Note]. *J Neurosurg* 1994;81: 629–633.
2. Olivier A, Alonso-Vanegas M, Comeau R, et al. Image-guided surgery of epilepsy. *Neurosurg Clin N Am* 1996; 7:229–244.
3. Olivier A, Cyr M, Comeau R, et al. Image-guided surgery of epilepsy and intrinsic brain tumors. In: Alexander E III, Maciunas RJ, eds. *Advanced neurosurgical navigation.* New York: Thieme Medical, 1999: 469–482.
4. Olivier A, Boling W. Diagnostic operative techniques in the treatment of epilepsy: stereotactic intracranial recording. In: Schmidek H, Sweet W, eds. *Operative neurosurgical techniques, indications, methods, and results.* Philadelphia: WB Saunders, 2000.
5. Blume WT. Occipital lobe epilepsies. In: Lüders HO, ed. *Epilepsy surgery.* New York: Raven Press, 1991: 167–171.
6. Blume WT, Whiting SE, Girvin JP. Epilepsy surgery in the posterior cortex. *Ann Neurol* 1991;29:638–645.
7. Cascino GD, Hulihan JF, Sharbrough FW, et al. Parietal lobe lesional epilepsy: electroclinical correlation and operative outcome. *Epilepsia* 1993;34:522–527.
8. Olivier A. Extratemporal resections in the surgical treatment of epilepsy. In: Spencer SS, Spencer SS, eds. *Contemporary issues in neurological surgery: surgery for epilepsy.* Boston: Blackwell Scientific, 1991:150–167.
9. Rasmussen T. Focal epilepsies of nontemporal and nonfrontal origin. In: Wieser HG, Elger CE, eds. *Presurgical evaluation of epileptics.* Berlin: Springer-Verlag, 1987:300–305.
10. Rasmussen T. Surgery for central, parietal, and occipital epilepsy. *Can J Neurol Sci* 1991;18:611–616.
11. Salanova V, Andermann F, Olivier A, et al. Occipital lobe epilepsy: electroclinical manifestations, electrocorticography, cortical stimulation, and outcome in 42 patients treated between 1930 and 1991. *Brain* 1992; 115:1655–1680.
12. Salanova V, Andermann F, Rasmussen T, et al. Parietal lobe epilepsy: clinical manifestations and outcome in 82 patients treated surgically between 1929 and 1988. *Brain* 1995;118:607–627.
13. Salanova V, Andermann F, Rasmussen T, et al. Tumoral parietal lobe epilepsy: clinical manifestations and outcome in 34 patients treated between 1934 and 1988. *Brain* 1995;118:1289–1304.
14. Sveinbjornsdottir S, Duncan JS. Parietal and occipital lobe epilepsy: a review. *Epilepsia* 1993;34:493–521.
15. Takeda A, Bancaud J, Talairach J, et al. Concerning epileptic attacks of occipital origin. *Electroencephalogr Clin Neurophysiol* 1970;28:647–648.
16. Williamson PD, Boon PA, Thadani VM, et al. Parietal lobe epilepsy: diagnostic considerations and results of surgery. *Ann Neurol* 1992;31:193–201.
17. Williamson PD, Thadani VM, Darcey TM, et al. Occipital lobe epilepsy: clinical characteristics, seizure spread patterns, and results of surgery. *Ann Neurol* 1992; 31:3–13.
18. Horsley SV. The function of the so-called motor area of the brain: the Linacre lecture. *BMJ* 1909;2:125–132.
19. Cushing H. A note upon the Faradic stimulation of the postcentral gyrus in conscious patients. *Brain* 1909;32: 3–12.
20. Foerster O. Die Pathogenese des epileptischen Krampfanfalles. Sonderabdruck aus den Verhandlungen der Gesellschaft deutscher *Nervenärzte* 1925:15–56.
21. Foerster O, Penfield W. Der Narbenzug am und im Gehirn bei traumatischer Epilepsie in seiner Bedeutung für das Zustandekommen der Anfälle und für die therapeutische Bekämpfung derselben. *Zeitschrift für die gesamte Neurologie und Psychiatrie* 1930;125:475–572.
22. Foerster O, Penfield W. The structural basis of traumatic epilepsy and results of radical operation. *Brain* 1930;53:99–119.
23. Penfield W, Erickson TC. *Epilepsy and cerebral localization.* Baltimore: Charles C. Thomas, 1941.
24. Penfield W, Steelman H. The treatment of focal epilepsy by cortical excision. *Ann Surg* 1947;126:740–762.
25. Penfield W, Paine KWE. The results of surgical therapy for focal epileptic seizures. International Conference, Lisbon, 1954.
26. Rasmussen T. Surgery of epilepsy associated with brain tumors. In: Purpura DP, Penry JK, Walter RD, eds. *Neurosurgical management of epilepsies. Advances in neurology,* vol 8. New York: Raven Press, 1975:227–239.
27. Bastos AC, Korah IP, Cendes F, et al. Curvilinear reconstruction of 3D magnetic resonance imaging in patients with partial epilepsy: a pilot study. *Magn Reson Imaging* 1995;13:1107–1112.
28. Clark E, O'Malley CD. *The human brain and spinal cord.* Berkeley-Los Angeles: University of California Press, 1968:409–412.
29. Dejerine J. *Anatomie des centres nerveux.* Paris: Rueff et Cie, 1895.
30. Parent A. *Carpenter's human neuroanatomy.* Philadelphia: Williams & Wilkins, 1996.
31. Poirier P, Charpy A. *Traité d'anatomie humaine.* Paris: Masson, 1898.

32. Yasargil MG. *CNS tumours:* surgical anatomy, *neuropathology, neuroradiology, neurophysiology—clinical considerations, operability, treatment options.* New York: Thieme Medical, 1994:14–79.

33. Testut L, Latarjet A. *Traité d'anatomie humaine. Tome deuxième.* Paris: Gaston Doin & Cie, 1929.

34. Larsell O. *Anatomy of the nervous system.* New York: Appleton-Century-Crofts, 1951.

35. Schäfer EA, Symington J, Bryce TH. *Quain's elements of anatomy,* Vol. III. London: Longmans, Green, 1909.

36. Broca P. *Memoires sur le cerveau de l'homme et des primates.* Paris: C Reinwald, 1888:739–804.

37. Gratiolet LP. *Anatomie comparée du système nerveux considéré dans ses rapports avec l'intelligence,* II. Paris: Baillière, 1857.

38. Crosby EC, Humphrey T, Lauer EW. *Correlative anatomy of the nervous system.* New York: Macmillan, 1962:343–518.

39. Mauguière F, Courjon J. Somatosensory epilepsy: a review of 127 cases. *Brain* 1978;101:307–332.

40. Palmini A, Gloor P. The localizing value of auras in partial seizures: a prospective and retrospective study. *Neurology* 1992;42:801–808.

41. Geier S, Bancaud J, Talairach J, et al. Ictal tonic postural changes and automatisms of the upper limb during epileptic parietal lobe discharges. *Epilepsia* 1977;18:517–524.

42. Ajmone-Marsan C, Goldhammer L. Clinical ictal patterns and electrographic data in cases of partial seizures of fronto–central–parietal origin. In: Brazier MAB, ed. *Epilepsy: its phenomena in man.* New York: Academic Press, 1973:236–258.

43. Palmini A, Andermann F, Dubeau F, et al. Occipitotemporal epilepsies: evaluation of selected patients requiring depth electrodes studies and rationale for surgical approaches. *Epilepsia* 1993;34:84–96.

44. Olivier A, Gloor P, Andermann F, et al. Occipitotemporal epilepsy studied with stereotaxically implanted depth electrodes and successfully treated by temporal resection. *Ann Neurol* 1982;11:428–432.

45. Russell WR, Whitty CWM. Studies in traumaic epilepsy 3. Visual fits. *J Neurol Neurosurg Psychiatry* 1955;18:79–96.

46. Collins RC, Caston TV. Functional anatomy of occipital lobe seizures: an experimental study in rats. *Neurology* 1979;29:705–716.

47. Bancaud J, Bonis A, Morel P, et al. Epilepsie occipitale à expression "rhinencéphalique" prévalente (corrélations électrocliniques à la lumière des investigations fonctionnelles stéréotaxiques). *Rev Neurol (Paris)* 1961;105:219.

48. Kuzniecky R, Gilliam F, Morawetz R, et al. Occipital lobe developmental malformations and epilepsy: clinical spectrum, treatment, and outcome. *Epilepsia* 1997;38:175–181.

49. Klein D, Olivier A, Milner B, et al. Obligatory role of the LIFG in synonym generation: evidence from PET and cortical stimulation. *Neuroreport* 1997;8:3275–3279.

50. AbouMadi M. Anesthesia considerations in epilepsy surgery. In: Gildenberg PL, Tasker R, eds. *Textbook of stereotactic and functional neurosurgery.* New York: McGraw-Hill, 1996;1875–1881.

51. Trop D, Olivier A, Dubeau F, et al. Seizure surgery: anesthetic, neurologic, neurobehavioral considerations. In: Albin MS, ed. *Textbook of neuroanesthesia with neurosurgical and neuroscience perspectives.* New York: McGraw-Hill, 1997;643–696.

52. Palmini A, Andermann F, Olivier A. Focal neuronal migration disorders and intractable partial epilepsy: results of surgical treatment. *Ann Neurol* 1991;30:750–757.

53. Palmini A, Gambardella A, Andermann F, et al. Outcome of surgical treatment in patients with localized cortical dysplasia and intractable epilepsy. *Ann Neurol* 1995;37:476–487.

54. Palmini A, Gambardella A, Andermann F, et al. The human dysplastic cortex is intrinsically epileptogenic. In: Guerrini R, et al. *Dysplasia of cerebral cortex and epilepsy.* Philadelphia: Lippincott–Raven, 1996:43–52.

55. Prayson RA, Estes ML. Cortical dysplasia: a histopathologic study of 52 cases of partial lobectomy in patients with epilepsy. *Hum Pathol* 1995;26:493–500.

56. Andermann F, Olivier A, Melanon D, et al. Epilepsy due to focal cortical dysplasia with macrogyria and forme fruste of tuberous sclerosis: a study of 15 cases. In: Wolf P, Dam M, eds. *Advances in epilepsy,* vol 16. New York: Raven Press, 1987:35–38.

57. Perot P, Weir B, Rasmussen T. Tuberous sclerosis: surgical therapy for seizures. *Ann Neurol* 1966;15:498–506.

58. Clarke DB, Olivier A, Andermann F, et al. Surgical treatment of epilepsy: the problem of lesion/focus incongruence. *Surg Neurol* 1996;46:579–585.

59. Sisodiya SM, Moran N, Free SL, et al. Correlation of widespread preoperative magnetic resonance imaging changes with unsuccessful surgery for hippocampal sclerosis. *Ann Neurol* 1997;41:490–496.

Neocortical Epilepsies.
Advances in Neurology, Vol. 84,
edited by P. D. Williamson, A. M. Siegel,
D. W. Roberts, V. M. Thadani, and M. S. Gazzaniga.
Lippincott Williams & Wilkins, Philadelphia © 2000.

44

Quantitative Temporal Lobe Volumetrics in the Surgical Management of Nonlesional Frontal and Temporal Neocortical Epilepsies

Sunghoon Lee, Kenneth Vives, Michael Westerveld, and Dennis Spencer

*Department of Neurosurgery, Yale University School of Medicine,
New Haven, Connecticut 06520-8082*

The advent of magnetic resonance imaging (MRI) has provided neuroanatomic details that have engendered a reclassification of neocortical partial epilepsies according to their related substrates. The substrates in the neocortical epilepsies, characterized by the respective underlying epileptogenic pathology and the associated anatomic localization, can be separated into neoplastic, vascular, gliotic, and developmental types. More recent scrutiny of gliotic substrates that are not clearly of traumatic, ischemic, or infectious etiology suggests that they also are developmental, consisting primarily of heterotopic neurons in the subcortical or molecular regions. For the purposes of this chapter, we have restricted our scope of investigation to neocortical epilepsy of gliotic and developmental origins from the temporal and frontal lobes. In addition, with the exception of traumatic gliosis, these patients have normal MRI scans. Mass lesions, including masses of developmental origin, such as cortical dysplasia, hematoma, and tuberous sclerosis, have been excluded so that a more uniform group requiring invasive electrophysiologic localization constitutes the study population.

We examined a group of 37 patients meeting these criteria who have undergone surgical treatments of their epilepsy in our institution. Preoperative evaluations consisted of a detailed history and neurologic examination, high-resolution MRI, scalp and intracranial electroencephalographic (EEG) monitoring, angiography, intracarotid amytal (Wada) tests, neuropsychologic testing, and hippocampal and temporal lobe volumetrics. The results from each diagnostic modality are considered and examined statistically in relation to the applied surgical strategies, including the anatomic locations and the volumes of resection. Postoperative outcomes such as changes in neuropsychological testing and seizure control are correlated to the volumetrics, resection volume, and other preoperative diagnostics. Finally, we speculate regarding the potential for improved understanding of nonlesional developmental neocortical epilepsies and strategies for better diagnosis and treatment.

The surgical substrate in our study population is electrographically defined to be of frontal and temporal neocortical onset from invasive intracranial monitoring; patients with mass lesions apparent on the preoperative MRI were excluded. These selection criteria excluded developmental lesions seen on the MRI, such as macroscopic cases of gray matter heterotopias, cortical dysplasias, and disorders of gyration. With these cases excluded, the study population consists of nonlesional neocortical epilepsies of frontal and temporal origin that may be otherwise considered cryptogenic if histopathologic findings of microdysgenesis and microscopic gray matter heterotopia are not taken into account. In this study, we examined postsurgical seizure control and neuropsychological outcome in this select group of patients. We found that temporal lobe volumetrics is a significant predictor of both seizure and neuropsychological outcome.

The identification of accurate predictors of surgical outcome is critical in the guidance of appropriate case selection. Retrospective studies from prominent epilepsy surgery centers reported large-volume analyses of surgical outcome that showed variable rates of success from neocortical resections. Haglund and Ojemann (1) reported their experience from the University of Washington Epilepsy Center in which 48% of the patients who had undergone cortical resections remained seizure free after a 4 to 5 years' follow-up. These investigators also reported that a total of 68% of their study group experienced significant reductions in seizure frequency postoperatively. Haglund and Ojemann (2) also reported a retrospective survey from multiple epilepsy surgery centers of outcomes in extratemporal resections during the years 1945 to 1984. They calculated a surgical cure rate of this era to be 43.2% and then noted the cure rate of the more recent era, from 1986 to 1990, to be 44.5%, showing no significant historical improvement in outcome. They noted the difficulties involved in the surgical treatment of extratemporal epilepsy, namely, the heterogeneity of underlying pathology and the inadequacy of electrophysiologic localizations.

Outcomes from the surgical treatment of neocortical epilepsies can be distinguished by whether or not the epileptogenic substrate is a structural abnormality. Cuckiert et al. (3) reported surgical cures in five of six patients with frontal lobe epilepsy caused by posttraumatic gliosis. These researchers noted the importance of a ready visualization of structural abnormalities by preoperative imaging in the guidance of the surgical resection. Davies and Weeks (4) studied postsurgical seizure outcome in 15 patients with structural abnormalities noted on preoperative imaging. The structural abnormalities were widely heterogeneous, including primary neoplasms, vascular pathologies, infectious lesions, and gliotic scars. Forty percent of these patients were seizure free, and another 47% experienced significant reductions in the frequency of their seizures. The authors noted that the presence of structural lesions seems to be a predictor of favorable postsurgical seizure outcome.

Smith et al. (5) performed comparative analysis of seizure outcome in the surgical treatment of lesional versus nonlesional frontal lobe epilepsy. In this study, 66% of the patients treated surgically for lesional epilepsy were seizure free, whereas only 29% of the patients with nonlesional substrates remained seizure free. Further evidence is noted by Lorenzo et al. showing that favorable surgical outcome in intractable frontal lobe epilepsy is marked by focal structural abnormalities on MRI and associated pathological abnormalities (6).

It is apparent that although surgical therapies for neocortical epilepsies have improved in the cases of lesional substrates, seizure outcomes from surgery for nonlesional frontal substrates have remained suboptimal. Surgical outcome may be improved in nonlesional neocortical substrates by better patient selection criteria and better definition of the epileptogenic substrate for surgical resection. Quantitative lobar volumetric measurements, along with invasive EEG, examine regional changes and may predict outcome and guide surgical planning. Surgical treatment of neocortical epilepsies will also benefit from improved predictability of potential postsurgical neuropsychological deficits. In the assessment of the neuropsychological outcome in our study population, we sought to determine subgroups of patients who might be at increased risk for postsurgical neuropsychological decline. In particular, we examined the role of quantitative temporal lobe volumetrics as a predictor of neuropsychological outcome.

METHODS

The patients studied were selected from a consecutive series of patients from 1987 to 1997 who underwent evaluation in the Yale Epilepsy Surgery Program. Each patient underwent standard phase I evaluation, including MRI, continuous audiovisual and EEG monitoring, neuropsychological evaluation, positron emission tomography (PET) scanning, and intracarotid amytal language and memory testing. Based on this evaluation, a subset of patients was recommended for intracranial EEG monitoring. Following this monitoring, a further subset of patients was recommended for resective surgery based on intracranial ictal onset. Those patients in whom the epileptogenic focus was found to involve functionally critical areas, in which resection would result in unacceptable deficits were not recommended for primary resective surgery and are not included in this analysis.

Inclusion criteria for this study included (a) the absence of structural lesion on MRI, (b) the necessity of intracranial monitoring for seizure evaluation, (c) the finding of a defined epileptogenic focus in either the frontal lobe or temporal neocortex based on intracranial EEG monitoring, and (d) the performance of resective surgery in either the frontal or temporal lobes with the goal of seizure relief. Thirty-seven patients met these requirements and were included for further analysis in the study.

Patient-related data were obtained retrospectively from chart review and, for more recent patients, prospectively from the Yale Epilepsy Surgery Database. MRI studies were reviewed individually. Surgical volumes were estimated based on measurements of the surgical defect on the postoperative MRI or by the dimensions of the resected surgical specimen as defined by the operative dictation. In cases in which data were available from both postoperative MRI and operative dictations,

the estimated volumes were averaged. We chose the postoperative MRI with the least delay from the date of the surgery for volume estimation. The surgical volume was estimated based on its dimensions in the axial, sagittal, and coronal planes. The formula $[(A*B*C)*\pi]/2$, which configures the volume of an ellipsoid, was applied with the derived dimensions to estimate the surgical volume. In temporal resection cases, we derived the lengths of the temporal neocortical resection (in centimeters) from postoperative MRI or operative dictations. The extent of the temporal resection was used as a variable for statistical comparison in outcome analysis.

For details of the volumetric procedures, see McCarthy and Luby (7). Briefly, preoperatively, a three-dimensional (3-D) volume set of coronal MRI images (SPGR 3-mm slices; repetition time/echo time [TR/TE] = 25/5; FOV 16) was obtained. These images then were reformatted into oblique images perpendicular to the long axis of the hippocampus, and adjustments were made for head rotation if needed. The hippocampus was carefully outlined on each of the five images starting 3 mm anterior to the superior colliculus. The volume of the hippocampus was taken as the sum of the outlined areas on each of these images. Temporal lobe volumes were obtained in a similar fashion. The temporal lobe was outlined on each image starting anteriorly from the temporal pole to, posteriorly, the same level of termination as detailed for the hippocampus. Superomedially, the temporal stem was used as the boundary. The volume was taken as the sum of the outlined areas on each of these images. Each volumetric measurement was compared with the mean and SD of the volumes of nonepileptic normal subjects, and a z-score was generated. Further classification of patients was performed based on deviation of the z-score greater than 1.96 SD from normals. All data were analyzed with Statview 5.0 (SAS Institute, Inc., Cary, NC, U.S.A. 1998). Appropriate univariate tests were chosen based on the type of data being analyzed. A p value of less than 0.05 was selected to represent statistical significance. Multivariate analysis was not carried out because of the relatively small number of patients in the study.

All patients underwent comprehensive neuropsychological examination as part of the presurgical workup. The test battery consisted of measures of language competency, intellectual functioning, verbal and visuospatial memory, and Wada testing. Each of the tasks are described in more detail in the following section.

All patients were administered a language battery that included measures of visual confrontation naming (8) and rapid word generation (cued fluency). The Boston Naming Test is a visual confrontation naming test that consists of 60 line drawings of common items. The items are arranged in order of decreasing frequency of occurrence of the word, from most common (e.g., bed, pencil) to least common (e.g., trellis, abacus). Patients are asked to provide verbal responses with varying levels of semantic and phonemic cues. The score included for analysis herein is the number of items correctly named without cueing. Cued-word fluency is the rapid generation of names that are cued with either semantic (e.g., animals, fruits, vegetables) or phonemic (e.g., F, A, S or C, F, L) cues. Impaired verbal fluency is associated with frontal lobe damage, particularly on the left, and is evident on spontaneous word production, oral reading, and writing tasks (9). The task used in the present study is a written fluency task requiring the patient to generate as many words beginning with the letter "H" as possible in a 2-minute period without using proper nouns. The raw score is the number of unique words generated, not including proper nouns.

All patients were administered the Wechsler Adult Intelligence Scale–Revised (WAIS-R)(10), a battery of tasks that provides estimates of ability in various domains of cognitive functioning. The WAIS-R contains two scales, the Verbal Scale and the Performance Scale. The Verbal Scale measures language expression, comprehension, listening, and the ability to apply these skills to solving problems. The examiner gives the questions orally, and a spoken response is required. The Perfor-

mance Scale assesses nonverbal problem solving, perceptual organization, speed, and visual–motor proficiency. Included are tasks like puzzles, analysis of pictures, imitating designs, and copying. Composite intelligence quotient (IQ) indexes were calculated based on complete administration of the WAIS-R in accordance with standardized instructions.

Verbal memory was examined using the Russell adaptation (11) of the Wechsler Memory Scale (12) logical memory subtest. This involves presentation of two separate prose passages, with each presentation followed by the patient providing immediate recall. After a delay of 30 minutes, the patient is asked to recall again the content of each prose passage. Three scores are calculated, one each for the immediate and delayed recall based on accuracy of recitation of story details. A third score is calculated to assess the amount of information forgotten over the period of delay (percent retention score). Each patient also was administered the verbal selective reminding test to evaluate verbal learning. The selective reminding procedure (13) is designed to assess verbal learning over multiple presentation trials. The unique presentation allows for scoring of long-term storage, long-term retrieval, and consistency of recall. Following initial presentation of the entire word list, the patient is asked to recall as many words as possible. Following the initial trial, the patient is reminded only of those words that were not recalled on the immediately preceding trial. The test continues in this manner until 12 trials have been completed or until the patient has recalled the entire word list on at least two successive trials.

Visual–spatial memory was assessed using the Wechsler Memory Scale (WMS) Figural Reproduction subtest. This task requires the patient to reproduce a simple line drawing from memory following a 10-second exposure of the stimulus card. Like the verbal portion of the WMS, scoring procedures resulted in an immediate recall score, delayed recall score, and percent retention score. The visual–motor selective reminding test also was used to assess nonverbal learning and recall.

This procedure involves brief (3 seconds) exposure of a series of 12 simple line drawings. The patient is required to reproduce as many as possible from memory. After the initial trial in which all 12 items are exposed, only the forgotten items are exposed on subsequent trials following the same procedure as the verbal selective reminding. This continues until the patient correctly reproduces all 12 items on 2 successive trials or until 12 trials have been completed, whichever comes first.

RESULTS

Seizure Outcome

All patients, with one exception, were assessed for seizure control at greater than 1-year follow-up. In one patient, only a 6-month follow-up was available. Patients' outcomes were graded as being either "seizure free" or "not seizure free." Thirty-one percent of our patients remained seizure free following surgery (n = 12); 69% of the patients continued to have seizures (n = 25) (Fig. 44.1). We found 31% of the patients to be Engel grade I, 41% Engel grade II, and 28% Engel grade III. No patients were found to be Engel grade IV.

Demographic and EEG Variables

We analyzed a spectrum of demographic variables that included age, gender, duration of seizures, and language dominance to examine whether they were statistically significant predictors of seizure outcome in nonlesional neocortical epilepsy. The mean age of the patients at surgery, the duration of the seizure disorder, and the age at seizure onset were examined for the seizure and the seizure-free group and analyzed using the two-tailed student's *t*-test. No statistical significant differences in seizure outcome were found based on these variables; mean age at surgery for the seizure group was 29 versus 33 for the seizure free group ($p = 0.334$). Mean duration of seizure disorder for the seizure group was 15.0, whereas that of the seizure free group was 13.7 ($p = 0.743$). Mean age of onset for the seizure group was 12.2 and 15.3 for the seizure free group ($p = 0.409$). No statistically significant differences in seizure outcome were observed based on language dominance or by gender by chi-square analysis (language dominance $p = 0.564$, gender $p = 0.295$).

All patients underwent phase III intracranial EEG monitoring for seizure localization. The EEG characteristics were determined and categorized based on their frequency and their focality. The ictal EEG frequency was categorized as follows. The patients with predominant alpha, beta, or theta frequency events were grouped as having *fast frequency*. The patients with predominant gamma fre-

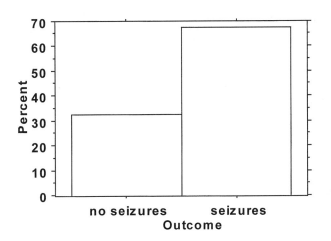

FIG. 44.1. Postoperative seizure outcome. The graph represents the postoperative seizure outcome in our study population. Thirty-one percent of the patients remained seizure free (n = 12), and 69% of the patients continued to have seizures (n = 25).

quency events were grouped as having *slow frequency*. The focality of ictal EEG for each patient was determined and characterized as having a predominant *focal onset* as opposed to a more diffuse *regional onset*. A statistically significant relationship was found between the frequency of seizures and the focality of their onset. Chi-square analysis revealed that patients with predominantly fast frequency seizures had a regional localization, whereas the patients with slow frequency seizures onset had a more focal localization ($p = 0.028$); however, neither EEG frequency nor focality were found to predict seizure outcome (frequency $p = 0.47$, and focality $p = 0.70$).

Volumes of Resection and the Extent of Temporal Neocortical Resection

We quantified surgical volumes in our study population by either measuring the dimensions of the postoperative MRI defect or by the dimensions of the surgical specimen as dictated in the operative reports. In cases where both data were available, the MRI and the dictated dimensions were averaged for volume derivation (Fig. 44.2). There are inherent limitations of this analysis in the standard estimations of the resection volumes to an ellipsoid ($A*B*C)*\pi/2$. The result is a crude estimation of resection volume when the conformation strays from the ellipsoid. Current technology does enable rigorous quantitative volumetric measurements of resection volumes based on MRI imaging. Such a technique may be worthwhile for future investigations.

We pursued the hypothesis that larger surgical resections might lead to improved seizure control; however, we found a trend for the larger surgical resection volumes to have poorer seizure outcome. The estimated resection volumes for the seizure free group was 20.26 mL (n = 12) compared with that of the seizure group with a volume of 38.48 mL (n = 24). The associated mean difference had a p value of 0.089 by t test analysis (Fig. 44.3). This trend may be significant with a larger

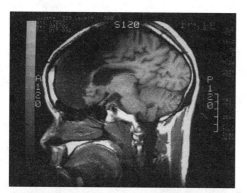

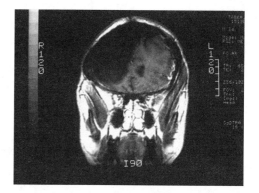

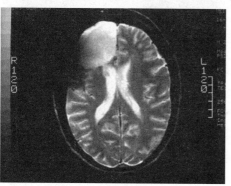

FIG. 44.2. Estimations of surgical volumes. The figure illustrates saggital, axial, and coronal postoperative MRI from a patient who had a right frontal lobectomy for the control of medically refractory seizures. The formula [(A*B*C)*π]/2, which configures the volume of an ellipsoid, was applied with the derived dimensions to estimate the surgical volume.

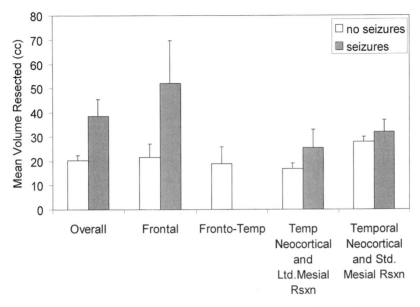

FIG. 44.3. Relationship of seizure outcome and resection volumes. The estimated resection volumes for the seizure-free group revealed a resection volume of 20.26 mLs (n = 12) compared with that of the seizure group with a resection volume of 38.48 mL (n = 24) $p = 0.089$ by t test analysis, shown under label *overall*. Analyses based on resection volumes were stratified by the location of the resection. These comparisons, labeled in the figure by the location (e.g., frontal) were not statistically significant.

study population. We studied the relationship of volume and seizure outcome based on the location of the presumed substrate, stratifying the analysis by the location of resection. With the exception of the group with both frontal and temporal resections (n = 2), in which both patients remained seizure free, the remaining three groups (frontal, temporal with *standard* mesial resection, temporal with *limited* mesial resection) followed a similar trend: Those that remained seizure free had smaller volumes of resection (Fig. 44.3).

In patients who had temporal resections, the extent of lateral temporal neocortical resection was not a statistically significant predictor of continued seizures. The same trend was noted, however, between volumes of resection and seizure outcome. The mean temporal neocortical resection in the seizure group was 6.53 cm, (n = 15, SE = 0.73), whereas it was 5.00 cm (n = 7, SE = 0.50) for the seizure-free group. The difference in the means revealed a p value of 0.190. The trend of larger temporal resection

correlating with relatively poor seizure control applied to both the group with *limited* mesial resections as well as those with *standard* mesial resections, although neither was statistically significant (*limited* mesial resection, $p = 0.293$; *standard* mesial resection, $p = 0.238$).

Seizure Outcome by Substrate: Locations of Resection

Seizure outcome was examined by the location of surgical resection. Seizure outcome did not differ when frontal resections were compared with temporal resections. Of the temporal resection patients (n = 22), 33.3% remained seizure free, whereas 31.8% of the patients with frontal resection (n = 15) were seizure free. Chi-square analysis revealed no significant differences in seizure outcome ($p = 0.923$). Seizure outcome also was examined within the temporal resection group between the patients who had neocortical plus *standard* mesial resections versus *limited* mesial resections. In the

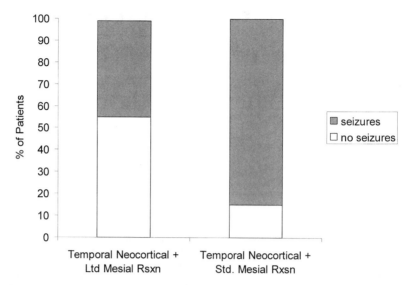

FIG. 44.4. Seizure outcome based on the extent of mesial resection. The patients who had temporal resections were stratified based on whether they had limited versus standard mesial resection. The seizure outcomes of these subgroups were compared with chi-square analysis. In the temporal resection group with standard mesial resection (n = 13), only 15.4% of the patients remained seizure free, whereas in the temporal resection group with limited mesial resections (n = 9), 55.6% of the patients had seizure-free outcomes (p = 0.047).

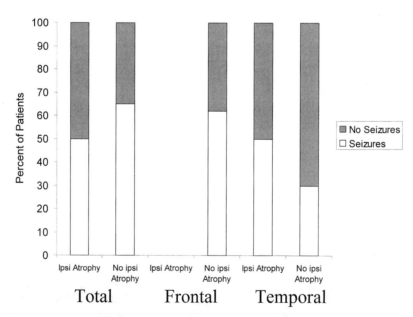

FIG. 44.5. Seizure outcome based on hippocampal volumetrics. Hippocampal volumetrics were obtained for 29 patients. Six of the 29 patients (20.7%) had significant hippocampal atrophy (z-score > 1.96) ipsilateral to the side of resection. Fifty percent (n = 6) of patients who had hippocampal atrophy became seizure free compared with 34.8% (n = 23) of patients without significant atrophy who became seizure (p = 0.82). Of the patients who had temporal resections, 50% of the patients with ipsilateral hippocampal atrophy (n = 6) remained seizure free, whereas 30% of those without ipsilateral hippocampal atrophy (n = 10) were seizure free (p = 0.424). Similar analysis of seizure outcome based on hippocampal volumetrics in the frontal resection patients could not be performed because none of the frontal resection patients was found to have ipsilateral hippocampal atrophy.

temporal resection group with *standard* mesial resection (n = 13), only 15.4% of the patients remained seizure free, whereas in the temporal resection group with *limited* mesial resections (n = 9), 55.6% of the patients had seizure-free outcomes ($p = 0.047$) (Fig. 44.4).

Hippocampal Volumetrics and Seizure Outcome

Hippocampal volumetrics were obtained for 29 patients in our study population. Six of the 29 patients (20.7%) had significant hippocampal atrophy (z-score > 1.96) ipsilateral to the side of resection. The presence of ipsilateral hippocampal atrophy was not predictive of seizure outcome. We found that 50% (n = 6) of patients who had hippocampal atrophy became seizure free compared with 34.8% (n = 23) of patients without hippocampal atrophy (p =

0.494) (Fig. 44.5). The predictive value of hippocampal atrophy was examined specifically in temporal resections. Fifty percent of these patients with ipsilateral hippocampal atrophy (n = 6) remained seizure free, whereas 30% of those without ipsilateral hippocampal atrophy (n = 10) were seizure free ($p = 0.424$) (Fig. 44.5). None of the frontal resection patients had ipsilateral hippocampal atrophy.

Temporal Lobe Volumetrics and Seizure Outcome

Temporal lobe volumetrics were obtained for 22 patients in our study. Sixteen patients (72.7%) had significant temporal neocortical atrophy (z-score > 1.96 or 2 SD) ipsilateral to the side of resection. Temporal lobe atrophy is a statistically significant predictor of seizure outcome (Fig. 44.6). None of the six patients

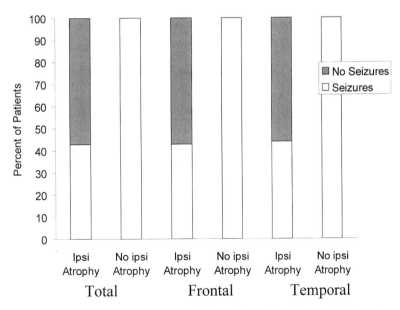

FIG. 44.6. Seizure outcome based on temporal lobe volumetrics. Temporal lobe volumetrics were obtained for 22 patients, of whom six did not have volumetric atrophy ipsilateral to the side of the surgical resection. None of these six patients were seizure free postoperatively. Nine of the 16 patients with significant ipsilateral temporal atrophy (56%) were seizure free postoperatively ($p = 0.017$). Comparison of seizure outcome was also further stratified by site of resection. In the frontal cases, four of the seven patients with significant temporal atrophy remained seizure free (57.1%); none of the four patients without temporal atrophy were seizure free ($p = 0.058$). In the temporal cases, five of the nine patients with significant temporal atrophy remained seizure free; the two patients without temporal atrophy continued to have seizures ($p = 0.153$).

who did not have ipsilateral temporal lobe at-rophy were seizure free postoperatively. Nine of the 16 patients with significant ipsilateral temporal atrophy (56%) were seizure free. Chi-square analysis found this to be statisti-cally significant ($p = 0.017$). Interestingly, the absence of ipsilateral temporal lobe atrophy was a predictor of poor seizure outcome in the frontal cases as well as in the temporal cases. In the frontal cases, four of the seven patients with significant temporal atrophy remained seizure free (57.1%), but none of the four pa-tients without temporal atrophy were seizure free ($p = 0.058$). In the temporal cases, five of the nine patients with significant temporal at-rophy remained seizure free, whereas the two patients without temporal atrophy continued to have seizures ($p = 0.153$).

Neuropsychological Outcome: Preoperative Profiles

A standard battery of neuropsychological tests was performed both preoperatively and postoperatively as described in the "Methods" section. As a broad indicator of cognitive out-come following frontal and temporal neocor-tical resections for medically intractable epilepsy, we compared the preoperative and postoperative IQs (Fig. 44.7). Postoperatively, no statistically significant changes were found in verbal, performance, and full-scale

IQs from the preoperative performance. The preoperative mean full-scale IQ was 86.70 compared with the postoperative full-scale IQ of 86.76.

Characteristic preoperative neuropsycho-logical profiles correlated well with the loca-tion of subsequent resection, however, sug-gesting that preoperative neuropsychological deficits may correlate with the location of the electrophysiologic focus. The performance of our study population based on the WMS and its battery of subtests, (logical memory sub-test, delayed logical memory subtest, percent retention of logical memory subtest, and per-cent retention for pictures subtest) showed a consistently better performance in the frontal group compared with the temporal group. This trend also was noted in the preoperative performance of the Boston Naming Test. Sta-tistical significance also was found in the de-layed retention subtest ($p = 0.017$) and the percent retention of the logical memory sub-test ($p = 0.002$). Although not statistically sig-nificant, this relationship was reversed in the preoperative performance of the Cued Flu-ency Test, which is more specific for frontal lobe function.

Neuropsychological Outcome: Volumetrics

The presence or the absence of temporal lobe atrophy may be an important predictor of

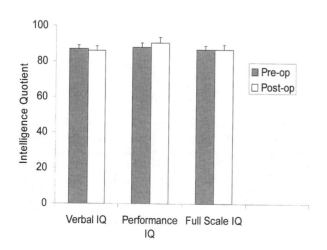

FIG. 44.7. Comparisons of preoper-ative IQ to postoperative IQ. Compar-isons of preoperative to postopera-tive verbal, performance, and full-scale IQs did not yield statistically significant differences of the means. The mean preoperative verbal IQ for the study population was 86.94 (SE = 2.09), and the postoperative verbal IQ was 86.11 (SE = 2.43). The mean preoperative performance IQ was 88.03 (SE = 2.44), and the postoper-ative performance IQ was 90.37 (SE = 3.2). The mean full-scale IQ preop-eratively was 86.7 (SE = 2.21) com-pared with the mean postoperative full-scale IQ of 86.8 (SE = 2.75).

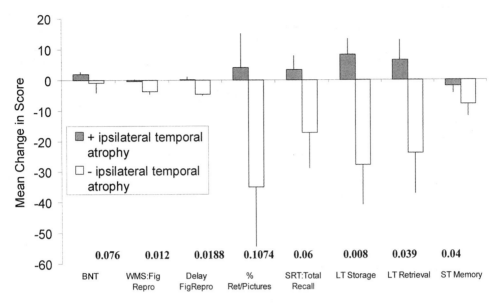

FIG. 44.8. The influence of temporal lobe atrophy on neuropsychological outcome. The changes in neuropsychological performance from preoperative to postoperative scores are compared for the group of patients with ipsilateral temporal atrophy and the group of patients without temporal atrophy. The group without temporal atrophy showed significantly larger postoperative deficits on the following neuropsychological tests: Wechsler Memory Scale *(WMS)*, figural reproduction subtest ($p = 0.019$), Selective Reminder Test *(SRT)*, long-term storage subtest ($p = 0.008$), SRT long-term retrieval subtest ($p = 0.039$), and SRT short-term memory subtest ($p = 0.04$). Although not statistically significant, other neuropsychological tests corroborated this trend: Boston naming test ($p = 0.076$), WMS% retention for picture subtest ($p = 0.107$), and SRT total recall subtest ($p = 0.06$). In the group with ipsilateral temporal atrophy, the mean postoperative performance was improved from the mean preoperative performance for the following tests: Boston naming test, WMS delayed figural reproduction subtest, WMS% retention of pictures subtest, and SRT total recall subtest, SRT long-term storage subtest, SRT long-term retrieval subtest, and SRT short-term memory subtest.

postoperative neuropsychological outcome. The patient group who had surgical resections without ipsilateral temporal lobe atrophy had greater postoperative deficits compared with the group with ipsilateral temporal lobe atrophy. Statistical significance was found in the figural reproduction and percent figural reproduction subsets of the WMS and the long-term retrieval, long-term storage, and short-term memory subtest of the Selective Reminding Test (Fig. 44.8). The patients who had surgical resections with ipsilateral temporal lobe atrophy showed either improved scores postoperatively from their preoperative scores or showed smaller declines of neuropsychological performances relative to the patients who had no ipsilateral atrophy.

DISCUSSION

Seizure Outcome

Studies of surgical outcome in frontal and temporal neocortical intractable epilepsies have reported inferior cure rates compared with those for mesial temporal sclerosis. Longitudinal analysis of seizure outcome in a patient population of mostly frontal and temporal neocortical epilepsies by Rougier et al. reported a long-term cure rate of 62% in a 5-year follow-up (14) in which patients with temporal neocortical epilepsy had a better outcome (68% seizure free) compared with patients with frontal neocortical epilepsy (42% seizure free). Davies and Weeks (4) reported their experience in the surgical treatment of extratemporal epilepsy (frontal, parietal, and occipital origin); these researchers found a cure rate of 40% among 17 patients in long-term follow-up. Laskowitz et al. (15) reported a seizure-free rate of 67% in surgical resections for the treatment of intractable frontal lobe epilepsy, with an average follow-up of 46 months.

We found a seizure-free rate of 31% in our study population; 69% of the patients continued to have seizures. We believe this discrepancy with some of the literature can be explained by our patient selection criteria. Many of the cited outcomes reported from the surgical management of neocortical epilepsies (4,14,15) represent the experience from the management of both lesional and nonlesional substrates. In our study, we excluded all patients who had lesional neocortical epilepsy, thus obtaining a selection of patients whose surgical substrate is not identified by imaging, but rather by phase III intracranial electrophysiological ictal onset. Our seizure-free rates are comparable to those reports in the literature examining outcome for resective surgery in nonlesional neocortical epilepsy (5,6). In fact, the poor seizure cure rate suggested by our study may give further support to the idea that nonlesional neocortical epilepsy is a fundamentally different disease from lesional neocortical epilepsy. Rather than focal mass lesions of neoplastic, vascular, or developmental origin, nonlesional neocortical epilepsy likely represents more diffuse alterations of development, as suggested by the frequent finding of microdysgenesis in the resected specimens.

Statistical analysis of a battery of preoperative variables (age, gender, duration of seizure disorder, and language dominance) failed to yield significant predictions of postoperative seizure outcome. Although ictal EEG patterns had a correlation between its frequency characteristics and its focality, we found that neither the frequency nor the degree of focality independently was predictive of seizure outcome. In exploring the potential relationship between the extent of resection and the subsequent surgical outcome, surgical volumes and the extent of temporal neocortical resection were estimated and analyzed in relation seizure outcome. Although the analysis was not statistically significant, we noted a trend suggestive of increasing surgical volumes being associated with relatively worse seizure outcome ($p = 0.089$). This relationship may reflect the lack of focality in nonlesional neocortical substrates, where the diseased substrate may be more diffuse and less amenable to surgical therapy.

Quantitative hippocampal volumetrics has been shown to be an excellent predictor of post surgical seizure outcome in patients with mesial temporal sclerosis. Luby et al. (16) reported that both seizure outcome and quantitative hippocampal cell counts are highly correlated with quantitative hippocampal volumetrics. Others have shown similar correlative evidence illustrating the efficacy of quantitative hippocampal volumetrics in predicting qualitative hippocampal pathology (17–20). Previous studies also noted the presence of temporal neocortical atrophy in patients with mesial temporal sclerosis (21–24).

Here we applied rigorous quantitative measurements of temporal lobe volume to patients with intractable neocortical epilepsies. We found that the presence of ipsilateral temporal lobe atrophy was a predictor of improved postsurgical seizure control. Although 56% of the patients who had volumetric temporal atrophy ipsilateral to the side of surgical resection remained seizure free, none of the patients who did not have ipsilateral temporal atrophy was seizure free. It is significant that in our study population of patients with neocortical epilepsies, hippocampal volumetrics were not predictive of seizure outcome. This finding may reflect the focality of the underlying diseased substrate. More focal lobar epileptogenic neocortical substrates may result in atrophy measured by quantitative MRI of temporal volumes, and these may be more amenable to control from surgical resection.

The finding that ipsilateral temporal lobe atrophy also predicts improved seizure outcome in patients undergoing frontal lobe resection merits further discussion. The volumetric studies performed were limited to temporal lobe and hippocampal volumetrics. Frontal lobe or hemispheric volumetrics were not performed. The predictive ability of temporal lobe volumetrics in these patients may reflect a larger bilobar or multilobar atrophy. We predict that these other volumetric measurements would have similarly predictive value. Segmentation analysis of the gray and white matter volumes individually also may provide additional insight to the anatomic substrate and the related seizure outcome in these patients.

In accordance with the correlation of hippocampal volumetrics and the mesial temporal sclerosis (MTS) substrate, lobar atrophy may indicate epileptogenic substrate involving cortically based circuits. The anatomy of the hippocampus lends itself to relatively simple quantitative study of cell counts and sprouting as a result of its laminar arrangement. It can be envisioned that a similar process in the cortex may take place, perhaps involving corticocortico or corticothalamic circuits. Because of the complex histology of the cortex, pathoanatomic changes similar to those in the hippocampus may be more subtle and difficult to detect. The syndrome of medial temporal lobe epilepsy associated with MTS may exist as an end result of an underlying developmental process. This may be similarly true in nonlesional cortical epilepsy. The findings of microdysgenesis in some studies may be a clue to diffuse developmental abnormalities in this disorder.

Microdysgenesis describes the disturbances in cortical architecture originally found in children with generalized epilepsy and then later described in association with the Lennox–Gastaut syndrome and West syndrome (25). Histopathological characteristics include the presence of neurons in the molecular layer, the presence or the increased numbers of neurons in the subcortical white matter, and the presence of Purkinje's cells in the granular and molecular layers and white matter. Microdysgenesis is further characterized by blurring of the borders between layers I and II and the gray–white junction, columnar arrangements of the neurons, and the protrusion of cortical gray matter into the adjacent pia (25,26). The clinical significance of these findings remains in debate. Meencke and Janz, in 1984, published findings consistent with microdysgenesis in eight patients with primary generalized epilepsy, developing a hypothesis that morphologic disturbances resulting from microdysgenesis may have dysfunctional and epileptogenic potential (27).

The functional significance of cortical microdysgenesis and the specificity of microdysgenesis were challenged by Lyon and Gastaut, who noted that the dysmorphic characteristics described by Meencke and Janz are found in normal controls (28). The pathological significance of microdysgenesis depends on quantitative studies. Comparative neuropathological studies of Meencke and Janz found changes of microdysgenesis associated with about half of the cases in West syndrome and Lennox–Gastaut syndrome (25). Morphometric comparisons found increased densities of neurons in the stratum moleculare and in the subcortical white matter in the patients with primary generalized epilepsy compared with normal controls (29). Meencke and Janz found these changes in 12.3% of the 591 epileptic patients compared with 2% of the 7,374 control brains.

Although these quantitative morphometric studies confirmed the disproportionate presence of misplaced neurons in the brain tissue of epileptic patients, the question as to their functional and physiological contribution to epileptogenesis remains unresolved. It is significant that increased frequencies of ectopic neurons also have been found in the brains of patients with focal epilepsies as well as in patients with generalized epilepsies. Hardiman et al. found an increased presence of ectopic neurons from temporal neocortex removed from patients who had superficial temporal lobectomies for intractable epilepsy (30). They also noted that the presence of ectopic neurons in the removed neocortical specimen was a statistically significant predictor of improved seizure outcome.

Neuropsychological Outcome

To assess the cognitive consequences of surgery for neocortical epilepsy, both preoperative and postoperative formal neuropsychological testings were obtained. Comparisons of the mean preoperative intelligence quotient did not differ significantly from the mean postoperative intelligence quotient. Preoperatively, we found that the lobe of resection (frontal versus temporal) correlated with the neuroanatomic localization of the neuropsychological deficits. This finding is not surprising in that the location

of the cortical region to be invasively studied is guided by the neuroanatomic localization of cognitive deficits as well as by scalp electrophysiologic localization and seizure semiology. Also, not surprisingly, we found that the colateralization of language dominance and the epileptic were found to be correlated with neuropsychological deficits of language function.

In the evaluation of postoperative neuropsychological performance, we found that the presence of temporal lobe atrophy by quantitative MRI, ipsilateral to the frontal or temporal resection, was a strong predictor of outcome. Patients with ipsilateral temporal lobe atrophy had significantly better neuropsychological outcome compared with patients who did not have ipsilateral temporal lobe atrophy. We considered two possible ex-

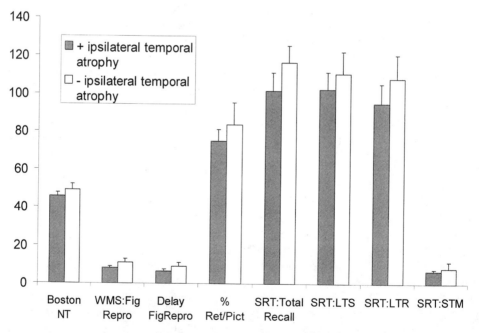

FIG. 44.9. Preoperative neuropsychological performance based on temporal atrophy. In the eight neuropsychological measures noted in Fig. 44.8 (Boston naming test, WMS figural reproduction subtest, WMS delayed figural reproduction subtest, WMS% retention of pictures subtest, SRT total recall subtest, SRT long-term retrieval, SRT long-term storage, SRT short-term memory), examination of the mean preoperative performances revealed that the group with ipsilateral temporal atrophy had relatively higher preoperative scores compared with the scores of the group without temporal atrophy. None of these comparisons, however, were significant by t test analysis.

planations for these differences in neuropsychological outcome based on temporal lobe volumetrics. First, we considered that the favorable postoperative neuropsychological performance could be secondary to improved seizure control. As discussed previously, the patient group with ipsilateral temporal lobe atrophy also had relatively favorable seizure outcome compared with the patient group without ipsilateral temporal lobe atrophy. The second explanation may be that the group of patients without temporal lobe atrophy ipsilateral to the side of the surgical resection had relatively better preoperative neuropsychological performance and thus were "at risk" from the surgical resection. Statistical comparison of preoperative neuropsychological tests revealed a consistently superior performance of the patient group without temporal lobe atrophy (Fig. 44.9).

Several studies showed a significant relationship between focal atrophy by quantitative MRI and functional neuropsychological deficits (31–37). Soininen et al. (36) showed that volumetric MRI of amygdala and hippocampus is predictive of age-associated deficits in visual and verbal memory. Baxendale et al. (32) showed that hippocampal volumetric measurements may be predictive of specific memory deficits, but also suggested that a number of demographic and epilepsy-related variables may influence this relationship. Quantitative MRI has been demonstrated to have correlative relationships with neuropsychological measures in schizophrenia and Alzheimer's disease (33,34). Little is known, however, about the predictive value of temporal lobe volumetrics for both preoperative neuropsychological profiles and postoperative neuropsychological change. Our data suggest that the presence of temporal lobe atrophy, on the side of resection, may be predictive of relatively lesser decline in postoperative neuropsychological performance. The absence of ipsilateral temporal lobe atrophy may lead to significantly larger declines in the postoperative neuropsychological performance.

CONCLUSION

We performed analyses of postsurgical seizure and neuropsychological outcomes in patients treated surgically for nonlesional, neocortical epilepsies from frontal and temporal regions. We examined demographic and electrographic variables in relation to seizure outcome and found that these variables were not predictive of seizure outcome. Analyses of seizure outcome in relation to estimated volumes of surgical resection or the degree of lateral temporal resection revealed no statistically significant findings; however, a trend suggests that larger surgical volumes may correlate with poorer seizure outcome. A similar trend is also noted in the finding that longer lateral temporal resections are correlated with poorer postsurgical seizure control. These findings may be consistent with the interpretation that larger surgical resections are attempted when the diseased substrates lack focality and are thus incompletely removed.

Hippocampal volumetric measurements were not predictive of seizure outcome; however, the presence of volumetric temporal lobe atrophy on the side ipsilateral to the surgical resection was predictive of significantly better outcome. The presence of ipsilateral temporal lobe atrophy was also predictive of relatively limited postoperative neuropsychological decline. In summary, we found that the patients who have surgical resections on the same side as significant temporal atrophy have better seizure and neuropsychological outcomes. In light of the strong predictive value of temporal lobe quantitative volumetrics with regard to postoperative seizure outcome and neuropsychological outcome, we propose that temporal volumetrics may represent a critically important tool in the preoperative assessment of nonlesional, neocortical epilepsy.

Finally, it is important to recognize the inherent limitations of our analyses. The most important limitation may be the small number of patients enrolled in our study (n = 37). This is the natural consequence of a rigorously defined study population designed to bring to examination, a group of patients with a clinically uniform and meaningful substrate. The statistical power is further limited as the study population is stratified into subgroups in outcome analysis. The strong predictive value of temporal lobe volumetrics in relation to outcome justifies its application and analysis prospectively in a larger study population. It is also useful to revisit the application of volumetrics in cases in which the defined epileptogenic substrate is extratemporal. In these cases, it may be more meaningful to obtain volumetric measurements of the lobe involved for comparative analysis. Nevertheless, we found that, even in patients who had frontal lobe resections, temporal lobe volumetrics were significantly predictive of postsurgical seizure outcome.

ACKNOWLEDGMENTS

We acknowledge the contributions of Ms. Marie Luby and Dr. Gregory McCarthy for the acquisition of the quantitative volumetric measurements. We recognize the contribution of Ms. Judith Hess in clinical data collection and database management.

REFERENCES

1. Haglund MM, Ojemann GA. Extratemporal resective surgery for epilepsy. *Neurosurg Clin N Am* 1993;4:283–292.
2. Haglund MM, Ojemann LM. Seizure outcome in patients undergoing temporal lobe resections for epilepsy. *Neurosurg Clin N Am* 1993;4:337–344.
3. Cukiert A, Olivier A, Andermann F. Post-traumatic frontal lobe epilepsy with structural changes: excellent results after cortical resection. *Can J Neurol Sci* 1996;23:114–117.
4. Davies KG, Weeks RD. Cortical resections for intractable epilepsy of extratemporal origin: experience with seventeen cases over eleven years. *Br J Neurosurg* 1993;7:343–353.
5. Smith JR, Lee MR, King DW, et al. Results of lesional vs. nonlesional frontal lobe epilepsy surgery. *Stereotact Funct Neurosurg* 1997;69:202–209.
6. Lorenzo NY, Parisi JE, Cascino GD, et al. Intractable frontal lobe epilepsy: pathological and MRI features. *Epilepsy Res* 1995;20:171–178.
7. McCarthy G, Luby M. Imaging the structural changes with human epilepsy. *Clin Neurosci* 1994;2:82–88.
8. Kaplan E, Goodglass H, Weintraub S. In: Febinger L, ed. *The Boston naming test,* 2nd ed. Philadelphia: 1983.
9. Lezak M. *Neuropsychological assessment,* 3rd ed. New York: Oxford University, 1995:544.
10. Wechsler D. *WAIS-R manual.* New York: The Psychological Corporation, 1981.
11. Russel E. A multiple scoring method for assessment of complex memory functions. *J Consult Clin Psychol* 1975;43:800–809.
12. Wechsler D. *Wechsler memory scale manual.* San Antonio, TX: The Psychological Corporation, 1974.
13. Buschke H, Fuld PA. Evaluation of storage, retention, and retrieval in disordered memory and learning. *Neurology* 1974;11:1019–1025.
14. Rougier A, Dartigues JF, Commenges D, et al. A longitudinal assessment of seizure outcome and overall benefit from 100 cortectomies for epilepsy. *J Neurol Neurosurg Psychiatry* 1992;55:762–767.
15. Laskowitz DT, Sperling MR, French JA, et al. The syndrome of frontal lobe epilepsy: characteristics and surgical management. *Neurology* 1995;45:780–787.
16. Luby M, Spencer DD, Kim JH, et al. Hippocampal MRI volumetrics and temporal lobe substrates in medial temporal lobe epilepsy. *Magn Reson Imaging* 1995;13:1065–1071.
17. Cascino GD, Jack CR Jr, Parisi JE, et al. Magnetic resonance imaging–based volume studies in temporal lobe epilepsy: pathological correlations. *Ann Neurol* 1991;30:31–36.
18. Cascino GD. Clinical correlations with hippocampal atrophy. *Magn Reson Imaging* 1995;13:1133–1136.
19. Van Paesschen W, Sisodiya S, Connelly A, et al. Quantitative hippocampal MRI and intractable temporal lobe epilepsy. *Neurology* 1995;45:2233–2240.
20. Van Paesschen W, Revesz T, Duncan JS, et al. Quantitative neuropathology and quantitative magnetic resonance imaging of the hippocampus in temporal lobe epilepsy. *Ann Neurol* 1997;42:756–766.
21. Kuzniecky R, Murro A, King D, et al. Magnetic resonance imaging in childhood intractable partial epilepsies: pathologic correlations. *Neurology* 1993;43:681–687.
22. Bronen RA, Fulbright RK, Kim JH, et al. Regional distribution of MR findings in hippocampal sclerosis. *Am J Neuroradiol* 1995;16:1193–1200.
23. Jack CR Jr, Gehring DG, Sharbrough FW, et al. Temporal lobe volume measurement from MR images: accuracy and left–right asymmetry in normal persons. *J Comput Assist Tomogr* 1988;12:21–29.
24. Jack CR Jr, Twomey CK, Zinsmeister AR, et al. Anterior temporal lobes and hippocampal formations: normative volumetric measurements from MR images in young adults. *Radiology* 1989;172:549–554.
25. Meencke HJ, Janz D. The significance of microdysgenesia in primary generalized epilepsy: an answer to the considerations of Lyon and Gastaut. *Epilepsia* 1985;26:368–371.
26. Meencke HJ. Pathology of childhood epilepsies. *Cleve Clin J Med* 1989;56(Suppl Pt 1):S111–S120;discussion S121–S123.
27. Meencke HJ, Janz D. Neuropathological findings in primary generalized epilepsy: a study of eight cases. *Epilepsia* 1984;25:8–21.
28. Lyon G, Gastaut H. Considerations on the significance attributed to unusual cerebral histological findings re-

cently described in eight patients with primary generalized epilepsy. *Epilepsia* 1985;26:365–367.

29. Meencke HJ. Neuron density in the molecular layer of the frontal cortex in primary generalized epilepsy. *Epilepsia* 1985;26:450–454.
30. Hardiman O, Burke T, Phillips J, et al. Microdysgenesis in resected temporal neocortex: incidence and clinical significance in focal epilepsy. *Neurology* 1988;38: 1041–1047.
31. Andersen C, Dahl C, Almkvist O, et al. Bilateral temporal lobe volume reduction parallels cognitive impairment in progressive aphasia. *Arch Neurol* 1997;54: 1294–1299.
32. Baxendale SA, van Paesschen W, Thompson PJ, et al. The relationship between quantitative MRI and neuropsychological functioning in temporal lobe epilepsy. *Epilepsia* 1998;39:158–166.
33. Jeste DV, McAdams LA, Palmer BW, et al. Relationship of neuropsychological and MRI measures to age of on-set of schizophrenia [in Process Citation]. *Acta Psychiatr Scand* 1998;98:156–164.
34. Laakso MP, Soininen H, Partanen K, et al. Volumes of hippocampus, amygdala, and frontal lobes in the MRI-based diagnosis of early Alzheimer's disease: correlation with memory functions. *J Neural Transm Park Dis Dement Sect* 1995;9:73–86.
35. Pantel J, Schroder J, Schad LR, et al. Quantitative magnetic resonance imaging and neuropsychological functions in dementia of the Alzheimer type. *Psychol Med* 1997;27:221–229.
36. Soininen HS, Partanen K, Pitkanen A, et al. Volumetric MRI analysis of the amygdala and the hippocampus in subjects with age-associated memory impairment: correlation to visual and verbal memory. *Neurology* 1994;44:1660–1668.
37. Trenerry MR, Westerveld M, Meador KJ. MRI hippocampal volume and neuropsychology in epilepsy surgery. *Magn Reson Imaging* 1995;13:1125–1132.

Neocortical Epilepsies.
Advances in Neurology, Vol. 84,
edited by P. D. Williamson, A. M. Siegel,
D. W. Roberts, V. M. Thadani, and M. S. Gazzaniga.
Lippincott Williams & Wilkins, Philadelphia © 2000.

45

Surgery for Neocortical Temporal and Frontal Epilepsy

J. Schramm, T. Kral, I. Blümcke, and C.E. Elger

Medical Centerx, University of Bonn, D-53105 Bonn, Germany

This chapter reviews the evaluation, surgical strategy, and results of a series of patients with neocortical frontal lobe epilepsy (NFLE) and of temporal lobe epilepsy with neocortical origin (NTLE). For the purpose of this chapter, *temporal neocortical epilepsy* is defined as present in all cases with a lateral neocortical seizure origin, with or without lesion, and without resection of the hippocampus. By using this definition, we excluded some cases that might have represented purely neocortical epilepsy, because in the first few years, anterior temporal lobectomy, mesial and lateral, was the standard procedure for temporal lobe epilepsy at the Bonn epilepsy surgery center. By not including the temporal lobectomy cases, all ambiguity in separating these into purely lateral or mesial temporal lobe epilepsy (MTLE) was avoided.

The growing awareness of NTLE as an entity that can be differentiated from MTLE (1,2) is reflected in the slowly growing literature on NTLE outcome. Although early epilepsy surgery was done mostly in cases with neocortical epilepsy (3), because in these extratemporal neocortical cases the clinical picture helped to localize the epileptogenic area, NTLE series were scarce in a recent review of the surgical outcome for neocortical extrahippocampal focal epilepsy (4). In the recent past, however, some studies not only differentiated NTLE from MTLE but also

gave indications that the surgical results for NTLE improved since the widespread use of modern diagnostic techniques such as magnetic resonance imaging (MRI), invasive recordings with simultaneous video electroencephalographic (EEG) monitoring and stimulation and mapping studies.

PATIENTS AND METHODS

Seventy-nine NFLE cases and 51 NTLE cases were included in this study. Only patients who fulfilled the following three criteria were included: a minimum 1-year history of medically intractable epilepsy, adequate trials of at least two first-line antiepileptic drugs, and continuous noninvasive video scalp EEG monitoring, including sphenoidal electrodes. Follow-up information was taken from a database collected in a prospective fashion and based on regular outpatient visits to the hospital at 3- to 12-month intervals.

The following figures allow a better perspective on the relationship between neocortical and other types of epilepsy in the Bonn series. Between September 1988 and June 1997, 79 NFLE cases were operated on compared with 443 cases of temporal lobe epilepsy, 52 of which were NTLE cases (12%) and 391 (88%) had a resection including mesial structures. Of these 391 resections including mesial structures, 156 were selective amygdalohippocampectomies (i.e., MTLE cases), 202 were anterior two-thirds lobectomies including hippocampectomy, and 33 were topectomies with added hippocampectomy.

Presurgical Evaluation and Indication

The indication for invasive recordings was based on conflicting or noncongruent MRI, EEG, and seizure semiology findings. A detailed history of the seizures and their semiology as well as neuropsychological studies provided basic clinical facts; neuropsychologic evaluation was used routinely in all patients (5). In all patients, interictal activity and a minimum of two seizures were recorded before the indication for surgery was established.

Functional mapping with evoked potentials and cortical stimulation and the Wada test were used as adjuncts when needed. Functional mapping in particular was for frontal lesions encroaching on the motor or language cortex and for temporal lesions encroaching on the speech areas. The type of electrodes used, implantation procedures, and details of our presurgical evaluation protocol were published previously (5–7). In NTLE cases, invasive recordings were used in 49% of the cases and in NFLE cases in 56%. A decision for an invasive evaluation was supported, for example, by finding one or more of the following: (a) seizure onset in the hemisphere opposite to an MRI-detectable lesion, (b) seizure onset two or more electrodes away (in the international 10/20 system) from the location of the tumor or lesion, (c) generalized ictal activity, (d) or the impossibility of detecting seizure onset due to artifacts. As previously described, subdural strip electrodes or depth and subdural grid electrodes could either be used alone or in various combinations (7). The morbidity of invasive recordings also has been previously described (6,8,9).

Intraoperative electrocorticography (ECoG) was used in 27% of NFLE cases. If intraoperative electrocorticography was necessary, induction of anesthesia was by thiopental (4 mg/kg) and fentanyl (0.15 mg/kg);

maintenance was with fentanyl and isoflurane.

The site and the extent of resection finally were based on ictal and interictal EEG and the lesion seen on MRI. In NTLE cases with a tumor or other structural lesion, a combination of intrahippocampal electrodes plus subdural electrodes was occasionally necessary to discriminate between hippocampal seizure origin and perilesional seizure origin. Further details of the interpretation of ECoG and EEG findings were described previously (10). MRI examinations were done in all patients, usually with and without contrast and, if at all possible, at our own institution. The parameters of own MRI examinations were described previously (11,12).

Surgical Technique

All surgeries were performed with the patient under general anesthesia. If an MRI lesion was present, complete removal of that lesion was the goal. Lesionectomies in most cases were accompanied by corticectomy of the surrounding cortex to a breadth of about 1 cm if the lesion was not close to a functionally important (i.e., eloquent) area. The types of surgical procedure are described in Tables 45.1 and 45.2. As can be seen, topectomies (or corticectomies) and lesionectomies were the most common types of resection in both NFLE and NTLE. Multiple subpial transection (MST) was used much more frequently as an add-on surgical treatment in frontal lobe cases.

TABLE 45.1. *Neocortical frontal lobe epilepsy: surgical procedures*

Procedure	Number
Lobe resection	12
Lobe resection plus MST	2
Front. topectomy/lesionectomy	46
Front. topectomy plus MST	15
Total	75
Pure MST	4
Total	79

MST, multiple subpial transection.

TABLE 45.2. *Neocortical temporal lobe epilepsy: surgical procedures*

Procedure	Number
Ant 2/3 lateral resection (i.e., lobectomy w/o hippocampus)	13
Temp. topectomy/lesionectomy w/o hippocampus	26 (1)
Temporodorsal topectomy w/o hippocampus	12
Total	51
Pure MST	1
Additional MST	(1)
Total	52

Ant, anterior; MST, multiple subpial transection; w/o, without.

Lateral lobectomy in the nondominant hemisphere had a resection line after 4.5 cm to 5.5 cm from superior to inferior temporal gyrus in the nondominant hemisphere and a 4- to 5-cm line in the dominant hemisphere; that is, the measures were the same as in classic anterior two-thirds lobectomy: however, the mesial structures were left behind (parahippocampal gyrus and hippocampus). In frontal lesions close to the motor strip, resection usually was done under monitoring of motor-evoked potentials as an aid to minimize postoperative motor defects, using the technique previously described (13–15).

In topectomies or corticectomies, as compared with lesionectomies, the goal was to remove the epileptogenic cortex around the lesion together with the lesion while guided by the results of a previous invasive recording or ECoG. Usually, the aim was to remove the seizure-onset zone completely. In NFLE, over the years, development away from frontal lobectomy to more tailored resections occurred. Frontal lobectomy was done in the standard fashion, whereas lesionectomies were oriented according to the MRI, and topectomies were guided by preoperative or intraoperative invasive EEG recording with the inclusion of the results of functional mapping of eloquent brain areas in cases studied with strip and grid-electrodes. The corticectomies around a lesion and the nonlesional topectomies usually were done with preservation of the arachnoid layer around the sulci.

This was achieved by removing the cortical tissue in the gyri with suction, and particular care was taken to spare the vascular supply between the two pial layers. In MST cases, the surgical technique described by Morrell et al. (16) was used initially, and later in the series a modified dissection technique as described by Wyler et al. (17) was used instead.

The postoperative seizure state was classified according to four outcome classes (18):

Class I: Seizure free (may have included auras or rare seizures in the immediate postoperative period)
Class II: Rare seizures (<2/year);
Class III: Marked reduction in seizure frequency (>75%);
Class IV: Little reduction of seizure frequency or unchanged (<75% reduction of seizure frequency).

The neuropathological techniques used have been described in detail previously (11, 12,19,20). In summary, slides stained with hematoxylin–eosin were available from all cases. For most of the cases, hematoxylin–eosin–luxol–fast blue stains and Nissl stains also were available. Various immunohistochemical reactions, and in selected cases, special stains (Bodian, van Gieson's, and others) also were used.

RESULTS

Demographic Data and Clinical Findings

In the 79 NFLE cases, simple or complex partial seizures were most frequent, and in 45 cases, they were associated with grand mal seizures. In 58 NTLE cases, complex partial seizures were most frequent, followed by a combination of complex partial seizures with grand mal, and then by simple partial seizures.

Postoperative follow-up had a mean duration of 30.9 months ± 15.8 months (range, 2–85 months) in NFLE and 26.1 months ± 15.7 months (range, 3–72) in NTLE. In the NFLE group, the mean age at operation was 27.0 years, ranging from 2 to 60 years and

26.5 (6–60 years) in the NTLE group. The age at seizure onset was 12.8 years (range, 1.0–36). The duration of the seizure disorder was 14.0 years (range, 0.5–53). The female:male ratio was 44:82.

The small subgroup of five patients who had pure MST as their surgical procedure had a mean age at seizure onset of 7.6 years (range, 5–9); the mean age at operation was 26.9 years (range, 7– 46), and the duration of the seizure disorder was a mean of 24 years with a range of 0.5 to 38 years. All had either invasive recordings or ECoG.

Neuropathological Findings

The neuropathologic classification of these cases according to revised World Health Organization (WHO) criteria as shown in Table 45.1 reveals three important facts. The number of cases that had no neuropathologic lesion was small (4 of 75 in the frontal group and 2 of 51 in the temporal group). In four frontal lesions and one temporal lesion, no histology was obtained because only MSTs were performed. In frontal cases, 35% of the patients had neoplastic lesions, and in temporal lobe cases, more than half (61%) had neoplastic lesions. Among the nonneoplastic lesions, dysgenesis was most common, both in frontal and temporal lobes (Table 45.3). The dysgenesis cases included hamartias, cortical heterotopias, ectopic neurons, hamartomas, and cortical subcortical disorganization. Of the 20 gliosis cases, 11 occurred following a lesion to the brain. Table 45.4 shows the various diagnoses in the neoplastic lesions group. Three of 57 glial tumors were high grade. Most likely, these developed

TABLE 45.4. *Diagnoses in neoplastic lesions*

Diagnosis	NFLE	NTLE	All
Ganglioglioma I, II	9	16	25
Astrocytoma I, II	3	8	11
Oligoastrocytoma I, II	3	1	4
Pleomorphic xanthoastrocytoma		1	1
Oligodendroglioma I, II	4	3	7
DNT	3	1	4
Miscellaneous	2		2
Astrocytoma III, IV	2	1	3
Total	26	31	57

DNT, dysembryonic neuroepithelial tumor; NFLE, neocortical frontal lobe epilepsy; NTLE, neocortical temporal lobe epilepsy.

out of indolent low-grade tumors. Not surprisingly, gangliogliomas formed the largest group of these tumors associated with long-term epilepsy, whereas DNTs were relatively rare. All together, 22 of 55 tumors belonged to the tumor groups of "ordinary" astrocytomas or oligodendrogliomas/mixed oligoastrocytomas "normally" encountered in nonepilepsy oncologic patients.

Seizure Outcome

Seizure outcome for the NTLE and NFLE groups as a whole is described in Table 45.5. Worthwhile improvement was achieved in 82% of the cases, with 70% in class I and 12% in class II. If NTLE and NFLE outcome are compared, worthwhile improvement could be achieved in 90% in NTLE versus 76% in NFLE; however, there are no significant differences between outcome class distribution in the NFLE and NTLE groups using the chi-square test.

The influence of the presence of a neoplastic or nonneoplastic lesion on seizure outcome is shown in Table 45.6. It is clear that outcome is better in the neoplastic cases compared with that of nonneoplastic lesional cases. In both NFLE and NTLE, freedom from seizures was achieved in more than 80% of the neoplastic cases but in nearly 60% of the nonneoplastic lesional cases. If outcome classes I and II are combined to assess worthwhile improvement, this difference is still

TABLE 45.3. *Diagnoses in nonneoplastic lesions*

Diagnosis	NFLE	NTLE	All
Dysgenesis	19	8	27
Vascular malformative	10	7	17
Gliosis	15	3	18
No lesion	4	2	6
Total	48	20	68

NFLE, neocortical frontal lobe epilepsy; NTLE, neocortical temporal lobe epilepsy.

TABLE 45.5. *Neocortical epilepsy: outcome*

Location	Follow-up (Months)	Outcome class							
		I		II		III		IV	
		%	n	%	n	%	n	%	n
NFLE (n = 75)	30.9 ± 15.8	64	48	12	9	16	12	8	6
NTLE (n = 51)	26.1 ± 15.7	78	40	12	6	2	1	8	4
Total (n = 126)		70	88	12	15	10	13	8	10

NFLE, neocortical frontal lobe epilepsy; NTLE, neocortical temporal lobe epilepsy.

quite clear: In NFLE, 89% of neoplastic cases had worthwhile improvement, and in NTLE, 97%. Comparing worthwhile improvement (i.e., combined outcome class I and II in neoplastic versus nonneoplastic lesional cases), the relationship was 89% to 73% in NFLE and 97% to 78% in NTLE. Using the chi-square test with alpha = 0.05, the difference between neoplastic and nonneoplastic lesional groups in NFLE was not significant, but there was a significant difference in outcome for the neoplastic versus the nonneoplastic lesional group in NTLE. Neocortical neoplastic lesions in the temporal lobe thus fared much better than neoplastic lesions in the frontal lobe, whereas a variety of other lesions had the same overall good outcome in the temporal and frontal lobe groups.

The number of cases without a histopathological lesion is too small to allow safe conclusions, although it is surprising that four of six cases were in outcome class I. An analysis of the 8 temporal and 19 frontal dysgenesis cases showed that freedom from seizures could be achieved in 60% of the temporal cases and in 68% of the frontal lobe cases. The group with only MST as the surgical procedure had a worthwhile improvement in their seizures in two of the five (one in class I, one in class II) and three patients in class III.

Complications

Complications in both groups combined were divided into surgical and neurologic complications. There was no mortality, and all complications resolved without permanent morbidity. Seven surgical temporary complications were observed (5.3%): two cases with meningitis, three wound infections, one pul-

TABLE 45.6. *Outcome and histology*

Histology[a]		Outcome class							
		I		II		III		IV	
		%	n	%	n	%	n	%	n
NFLE									
Neoplastic	(n = 26)	81	21	8	2			11	3
Lesional	(n = 44)	57	25	16	7	23	10	5	2
No lesions	(n = 4)	50	2			25	1	25	1
Total	(n = 75)[b]	64	48	12	9	16	12[b]	8	6
NTLE									
Neoplastic	(n = 31)	87	27	10	3	3	1		
Lesional	(n = 18)	61	11	17	3			22	4
No lesions	(n = 2)	100	2						
Total	(n = 51)	78	40	12	6	2	1	8	4

NFLE, neocortical frontal lobe epilepsy; NTLE, neocortical temporal lobe epilepsy.
[a]Histologic diagnoses not available for four multiple subpial transection (MST) cases in NFLE group and one MST case in NTLE group. Percentages for total number in NFLE group include one case with a cyst that was not included in the detailed figures for the three subgroups.
[b]One cyst.

monary embolism, and one diabetic coma. Six neurologic temporary complications were observed (4.5%): two patients with dysphasia, one with hemiparesis, two with brachial monoparesis, and one with hemihypesthesia.

DISCUSSION

The definition of neocortical epilepsy poses a problem in temporal lobe epilepsy (21). In the past, when so-called standard temporal lobe resection was the most frequently performed operative procedure, clear differentiation between mesial and lateral NTLE was frequently not made; it was not a high priority because of the type of resection. With limited resection becoming more common, however, the differentiation between a syndrome of epilepsy resulting from mesial temporal lobe sclerosis and NTLE located in the lateral part of the temporal lobe has been made (1,2), and several recent reports on NTLE have appeared (22–25).

Fried and Spencer (21) described the two approaches that can be taken in the study of NTLE: One is the study of temporal lobe pathology in individual patients with invasive recordings of ictal events extraoperatively or by intraoperative mapping of interictal discharges. The other approach is the systematic classification of seizures proposed by Wieser et al., who based the classification on the relation of ictal semiology to ictal localization and thus described five subtypes of lateral temporal lobe epilepsy compared with temporobasal limbic epilepsy (2). The selection of cases for this study was not based on the systematic use of the classification used by Wieser et al., but it corresponds to the definition they used for neocortical epilepsy, as a contrast to MTLE, "meaning lesions outside the limbic system with ictal discharges that rapidly propagate into the limbic system causing identical ictal semiology...."

Differential Diagnosis

As pointed out by various researchers (21,22,25–30), the differentiation between

MTLE and NTLE can be difficult; therefore, invasive presurgical evaluation is frequently necessary. This has been pointed out in other neocortical epilepsy series (11,12,25,28), and it is justified to reflect on the merits and disadvantages of invasive electrode recordings. The complication rates of invasive recordings have been mentioned by several authors and have been discussed in our own articles (6–9). In the Bonn series, electrode-related complications occurred in 4% to 5% of patients (6,8,9), and permanent sequelae were rare exceptions as described in a recent subseries (6). It is generally agreed in most series of NTLE that invasive recording is unavoidable in a large proportion of cases, usually much more frequently than in classic cases of MTLE, in which, as a result of modern MRI, volumetry, and long-term EEG recording, including sphenoidal electrodes, the proportion of cases coming to surgery without invasive recording is much higher.

The value of invasive recordings was emphasized in a study of 82 patients by Brekelmans et al. (26), who concluded that the use of subdural and intracerebral electrodes together usually gives a better yield in terms of localizations and that the exclusive use of either electrode type may result in erroneous diagnosis. The problems in differential diagnosis have been highlighted by a recent report from Seattle showing that even the identification of a focal structural or neocortical lesion, followed by resection based on ictal onsets during EEG recordings, is not always a reliable indicator of the site of seizure origin (29).

A more recent approach regarding the noninvasive differentiation between lateral and mesial temporal epilepsy was described by Vermathen et al. (31). They showed in an MRI spectroscopy study on 20 lateral and 23 mesial TLE patients, with 16 control cases, that N-acetylaspartate is not reduced in the hippocampus of NTLE patients and suggested that this examination may help to distinguish NTLE from MTLE.

A preliminary study on the different neuropsychological sequelae of resective procedures for MTLE and NTLE has been done (32), but Walczak (1) has pointed out that a purely anatomic distinction between the two syndromes is unlikely to be adequate. In the series reported here, however, the definition used for NTLE coincides with his idea that the diagnosis of NTLE is more secure with lesions lateral to the collateral sulcus. This is exactly where our resection stopped in the NTLE cases included in this series.

Surgical Aspects

In the recent past, it has become easier to differentiate in the published literature between these two clinical syndromes (MTLE and NTLE) and to obtain surgical results differentiating them. In our own center, in the early years, the standard resection was temporal lobectomy in the so-called classic anterior two-thirds fashion, soon supplemented by a more tailored version of anterior temporal lobectomy. As pointed out by Fried and Spencer (20), however, the term *temporal lobectomy* has become an anachronism. This is also well reflected in our own series; we now differentiate between various types of temporal lobe surgery, such as standard anterior lobectomy, tailored lobectomy, lesionectomy, corticectomy, selective amygdalohippocampectomy (SAH), and combinations of lateral procedures with SAH (Tables 45.1 and 45.2).

If invasive recordings showed the hippocampus to be involved with seizure onset, we usually opted for a combined resection of the lateral neocortical areas of the lesion plus epileptogenic zone plus an additional hippocampectomy. This procedure was used in 31 of 385 resections, including mesial structures in the Bonn series that took place in the same period in which the 58 NTLE cases reported here underwent sugery.

The necessity for a well-differentiated surgical approach is underlined by the findings of Hajek et al. (28); in their series, none of five patients with NTLE became seizure free after SAH.

NTLE Seizure Outcome

In several small series, freedom from seizures was achieved in 72% of 11 patients

(22) and in 60% of 15 patients (25). In O'Brien's series (25), another 33% had a seizure reduction of 90%, leading to a worthwhile improvement in 93%. In a small series of four cases, no patient became seizure free (30). The results of this study do not vary significantly from those of Burgermann et al. (22), O'Brien and associates (25), or Rougier and colleagues (24). Some studies with a greater patient volume have shown that freedom from seizures can be achieved in NTLE cases in the 60% to 70% range with a high proportion of additional worthwhile improvement (24), thus confirming the findings of O'Brien's et al. (25) and Burgermann and colleagues (22).

The presence of a tumor increases the proportion of seizure-free cases considerably, both in NTLE and NFLE, as was the case in this series but also in other series: five of six tumor cases were seizure free in the series of Fried et al. (27), and 80% of the tumor cases of Smith et al. were seizure free (23). The presence of a nontumoral lesion has been associated with variable results: Smith et al. (23) reported that 66% of their patients were seizure free, and Rougier et al. (24) reported that 68% of their patients were seizure free; again, these percentages are similar to those of our series. Of the nontumoral, nonlesional cases in the series of Smith et al. (23), only 29% were seizure free, compared with a somewhat surprisingly high 66% (four of six cases) in our series.

In a small series of postinfectious lesional cases, Lancman and Morris (33) performed surgery in three cases, one of which became seizure free and one had a class II outcome. Six NTLE cases following central nervous system infection had poor results: Only two of six patients achieved class II outcomes as reported by Lee et al. (34).

The problem of NTLE associated with hippocampal histologic changes was addressed by Cascino et al. (35), Levesque et al. (36), and Hajek et al. (28). Cascino and colleagues indirectly confirmed Hajek's findings in that all the patients with NTLE who also had hippocampal formation atrophy had an unfavorable operative outcome (28).

An important conclusion from these reports (21,28,29) is that the distinction between purely NTLE and a combination of neocortical lesion plus hippocampal involvement (even if only in the morphologic sense) should be strictly established, if possible, because dual pathology obviously affects surgical outcome (21).

NFLE Outcome

The literature on NFLE outcome is somewhat more rewarding than that on NTLE. The review by Van Ness (4) described series from Montreal, Paris, Zürich, Cleveland, Yale, and Miami. It should be noted, however, that several of these series included cases from the era before computed tomography and MRI. The rate of achieving freedom from seizures is given as 30%, 23%, 49%, 18%, and 25%. In a previously published study on extratemporal epilepsy from this center (36), 36 frontal cases were included, with a seizure freedom rate of 50%. In another large tumor series (26), seven frontal cases were included, but no specific results for frontal lobe surgery were given. Rougier et al., in their series (24), described the probability of achieving freedom from seizures for NFLE at the fifth postoperative year of 42%, compared with 68% for NTLE; they calculated this difference to be statistically significant. Lorenzo et al. (37), in a series of 48 patients, pointed out the significance of the presence of a focal lesion. Six of eight patients with tumors were seizure free after surgery and two in class I. Patients with other focal lesions also had either class I or class II outcomes. This study demonstrated that a worthwhile improvement in seizure control can be achieved in frontal lobe epilepsy if a lesion is present. The article by Smith et al. (23) on 53 frontal lobe cases also outlined a significant difference between nonlesional and lesional frontal lobe cases in which 29% of the nonlesional cases were seizure free versus 66% of the lesional cases. In the same series, freedom from seizures was achieved in 80% of the patients who had tumors and in 59% of the nontumor lesional cases. These figures are similar to our own figures (30). Even in posttraumatic frontal lobe epilepsy, positive results have been described in six circumscribed lesional cases (38).

CONCLUSION

In neocortical epilepsies of frontal and temporal origin, patients without a clear-cut lesion are rare. Low-grade tumors form the largest group of lesions. Freedom from seizures can be achieved by surgery in a satisfactorily high proportion of frontal cases; outcome is slightly better for NTLE cases. The presence of a lesion is a prognostic indicator for a better outcome and the difference between lesional and nonlesional surgery being statistically significant in temporal lobe epilepsy.

ACKNOWLEDGMENTS

We acknowledge the contributions of the other epilepsy surgeons (J. Zentner, D. Van Roost, E. Behrens) and epileptologists (M. Kurthen, A. Hufnagel, T. Grunwald) involved. D. Haun has been helpful with the preparation of the data and the manuscript.

REFERENCES

1. Walczak TS. Neocortical temporal lobe epilepsy: characterizing the syndrome. *Epilepsia* 1995;36:633–635.
2. Wieser HG, Engel J Jr, Williamson PD, et al. Surgically remediable temporal lobe syndromes. In: Engel J Jr, ed. *Surgical treatment of the epilepsies,* 2nd ed. New York: Raven Press, 1993:49–63.
3. Gowers WR. *Epilepsy and other chronic convulsive diseases: their causes, symptoms, and treatment.* London: J & A Churchill, 1881:309.
4. van Ness PC. Surgical outcome for neocortical (extrahippocampal) focal epilepsy. In: Lüders HO, ed. *Epilepsy surgery.* New York: Raven Press, 1991: 613–624.
5. Elger CE, Hufnagel A, Schramm J. Epilepsy surgery protocol, University Hospital, Bonn, Germany. In: Lüders HO, ed. *Epilepsy surgery.* New York: Raven Press, 1992:783–784.
6. Van Roost D, Solymosi L, Schramm J, et al. Depth electrode implantation in the length axis of the hippocampus for the presurgical evaluation of medial temporal lobe epilepsy: a computed tomography-based stereotactic insertion technique and its accuracy. *Neurosurgery* 1998;43:819–827.

7. Behrens E, Zentner J, Van Roost D, et al. Subdural and depth electrodes in the presurgical evaluation of epilepsy. *Acta Neurochir* 1994;128:84–87.

8. Fernandez G, Hufnagel A, Van Roost D, et al. Safety of intrahippocampal depth electrodes for presurgical evaluation of patients with intractable epilepsy. *Epilepsia* 1997;38(8):922–929.

9. Behrens E, Schramm J, Zentner J, et al. Surgical and neurological complications in a series of 708 epilepsy surgery procedures. *Neurosurgery* 1997;41:1–20.

10. Zentner J, Hufnagel A, Wolf HK, et al. Surgical treatment of neoplasms associated with medically intractable epilepsy. *Neurosurgery* 1997;41:378–387.

11. Zentner J, Hufnagel A, Ostertun B, et al. Surgical treatment of extratemporal epilepsy: clinical, radiologic, and histopathologic findings in 60 patients. *Epilepsia* 1996;37:1072–1080.

12. Zentner J, Hufnagel A, Wolf HK, et al. Surgical treatment of temporal lobe epilepsy: clinical, radiological, and histopathological findings in 178 patients. *J Neurol Neurosurg Psychiatry* 1995;58:666–673.

13. Cedzich C, Taniguchi M, Schäfer S, et al. Somatosensory evoked potential phase reversal and direct motor cortex stimulation during surgery in and around the central region. *Neurosurgery* 1996;38:962–970.

14. Taniguchi M, Cedzich C, Schramm J. Modification of cortical stimulation for motor evoked potentials under general anesthesia: technical description. *Neurosurgery* 1993;32:219–226.

15. Pechstein U, Cedzich C, Nadstawek J, et al. Transcranial high-frequency repetitive electrical stimulation for recording myogenic motor evoked potentials with the patient under general anesthesia. *Neurosurgery* 1996; 39:335–344.

16. Morrell F, Whisler W, Bleck T. Multiple subpial transsections: a new approach to the surgical treatment of focal epilepsy. *J Neurosurg* 1989;70:231–239.

17. Wyler AR, Wikus RJ, Vossler DG. Multiple subpial transsections in sensori motor cortex. *Neurosurgery* 1995;37:1122–1127.

18. Engel J, van Ness P, Rasmussen TB, et al. Outcome with respect to epileptic seizures. In: Engel J Jr, ed. *Surgical treatment of the epilepsies,* 2nd ed. New York: Raven Press, 1993:609–621.

19. Wolf HK, Campos MG, Zentner J, et al. Surgical pathology of temporal lobe epilepsy: experience with 216 cases. *J Neuropathol Exp Neurol* 1993;52:499–506.

20. Wolf HK, Zentner J, Hufnagel A, et al. Surgical pathology of chronic epileptic seizure disorders: experience with 63 speciments from extratemporal corticectomies, lobectomies, and functional hemispherectomies. *Acta Neuropathol* 1993;86:466–472.

21. Fried I, Spencer DD. Temporal lobectomy: surgical aspects. In: Wyllie E, ed. *The treatment of epilepsy: principles and practice,* 2nd ed. Orlando, FL: Williams & Wilkins, 1997:1056–1057.

22. Burgerman RS, Sperling MR, French JA, et al. Comparison of mesial versus neocortical onset temporal lobe seizures: neurodiagnostic findings and surgical outcome. *Epilepsia* 1995;36:662–670.

23. Smith JR, Lee MR, King DW, et al. Results of lesional vs. nonlesional frontal lobe epilepsy surgery. *Stereotact Funct Neurosurg* 1997;69:202–209.

24. Rougier A, Dartigues JF, Commenges D, et al. A longitudinal assessment of seizure outcome on overall benefit from 100 cortectomies for epilepsy. *J Neurol Neurosurg Psychiatry* 1992;55:762–767.

25. O'Brien TJ, Kilpatrick C, Murrie V, et al. Temporal lobe epilepsy caused by mesial temporal sclerosis and temporal neocortical lesions: a clinical and electroencephalographic study of 46 pathologically proven cases. *Brain* 1996;119:213–2141.

26. Brekelmans GJ, van Emde Boas W, Velis DN, et al. Comparison of combined versus subdural or intracerebral electrodes alone in presurgical focus localization. *Epilepsia* 1998;39:1290–1301.

27. Fried I, Kim JH, Spencer DD. Limbic and neocortical gliomas associated with intractable seizures: a distinct clinicopathological group. *Neurosurgery* 1994;34:5: 815–824.

28. Hajek M, Antonini A, Leender KL, et al. Mesio–basal versus lateral temporal lobe epilepsy: metabolic differences in the temporal lobe shown by interictal 18 F-FDG positron emission tomography. *Neurology* 1993; 43:79–100.

29. Holmes MD, Wilensky AJ, Ojemann GA, et al. Hippocampal or neocortical lesions on magnetic resonance imaging do not necessarily indicate site of ictal onsets in partial epilepsy. *Ann Neurol* 1999;45:461–465.

30. Spencer SS, Spencer DD, Williamson PD, et al. Combined depth and subdural electrode investigation in uncontrolled epilepsy. *Neurology* 1990;40:74–79.

31. Vermathen P, Ende G, Laxer KD, et al. Hippocampal N-acetylaspartate in neocortical epilepsy and mesial temporal lobe epilepsy. *Ann Neurol* 1997;42:194–199.

32. Helmstaedter C, Elger CE, Hufnagel A, et al. Different effects of left anterior temporal lobectomy, selective amygdalohippocampectomy, and temporal cortical lesionectomy on verbal learning, memory, and recognition. *J Epilepsy* 1996;9:39–45.

33. Lancman ME, Morris HH III. Epilepsy after central nervous system infection: clinical characteristics and outcome after epilepsy surgery. *Epilepsy Res* 1996;25:285–290.

34. Lee JH, Lee BI, Park SC, et al. Experiences of epilepsy surgery in intractable seizures with past history of CNS infection *Yonsei Med J* 1997;38:73–78.

35. Cascino GD, Clifford RJ Jr, Parisi JE, et al. Operative strategy in patients with MRI-identified dual pathology and temporal lobe epilepsy. *Epilepsy Res* 1993;14:175–182.

36. Lévesque MF, Nakasato N, Vinters HV, et al. Surgical treatment of limbic epilepsy associated with extra-hippocampal lesions: the problem of dual pathology. *J Neurosurg* 1991;75:364–370.

37. Lorenzo NY, Parisi JE, Cascino GD, et al. Intractable frontal lobe epilepsy: pathological and MRI features. *Epilepsy Res* 1995;20:171–178.

38. Cukiert A, Olivier A, Andermann F. Post-traumatic frontal lobe epilepsy with structural changes: excellent results after cortical resection. *Can J Neurol Sci* 1996; 23:114–117.

Neocortical Epilepsies.
Advances in Neurology, Vol. 84,
edited by P. D. Williamson, A. M. Siegel,
D. W. Roberts, V. M. Thadani, and M. S. Gazzaniga.
Lippincott Williams & Wilkins, Philadelphia © 2000.

46

Analysis of Failures and Reoperations in Resective Epilepsy Surgery

Claudio Munari, Emilia Berta, Laura Tassi, Giorgio Lo Russo, Francesco Cardinale, Stefano Francione, *Philippe Kahane, and †Alim Louis Benabid

Centro Regionale per la Chirurgia dell'Epilessia, Niguarda Hospital, 20126 Milan, Italy;
*Clinique Neurologique, CHU Régionale, Cedex 09 Grenoble, France;
†Service de Neurochirurgie, INSERM U318, CHU Régional, Cedex 09 Grenoble, France

There is general agreement on the efficacy of surgical treatment of severe drug-resistant, partial epilepsies for either eliminating or decreasing the frequency of seizures. Evaluation of the results, however, varies greatly from one article to another: Some researchers clearly separate class IA of Engel (1) from the other classes (2); others consider that patients in class I (A + B + C + D) are seizure free (3); other investigators mix the classes I and II (4); and results are sometimes expressed only in terms of the percentage of seizure frequency reduction (i.e., >90% reduction) (5,6). Also, there are no homogeneous criteria for evaluating the surgical results. There are no accepted standardized criteria for defining *failure* following epilepsy surgery (7,8). Similarly, "there is no commonly accepted definition of reoperation in epilepsy surgery" (9): Only a few studies have examined the strategy and results of reoperations in epilepsy surgery failures (5,6,9–11). In this chapter, the authors present and discuss their experience of epilepsy surgery failures and reoperations.

PATIENTS AND METHODS

During the period from March 1990 through July 1998, we operated on 386 consecutive patients (270 in Grenoble, 116 in Milan).

Single Operations

Only one surgical intervention was performed in 344 patients (170 male, 174 female; age, 1–61 years; mean, 27 years). The age at operation was before the age of 16 years in 20% (12). Neurologic examination was normal in 260 (76%) patients. Magnetic resonance imaging (MRI) did not show anatomic alterations in 132 (38%). No antecedents were found in 191 (56%); febrile convulsions were reported in 71 (21%). The mean age at seizure onset was 9.5 years (range, 0–43). The mean epilepsy duration was 17.5 years (range, 1–49). Only a few children with catastrophic epilepsy were operated on within less than 2 years after the seizure onset. Twenty-five percent of the patients had fewer than three seizures per week, 22% had three to six seizures per week, 52% had more than one seizure per day, and 1% had a Kojewnikow's syndrome.

This group included three patients who had a second neurosurgical operation: one patient with tuberous sclerosis in class IA after removal of a right precentral tuber responsible for epilepsy had a second operation for a giant cell astrocytoma occluding the foramen of Monro without recurrence of the seizures; another patient, after being seizure free after the first partial lesionectomy, had a second surgery for recurrence of left temporal ganglioglioma, without recurrence of the seizures; and a third patient who presented in 1990 with three recognized cavernous angiomas (right temporal, pontine, and cerebellar) and was seizure free for 6 years after a right temporal lesionectomy, then he developed a left temporal epilepsy resulting from bleeding of another undiagnosed cavernous angioma on which surgery had also been done. At that time, other six cavernous angiomas were discovered by a fast field echo T2-weighted (FFET2) MRI sequence.

Presurgical Investigations

Video–electroencephalographic (EEG) ictal recordings (Computerized Video EEG system for prolonged monitoring, up to 128 channels, 256 Hz sampling frequency: Beehive, Telefactor Corporation, Conshohocken, Pennsylvania, U.S.A.), were performed in 244 patients (71%). Stereo EEG recordings (7–16 multilead intracerebral electrodes; Dixi-Besançon, France) were considered necessary in 205 of 344 patients (60%). In Grenoble, electrodes were implanted using a stereotactic robot (13,14) (NeuroMate, Integrated Surgical System Company, Bron, France). The methodology has been described in detail previously (15–17). The percentage of patients operated on without previous Stereo EEG was different in Grenoble (32%) and Milan (61%). The epileptogenic zone was defined according to the criteria of Munari and Bancaud (15); it was temporal in 211 patients (61%), unilobar extratemporal in 41 (12%), multilobar in 92 (27%) (18).

Surgical Treatment

Different kinds of surgical intervention were performed (Table 46.1) using two differ-

TABLE 46.1. *Single operation: different type of performed surgical intervention*

Intervention	No. of patients	%
Cortectomy	163	47
Lesionectomy + cortectomy	136	40
Lesionectomy	30	9
Partial lesionectomy	8	2
Partial lesionectomy + cortectomy	7	2
Total	344	100

ent Neuronavigation systems: SurgiScope (Dee-Med) (19) in Grenoble and MKM (Zeiss, Oberkochen, Germany) (20) in Milan. The intervention concerned the right hemisphere in 207 patients and the left in the remaining 137. The resection was limited to temporal lobe cortical areas in 228 (66%), unilobar extratemporal cortical areas in 59 (17%), and cortical areas of at least two lobes in 57 (17%).

All the obtained specimens were submitted for histopathologic examination (21). In several patients, immunohistochemical studies also were performed (22,23). A double pathology was found in 6% of the Grenoble patients and 34% of Milan patients. Principal histologic diagnoses are shown in Table 46.2.

TABLE 46.2. *Single operation: histological diagnosis*

Diagnosis	No. of patients	%
Cryptogenic	44	13
Glial tumor	23	7
Dysembryoplastic neuroepithelial tumor	37	11
Ganglioglioma	24	7
Hamartoma	22	6
Cryptic vascular malformation	28	8
Tuberous sclerosis	10	3
Neuronal migration disorders	53	15
Scar	14	4
Mesial temporal sclerosis	80	23
Other	9	3
Total	344	100

Postoperative Follow-up

The mean follow-up of Grenoble patients was 5 years (18–109 months). The mean follow-up of Milan patients was 18 months (7–33 months).

The effects of surgery on seizure frequency were assessed using Engel's classification (1), even if not all the Milan patients had 2 years of minimum follow-up. We separated the class IA patients (who did not have any kind of seizure after the operation) from the others. In this study, indeed, we considered as a failure every case in which seizures did not disappear immediately after the intervention, even if the persisting seizures were resumed in subjective manifestations only. We do not discuss the problem of the adequacy of the obtained result relative to the presurgical expectation. In our protocol, postoperative evaluations (neurologic and neuropsychological testing, interictal EEG, and MRI) were performed at 6, 12, 18, and 24 months and then yearly for at least 5 years.

Analysis of Failures

We identified five groups of patients with possible reasons for the persistence of seizures:

1. Patients in which the incomplete surgical resection was due to functional limits: In these cases, we thought the epileptogenic zone included highly functional cortical areas (speech, sensory–motor) that could not be removed. In such cases, we preoperatively informed the patients, their relatives, and the referring neurologist or neuropediatrician that we could not remove the entire epileptogenic zone and that surgical failure was possible.

2. Patients with incomplete definition of the epileptogenic zone: The information obtained during video EEG, and video stereo EEG recordings were considered sufficient for proposing an intervention in very severe cases, despite a lack of precise definition of the epileptogenic zone.

3. Patients with incomplete surgical resection: During the operation, the presurgically defined limits of the cortical removal were not respected for different reasons. The postoperative MRI confirmed in these cases that the presurgical plan was not entirely fulfilled.

4. Patients with "two-step" surgery: In some cases, we considered that the removal of the entire epileptogenic zone, mostly in multilobar cases, could increase the surgical risks. In some other cases that had a single limited lesion (e.g., focal cortical dysplasia), we proposed, to the clearly informed patient, a simple lesionectomy, reserving further resection of the defined extralesional epileptogenic zone only if seizures persisted.

5. Unexplained patients were included in this group when we unable to understand the reasons of the failure.

Reoperations

Forty-two patients underwent two operations. Patients were divided in two groups: 19 patients who had their first operation at another institution (group A); 23 patients who were operated on the first time by our team (group B). General characteristics are presented in Table 46.3. Group B included one patient who was operated on by the senior author 10 years earlier in another institution.

TABLE 46.3. *Reoperations: general characteristics*[a]

Characteristic	Group A	Group B
Male	12	13
Female	7	10
Age (mean, yr)	24.5	25.5
Age at onset (mean, yr)	9.5	9.5
Duration of epilepsy (yr)	13.5	11
Mean seizure frequency (per mo)	50	75
Normal neurological examination	11	17
Normal MRI	0	3
Interval between I and II surgery (yr)	1–20	1–10
Total	19	23

[a]Group A: first operation in another institution. Group B: first and second operation performed by our team.

TABLE 46.4. *Reoperations: characteristics of the first and second surgical procedures performed in the two groups of patients*

Surgical procedure	Group A (19 patients)		Group B (23 patients)	
	I	II	I	II
Cortectomy	0	3	3	4
Lesionectomy + cortectomy	1	14	3	10
Lesionectomy	5	1	3	2
Partial lesionectomy	13	0	6	1
Partial lesionectomy + cortectomy	0	1	8	6

Presurgical Investigations

In group A, obtained information did not allow one to identify precisely the noninvasive investigations preceding the first intervention. None had a stereo EEG, and several had perioperative corticography. Before reoperation, we performed video EEG ictal recordings in two patients and a stereo EEG in 11 patients.

In group B, 16 of 23 patients had a video EEG and 14 of 23 underwent a video–stereo EEG before the first operation. Before the second operation, four underwent a video EEG study. In four cases, we considered that a second stereo EEG would be useful. This investigation also was performed in three patients for whom invasive recordings were not judged necessary before the first operation.

Surgical Treatment

Characteristics of the first and of the second operation are shown in Table 46.4. Histo-

TABLE 46.5. *Reoperations: histological diagnosis*

Diagnosis	Group A	Group B
Cryptogenic	2	2
Glial tumor	4	5
Dysembryoplastic neuroepithelial tumor	4	7
Ganglioglioma	1	1
Cryptic vascular malformation	1	1
Tuberous sclerosis	1	0
Neuronal migration disorders	2	4
Scar	2	1
Mesial temporal sclerosis	2	0
Other	0	2
Total	19	23

logic data obtained at the second operation in both groups are presented in Table 46.5.

RESULTS

Seizure Outcome

Single Operation

The obtained results on seizures, as function of the location and the extent of the epileptogenic zone, are shown in Table 46.6. The results were better when the epileptogenic zone was *temporal* (class IA, 73%) than when it was unilobar *extratemporal* (57%) or multilobar (37%). Class IV outcomes were obtained in 2.5% of temporal patients compared with 15% of extratemporal and 32% of the multilobar. The mean duration of the presurgical epilepsy was 18 years (range, 1–48 years) in the 213 patients in Engel's class IA and 16.5 years (range, 2–49 years) in the others. The mean seizure frequency was much lower (48/month) in the IA group than in failures (148/month). Results were more favorable in the 139 patients operated on without presurgical invasive investigations (class IA, 70%; class I, 86%) (Table 46.7).

Reoperations

In group A patients (Table 46.8), after the second operation, 89.4% improved and nobody worsened: 68.4% are now in class IA, and two (10.5%) remain in class IV as before. In group B patients, (Table 46.9), 16 patients (69.5%) improved after the reoperation, and nobody worsened; however, only seven

TABLE 46.6. *Single operation: control of seizures as a function of the location and the extent of the epileptogenic zone*

Epileptogenic Zone	Engel outcome class						Total no. of patients
	IA	IB	ID	II	III	IV	
Temporal (%)	155 (73)	24 (12)	18 (8)	8 (4)	1 (0,5)	5 (2,5)	211
Extratemporal[a] (%)	24 (57)	1 (3)	2 (5)	2 (5)	6 (15)	6 (15)	41
Multilobar (%)	34 (37)	4 (4)	1 (1)	8 (9)	16 (17)	29 (32)	92
Total no. of patients (%)	213 (61)	29 (9)	21 (6)	18 (5)	23 (7)	40 (12)	344

[a]Extratemporal = unilobar extratemporal.

TABLE 46.7. *Single operation: control of seizures in relation to the presurgical investigations*

Investigation	Engel outcome class						No. of patients
	IA	IB	ID	II	III	IV	
SSEG+ (%)	115 (56)	8 (4)	21 (10)	14 (6)	16 (8)	31 (16)	205 (60)
SEEG− (%)	98 (70)	21 (16)	0	4 (3)	7 (5)	9 (6)	139 (40)
No. of patients (%)	213 (61)	29 (9)	21 (6)	18 (5)	23 (7)	40 (12)	344

+, performed; −, not performed; SEEG, stereo electroencephalography.

TABLE 46.8. *Reoperations: results on seizure frequency in group A*

	Outcome class	Second operation					Total
		IA	IB	II	III	IV	
First Operation	II	1	—	—	—	—	1
	III	—	—	—	—	—	—
	IV	12	2	1	1	2	18
	Total	13	2	1	1	2	19

TABLE 46.9. *Reoperations: results on seizure frequency in group B*

	Outcome class	Second operation					Total
		IA	IB	II	III	IV	
First operation	II	2	1	—	—	—	3
	III	2	—	—	—	—	2
	IV	3	—	3	5	7	18
	Total	7	1	3	5	7	23

(30.5%) reached class IA, and 7 of 18 remain in class IV as before.

Analysis of failures

Single Operation

As mentioned in this chapter, we consider *failures* as having occurred in all the 131 pa-tients whose seizures did not disappear imme-diately after the intervention. Because the group of 21 patients who presented with "atypical generalized convulsions with antiepileptic medication withdrawal only" (class ID) is still under critical evaluation, they are excluded from the analysis. There-fore, we present in Table 46.10 the analysis of the remaining 110 patients.

TABLE 46.10. *Supposed explanation of 110 failures after a single operation*

Reason for failure	Engel outcome class				
	IB	II	III	IV	Total
Functional limits	16	10	16	20	62
Incomplete surgical resection	10	2	3	3	18
Incomplete definition of EZ	—	—	1	5	6
Two steps	1	6	3	11	21
Unexplained	2	—	—	1	3
Total	29	18	23	40	110

EZ, epileptogenic zone.

The voluntary incomplete removal of the epileptogenic zone, for functional reasons, should explain the persistence of seizures in 62 of 110 cases (56%). In this group of 62 patients, 16 (26%) were in class IB, and 20 (32%) were in class IV. This same explanation applies to 20 of the 40 patients in class IV. Unintentional incomplete surgical resection was at the origin of the failure in 18 of 110 patients (16.4%), and three were in class IV (16.6%).

Definition of the epileptogenic Zone was incomplete in six cases, five (83%) of whom were in class IV. In 21 cases (19%), the pre-liminary program was in two steps; 11 (52%) were in class IV. The reason for the failure remained obscure in three of 110 patients.

Reoperations

In group A patients (Table 46.11), incomplete removal of the epileptogenic zone because of functional reasons was at the origin of the lack of improvement in the two class IV patients. In one patient, our surgical program was in "two steps" but, considering the first intervention, it is probably more correct to call it "three-step" surgery.

TABLE 46.11. *Reoperations: supposed explanation of the reoperation failures in group A*

Reason for failure	Engel outcome class				
	IB	II	III	IV	Total
Functional limits	—	1	—	2	3
Incomplete surgical resection	1	—	—	—	1
Incomplete definition of EZ	—	—	—	—	0
Three steps	—	—	1	—	1
Unexplained	1	—	—	—	1
Total					6/19

EZ, epileptogenic zone.

TABLE 46.12. *Reoperations: supposed explanation for the reoperation failures in group B*

Reason for failure	Engel outcome class				
	IB	II	III	IV	Total
Functional limits	1	3	3	3	10
Incomplete surgical resection	—	—	—	1	1
Incomplete definition of EZ	—	—	—	2	2
Unexplained	—	—	2	1	3
Total					16/23

EZ, epileptogenic zone.

In most group B patients (10/16) (Table 46.12), the failure was due to functional limits. Three of them were in class IV, as were the two patients in whom the definition of the epileptogenic zone was incomplete.

DISCUSSION

Williamson (25), while attempting to obtain "lessons from failures," defines five different categories of failure: (a) an inability to localize the epileptogenic region; (b) persistent seizures following surgery; (c) psychosocial failure; (d) communication failure; and (e) lost to follow-up. Polkey and Scarano (26) consider that "good" results include patients who are completely seizure free as well as those with persisting auras and those with a seizure frequency reduction >75% than the preoperative frequency. Criteria adopted by Olivier (27) are even less restrictive: Oliver considers as a success all patients with a seizure reduction of more than 50% seizure. More recently, Polkey (9) stated that "in general terms, for resective surgery, the goal should be complete freedom from seizures, that is, Engel class IA, with no additional neurologic, intellectual, or psychiatric disability-in short, preservation of, or improvement in, quality of life." Abou-Khalil and co-workers (28) compared statistically the results obtained in two series of patients, both with and without previous febrile convulsions, who underwent a temporal resection. In the first group, 16 of 19 (84%) were class I patients (84%), whereas in the group without previous febrile convulsions, only 9 of 28 cases (32%) were in class I. Results can be evaluated differently by comparing patients in class IA against the others: 7 of 19 (36.8%) in the first group, 4 of 28 (14.2%) in the second group. There are no doubts as to the efficacy of the surgical treatment in well-selected cases, but there are much bigger differences in the quality of life between class IA and class IB than between class IB and the other classes (29).

An easier way to define an epilepsy surgery failure could be the postoperative occurrence of seizures, more or less similar to the presurgical ones; however, this solution can be considered too simplistic. In a number of cases, when the epileptogenic zone also includes highly functional cortical areas, surgical removal of the neighboring less functional epileptogenic cortex often allows major relief from seizures, if not their total suppression. Theoretically, a surgical team aiming only to reach a success rate neighboring 100% could refuse surgical operations to patients who can be only *improved,* with all the negative effects of such a choice for the patients. Therefore, it seems to us that a better definition of a *failure* would be the persistence of postoperative seizures, but only when it is not foreseen, or a discrepancy between the obtained and the expected results, as suggested, among other criteria, by Wyler et al. (10).

In this vein, a patient who becomes seizure free after an operation presurgically considered only palliative should be included among failures, at least of the presurgical evaluation. This statement, which is at least partially provocative, raises the problem of the adequacy of correlation between the presurgical evaluation, the expected result, and the obtained result. In fact, in many reports, when the presurgical strategy is variable, it is difficult for the reader to identify correctly the possible relationships between the different modalities used and the obtained results.

Awad et al. (5) stated that seizures "persist or recur in 20 to 60% of patients who have undergone resection for intractable partial epilepsy," referring only to a small number of studies. In fact, it is difficult to formulate precise ideas about the frequency of this phenomenon because the duration of the studies may vary from a few years to several decades, and the duration of the postoperative follow-up is also very variable and sometimes is expressed only as a mean value. In our recent experience of 8 years, postoperative seizures occurred in 39% of 344 patients, with important differences correlated with the site and the extent of the epileptogenic zone. This rate falls to 27% in temporal lobe cases and rises to 63% in multilobar cases. Adopting the criteria of Abou-Khalil et al. (28), we obtained excellent results in 76% of the global series, 93% of temporal, 65% of unilateral extralobar, and 42% of multilobar cases. Applying Olivier's criteria (27), we obtained a success in 88% in the global series, 97.5% of temporal, 85% of unilobar extratemporal, and 68% of multilobar cases. These different evaluations clearly show how difficult it is to evaluate success and failure rates in the literature.

Usually, articles about the results of epilepsy surgery report only the rates of success and failures, as previously discussed, and rarely do they try to analyze the causes of failures. In a recent literature review concerning childhood epilepsy surgery, Lo Russo et al. (30) found that only in the article by Berger et al. (31), of 70 articles, were the causes of failure discussed: 4 of 45 patients with low-grade gliomas associated with intractable epilepsy, using electrocorticography during tumor resection, continued to have seizures; in three patients, failures were due to functional limits, and the last case was considered a surgical failure because of incorrect definition of the epileptogenic zone. Other researchers give general statements but do not discuss in details their data: Adler et al. (32) affirmed that "most failures in surgery for epilepsy, whether dictated by pathology and anatomy, or secondary to an intentional conservative surgical approach, have been ascribed to insufficient localization and/or inadequate resection. This is consistent with our experience." In other articles, the analysis of failures consists only of reporting multifactorial causes, obviously linked to the used investigational strategy. Cascino et al. (33), in a study of temporal lobe epilepsy, focused on long-term EEG monitoring, quantitative MRI, and operative outcome. They stated that "potential reasons for an unfavourable operative outcome" (class III or IV) were identified in 27 of 32 patients: (a) quantitative MRI was indeterminate for hippocampal volume loss in 20 patients and revealed bilateral symmetrical hippocampal atrophy in another three pa-

tients; (b) long-term monitoring showed bitemporal interictal discharges without lateralized predominance in 12 patients and predominantly frontal lobe epileptiform discharges in one patient." Wyllie et al. (34) analyzed, in an epilepsy surgery series, the "completeness" of resection based solely on chronic scalp and subdural EEG recording. They found that good outcome appeared to correlate with completeness of resection (39/61 patients, or 64%) independent of the presence or absence of computed tomography (CT)-detected structural lesions or of interictal epileptiform discharges during postresection intraoperative electrocorticography. Poor outcome (<90% reduction in seizure frequency) appeared to correlate with partial resection.

Reevaluation of surgical failures, when the rationale of the presurgical investigations and the consequent operative plan allows analysis of the failure, should include careful consideration of a second surgical intervention.

Polkey (9) proposed the following definition for *reoperation*: the performance of a further surgical procedure intended to relieve drug-resistant epilepsy when a previous procedure for the same purpose has failed. After reviewing the few articles available in the literature, he estimated reoperation rates to vary from 5.2% to 13.7%.

Penfield and Jasper (35) were among the first to describe reoperations (up to five) on patients who postoperatively continued to have seizures. They did not provide, however, a systematic analysis of the causes for failure or factors influencing successful reoperations.

Rasmussen (36) reported his experience with 1,145 patients with satisfactory follow-up duration: 416 (36%) became and remained seizure free, and overall 763 patients (64%) had a complete or nearly complete elimination of seizure activity. Moreover, he reported the results of a surgical seizure series of 129 patients with nontumoral lesions that had undergone one and occasionally two or three reoperations for inadequate reduction in seizure frequency after initial operation. Following the additional removal of epileptogenic cortex, 29 patients (25%) became seizure free, and overall 52% of these patients experienced a reasonably satisfactory reduction in seizure frequency. He concluded that the effectiveness of cortical resection correlated with the completeness of removal of the epileptogenic cortex. He did not explain how the initial operation might be improved, however, so that failures and reoperations could be prevented.

Polkey (9), in reviewing literature about reinterventions in epilepsy surgery, calculated that overall, 44.3% patients become seizure free, 30.5% significantly improved, and 25.2% did not improve; in temporal lobe reoperations, 55.7% became seizure free, and 16.5% did not improve, whereas for other resections, only 24.5% are seizure free, and 40% are not improved.

Only a few authors indicated how many patients in their series had been operated on elsewhere the first time. For example, Wyler et al. (10) reported this to be the case in 10 of 39 patients; Polkey (9), six patients; and Awad et al. (5), 5 of 15 patients. No author separated them when discussing their results. We divided our patients who had undergone reoperation for epilepsy according to whether the first operation was performed at our center or in another institution because presurgical studies and strategies and the surgical approach are not necessarily identical across institutions.

In our experience, the anatomo-electroclinical data collected during presurgical investigations allowed us to reach 68% class IA results after reoperation when the first intervention was performed in another institution. On the contrary, reoperation in patients who had been first operated on by us, using the same methods for presurgical investigations, allowed us to obtain an additional 30.5% class IA seizure-free outcome.

Failures that were foreseen are due to limited removal because of functional reasons in 62 of 110 failures (56%) among patients who had a single operation. The same was true of reoperation in 3 of 19 (6.3%) patients operated on the first time elsewhere and in 10 of 23 (43%) patients previously operated on at our institution.

Persistence of postoperative seizures should not necessarily be defined as a *failure*. It is a failure only when not foreseen. The possibility of presurgically informing the patient that his or her epileptogenic zone cannot be totally removed, allows the patient to be aware of the expected results and to give informed consent for surgery or to abstain from it.

Holmes and colleagues (37) identified, in a series of 21 patients, two factors that were significantly related to the outcome after reoperation: first, when central nervous system infections predated the epilepsy, no patient had a seizure-free outcome; second, when reoperation extended the previous resection, with the condition that new ictal EEG recordings showed seizure onset concordant with both previous EEG ictal onset and MRI findings, all the patients were seizure free or had a 95% reduction in seizures.

Analysis of failures should permit us to recognize patients in whom a more adequate and individualized evaluation of the anatomo-electroclinical correlations may lead to a more precise definition of the epileptogenic zone before the first intervention. Some evidence strongly suggests that the epileptogenic zone is often more extended than the lesion seen on MRI itself (23,24), but the relationship between them is not always immediately clear (38).

REFERENCES

1. Engel J Jr. Outcome with respect to epileptic seizures. In: Engel J Jr, ed. *Surgical treatment of the epilepsies.* New York: Raven Press, 1987:553–571.
2. Kahane P, Francione S, Tassi L, et al. Results of epilepsy surgery: criteria for validation of presurgical investigations. *Boll Lega It Epil* 1994;86/87:405–419.
3. Wyllie E, Comair YG, Kotagal P, et al. Epilepsy surgery in infants. *Epilepsia* 1996;37:625–637.
4. Broglin D, Landrè E, Chauvel P, et al. Epilepsy surgery in adolescent and children: stereotactic preoperative evaluation and results. *Epilepsia* 1991; 32(Suppl 1):21.
5. Awad IA, Nayel MH, Lüders HO. Second operation after failure of previous resection for epilepsy. *Neurosurgery* 1991;28:510–518.
6. Germano I, Poulin N, Olivier A. Reoperation for recurrent temporal lobe epilepsy. *J Neurosurg* 1994;81: 31–36.
7. Munari C, Francione S, Kahane P, et al. Surgical treat-

ment of partial "symptomatic" epilepsies: analysis of failures. *Bolet Epileps* 1996;2:13–16.

8. Wyler AR, Vossler DG. Reoperation for failed epilepsy surgery. *J Epilepsy* 1997;10:265–269.

9. Polkey CE. Reoperation. In: Engel J Jr, Pedley TA, eds. *Epilepsy: a comprehensive textbook.* Philadelphia: Lippincott–Raven, 1997:1859–1865.

10. Wyler AR, Hermann BP, Richey ET. Results of reoperation for failed epilepsy surgery. *J Neurosurg* 1989;71: 815–819.

11. Salanova V, Quesney LF, Rasmussen TB, et al. Reevaluation of surgical failures and the role of reoperation in 39 patients with frontal lobe epilepsy. *Epilepsia* 1994; 35:70–80.

12. Munari C, Lo Russo G, Minotti L, et al. Presurgical strategies and epilepsy surgery in children: comparison of literature and personal experiences. *Childs Nerv Syst* 1999;15:149–157.

13. Benabid AL, CInquin, Lavallée S, et al. Computer-driven robot for stereotactic surgery connected to CT scan and magnetic resonance imaging. *Appl Neurophysiol* 1987;50:153–154.

14. Benabid AL, Hoffmann D, Munari C, et al. Surgical robotics. In: Haines, Cohen, eds. *Minimally invasive techniques in neurosurgery: concepts in neurosurgery,* vol 7. Baltimore: Williams & Wilkins, 1995:85–97.

15. Munari C, Bancaud J. The role of the Stereo-EEG in evaluation of partial epileptic seizures. In: Morselli PL, Porter RJ, eds. *The epilepsies.* London: Butterworth, 1985:267–306.

16. Munari C, Giallonardo AT, Brunet P, et al. Stereotactic investigations in frontal lobe epilepsy. *Acta Neurochir* 1989(Suppl);46:9–12.

17. Munari C, Hoffmann D, Francione S, et al. Stereo-electroencephalography methodology: advantages and limits. *Acta Neurol Scand* 1994(Suppl);152:56–67.

18. Munari C, Francione S, Kahane P, et al. Multilobar resections for the control of epilepsy. In: Schmideck HH, Sweet WH, eds. *Operative neurosurgical techniques.* Philadelphia: WB Saunders, 1995:1323–1339.

19. Benabid AL, Hoffmann D, Ashraff A, et al. Robotic guidance in advanced imaging environments. In: Eben A, Maciunas RJ, eds. *Advanced neurosurgical navigation.* New York: Thieme Medical, 1999:571–583.

20. Pillary PK, Luber J. Image-guided neurosurgery with the stereotactic microscope. In: Gildenberg PL, Tasker RR, eds. *Textbook of stereotactic and functional neurosurgery.* New York: McGraw-Hill, 1998:357–371.

21. Pasquier B, Bost F, Peoc'h M, et al. Données neuropathologiques dans l'épilepsie partielle pharmaco-résistantes: rapport d'une serie de 195 cas. *Am Pathol* 1996;16:174–181.

22. Spreafico R, Pasquier B, Minotti L, et al. Immunocytochemical investigation on dysplastic human tissue from epileptic patients. *Epilepsy Research* 1998;32:34–48.

23. Garbelli R, Munari C, De Blasi S, et al. Taylor's cortical dysplasia: a confocal and ultrastructural immunohistochemical study. *Brain Pathology* (in press).

24. Munari G, Francione S, Kahane P, et al. Usefulness of stereo EEG investigations in partial epilepsy associated with cortical dysplastic lesions and grey matter heterotopia. In: Guerrini R, Andermann F, Canapicchi R, et al., eds. *Dysplasias of cerebral cortex and epilepsy.* Philadelphia: Lippincott–Raven, 1996:383–394.

25. Williamson PD. Lessons from failures. In: Engel J Jr, ed. *Surgical treatment of the epilepsies,* 2nd ed. New York: Raven Press, 1993:587–591.

26. Polkey CE, Scarano P. The durability of the result of anterior temporal lobectomy for epilepsy. *J Neurosurg Sci* 1993;37:141–148.

27. Olivier A. Risk and benefit in the surgery of epilepsy: complications and positive results on seizures tendency and intellectual function. *Acta Neurol Scand* 1988;117 (Suppl):114–121.

28. Abou-Khalil B, Andermann E, Andermann F, et al. Temporal lobe epilepsy after prolonged febrile convulsions: excellent outcome after surgical treatment. *Epilepsia* 1993;34:878–883.

29. Vickrey BG, Hays RD, Engel J Jr. Outcome assessment for epilepsy surgery: the impact of measuring health-related quality of life. *Ann Neurol* 1995;37: 158–166.

30. Lo Russo G, Minotti L, Leocata F, et al. Le epilessie parziali di interesse chirurgico in età pediatrica. *Epilepsy Rev* 1998;2:8–16.

31. Berger MS, Ghatan S, Haglund MM, et al. Low-grade gliomas associated with intractable epilepsy: seizure outcome utilizing electrocorticography during tumor resection. *J Neurosurg* 1993;79:62–69.

32. Adler J, Erba G, Winston KR, et al. Results of surgery for extratemporal partial epilepsy that began in childhood. *Arch Neurol* 1991;48:133–140.

33. Cascino GD, Trenerry MR, So EL, et al. Routine EEG and temporal lobe epilepsy: relation to long-term EEG monitoring, quantitative MRI, and operative outcome. *Epilepsia* 1996;37:651–656.

34. Wyllie E, Lüders HO, Morris HH, et al. Clinical outcome after complete or partial cortical resection for intractable epilepsy. *Neurology* 1987;37:1634–1641.

35. Penfield W, Jasper H. *Epilepsy and the functional anatomy of the human brain.* Boston: Little, Brown, 1954.

36. Rasmussen T. Cortical resections in the treatment of focal epilepsy. In: Purpura DP, Penry JK, Walter RD, eds. *Neurosurgical management of the epilepsies. Advances in neurology,* vol 8. New York: Raven Press, 1975: 139–154.

37. Holmes MD, Wilensky AJ, Ojemann LM, et al. Predicting outcome following reoperation for medically intractable epilepsy. *Seizure* 1999;8:103–106.

38. Munari C, Berta E, Francione S, et al. Clinical ictal symptomatology and anatomical lesion: their relationships in severe partial epilepsy. *Epilepsia* (in press).

Neocortical Epilepsies.
Advances in Neurology, Vol. 84,
edited by P. D. Williamson, A. M. Siegel,
D. W. Roberts, V. M. Thadani, and M. S. Gazzaniga.
Lippincott Williams & Wilkins, Philadelphia © 2000.

47

Interplay Between "Neocortical" and "Limbic" Temporal Lobe Epilepsy

George A. Ojemann

Department of Neurological Surgery, University of Washington, Seattle, Washington 98195-6470

Temporal lobe epilepsy (TLE) is commonly divided into *limbic* and *neocortical* forms. The exemplar of limbic TLE is the patient with medically refractory seizures associated with mesial temporal sclerosis (MTS). Indeed, patients with TLE who do not have MTS often are considered to be in the neocortical group; however, in many larger surgical series (including the author's), there is a group of patients with TLE and medial temporal epileptogenic zones by electrophysiologic criteria who do not have evidence of MTS (or other lesional pathology) either by imaging or by postoperative pathologic examination. More than half of these patients will be seizure free after resections encompassing the anterior and medial temporal lobes. In 141 consecutive patients with refractory TLE whom I treated with anteriomedial temporal resections tailored to epileptiform activity on the electrocorticogram and "en bloc" hippocampal removal, 45 (32%) did not have evidence of MTS (or other lesions), and yet 60% of those TLE cases with medial temporal epileptogenic zones but without MTS had Engel class I outcome with a minimum of 1 year follow-up (McKhann, Schoelfield-McNeill, and Ojemann, unpublished data). The anteriomedial temporal structures represent the epileptogenic zone in many patients who do not have MTS or other lesions. Thus, even "limbic" TLE is a heterogenous group with

different pathologic substrates, some of which are not presently well defined.

This chapter extends this concept of heterogeneity in TLE by examining the relation between neocortical and limbic forms. For the purposes of this chapter, *neocortical* is defined as evidence of lateral temporal involvement in the epileptogenic zone, and *limbic* is defined as medial temporal involvement. Pathologic findings in TLE not infrequently involve both neocortical and limbic structures. These findings include *dual pathology,* that is, lateral temporal lesions, usually tumors, associated with MTS (1), with evidence that a resection that is likely to control seizures needs to encompass both medial and lateral abnormalities (2,3). Lateral temporal cortical dysplasias and heterotopias also have been described in conjunction with MTS (4,5).

The interaction between neocortical and limbic structures in TLE also can be investigated from an electrophysiologic perspective. To this end, the sites of seizure onsets were identified in all TLE patients evaluated between 1991 and 1998 at the University of Washington Epilepsy Center with ictal recording through chronic lateral cortical subdural grids and basal temporal strip electrodes extending to medial structures and who had resections that included portions of temporal lobe.

Seventy patients met these criteria. They were selected from 470 patients who had undergone resective epilepsy surgery during the same period, about 80% with temporal lobe resections. Of the 470 patients, 130 had preoperative evaluation with intracranial grids. At our center, intracranial electrodes are placed in only the most complex cases, with most patients coming to epilepsy surgery selected on scalp electroencephalography (EEG) and imaging criteria and the surgery tailored to intraoperative EEG recording and stimulation mapping (6).

Additional electrophysiologic evaluation of the hippocampus was available for 42 of the 70 patients with temporal lobe grid recordings. In 15 patients in whom there was surgical access to the temporal horn of the lateral ventricle at the time of grid placement, a chronic strip electrode was placed on the surface of the hippocampus and ictal recordings were obtained. In another 27 patients in whom ictal recordings through chronic electrodes suggested medial temporal onsets, intraoperative recording of interictal activity in hippocampus was obtained through a similarly acutely placed strip electrode. We previously showed that the extent of hippocampal interictal discharges indicates the amount of hippocampus that must be resected and that the absence of hippocampal interictal discharges recorded intraoperatively after a hippocampal resection is highly correlated with a seizure-free outcome, whereas persisting dis-

charges presage a poor outcome, regardless of hippocampal pathology (7). Thus, the presence of hippocampal interictal discharges is evidence of involvement of that structure in the epileptogenic zone, the area requiring resection to control seizures.

PATIENTS WITH LESIONS

The 70 patients with ictal recording through chronic temporal lobe subdural electrodes were divided into three groups: 22 had various types of lesions, 20 had previous temporal resections with persisting seizures, and 28 had no previous lesions or resections. The 22 patients with lesions included 2 gliomas, 2 cavernous angiomas, 4 dysplasias, 1 subacute infarct and 13 with areas of encephalomalacia, most of them from previous trauma or stroke. These patients differed substantially from the patients with TLE and lesions in most series of grid recordings in that few of our patients had tumors. In our center, the resection of tumors, even when there are concerns about the relation to eloquent cortex, usually is based on intraoperative findings, including intraoperative mapping of eloquent cortex and intraoperative EEG to identify epileptogenic areas in tumor patients with intractible epilepsy (8,9).

Table 47.1 relates the location of ictal onset to the location of the lesions in these 22 patients. There were two interesting findings in this group. The location of the lesion does *not* indicate the site of seizure onset. Of the nine

TABLE 47.1. *Ictal recording, medial and lateral temporal subdural electrodes and temporal lobe resections in 22 patients with lesions[a,b]*

Ictal onset		Lesion location				Lat T	Med T	xT	xT + T
		Hippocampus evaluation[c]							
T neocortex only	10	3	3	0		5	2		
T + xT neocortex	1	0	0	0		1	0		
xT neocortex only	1	0	0	0		1	0		
Medial T only	5	4	1	1		0	3		
Widespread T	5	④				1	①	2	1
Total						5	2	9	6

lat, lateral; T temporal; xT, extra temporal.
[a]Of a total of 70 patients.
[b]Nature of lesions described in test.
[c]All positive for hippocampal interictal spikes except one patient, circled.

patients with lesions that were entirely extratemporal, only one had ictal onsets that were entirely extratemporal. Excluding the cases with encephalomalacia, the site of seizure onset and that of the lesion match in four cases but not in five. The site of seizure onset thus could not be identified reliably from the imaging studies showing the lesions. Holmes et al. (10) came to the same conclusion based on 20 of our cases in whom the lesion identified by imaging studies and the site of seizure onset differed. In some cases, the two were contralateral.

Lesions that involved lateral temporal neocortex often had seizure onsets in mesial structures, particularly when the lesion represented an area of encephalomalacia. On the other hand, mesial lesions with seizure onsets exclusively in lateral cortex were not observed. Further evidence of the involvement of mesial temporal structures, regardless of lesion location, comes from the findings from hippocampal recordings, in which interictal discharges were identified in 10 of the 11 patients who underwent such recordings, including all three patients with ictal onsets involving only temporal neocortex. The only patient with hippocampal recordings but no interictal discharges had a mesial temporal tumor. Thus, for the entire group of 22 cases, in at least seven patients evidence of dual pathophysiology was found: lateral lesions with medial limbic epileptic activity (four with mesial seizure onset and neocortical lesions and three with lateral seizure onsets and hippocampal interictal spikes).

PATIENTS WITH NO PREVIOUS LESIONS

The locations of ictal onset in the 28 cases with no lesion evident on imaging studies are indicated in Table 47.2. In 15 patients, the ictal onsets involved only lateral structures, but in four additional patients, seizure onsets involved both medial and lateral temporal lobe and in the remaining nine, only medial structures were involved. Recordings were obtained, however, from the hippocampus in 19,

TABLE 47.2. *Ictal recording, medial and lateral temporal subdural electrodes, and temporal lobe resections in 28 patients without previous lesions[a]*

	Ictal onset	Hippocampus evaluated[b]
T neocortex only	9	6
T + xT neocortex	4	0
xT neocortex only	2	1
Medial T only	9	9
Widespread T	4	4

T, temporal; xT, extratemporal.
[a]Of 70 patients.
[b]All positive for hippocampal interictal spikes.

and all, including seven patients with only lateral ictal onsets, had hippocampal interictal spikes. Including these seven, plus the four patients with widespread medial and lateral temporal ictal onsets, at least 11 of the 28 nonlesional patients also had evidence for dual pathophysiology.

PATIENTS WITH PREVIOUS TEMPORAL RESECTIONS

Particularly instructive are the remaining 20 patients who had previous temporal resections. The previous resections in those patients were based on scalp interictal or ictal recordings and intraoperative corticography, with either persistence or recurrence of seizures. In 19 of these cases there was evidence of mesial temporal involvement in the epileptogenic zone, and the previous resection included some mesial structures, including at least the pes portion of hippocampus. Table 47.3 indicates

TABLE 47.3. *Ictal recording, medial and temporal subdural electrodes, temporal lobe resections in 20 patients with previous temporal resection and persisting seizures*

	Ictal onset	Hippocampal strip ictal involvement
T neocortex	9	4–
T + xT neocortex	0	0
xT neocortex only	3	0
Medial T only	4	4+
Widespread T	4	2 + 1–

T, temporal; xT, extratemporal.

the sites of seizure onset in these patients. In 11 of these patients, a chronic strip electrode was placed on the residual hippocampus; the involvement of this strip in ictal onset is shown separately. Based on previous experience, we expected to find most seizure onsets in the residual hippocampus, but only four patients showed exclusively medial temporal onsets, and nine had exclusively lateral temporal onsets and three extratemporal onsets. In the 11 patients with hippocampal strips, five had no evidence of involvement in ictal onsets.

One of these cases is particularly illustrative. This patient had a left temporal resection at age 14, based on scalp interictal criteria and guided by intraoperative electrocorticography, with interictal discharges recorded from hippocampus and parahippocampal gyrus. The resection included 30 mm of hippocampus encompassing the portion of that structure with interictal spikes. The pathologic findings on that specimen was gliosis. The patient's seizure frequency was reduced by 75%, but she was never seizure free, despite trials of the newer antiepileptic drugs. She was reevaluated at age 19 with ictal recordings through a lateral temporal subdural grid and strip electrodes on the residual basal temporal lobe and residual hippocampus. Ictal onsets were in the superior temporal gyrus. Based on that finding, additional lateral temporal cortex was resected but no additional hippocampus. The patient has been seizure free in the 19 months since the second operation and off all antiepileptic drugs for the last 3 months.

Generally, MTS is considered a hallmark of limbic involvement in TLE. In nine of the cases with previous temporal resections but persisting seizures, hippocampal pathology was MTS. At reevaluation, ictal onsets in these patients were exclusively medial in three, exclusively lateral in three, and widespread in the remaining three. Holmes et al. (10) described seven cases with MTS by imaging criteria who had extratemporal neocortical onsets; three of these patients were seizure free after resection of a frontal site of seizure onset despite the presence of the unresected MTS.

OUTCOME

A seizure-free outcome after resection is the real gold standard for the location of sites of seizure generation. In general, my strategy has been to resect all sites of recorded seizure onset, medial temporal structures when there is electrophysiologic evidence of their involvement in the epileptogenic zone, and any resectable lesion, if present (areas of encephalomalacia are not resected). As might be expected, in the lesion group, outcome was less favorable in those with encephalomalacia (five seizure free, one worthwhile improvement, six not significantly improved, one lost to follow-up), compared with the remaining patients (four seizure-free, three significantly improved, one not significantly improved, and one lost to follow-up). Patients with evidence of dual pathophysiology, that is, evidence for involvement of both lateral and medial temporal structures in the epileptogenic zone, did somewhat less well in either group, with two seizure free, one with worthwhile improvement, four with no significant improvement, and one lost to follow-up, compared with the remaining patients, with seven seizure-free, three experiencing worthwhile improvement, three not significantly improved, and one lost to follow-up. Resections that included all sites of electrophysiologic epileptiform activity, regardless of whether the lesion was included, were most effective.

In the nonlesion group, all resections encompassed the site(s) of electrophysiologic epileptiform activity. Results were somewhat better when the epileptogenic zone involved only medial structures (six became seizure free, two had worthwhile improvement, one was lost to follow-up), than in those with exclusively lateral epileptogenic zones (two were seizure free, four had worthwhile improvement, three had no significant improvement, and one lost to follow-up) or those with dual pathophysiology (two seizure free, three with worthwhile improvement, four with no significant improvement).

Kutsy et al. (11) analyzed the relationship between the rate of seizure spread and outcome in a series of 26 patients with neocortical epilepsies evaluated by subdural grids at our institution, including 18 patients with temporal lobe electrodes who were part of the series reported in this chapter. Slow spread of seizure activity in neocortex was associated with a more favorable outcome, noncontiguous neocortical spread with a worse outcome, and rate of propagation to medial temporal lobe not related to outcome in that series.

CONCLUSION

There is a subset of patients with TLE in whom the distinction between limbic and neocortical does not apply. Rather, they appear to have epileptogenic pathophysiologic abnormalities in both limbic and neocortical structures, so-called dual pathophysiology. Dual pathophysiology was identified in patients both with and without lesions. It was present in at least a third of our patients with TLE that was particularly difficult to localize, requiring ictal recording through chronic subdural electrodes and who had lesions; it was present in 40% of those without lesions. In the lesional group, patients with encephalomalacia from previous trauma or stroke were particularly likely to show dual pathophysiology. In those cases, this dual pathophysiology always represented mesial involvement with lateral lesions and not the reverse. The presence of dual pathophysiology seems to be a generally unfavorable prognostic factor for the outcome of resective surgery, even when the resection includes all sites of identified epileptogenic pathophysiologic abnormalities and any resectable lesion; however, recognition of this process and resection of the neocortical component sometimes can salvage a less than optimal outcome after a standard temporal resection directed at medial structures.

ACKNOWLEDGMENTS

Dr. Donald Farrell interpreted most of the EEG recording in the cases reported here.

REFERENCES

1. Levesque MF, Nakasato N, Vinters HV, et al. Surgical treatment of limbic epilepsy associated with extra hippocampal lesions: the problem of dual pathology. *J Neurosurg* 1991;75:364–370.
2. Cascino GD, Jack CR Jr, Parisi JE, et al. Operative strategy in patients with MRI-identified dual pathology and temporal lobe epilepsy. *Epilepsy Res* 1993;14:175–182.
3. Li LM, Cendes F, Watson C, et al. Surgical treatment of patients with single and dual pathology: relevance of lesion and of hippocampal atrophy to seizure outcome. *Neurology* 1997;48:437–444.
4. Raymond AA, Fish DR, Stevens JM, et al. Association of hippocampal sclerosis with cortical dysgenesis in patients with epilepsy. *Neurology* 1994;44:1841–1845.
5. Ho SS, Kuzniecky RI, Gilliam F, et al. Temporal lobe developmental malformations and epilepsy: dual pathology and bilateral hippocampal abnormalities. *Neurology* 1998;50:748–754.
6. Ojemann GA. Intraoperative tailoring of temporal lobe resection. In: Engel J Jr, ed. *Surgical treatment of epilepsies,* 2nd ed. New York: Raven Press, 1993.
7. McKhann GM, Schoenfield-McNeill J, Born DE, et al. Intraoperative hippocampal electrocorticography predicts the extent of hippocampal resection in temporal lobe epilepsy surgery. *J Neurology* 2000 (in press).
8. Berger MS, Ojemann GA, Lettich E. Neurophysiological monitoring during astrocytoma surgery. *Neurosurg Clin N Am* 1990;1:65–80.
9. Pilcher WH, Silbergeld DL, Berger MS, et al. Intraoperative electrocorticography during tumor resection: impact on seizure outcome in patients with gangliogliomas. *J Neurosurg* 1993;78:891–902.
10. Holmes MD, Wilensky AJ, Ojemann GA, et al. Focal hippocampal or neocortical lesions on high resolution MRI do not necessarily indicate site of seizure onset in partial epilepsy. *Ann Neurol* 2000 (in press).
11. Kutsy R, Farrell D, Ojemann G. Ictal patterns of neocortical seizures monitored with intracranial electrodes: correlation with surgical outcome. *Epilepsia* 1999;40:257–266.

Neocortical Epilepsies.
Advances in Neurology, Vol. 84,
edited by P. D. Williamson, A. M. Siegel,
D. W. Roberts, V. M. Thadani, and M. S. Gazzaniga.
Lippincott Williams & Wilkins, Philadelphia © 2000.

48

Multiple Subpial Transection in Neocortical Epilepsy: Part I

Michael C. Smith and Richard Byrne

Rush-Presbyterian–St. Luke's Medical Center, Chicago, Illinois 60612-3833

Multiple subpial transection (MST) is a novel surgical technique that was designed for use in patients in whom the epileptic zone resides or encroaches on eloquent neocortex (1). *Eloquent neocortex* is defined as primary sensory, motor, and language cortex. The procedure is designed to transect horizontal nerve fibers while preserving the intrinsic columnar organization of the brain. This procedure disrupts the synchronization of epileptic neurons while sparing input, output and the vascular system.

We have performed MST in more than 100 cases, usually in combination with a cortical resection. The efficacy and morbidity of the procedures performed in these cases, all with follow-up for a minimum of 2 years, are described herein and include cases of pure transection of neocortical epileptic foci.

Multiple subpial transection was conceived and developed by Morrell and colleagues to allow operation on eloquent neocortex (1). Several independent scientific discoveries preceded and allowed for its development, including the demonstration that the vertically oriented cortical column is the functional organizational unit in the cerebral cortex (2–4); that damage to or interruption of the transverse fibers of the cerebral cortex does not eliminate the physiologic function of that cortex (5); and that the horizontal conductivity via the transverse fibers of neurons is critical for the development of epileptic discharges

(6–10). In addition, it was found that a minimum area of 12 to 25 mm^2 of synchronous firing neocortex was necessary for an epileptic spike to be recorded by surface electroencephalography (EEG). It was also found that independent epileptic foci produced by exposure to penicillin fired synchronously when the distance between them was 5 mm or less (11–13). Finally, it was demonstrated that the slow propagation of epileptic activity, the so-called *jacksonian march,* is dependent on the horizontal fiber system (7,8).

With these experimental observations in mind, Morrell and colleagues tested the hypothesis that subpial transection at 5-mm intervals would disrupt an experimental epileptic focus in the monkey without causing a significant functional deficit (1,14). Aluminum gel lesions were placed in the precentral gyrus of monkeys, producing spontaneous epileptiform discharges as well as clonic seizures of the forelimb. Transection of the established epileptic focus in precentral gyrus eliminated the epileptiform discharges and abolished the clinical seizures. Background rhythms, initially attenuated, returned to baseline over the next several months. Over this period, no evidence of epileptiform activity, clinical seizures, or paralysis was found. To prove that the transected cortex was responsible for motor function, the transected area was resected, producing the expected complete right hemiplegia. These observations were confirmed by the electrophysiologic and histologic studies of MST in experimental epilepsy in rabbits conducted by Sugiyama and colleagues. MST prevented neuronal synchronization and excitatory interneuronal conduction with little tissue disruption and preservation of neuronal cell bodies and vertical fiber system (15). With experimental proof of the safety and efficacy of multiple subpial transection, the procedure was taken from the laboratory into the operating room to treat intractable epilepsy arising from or involving eloquent neocortical areas.

It is important to note that the horizontal fiber network has a documented role in local recurrent inhibition and excitatory interac-tions. This fiber network underlies the flexibility and plasticity of cellular function in motor and in visual cortex (16,17). It may be that the horizontal fiber system is more important in the learning of new function than in the elaboration of previously learned behaviors. This is one of several critical unanswered questions about the effects of MST on neuronal function and plasticity.

OPERATIVE TECHNIQUE

The technical aspects of the MST procedure have been published in detail (1,14,18–19). Whereas in theory this procedure is relatively straightforward, its application requires a skilled and practiced touch by

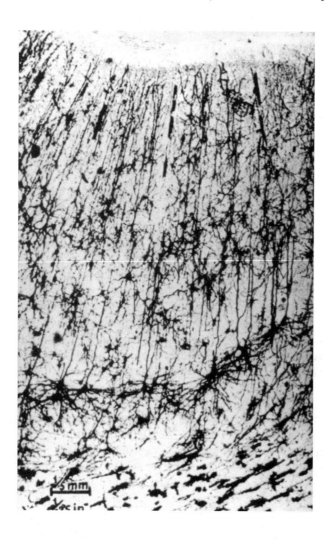

FIG. 48.1. Silver-stained section of neocortex demonstrating vertically oriented columnar organization.

the neurosurgeon. It is carried out using a specially designed instrument with a 4-mm bent tip, corresponding to the thickness of the neocortical gray matter (Fig. 48.1). The angle is turned to an angle of 105 degrees, which allows transection of the cortex without snagging of major blood vessels, a critical measure in preventing morbidity (18). The tensile strength of the wire is important to allow the tip to be pressed against the pial undersurface and drawn along the membrane without puncturing it. Preserving the pial membrane prevents fibroblastic scarring. It is critical to ensure that the instrument is kept in a vertical orientation to avoid additional damage to cortical columns and cortical function. Transections are performed perpendicular to the long axis of the gyrus. Transections parallel to the gyrus may compromise the blood supply.

A small hole is made with a 20-gauge needle at the sulci border of the gyrus, and the transector is introduced into this pial opening and swept forward in a vertical orientation. The tip is raised at the edge of the gyrus so that it is visible beneath the pial border without penetrating it (Fig. 48.2). The blade then is drawn back across the gyrus carefully to avoid snagging cortical vessels. Capillary bleeding is seen at the site of the transection, and thrombin-soaked Gelfoam is used to stop this oozing. The capillary bleeding provides a convenient marker for the next transection at a distance of 5 mm. The transections are repeated as often as necessary to eliminate the entire epileptogenic focus, as defined by electrocorticography (ECoG). This may include several gyri in a large area of neocortex. Other centers have modified the technique of sub-

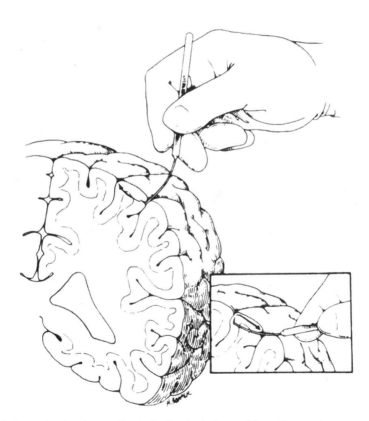

FIG. 48.2. Schematic drawing to illustrate the technique of insertion and movement of the subpial transector. (From Morrell F, Whisler WW, Bleck T. Multiple subpial transection: a new approach to the surgical treatment of focal epilepsy. *J Neurosurg* 1989;70:231–239, with permission.)

pial transections. Wyler et al (20) reported a modification of the transection itself. Changing the orientation of the tip of the transector so that it points away from the pia has been used with good results. The histologic effect that arises from this modified technique has not been reported but is not likely to be significantly different. This orientation of the transector has been used at our center in situations of deep sulcal transection, sylvian fissure transection, or midline transection of precentral and postcentral gyrus. The morbidity of our midline transection of sensorimotor foot neocortex is higher, but this is not related to the orientation of the transector. Some centers are performing MST with the aid of the operating microscope. Others open the sulci prior to the MST procedure. We have used all these techniques as dictated by the unique clinical and neuroanatomical situation. These modifications are most commonly used with intrahemisphere MST or transection within the sylvian fissure.

A critical component of multiple subpial transection is intraoperative ECoG. Analysis of epileptic activity and background activity allows the demarcation of the area to be transected and provides confirmation of the success in disrupting the synchrony of the paroxysmal process and eliminating the epileptic activity. Whereas preoperative subdural grid studies would also identify the epileptic zone, intraoperative ECoG provides confirmation of success. If initial MST is unsuccessful, other options, including further transection, are pursued.

Although this technique is simple in principle, experience is necessary to ensure that blood vessels are not injured and that the transections are perpendicular to the pial surface to prevent disruption or undercutting of the vertical columns (21). When larger vessels are transected, hemorrhaging into the neocortex and underlying white matter may occur, resulting in large cystic lesions and focal atrophy. The experienced touch of the neurosurgeon allows one to bypass these hidden vessels as they are encountered. Occasionally, persistent spikes are seen after transection.

The origin of these discharges are in areas where the transections were too far apart or from a projected site at the depth of the sulcus or transmitted from a distant source. When it appears that the discharges are coming from a sulcus, transections into the sulcus with the tip facing away from the sulcus can be done cautiously.

We have seen epileptiform discharges at the depth of the sulcus from infiltrating tumors and Rasmussen's encephalitis (1,14). In cortex with abnormal architecture and thickness, as seen in heterotopias and other neuronal migration abnormalities, MST may be unsuccessful in interrupting the epileptic activity as a result of the inability to disrupt the horizontal fiber system in the abnormal neuropile. In cases where the epileptic activity is not eliminated, small cortical resections may be combined with MST, producing a favorable outcome with minimal morbidity.

Electrocorticography

Electrocorticography is critical in demarcating the area to be transected. Eloquent cortical areas, mediating primary sensory, motor, or language function, are identified by functional mapping utilizing electric stimulation, either intraoperatively in an alert and cooperative patient or by means of extraoperative stimulation via subdural grid. The behavioral effects need to be reproducible at a threshold voltage and are discounted if an extensive afterdischarge occurs. The central sulcus also is identified intraoperatively by median or tibial nerve somatosensory-evoked potentials (SSEPs) (22). Methohexital is the anesthetic used in patients who require general anesthesia. Although it is established that methohexital may activate interictal epileptiform activity, this activity is restricted to the epileptogenic zone (23). Our ECoG protocol requires the electroencephalographer to analyze the morphology, voltage, frequency, and distribution of recorded spikes as well as background rhythms. These data allow distinction of whether the recorded epileptiform activity arises from the local epileptogenic trigger zone or from a distant source seen by volume conduction or from transynaptic propagation. The aim of the MST procedure with ECoG is to eliminate the source of the epileptic process and not to chase spikes. Experience with electrocorticography in normal and abnormal neocortex is critical to the success of MST (Figs. 48.3 and 48.4).

Transection of an epileptogenic area usually results in immediate elimination of the recorded epileptic activity and marked attenuation of normal background rhythms (1,14,19). High-voltage delta focal slowing is not commonly seen and suggests vascular injury. The attenuation of the background activity returns to normal frequency and amplitude over the following few months. Likewise, transection of the primary somatosensory cor-

tex will result in an immediate decrease of the amplitude of the SSEP by up to 50% without affecting its latency (22). Like background rhythms, the amplitude of the SSEP returns toward baseline over time.

Neuroradiology

The acute effects of MST, as documented by postoperative computed tomography (CT) scan within days of surgery, show mild cortical edema, subarachnoid blood, and lines of intracortical bleeding at the transection site. The permanent magnetic resonance imaging (MRI) changes, 6 months postoperatively, show a number of common findings (Fig. 48.5). Most patients display fine microcystic transection lines at the site of operation. In

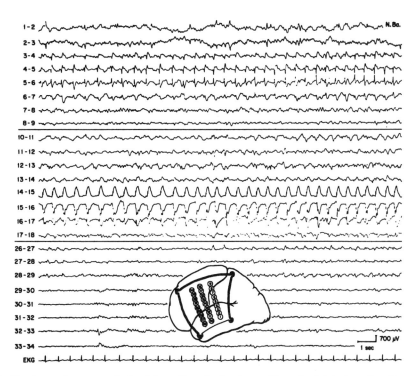

FIG. 48.3. Electrocorticogram derived from the electrode positions indicated on the diagram during craniotomy of a 23-year-old woman with intractable seizures arising in the lower portion of the precentral gyrus. Note that the abnormality was localized to the precentral and postcentral gyri and did not encroach on the temporal lobe or the frontal cortex anterior to the precentral gyrus. (From Smith MC, Whisler WW, Morrell F. *Seminars in Neurology, Neurosurgery of Epilepsy* 1989;9;244, with permission.)

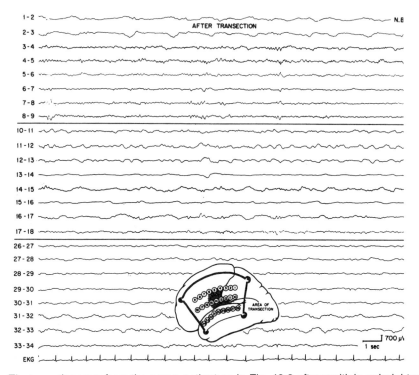

FIG. 48.4. Electrocorticogram from the same patient as in Fig. 48.3 after multiple subpial transection of a portion of the precentral gyrus and the anterior segment of the postcentral gyrus. Note the elimination of the epileptiform activity and attenuation of background rhythms. (From Smith MC, Whisler WW, Morrell F. *Seminars in Neurology, Neurosurgery of Epilepsy* 1989;9;245, with permission.)

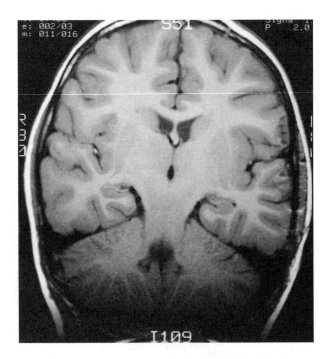

FIG. 48.5. Coronal MRI in patient 6 months after extensive MST of frontotemporal and parietal cortex. Whereas many of the transection sites cannot be visualized, some *(arrows)* are seen.

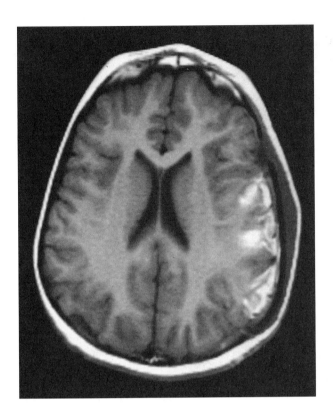

FIG. 48.6. Even in the most experienced hands, injury to vascular supply may occur as a result of snagging and injury to small venules and arterioles during MST. Immediate postoperative MRI of patient who underwent extensive MST of the frontotemporal parietal cortex who suffered cortical and subcortical hemorrhage.

some patients, larger cystic changes and focal atrophy of the transected gyrus are seen. There is some correlation with the amount of acute cortical blood as documented on CT (especially if it extends into white matter) and larger cystic changes and gyral atrophy. Presumably, these changes are due to interruption of the vascular supply and venous drainage. MRI low-intensity signal changes, produced by the paramagnetic effect of hemosiderin and iron, are not seen unless a larger hemorrhage has occurred (Figs. 48.6 and 48.7). Functional outcome, as determined by clinical examination and activities of daily living, does not appear to correlate with MRI changes (24).

Neuropathology

Two studies of the acute and one of the chronic neuropathological changes associated with MST have been reported (19,25). In the first study, we examined neocortex subjected

to MST from the lateral temporal lobe removed during a temporal lobectomy. The acute effects of MST included intracortical hemorrhage, inflammatory response, and acute neuronal injury in the areas immediately adjacent to the transection (22).

The second study of acute histologic effects of MST was reported by Kaufmann and colleagues (21), who found that 30% of the transections reached into the subcortical white matter, 35% were oblique, and another 17% were horizontal to perpendicular cortical columns. These types of transections would be expected to interfere with cortical function of the transected columns. They believed this to be due to the observed patient variability in cortical mantle thickness and microscopic cortical gyration (25,26). It is clear that without experience with MST, extension into the subcortical white matter may occur. This has been observed with our neurosurgical residents' attempts at MST on lateral temporal neocortex prior to resection.

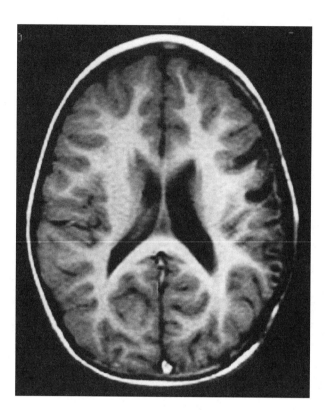

FIG. 48.7. MRI (6 months postoperative) of same patient. Although MRI cuts are not identical, large cystic changes and gyral atrophy are seen in the region of cortical and subcortical hemorrhage.

The one example of the chronic effects of MST comes from a patient who died many years after his seizures had been successfully treated by MST. The chronic microscopic effects of MST revealed a small, full-thickness breach of the neuropile with gliosis, hemosiderin staining, and neuronal dropout in the area immediately adjacent to the transection (27). Neovascularization and severe gliosis were not seen. Most importantly, the transection zone was not bridged over time by neuronal processes, providing proof of the permanence of the transection in disrupting neuronal continuity and, therefore, neuronal synchronization. Whereas MST was designed to transect only transverse fibers, a certain amount of neuronal injury and death occur.

Importantly, the neuronal injury and loss is mild and occurs in the area immediately adjacent to the transection. Additional studies with quantitative measures and neuronal counts are necessary to document neuronal loss due to MST.

EFFICACY

The efficacy of MST in the elimination of epileptic activity and resolution of seizures was documented previously in a number of publications, both from our center and others (1,14,19–20,28–31). In evaluating efficacy results of MST, a distinction must be made between those with MST plus cortical resection and those with MST alone. Of the 100 cases of MST performed at our center, with at least 2 years' follow-up, two thirds had a combination of resection and transection (1,14,18,22).

The most common clinical situation requiring a combination resection/transection is a patient undergoing a temporal lobectomy in the dominant hemisphere. Persistent epileptiform activity in the posterior temporal neocortex language area after anterior temporal lobectomy and hippocampal resection is subjected to MST. A less frequent situation is the combination of a dominant frontal lobectomy with transection of Broca's area when persistent epileptiform activity is seen following resections. A number of patients have had more than one eloquent area transected at operation. The results for seizure outcome in the combination resection and transection group are quite good. The efficacy in this group, according to Engel's classification, is displayed in Table 48.1. Forty-nine percent of the group were seizure free, 10% had rare seizures, and 24% had a 90% reduction in seizure frequency. Eighteen percent were unchanged or worse. Half of the group who failed surgery suffered from progressive pathological processes with 25% having biopsy-proven Rasmussen's encephalitis (1,14,18). We have found that MST will eliminate seizures temporarily in patients with Rasmussen's encephalitis but that adjacent neocortex not transected becomes involved over time (14). MST may be used in Rasmussen's patients in whom hemispherectomy is not yet indicated as a result of continued functional use of the hand and functional language (14,33) dependent on this hemisphere. MST may postpone the necessity of performing a hemispherectomy in some patients with Rasmussen's encephalitis (14,33) involving the dominant hemisphere.

Of the 32 patients in whom MST was performed without cortical resection, half were children with acquired epileptic aphasia. These patients have been reported previously (19). Efficacy as measured by seizure frequency is not a relevant measure because of the low baseline frequency of clinical

seizures. The goal of MST in these children is to eliminate the source of the continuous spike and wave discharge that is affecting the primary auditory and language cortex. With this caveat, at 2-year follow-up, 79% were seizure free; 21% suffered recurrent seizures (19). Recurrence of epileptiform activity occurred in 36%, including all with recurrent seizures (19). At the time of surgery, all patients had not displayed functional, useful language for at least 2 years, and most were mute. At the 2-year postoperative evaluation, 7 of 16 (44%) displayed age-appropriate language; another 6 of 16 (38%) had a significant improvement of functional language but still were undergoing speech therapy. Three patients (18%) failed to improve. Two of six patients (33%), in whom the sylvian fissure was opened to expose the epileptogenic zone within the planum temporale, experienced subcortical infarcts as a result of manipulation of the vascular supply in the opening (19).

Sixteen patients underwent primarily transection alone for the treatment of their intractable partial epilepsy. In some, a biopsy or small gyral resection was performed to facilitate transection (18). The MST involved the frontal lobe in six, frontoparietal in four, parietal lobe in three, and parieto–tempo–occipital in two. The efficacy of MST is displayed in Table 48.1. Six of the patients (37.5%) are seizure free, and another six patients have only rare seizures, with a greater than 90% reduction in seizure frequency. Thus, 75% of these patients had a worthwhile outcome with

TABLE 48.1. *Postsurgical outcome*

| | | Engel's Classification | | | | | |
| | | Significant, worthwhile improvement | | | No significant improvement | Neurologic Complications | |
Surgical Procedure	N	Class I (%)	Class II (%)	Class III (%)	Class IV (%)	Transient (%)	Permanent (%)
MST only partial seizures	16	6 (37.5)	4 (25)	2 (12.5)	4 (25)	1 (6)	3 (19)
MST only LKS	16	9 (57.7)	2 (12.5)	2 (12.5)	3 (18)	2 (12.5)	—
MST/RESECTION	68	33 (48.5)	7 (10)	16 (23.5)	12 (18)	7 (10)	4 (6)
Total	100	48	13	20	19	10	7

LKS, Landau Kleffner syndrome; MST, multiple subpial transection.

MST. Permanent neurologic deficit of aphasia or weakness was seen in three patients, with another two patients suffering transient weakness (1,14,18).

The success of MST in the treatment of intractable partial epilepsy arising from eloquent cortex had been confirmed by surgical centers worldwide (20,28–32,34–35). Table 48.2 lists the success rate judged as significant improvement (Engels' class I, II, or III) or not worthwhile (Engel's class IV) (18,20,28–32,34–35). Combined analysis of these studies suggests that MST alone is successful in treating the intractable epilepsy in 76% of patients, whereas a combination of MST and resection shows significant improvement in 104 of 110 (86%) of patients. Neurologic complications are seen in 15% of patients, with half being transient (18).

The success of MST, judged by functional outcome, also has been well documented in previous publications, both from our center and from others (1,14,18–20,28–36). These studies showed that MST does not interfere significantly with the function of the transected area. Activities of daily living that re-quire the function of the eloquent cortex transected are well preserved; that is to say, patients with transected primary sensorimotor cortex have functional use of the hand with adequate strength, dexterity, and sensory function to perform activities of daily living without difficulties. In the immediate postoperative period, clear and demonstrable deficits are seen in the function of the transected cortex as a result of multiple factors, including cerebral edema. These deficits are maximal at 48 to 72 hours and then resolve, typically within a few weeks. The deficits are typically mild to moderate; a dense hemiplegia or hemisensory loss within 24 hours of transection suggests some complicating factor, such as ischemia or hemorrghage. Functional outcome after MST in specific neocortical areas is detailed.

Anterior Speech Cortex

At the Rush Epilepsy Center, 23 patients have undergone subpial transection of Broca's area (1,14,18–19,22). At 6 months postoperatively, each patient has continued to speak and

TABLE 48.2. *Postsurgical outcome following MST at epilepsy centers (18)*

| Author (ref. no.) | No. of patients | Significant improvement | | No worthwhile improvement | | | Neurologic complications | |
		MST only	MST + RES	MST only	MST + RES	Number	Type
Shimizu et al., 1991 (31)	12	12	—	0	0	0	—
Sawhney et al., 1995 (33)	21	8	12	1	0	0	—
Zonghkil, et al., 1995 (35)	50	32[a]	—	18[a]	0	—	
Wyler et al., 1995 (20)	6	6	—	0	—	1	Mild motor (1)
Hufnagel et al., 1997 (28)	22	4	15	2	1	7	Mild speech deficits (2) Mild motor deficits (3) Overt speech deficits (2)
Pacias et al., 1997 (30)	21	3	18	0	1	9	Mild dysnomia (7) Moderate dysphasia (1) Loss of proprioception in hand (1)
Rougier et al., 1934 (34)	7	2	0	5	0	0	
Patil et al., 1997 (36)	19	4	13	1	1	0	
Rush Epilepsy, Center	100	25	56	7	12	17	Permanent (7) Transient (8) Sensorimotor (13)
Total	258	96	114	34	15	34	

[a]In this study, it was not clear whether MST alone versus MST and resection were performed.
MST, multiple subpial transection; RES, resection.

to write spontaneously, both to dictation and to copy. There is a demonstrable decrease in verbal fluency in these postoperative patients compared with age-matched controls. Their scores remained unchanged postoperatively, however, and reflect their abnormal baseline language function. This suggests that MST does not measurably affect expressive verbal function. In patients with the diagnosis of Landau–Kleffner syndrome (LKS), all except three patients reacquired expressive language. Half of these children have recovered age-appropriate speech and, at 2 years postoperatively, no longer require speech therapy. Thirty percent of the group, although showing marked improvement in language function, are still receiving speech therapy (19).

Posterior Language Area

Wernicke's area, the angular gyrus, and supermarginal gyrus have been subjected to transection in 45 cases (1,14,18–19,22). Receptive language function, including comprehension of written and spoken language, has remained intact in 41 of 45 patients postoperatively.

One patient suffered a subcortical hemorrhage, and three of these patients carried the diagnosis of LKS and remained mute at 6-month follow-up. Two remained mute after surgery, and the third recovered speech transiently and then deteriorated (19).

Precentral Gyrus

Transection of the primary motor cortex of the precentral gyrus was carried out in 51 patients (1,14,16,19,22). In the vast majority (44/51), MST was performed in the face and hand area as demarcated by functional mapping. There was no functional effect of the MST in the use of the hand in activities of daily living or in strength once postoperative edema resolved. In patients with transection of the motor sensory foot area and other mesial frontoparietal cortex, however, morbidity for MST increased to almost 30% (2/7). Two patients suffered permanent foot

drop and mild leg weakness as a result of venous hemorrhage as documented by CT/MRI. Transection of the mesial cortex presents significant technical difficulties to the neurosurgeon in both exposure and avoidance of the extensive vascular supply while remaining perpendicular to the long axis of the gyrus. Transection in this area should be performed with caution.

Postcentral Gyrus

Transection of the postcentral gyrus (sensorimotor) has been performed in 56 patients (1,14,18,21,27). Postoperatively, a sensory deficit to primary sensory modalities was seen. At 6-month follow-up, no measurable evidence of a parietal sensory loss as characterized by loss of stereognosis or graphaesthesia was seen; however, in 29 of 56 patients (52%), a mild but clear decrease in rapid skilled movements was noted, although it did not significantly affect activities of daily living. We now tell the patient that if postcentral gyrus requires transection, sensorimotor deficits are expected postoperatively and may be permanent.

Morbidity

Neurologic complications were seen in 17% (17/100). In seven patients, this complication was permanent, and in the remainder, it was transient (1,14,16,19,22). No mortality has been associated with the procedure. The complications include residual aphasia, residual weakness, parietal sensory loss, visual-field deficit, and worsening of a preexisting language disorder. The transient complications included mild weakness in five, transient cortical sensory loss in one, and a transient dyslexia in another. Four complications were related to the operative event and were not related to the transection itself. These included meningitis, phlebitis, orchitis, and a sixth nerve palsy. The total complication rate was 17% in the perioperative period, with only 7% permanent (18,22). This complication rate should be compared with the expected complication rate of resection of the involved eloquent cortex, the only other surgical option available in these patients. In a number of surgical situations, one might predict technical difficulties with MST. Transection of the mesial frontal/parietal cortex is fraught with technical difficulties as a result of poor visual exposure and the presence of bridging veins. Retraction of the mesial cortex to gain proper exposure, risks both temporary and permanent deficits. Patients with a prior craniotomy often have extensive adhesions from neovascularization and adhesions between cortex and dura. This makes it difficult, if not impossible, to expose the neocortex sufficiently and safely without injury to the underlying pia membrane or brain substance itself. Adhesions and neovasculation must be kept in mind when MST is to be used following diagnostic grid placement. The definitive surgical procedure should be performed at grid removal, decreasing the chance of adhesions. Transection of neocortex in areas of neuronal migration abnormalities may not be successful either because of the abnormal thickness or architecture of the involved cortex. A combination of resection and transection has been more successful in eliminating the epileptic zone. Patients with inflammatory processes affecting the neocortex or pia present difficulties for transecting because of the integrity of the pia and neocortex. Neurologic deficits are more likely to be seen in these patients.

Whereas in principle the procedure of MST sounds simple, technical expertise and experience of the neurosurgeon are critical for successful outcome. An experienced neurosurgeon can detect by the feel of the transector pulling through the tissue whether the underlying cortex is abnormal. This same feel allows our colleagues to avoid and go around the small vessels buried in the neuropile, thus minimizing hemorrhage and ischemic changes in the area of transection. Even in the most experienced neurosurgeon's hands, focal atrophy and cystic changes are seen at times in postoperative MRIs, suggesting more extensive vascular injury to the underlying neocortex.

CLINICAL AND SCIENTIFIC ISSUES

The documented success of MST in eliminating epileptiform activity provides direct evidence that neuronal synchronization via the horizontal fiber system is critical in the genesis and clinical expression of seizures. Synchronization remains a poorly characterized factor in epilepsy. Remarkably, transection of less than a third of the surface area of the entire affected gyrus eliminates epileptiform activity throughout, thus providing direct evidence for the critical role of neuronal synchronization in the genesis of seizures.

Another question is which neuronal structures and what neocortical layers participate in neuronal synchronization? Most experimental evidence suggests that deep axonal processes in layers IV/V mediate neuronal synchronization (7–13); the superficial entwined dendritic mesh also may participate in this process. Experimental studies in partial transection of cortex in models of epilepsy, in both normal and epileptic animal cortex, coupled with intraoperative observation, may provide important information about this critical issue. If superficial disruption of the dendritic mesh would successfully disrupt epileptiform activity, this modification could be performed and be expected to cause less functional morbidity.

Finally, the success of MST in operating on eloquent cortex without clear functional sequelae is not fully understood and is probably due to a number of factors, including the insensitivity of the bedside neurologic examination to document dysfunction of transected cortex, poor understanding of the localized function of large areas of neocortex, and the functional redundancy in the activity of cortical columns, allowing loss of neurons to some critical point before function deteriorates. Patients undergoing MST offer a unique opportunity to study localized cortical function and the subtle but measurable effects of disconnection.

More careful innovative and quantitative assessment of cortical function is necessary to judge the morbidity of the procedure. Unfor-

Neocortical Epilepsies.
Advances in Neurology, Vol. 84,
edited by P. D. Williamson, A. M. Siegel,
D. W. Roberts, V. M. Thadani, and M. S. Gazzaniga.
Lippincott Williams & Wilkins, Philadelphia © 2000.

49

Multiple Subpial Transections in Neocortical Epilepsy: Part II

Allen R. Wyler

Neuroscience Institute, Swedish Medical Center, Seattle, Washington 98122

Multiple subpial transections (MST) is a nonresective surgical technique for eradicating epileptiform discharges and seizures from epileptogenic cortex. This chapter discusses the rationale and indications for MST and defines the syndrome of central neocortical epilepsy (CNE).

RATIONALE

Partial seizures originate from a restricted region of cortex considered to be the focus. Although incompletely understood, the mechanisms underlying the initiation of a focal seizure are believed to involve abnormally discharging neurons and an abnormal degree of interneuronal synchrony (1,2). Whether neurons fire abnormally in bursts of action potentials solely as a result of abnormal interneuronal synchrony or intrinsic abnormalities, or a combination of both, is not known with certainty; however, recordings from chronic animal models as well as human cortex have shown that seizures are associated with periods of increased synchrony (3) between cortical neurons as well as between cortex and subcortical nuclei. Theoretically, if this intracortical synchronization can be disrupted, the epileptogenic potential of the focus can be reduced or eliminated. Parallel slices through cortex would be expected to disrupt permanently side-to-side intraneu-

ronal synchronization. Because neocortex is organized in linear functional columnar units (4,5), MST cuts at right angles to the pial surface, should spare cortex–subcortical input–output interactions. Thus, MST is theoretically ideal for treating epileptogenesis while preserving intrinsic cortical function.

INDICATIONS

1. For epileptogenic foci in cortex serving indispensable function such as speech or motor control, MST is the only acceptable surgical treatment.
2. Patil et al. (6) have used MST to treat bilateral seizure foci for cases otherwise considered nonsurgical. (Whether this will become a standard practice remains to be determined.)
3. MST has been used as surgical treatment for Landau–Kleffner syndrome (LKS), a form of acquired aphasia associated with epileptiform spiking (but not necessarily seizures) in central neocortex.

EXPERIMENTAL STUDIES

Sugiyama et al. (7) studied MST-induced histologic changes and effects on cortical seizure spread in acutely kindled rats. MST severed horizontal fibers but preserved vertical fibers and neuronal cell bodies. Cortical hypereactivity across the transected zone was reduced. Kindling-induced afterdischarge propagation also was inhibited. These results suggest that MST interrupts both neuronal synchronization and excitatory interneuronal conduction.

Using a cat kainic acid model, Tanaka et al. (8) showed that MST suppressed epileptic activity at the cortical surface; however, using ^{14}C-deoxyglucose autoradiography, residual hypermetabolic areas were observed not only in the deep cortical layers and caudate nucleus but also in contralateral sensorimotor cortex. These results suggest that in neocortical epilepsy, seizure propagation relies more on side-to-side propagation than on vertical (cortical–subcortical) propagation.

CLINICAL STUDIES

Morrell et al. (10) were the first to publish results of using the MST technique and the outcome. Thirty-two cases were reviewed. Because of a 5-year follow-up requirement to assess seizure outcome, those data were available in only 20 cases. Complete seizure control occurred in 11 (55%) cases. Taken in the context of neocortical epilepsy, these results are comparable with those of cortical resection. With respect to neurologic outcome, no major complications occurred in 16 cases involving precentral gyrus, six in postcentral cortex, five in Broca's area, and five in Wernicke's area. Evaluation of antiseizure effects of MST was compromised by the inclusion of patients with progressive neurologic diseases (e.g., chronic encephalitis) and patients in whom structural lesions (such as tumors) also were removed. For example, did continued seizures in a chronic encephalitis patient represent a failure of MST or progression of the underlying disease? Was seizure control after lesionectomy plus MST the result of the lesionectomy or of MST? On the other hand, this pioneering report helped document possible cognitive/behavioral sequelae of MST. A longer-term follow-up of this ongoing series was recently presented by Smith (11).

Subsequent papers supported Morrell's findings. Shimizu et al. (12) reported 12 cases of MST with fair results. Sawhney et al. (13) reviewed 21 cases of MST, 18 with epilepsy and 3 with LKS. Of the 18 with epilepsy, 8 demonstrated focal abnormalities on magnetic resonance imaging (MRI), including 6 with chronic encephalitis and one with a tumor. Cortical resection plus MST was done in 12 patients, with 11 showing "worthwhile" seizure frequency decreases. None of the 21 patients developed chronic neurologic deficits attributable to MST. Devinsky et al. (14) reported results of MST in language cortex of three patients. Pacia et al. (9) reported 21 patients, only three of whom underwent MST alone; the other 18 had additional cortical resections. Hufnagel et al. (15) reported a series of 22 patients with less encouraging outcomes. A mixture of these patients had resection and MST. Devinsky et al. (16) reported 13 patients with transections in language cortex (11 patients had additional resective surgery). Although 11 of 13 patients had greater than 90% seizure reduction, MST patients had significantly poorer postoperative naming, verbal fluency, and oral reading than patients with dominant temporal lobe resections that spared language function.

In many of these reports, it is impossible to quantify the antiseizure effect of MST because (1) some patients' pathology included tumors or progressive neurodegenerative diseases, and (2) many patients were treated with lesionectomy or cortical resection plus MST.

Wyler et al. (17) described six patients without structural lesions who underwent only precentral or postcentral MST. In longer follow-up of that series, two patients (33%) are seizure free, whereas three (50%) showed greater than 90% seizure reduction. Two patients showed no benefit from operation. Four of these patients underwent MST in primary language cortex. MST of precentral language areas resulted in subjectively improved fluency, whereas MST in postcentral language areas showed no postoperative improvements or deficits. Also, Wyler et al. (17) modified the technique from Morrell's original description by pointing the instrument tip downward, away from the pia, rather than toward the pia

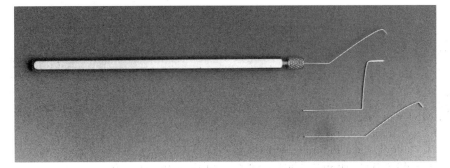

FIG. 49.1. Ad-Tech MST knife with various angled blades.

in the belief this is technically easier and results in less subpial hemorrhage because of less pial tearing at the point of instrument insertion. A special knife was developed (Ad-Tech, Racine, Wisconsin) for this purpose (Fig. 49.1).

Patil et al. (18) reported on patients who were subjected to MST in large multilobar areas or bilateral areas of cortex with good results. They also reported (19) patients with bilateral foci treated with MST plus other "minimally resective" procedures.

MST Applied to Landau–Kleffner Syndrome

Perhaps the most sensitive method to validate an antiepileptic effect without damage to underlying cortical function is MST applied to LKS (20–22), which is a verbal auditory agnosia acquired in childhood and associated with epileptiform discharges recorded from central regions in most cases and superior temporal regions in some. Children often become mute and unresponsive to verbal commands after initially acquiring rudimentary language. What is particularly interesting is that these children seldom show overt seizures in spite of obvious epileptiform discharges, which become more frequent during sleep. At times, these discharges are so diffuse and continuous that they resemble the epilepsy syndrome of continuous spike waves in slow-wave-sleep. Treatment with antiepileptic drugs alone seldom regains speech. Steroid

therapy, on the other hand, may provide temporary improvement but seldom any long-lasting benefit. It is tempting to theorize that LKS provides a pure clinical model of "neural noise" (the disruptive effect of epileptiform discharges on brain function).

Sawhney et al. (13) described three preoperatively mute LKS patients with "substantial recovery of speech" months after MST. Morrell et al. (23) reported on 14 LKS children treated with MST. Seven recovered age-appropriate speech and were taking regular classes in school. Four have shown marked improvement. Thus, 11 of 14, none of whom possessed communicative language for at least 2 years preoperatively, are now speaking. These results have several important implications: First, they add evidence that this novel technique is effective in eliminating epileptiform electrical activity from cortex while preserving intrinsic function. Second, they support the concept of early surgical intervention in well-defined epileptic childhood syndromes to prevent negative cognitive or behavioral sequelae (24,25) associated with epileptiform discharges.

TECHNIQUE

Defining the Focus

As in all cases of surgery for partial epilepsy, the location and margins of the epileptic focus must be clearly defined. Although LKS foci must be defined on the basis of interictal recordings (because most LKS children do not have seizures), all other cases should be carefully documented by long-term ictal recordings using a subdural grid electrode. The value of these recordings depends on the accuracy with which the grid electrode covers the focus. Because most cases considered for MST will involve primary motor cortex, the focus will be either near central sulcus or, more commonly, near the junction of central sulcus with sylvian fissure. Thus, a craniotomy providing adequate exposure of this area is required. A 64-electrode (8 × 8) contact subdural grid centered over the suspected region of ictal onset is recommended.

To orient the grid with respect to the sensorimotor cortex once long-term monitoring has started, our preference is to map somatosensory-evoked potentials (26) within hours of surgery. Direct cortical mapping by electric stimulation can be accomplished later as needed for individual cases. Once sufficient ictal recordings have identified the zone of

seizure onset, the patient can be returned to surgery for grid removal and MST.

Often the ictal region is no more than a few square centimeters and usually is bordered by sulci (i.e., the focus is contained within one or two gyri). Seizure propagation is commonly seen along the long axis of the involved gyri. The entire region of ictal onset should undergo MST as well as 1 to 2 cm to either side of the ictal zone. It is our belief that if a discrete ictal zone is not evident from long-term recordings results, MST outcome is not good.

My preference is to use a specially designed MST knife (AD-TECH, Racine, WI, U.S.A.) with the point angled downward (Fig. 49.1) rather than upward as originally described (10). Also, the cutting portion of this knife is sharpened to a blade to minimize the excessive damage (Fig. 49.2) incurred from using blunt instruments like bent wire or a right-angled dissector. Manipulation of the knife should be done only under direct vision

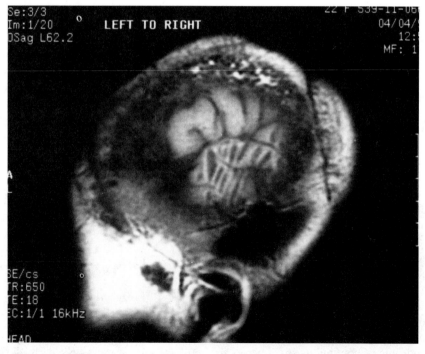

FIG. 49.2. Tangential MRI scan through left temporal neocortex that has been subjected to MST using a bent orthopedic wire held by a hemostat. Scan was taken 4 months after surgery revealing surprisingly wide cuts.

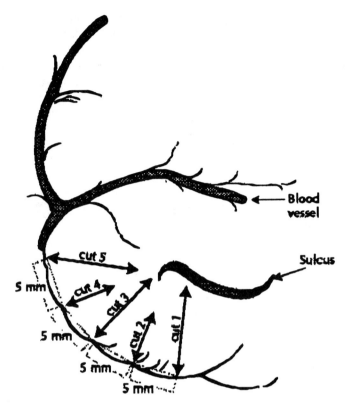

FIG. 49.3. View looking down on curving gyrus to show the variation of MST lengths to preserve the cortex at the convergence point.

through the operating microscope rather than through loupes.

After protecting surrounding cortex with cotton patties, the point of insertion can be either at the side of the gyrus or at the crest. I prefer the crest, but this requires two cuts (in opposite directions) for each entrance point. First, a small pial point is cauterized with the bipolar. The MST knife blade is used to puncture the pia. It is inserted to the proper angle and then is pushed subpially toward the sucal margin, making a right-angled cut to the long axis of the gyrus. The horizontal arm to the MST knife blade should be barely visible through the pia at all times. If the insertion point is made in the center (rather than to one side) of the gyrus, after the first half-cut, the instrument is removed and replaced (aiming in the opposite direction), and the remainder of the slice is completed. Parallel cuts (spaced 4 mm apart) then are made

from this cut until the entire proposed ictal zone and surrounding area have been sliced.

Care must be taken when encountering curves in a gyrus because the outer length of the curve is much longer than the inner length. When this is encountered, I suggest staggering the cut lengths (Fig. 49.3) so that slices converging at the center of the curve do not all join at a common point or come so close together as to damage cortex severely.

Usually, pial bleeding at the blade insertion point can be controlled with a bipolar or a small square of thrombin-soaked Gelfoam. Significant subpial hemorrhage should not occur.

SYNDROME OF CENTRAL NEOCORTICAL EPILEPSY

I have treated with MST several patients with similar histories, similar MRI scans, and a similar location of epileptic focus. All these patients had normal-appearing MRI scans despite having an epileptogenic focus in suprasylvian neocortex. In 1996, Wyler et al. (27) suggested that these cases form a syndrome of central neocortical epilepsy. These patients have the following clinical characteristics:

1. Their first seizure occurred in childhood.
2. As is the case with hippocampal sclerosis, there was an association with an early event (usually before the age of 4 years), such as prolonged febrile seizure.
3. A latent period of variable length is followed by the appearance of clinical seizures with characteristic sequelae.
4. Patients are usually neurologically normal.
5. Cortical biopsy at the site of ictal onset (determined by subdural grid electrode) is negative for cortical dysplasia or tumor.
6. These biopsies show only gliosis and neuronal cell loss in excess of what would be expected from a random biopsy of a brain in a person with epilepsy.
7. Ictal foci are found in the central neocortical region, most commonly above the sylvian fissure near the junction with the Central Sulcus.
8. The spectrum of seizure activity ranges from simple partial to complex partial with secondary generalization.
9. Foci not primarily involving motor strip may demonstrate secondary bilateral synchrony on long-term scalp EEG monitoring, and seizure semiology may superficially look generalized from onset.

Under the recently published Spencer classification system (28), these cases fall into the developmental acquired type of localization-related epilepsy.

The hypothesized etiology is a vascular event, suspected to be similar to whatever mechanism underlies the generation of hippocampal sclerosis (HS) in mesial temporal lobe epilepsy (MTLE). The basis of this hypothesis rests primarily on the following observations:

1. If one examines the infarcts of patients with infantile hemiplegia [Ford and Schaffer (29), hemiconvulsions–hemiplegia–epilepsy (HHE) syndrome of Gastaut et al. (30)], one finds considerable variability ranging from three-vessel [posterior cerebral artery (PCA), middle cerebral artery (MCA), and anterior cerebral artery (ACA)] distributions to infarcts limited to one or two suprasylvian MCA branches.
2. As these infarcts become more specific to one or two MCA branches, they tend to involve syprasylvian branches more frequently than infrasylvian branches.
3. Smaller infarcts tend to involve a more posterior suprasylvian distribution than anterior.
4. Given these characteristics, if one extrapolates this spectrum toward the point of being MRI negative, one finds cases previously reported in our MST series.
5. In all our MRI-negative perisylvian foci, the cortical biopsy has shown gliosis compatible with, but not diagnostic of, cortical ischemic damage.

Put another way, our patients with MRI-normal perisylvian epileptogenic foci have ictal foci within a distribution that is similar, but smaller, to those patients with MRI-apparent vascular lesions. Anatomically, this ictal region coincides with the distribution of foci in patients with surgically corrected LKS. Cortical biopsies from our cases of LKS have shown gliosis and neuronal cell loss indistinguishable from our CNE cases.

Because of these similarities, I hypothesize that cases of CNE represent one end of a wide spectrum of middle cerebral vascular insults as shown in Fig. 49.4. The most severe end of this spectrum is represented by the cystic cavitating infarctions associated with infantile hemiplegia. Milder cases are restricted to just one or two suprasylvian MCA branches. The mildest end of the spectrum might be exemplified by cases devoid of MRI-obvious lesions but having foci in a perisylvian distribution. This perisylvian distribution has a peak

Central Neocortical Epilepsy
Spectrum of vascular insults

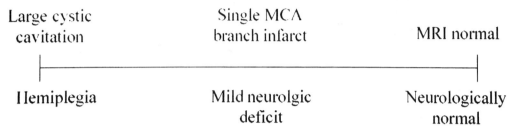

FIG. 49.4. Spectrum of cortical infarcts ranging from severe hemispheric cavitation with hemiplegia to MRI-negative lesions without neurologic deficit.

incidence at the junction of the central and sylvian fissures. Excellent examples of such cases were presented in our initial report of MST. Other examples could be some cases of LKS.

REFERENCES

1. Schwartzkroin PA, Turner DA, Knowles WD, et al. Studies of human and monkey "epileptic" neocortex in the in vitro slice preparation. *Ann Neurol* 1983;13:249–257.
2. Schwartzkroin PA, Wyler AR. Mechanisms underlying epileptiform burst discharge. *Ann Neurol* 1980;7:95–107.
3. Miles R, Wong RKS, Traub RD. Synchronized afterdischarges in the hippocampus: contribution of local synaptic interactions. *Neuroscience* 1996;12:1179–1189.
4. Hubel DH, Wiesel TN. Receptive fields, binocular interaction, and functional architecture in the cat's visual cortex. *J Physiol* 1962;160:106–154.
5. Mountcastle VB. Modality and topographic properties of single neurons of cat's somatic sensory cortex. *J Neurophysiol* 1957;20:408–434.
6. Patil AA, Andrews RV, Torkelson R. Surgical treatment of intractable seizures with multilobar or bihemispheric seizure foci (MLBHSF). *Surg Neurol* 1997;47:72–78.
7. Sugiyama S, Fujii M, Ito H. The electophysiological effect of multiple subpial transection (MST) on experimental epilepsy model. *Epilepsy Res* 1995;21:1–9 (abst).
8. Tanaka T, Kunimoto M, Hashizume K, et al. Multiple-subpial transections in animal experiments: behavioral, neurophysiological, metabolic, and pathological

changes. In: Tuxhorn I, Holthausen H, Lüders HO, eds. *Pediatric epilepsy syndromes and their surgical treatment.* London: John Libbey Eurotext, 1997.
9. Pacia SV, Devinsky O, Perrine K, et al. Multiple subpial transection for intractable partial seizures: seizure outcome. *J Epilepsy* 1997;10:86–91.
10. Morrell F, Whisler WW, Bleck TP. Multiple subpial transection: a new approach to the surgical treatment of focal epilepsy. *J Neurosurg* 1989;70:231–239.
11. Smith MC. Multiple subpial transection in patients with extratemporal epilepsy. *Epilepsia* 1998;39(Suppl 4):S81–S89.
12. Shimizu H, Suzuki I, Ischijima B. Multiple subpial transection for the control of seizures that originated in unresectable cortical foci. *Japanese Journal of Psychiatry and Neurology* 1991;354–356.
13. Sawhney IMS, Robertson IJ, Polkey CE, et al. Multiple subpial transection: a review of 21 cases. *J Neurol Neurosurg Psychiatry* 1995;58:344–349.
14. Devinsky O, Perrine K, Vazquez B, et al. Multiple subpial transections in language cortex. *Brain* 1994;117:225–265.
15. Hufnagel A, Zentner J, Fernandez G, et al. Multiple subpial transection for control of epileptic seizures: effectiveness and safety. *Epilepsia* 1997;38:678–688.
16. Devinsky O, Perrine K, Pacia S, et al. Multiple subpial transections in language cortex: effects on language functions. *J Epilepsy* 1997;10:247–253.
17. Wyler AR, Wilkus RJ, Vossler DG, et al. Multiple subpial transections for partial seizures in sensory–motor cortex. *Neurosurgery* 1995;37:1122–1128.
18. Patil AA, Andrews R, Torkelson R. Multiple subpial cortical transection (MST) for the treatment of extensive seizure foci. *J Epilepsy* 1997;10:198–202.
19. Patil AA, Andrews R. Surgical management of independent bihemispheric seizure foci. *J Epilepsy* 1997;10:203–207.

20. Deonna TW. Acquired epileptiform aphasia in childern (Landau–Kleffner syndrome). *J Clin Neurophysiol* 1991;8:288–298.

21. Hirsch E, Marescaux C, Maquet P, et al. Landau–Kleffner syndrome: a clinical and EEG study of five cases. *Epilepsia* 1990;31:756–767.

22. Paquier PF, Van Dogen HR, Loonen CB. The Landau–Kleffner syndrome or 'aquired aphasia with convulsive disorder.' *Arch Neurol* 1992;49:354–359.

23. Morrell F, Whisler WW, Smith MC, et al. Landau–Kleffner syndrome: treatment with subpial intracortical transection. *Brain* 1996;118:1529–1546.

24. Chugani HT, Shields WD, Shewmon DA, et al. Infantile spasms: I. PET identifies focal cortical dysgenesis in cryptogenic cases for surgical treatment. *Ann Neurol* 1990;27:406–413.

25. Shields WD, Shewmon DA, Chugani HT, et al. Treatment of infantile spasms: medical or surgical. *Epilepsia* 1992;33(Suppl 4):S26–S31.

26. Wood CC, Spencer DD, Allison T, et al. Localization of human sensorimotor cortex during surgery by cortical surface recording of somatosensory evoked potentials. *J Neurosurg* 1988;68:99–111.

27. Wyler AR, Vossler DG, Wilkus RJ, et al. Central neocortical epilepsy: hypothesis and surgical approach. *J Epilepsy* 1996;9:128–134.

28. Spencer SS. Substrates of localization-related epilepsies: biologic implications of localizing findings in humans. *Epilepsia* 1998;39:114–123.

29. Ford FR, Schaffer AJ. The etiology of infantile (acquired) hemiplegia. *Arch Neurol Psych* 1927;18:323–327.

30. Gastaut H, Poirier F, Payan H, et al. H.H.E. syndrome: hemiconvulsions, hemiplegia, epilepsy. *Epilepsia* 1959; 1:418–447.

Neocortical Epilepsies.
Advances in Neurology, Vol. 84,
edited by P. D. Williamson, A. M. Siegel,
D. W. Roberts, V. M. Thadani, and M. S. Gazzaniga.
Lippincott Williams & Wilkins, Philadelphia © 2000.

50

Technical Advances in the Surgical Treatment of Epilepsy

David W. Roberts

Section of Neurosurgery, Dartmouth–Hitchcock Medical Center, Lebanon, New Hampshire 03756

The past decade has seen tremendous advances in the clinical neurosciences, perhaps the most apparent of which have been in neuroimaging. Parallel to these radiologic developments, however, has been the digitization of the operating room, enabled by the same rapid growth in computing capability. This process has brought together a methodology by which increasingly sophisticated patient databases can be developed, archived, and analyzed. Using these databases, treatment plans can be developed by a multidisciplinary epilepsy team, and, not least importantly, computer-assisted surgery makes it possible to execute these treatment plans in the operating room with an accuracy and precision not previously possible (1–6). The great strides of the past decade in the treatment of epilepsy refractory to medical management have been made possible by both imaging and surgical achievements. This overview focuses on the pervasive although less well-known technical advances driven by computer assistance in the operating room.

IMAGE-GUIDED SURGERY

The concept of image-guided surgery arose from a background of frame-based stereotaxy and was enabled by emerging computing power that facilitated coregistration of radiologic studies with the surgical field. Traditional stereotactic frames essentially perform three principal functions: establish a coordinate space for the region of surgical interest; provide a mechanism by which coregistration of an imaging study (obtained with the frame in place) with the surgical field can be accomplished; and, using this coregistered information, provide a guide for an effector tool. A computer within the operating room can perform all these tasks and, in doing so, eliminate the need for the frame.

The coordinate defining hardware for image-guided surgery, known as *three-dimensional digitizers,* comes in a variety of forms, but all perform the same function of providing unique coordinate addresses for each point within their working volume. Our first prototype at Dartmouth (7) adapted a sonic digitizer consisting of a spark gap, which emitted a broad bandwidth ultrasonic click and an array of three microphones. From the time of flight of the acoustic impulse to each of the microphones, the respective distances could be calculated, and from these slant ranges, the location of the spark gap could be determined. There are a number of alternative digitizing technologies, but the most common ones for surgical purposes have been articulated arms (the location of its tip determined through knowledge of the length of each link and the angles between those links), camera-based systems detecting arrays of light-emitting diodes (LEDs), and electromagnetic transmitter–receiver systems (8). Each has respective advantages and disadvantages, but each has been employed in clinically used systems (9).

Coregistration of preoperative imaging with the surgical field is achieved most commonly by using three or more reference points on the head. Employing either imaging-appropriate markers or natural landmarks, such as the tragus or lateral canthi, these algorithms use the paired sets of coordinates derived for those respective points first in the imaging study and then, through use of the digitizer just described, in operating room space. Alternative strategies, such as matching the contour of the scalp with that in the imaging study, also have been developed and implemented (10).

The final task, that of making this imaging useful to the surgeon, is generally accomplished by a computer graphic showing the location of the tip of a tool within the surgical field on the appropriate preoperative imaging study (Fig. 50.1). Alternatively, a heads-up display within the operating microscope allows a guiding graphic to be superimposed on the surgical field. With the introduction of robotic technology into the operating room, such as the SurgiScope stereotactic operating microscope system (Elekta AB, Stockholm, Sweden) (Fig. 50.2) or the MKM microscope system (Zeiss Inc., Oberkochen, Germany), the effector function may be served by the ability to drive the operating microscope's op-

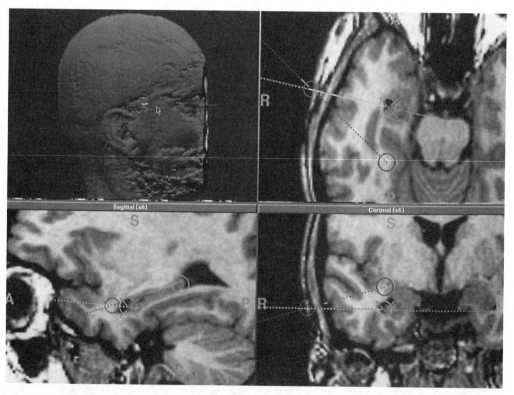

FIG. 50.1. This composite computer graphic, shown on a monitor adjacent to the surgical field during surgery, provides a triplanar display with the focal point of the operating microscope depicted by the light-colored *X*. The optical axis of the microscope is represented by the light-colored *dotted line;* preoperatively selected targets, to which the microscope may be driven robotically and corresponding to the anterior hippocampus and a point on the hipppocampus 3 cm posteriorly, are represented by the *darker circles.*

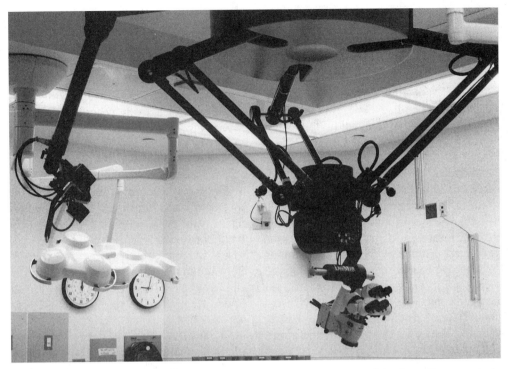

FIG. 50.2. The SurgiScope stereotactic operating microscope system consists of a ceiling-mounted robotic microscope holder that can direct the microscope to any location selected on the imaging studies. It also tracks the position of the microscope's focal point and optical axis on the imaging studies when it is independently positioned by the surgeon. (Reprinted with permission from Roberts DW. Stereotactic guidance with the operating microscope: SurgiScope. In: Alexander E III, Maciunas RJ, eds. *Advanced neurosurgical navigation.* New York: Thieme Medical, 1999:333–338.)

tical focal point to a target previously chosen on the preoperative imaging study.

Multiple image-guidance, or frameless stereotaxy, systems are commercially available today. They are increasingly user friendly, reliable, and accurate to within several millimeters. As surgery for the treatment of epilepsy is inherently a stereotactic procedure—first to identify the seizure focus and then to remove it surgically—it is hardly surprising that image-guided techniques have proven especially invaluable in this area.

SurgiScope Operating System

The SurgiScope combines a robotic operating microscope holder with an intraoperative computer workstation by which coregistration with preoperative imaging and graphic display of the microscope's focal point in that imaging are made possible. It consists of the DeeMed ceiling-mounted robot that supports a Leica operating microscope, a Hewlett-Packard workstation, an LED-based digitizer, a microterminal within the surgical field, and a joystick. Computed tomography (CT) and magnetic resonance imaging (MRI) studies may be imported into the workstation, and coregistration of the patient and those studies is accomplished at the start of the procedure by holding an LED probe at each of three or more points that have been identified on both the patient and the imaging study. At any subsequent time during the surgery, the position of the focal point of the microscope in the surgical field may be followed on the images, where its location is depicted; alternatively, the microscope's focal point may be directed robotically to a preselected object of interest. Typical accuracy of the system is on the order of a few millimeters, and no additional personnel are required during the surgery.

Dartmouth Clinical Experience

Between March 1995 and March 1999, 144 procedures for the diagnostic evaluation and surgical treatment of medically intractable epilepsy were performed at Dartmouth. These included 69 procedures for the implantation of intracranial electrodes, 21 temporal lobe resections, 20 selective amygdalohippocampectomies, 25 extratemporal resections, 8 callosal sections, and 1 multiple subpial transection. The mean age of patients operated on was 32 years (range, 4–59). High-resolution MRI imaging, obtained per our institution's epilepsy protocol, was available in all patients, and coregistration was performed using natural fiducial landmarks, most commonly the tragus, the superior aspect of the pinna, and the lateral canthi.

Electrode Implantation

It was not anticipated initially that the addition of image guidance to the relatively simple procedure of subdural strip and grid implantation (11–15) would offer particular advantage over unguided placement. In practice, however, it has improved our standard procedure and in selected cases has proven invaluable. Subdural strip placement, most commonly through burr holes, has been accomplished in the awake patient by temporarily immobilizing the gelpad-supported head with tape and using the robotically directed but undraped microscope's laser light indicator to guide both the entry site and the trajectory of the electrode. Inadvertent movement of the head during the 5 minutes necessary for such guidance has not occurred in 35 procedures, and improved reliability of final electrode location has resulted. If placement over a particular subcortical structural lesion has been desired, the ability to direct such an electrode more precisely than by the freehand method is particularly attractive.

Subdural grid placement obviously requires a larger craniotomy, and in such an instance, optimization of final electrode location is also achievable. Typically, the desired location of several points on the grid, such as its center and an additional orienting contact, are programmed before the surgery, and the final electrode position is appropriately adjusted with the actively positioned laser.

Selective Amygdalohippocampectomy

The increasingly common practice of resecting selectively the amygdala and hippocampus, with sparing of the temporal neocortex, has been supported by recognizing that about 90% of temporal lobe epilepsy arises from mesial structures. Although this more limited procedure has been performed for many years (16), the application of image-guided technique has refined this procedure considerably.

A trajectory through either the anterior middle temporal gyrus or the sulcus between the middle and inferior temporal gyri down to the anterior temporal horn is planned preoperatively, and at surgery a linear scalp incision and 2-cm craniotomy are used to expose the corticotomy site. With the microscope's laser guide positioned along this trajectory, a 15-mm corticotomy and dissection down to the temporal horn are executed. As the ventricle is approached, the laser beams converge until they are one as the ventricle is entered. A subpial dissection is carried out lateral to the hippocampus in either the parahippocampal or fusiform gyrus, first anteriorly around to the region of the uncus, and then posteriorly to the desired extent of hippocampal resection. Image feedback can be used both anteriorly and posteriorly, but it is particularly useful along the superior resection line of the amygdala. The choroidal fissure is identified posteriorly, and the tail of the hippocampus then is transected, joining the previous lateral dissection with the fissure. Standard technique, aided by the joystick's spherical rotation of the microscope, then is used to identify and divide the sequential vascular supply to the hippocampus medially. At the anterior extent of the fissure, the head of the hippocampus is resected and the dissection is joined to the previously resected uncal region. The remaining parahippocampal gyrus now is resected, and the hippocampal specimen, typically 3.5 cm long, is delivered en bloc. Closure follows standard surgical practice.

Lesionectomy

Seizure outcomes in resections associated with structural lesions are generally favorable (17–22), and frameless technique has facilitated such operative procedures much as it has tumor surgery (23). Small subcortical as well as deeper pathology, including cavernous angioma and low-grade glial tumors, is efficiently localized, and sufficient but not excessive exposure is enabled. In addition, both the extent of resection of surrounding cortex and the location of functional cortex can be identified by either imaging or stimulation intraoperatively for the surgeon. With the operating microscope, all these can be actively located and demonstrated with the laser, but handheld systems using any of the available digitizing technology also may be useful in this application.

Neocortical Resection

The resection of neocortical epileptogenic foci, an area of increasing attention today, especially benefits from guidance because of its less stereotypical and more individualized nature and its reliance on a multimodality database and preoperative treatment plan. The integration of one or more sequence from MRI, often coupled with functional MRI data, interictal and ictal single-photon emission tomography (SPECT), and CT demonstrating intracranial electrode positions into a resection strategy that takes into account a seizure focus, the extent of surrounding resection, and critical functional cortex to be preserved illustrates well the powerful role played by computer databases in the operating room (2–4,24).

The actual surgical procedure follows standard operative technique. Localization of re-

section margins and of tissue to be spared is incorporated directly into the procedure, however, as outlined previously. The positions of previously implanted electrodes and associated regions of pathology or normal function are followed either on the adjacent monitor image or demarcated by the microscope's laser. In those instances in which there is no visible structural pathology to follow during the surgery, the resection itself is dictated entirely by the image guidance.

Corpus Callosotomy

Commissurotomy does not require image guidance, but if it is available, its assistance can facilitate and assure the desired extent of resection (1,25). With any digitizing system, one simply may follow during the section how much of the callosum has been sectioned, thereby avoiding an inadvertently too modest section. We do this as well but, in addition, usually direct the robotic scope to the posteriormost point of division as it is approached and then complete the section without having to look away from the field. Similar to following a neocortical resection plan, a preoperative intent to divide, for example, the anterior 80% of the corpus callosum can be reliably carried out in the operating room.

REOPERATION

Most epilepsy surgery procedures are facilitated with guidance, but with the often rewarding procedure of reoperation (26,27), computer assistance becomes invaluable. The obscuring of normal landmarks and the presence of difficult gliotic tissue can be regularly overcome by guidance to the limits of planned resection; in a number of cases, this has been essential. As with the opposite but similar problem of operating on an MRI-normal brain, operating along computer-guided lines of resection has become standard procedure. Familiarity with and confidence in the accuracy of the particular system employed as well as the methodology are obviously necessary in such applications; once gained from other procedures, however, more difficult reoperations are aided considerably.

OVERVIEW

The advantages derived from image guidance in epilepsy surgery are considerable and straightforward. Fundamentally, these advantages include first the ability to integrate through coregistration an increasingly more sophisticated multimodality database and to develop preoperatively, in collaboration with colleagues from the entire epilepsy team, a surgical treatment strategy. Second, image-guided technology enables reliable execution of that plan in the operating room with accuracy, safety, and confidence.

Certain costs are associated with the introduction of this technology, but these costs are primarily in the form of initial equipment acquisition and are balanced by the enhanced capabilities and efficiencies it brings. All such systems have limitations of accuracy, typically in the range of a few millimeters, but in instances of shift in the later stages of resection, this may be considerably poorer (28). Awareness of the limitations of such technology and attention to steps that may minimize the risk of associated errors are essential. What role intraoperative imaging may come to play in an attempt to update the imaging database remains to be determined. It is important to state, however, that these limitations are not presently preventing real benefit from being derived today.

Areas of development and investigation in frameless stereotaxy include continued refinement of digitizing and display components and enhancements in planning and graphics software. Automation of many current steps required by these systems will render their employment increasingly transparent. Updating of the database, alluded to earlier, will likely draw from intraoperative data to improve both diagnostic ability and system accuracy (29–31). As neuroimaging, neurophysiological understanding, and surgical precision all continue to evolve, success-

ful intervention will be enabled for increasingly difficult seizure disorders.

CONCLUSION

Few areas of neurosurgery have benefited as much as epilepsy surgery from the advent of computer-assisted, image-guided methodology. Systems approved by the U.S. Food and Drug Administration that are user friendly are available today, and these can be incorporated into regular neurosurgical practice with efficiency and safety.

REFERENCES

1. Bucholz RD, Baumann CK. The use of image-guided frameless stereotaxy during epilepsy surgery. San Diego: *Scientific Program for the 62nd Annual Meeting of the American Association of Neurological Surgeons,* 1994:348.
2. Olivier A, Germano IM, Cukiert A, et al. Frameless stereotaxy for surgery of the epilepsies: preliminary experience (technical note). *J Neurosurg* 1994;81: 629–633.
3. Olivier A, Lacertee D, Cukiert A, et al. Frameless stereotactic craniotomies in the surgical treatment of epilepsy: preliminary experience in 70 patients. San Diego: *Scientific Program for the 62nd Annual Meeting of the American Association of Neurological Surgeons,* 1994:352.
4. Roberts DW, Darcey TM. The evaluation and image-guided surgical treatment of the patient with a medically intractable seizure disorder. *Neurosurg Clin N Am* 1996;7:215–227.
5. Uematsu S, Lesser RP, Gordon B, et al. Total resection of perioccipital epileptogenic area with preservation of visual function: the advantage of preoperative subdural grid mapping. San Diego: *Scientific Program for the 62nd Annual Meeting of the American Association of Neurological Surgeons,* 1994:357.
6. Watson V, Xei J, Wilson C, et al. MR stereotactic procedure planning with vascular and cortical guidance: comparison and correlation of MRA, 3-D MRI, digital subtraction angiography (DSA), and intracerebral electrodes. San Diego: *Scientific Program for the 62nd Annual Meeting of the American Association of Neurological Surgeons,* 1994:351.
7. Roberts DW, Strohbehn JW, Hatch JF, et al. A frameless stereotaxic integration of computerized tomographic imaging and the operating microscope. *J Neurosurg* 1986;65:545–549.
8. Bucholz RD, Smith KR. A comparison of sonic digitizers versus light emitting diode-based localization. In: Maciunas R, ed. *Interactive image-guided neurosurgery.* Park Ridge, IL: American Association of Neurological Surgeons, 1993:179–200.
9. DeSalles AAF, Hoebel B, Bhenke E, et al. Frameless stereotaxy validation in general neurosurgery. San

Diego: *Scientific Program for the 62nd Annual Meeting of the American Association of Neurological Surgeons,* 1994:357.

10. Pelizzari CA, Chen GTY. Registration of multiple diagnostic imaging scans using surface fitting. *Proceedings of the 9th International Conference on the Use of Computers in Radiation Therapy.* North Holland: Elsevier, 1987:437–440.

11. Blom S, Flink R, Hetta J, et al. Interictal and ictal activity recorded with subdural electrodes during preoperative evaluation for surgical treatment of epilepsy. *J Epilepsy* 1989;2:9–20.

12. Devinsky O, Sato S, Kufta CV, et al. Electroencephalographic studies of simple partial seizures with subdural electrode recordings. *Neurology* 1989;39:527–533.

13. Lesser, RP, Gordon B, Fisher R, et al. Subdural grid electrodes in surgery of epilepsy. In: Lüders HO, ed. *Epilepsy surgery.* New York: Raven Press, 1991: 399–408.

14. Rosenbaum TJ, Laxer KD, Vessely M, et al. Subdural electrodes for seizure focus determination. *Neurosurgery* 19:73–81.

15. van Veelen CWM, Debets RMChr, van Huffelen AC, et al. Combined use of subdural and intracerebral electrodes in preoperative evaluation of epilepsy. *Neurosurgery* 1990;26:93–101.

16. Weiser HG, Yasargil MG. Selective amygdalohippocampectomy as surgical treatment of mediobasal limbic epilepsy. *Surg Neurol* 1984;17:445–457.

17. Awad IA, Rosenfeld J, Ahl J, et al. Intractable epilepsy and structural lesions of the brain: mapping, resection strategies, and seizure outcome. *Epilepsia* 1991;32: 179–186.

18. Cascino GD, Kelly PJ, Sharbrough FW, et al. Long-term follow-up of stereotactic lesionectomy in partial epilepsy: predictive factors and electroencephalographic results. *Epilepsia* 1992;33:639–644.

19. Cohen DS, Zubay BA, Goodman RR. Seizure outcome after lesionectomy for cavernous malformations. *J Neurosurg* 1995;83:237–242.

20. Jooma R, Yeh H-S, Privitera MD, et al. Lesionectomy versus electrophysiologically guided resection for temporal lobe tumors manifesting with complex partial seizures. *J Neurosurg* 1995;83:231–236.

21. Montes JL, Rosenblatt B, Farmer J-P, et al. Lesionectomy of MRI detected lesions in children with epilepsy. *Pediatr Neurosurg* 1995;22:167–173.

22. Moore JL, Cascino GD, Trenerry MR. A comparative study of lesion resection with corticectomy with stereotactic lesionectomy in patients with temporal lobe lesional epilepsy. *Epilepsia* 1992;33(Suppl 3):96.

23. Matz P, McDermott M, Gutin P, et al. Cavernous malformations: results of image-guided resection. *Journal of Image-Guided Surgery* 1995;1:273–279.

24. Krombach GA, Spetzger U, Rohde V, et al. Intraoperative localization of functional regions in the sensorimotor cortex by neuronavigation and cortical mapping. *Computer Aided Surgery* 1998;3:64–73.

25. Awad IA, Wyllie E, Lüders HO, et al. Intraoperative determination of the extent of corpus callosotomy for epilepsy: two simple techniques. *Neurosurgery* 1990; 25:102–106.

26. Awad IA, Nayel MH, Lüders HO. Second operation after failure of previous resection for epilepsy. *Neurosurgery* 1991;28:510–518.

27. Polkey CE, Awad IA, Tanaka T, et al. The place of reoperation. In: Engel J Jr, ed. *Surgical treatment of the epilepsies,* 2nd ed. New York: Raven Press, 1993: 663–667.

28. Roberts DW, Hartov A, Kennedy FE, et al. Intraoperative brain shift and deformation: a quantitative analysis of cortical displacement in 28 cases. *Neurosurgery* 1998;43:749–760.

29. Miga MI, Paulsen KD, Lemery JM, et al. Model-updated image-guidance: initial clinical experience with gravity-induced brain deformation. *IEEE Transactions on Medical Imaging* 1999;18:866–874.

30. Paulsen KD, Miga MI, Kennedy FE, et al. A computational model for tracking subsurface tissue deformation during stereotactic neurosurgery. *IEEE Transactions on Biomedical Engineering* 1999;46:213–225.

31. Roberts DW, Miga MI, Hartov A, et al. Intraoperatively updated neuroimaging using brain modeling and sparse data. *Neurosurgery* 1999;45:1199–1207.

Subject Index

Page numbers in *italics* indicate figures; those followed by *t* indicate tabular material.

A

A[^{11}C]methyl-L-tryptophan positron emission tomography, 451–454, *453*

Abdominal pain, in parietal lobe epilepsy, 191

Absence seizures, frontal lobe, 218–219, 232–236

N-Acetylaspartate, magnetic resonance spectroscopy of, 408, 409, 410, *411, 412*

Achromatopsia, 211

Adenosine triphosphate, magnetic resonance spectroscopy of, 406

Ad-Tech multiple subpial transection knife, 637, *637*
  epileptic focus and, 638–639

Affective disorders, 470–473

Age-specific epilepsy, classification of, 122, 123

Agnosia
  apperceptive, 79, *79*
  in Landau-Kleffner syndrome, 637
  mirror, 68–69, *70*
  visual form, 79–82

Agranular frontal lobe
  anatomy of, *52*, 53
  functional motor representations in, 53, 54t
  parietofrontal circuits and, 51, 53–60

Agyria, 156–161, *157, 159, 160*

AIP-F5 bank circuit, 54–56, *55,* 59

α band desynchronization, 34
  in memory function assessment, 338, *338*
  in sensorimotor localization, 333
  in visual area localization, 335

Alpha-methyl-tryptophan uptake, in cortical dysplasia, 485, *486*

Amaurosis, in parietal lobe epilepsy, 194

Amobarbital, intracarotid injection of, in cerebral dominance determination, 460–461

Amygdala
  in neurologic/psychiatric disorders, 104
  projections of to prefrontal cortex, *93,* 93–95, 99–100, 102, *102*
  seizure propagation to/from, 302–304

Amygdalohippocampectomy, selective, 646–647

Anesthesia
  for image-guided craniotomy, 545, *546*
  for intraoperative electrocorticography, in neocortical temporal and frontal epilepsy, 596

Angular gyrus, transection of, 631

Anterior cingulate gyrus seizures, 219

Anterior intraparietal sulcus lesions, tactile apraxia and, 65, *65*

Anterior parietal lobe, functional anatomy of, 63–64

Antiepileptic drugs, 525–530
  L* maps and, 319, *322*
  mechanisms of action of, 529t, 529–530
  pharmacology of, 525–528
  for status epilepticus, 248–249

Aphasia
  in parietal lobe epilepsy, 194
  sign language, 66

Apperceptive agnosia, 79, *79*

Apraxia
  constructional, 66–67
  ideational, 66
  ideokinetic, 66
  inferior parietal lobule lesions and, 66–67
  tactile, 65

Areas of reduced complexity, 319, *321*

Arteriovenous malformations, MRI of, *379,* 380–381

Artificial neural networks, in seizure detection, 310–314

Asomatognosia, in parietal lobe epilepsy, 190

Asperger's syndrome, 469–470

Astereognosis, 64, 211

Astrocytoma
  frontal lobe epilepsy and, 598t
  temporal lobe epilepsy and, 598t

Asymmetric tonic posture, in supplementary motor area seizures, 217–218, 223

Asymmetric tonic seizures
  case report of, 132
  classification of, 130–132

Ataxia
  mirror, 69
  optic, 67, 71, 77
  visuomotor, 67–69

Atlases, cerebral, surface-based, 26–28, *29*

ATP, magnetic resonance spectroscopy of, 406

Attentional processing
  event-related potentials and, 35–38. *See also* Event-related potentials
  eye movements and, 69–71
  functional anatomy of, 37–48
  functional neuroimaging and, 35–48
  gain-control model for, 36–37
  inferior parietal lobule in, 69
  inverse model for, 37–38, *41*
  neglect and, 72–73
  P1 component and, 35–36, *36,* 37
  postural movements and, 71
  seeded forward model of, 40, *41*
  superior parietal lobule in, 69

Auditory cortex
  emotional vocalization and, 94–95
  localization of, 336, *336*
  projections of to prefrontal cortex, 89–93, *90, 93*

Auditory hallucinations, 94–95
  in neocortical temporal lobe epilepsy, 211

Auditory oddball responses, in functional mapping
  of auditory association cortex, 336, *336*
  of medial temporal lobe, 336, *336*

Augmenting response, 147–148, *148*